Register Now for Online Access to Your Book!

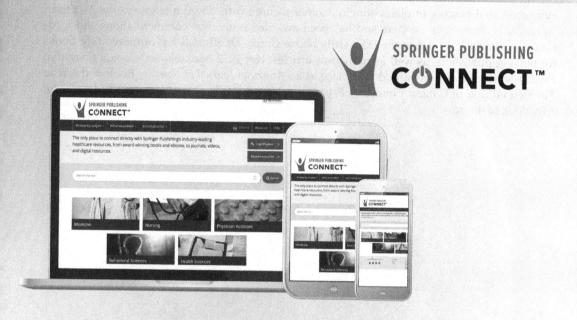

SPRINGER PUBLISHING CONNECT™

Your print purchase of *Clinical Consult to Psychiatric Mental Health, Second Edition,* **includes online access to the contents of your book—** increasing accessibility, portability, and searchability!

Access today at:
http://connect.springerpub.com/content/book/978-0-8261-6184-0
or scan the QR code at the right with your smartphone and enter the access code below.

8LETDWBK

Scan here for quick access.

If you are experiencing problems accessing the digital component of this product, please contact our customer service department at cs@springerpub.com

The online access with your print purchase is available at the publisher's discretion and may be removed at any time without notice.

Publisher's Note: New and used products purchased from third-party sellers are not guaranteed for quality, authenticity, or access to any included digital components.

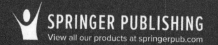

SPRINGER PUBLISHING
View all our products at springerpub.com

Jacqueline Rhoads, PhD, ACNP-BC, ANP-C, PMHNP-BE, CNL-C, FAANP, has held many faculty positions during her career and has taught in nurse practitioner programs since 1994. Dr. Rhoads has been awarded major research funding for a variety of research projects and continues to foster an evidence-based practice implementing outcomes-focused care. She is a fellow in the American Academy of Nurse Practitioners and has been awarded numerous commendations and medals for meritorious service in the U.S. Army Nurse Corps. Dr. Rhoads has authored four books for nursing publishers, as well as numerous articles. Her 2012 book *Nurses' Clinical Consult to Psychopharmacology* was awarded first place as an *American Journal of Nursing* Book of the Year. The first edition of *Clinical Consult to Psychiatric Mental Health Care* won second place as an AJN Book of the year.

Register Now for Online Access to Your Book!

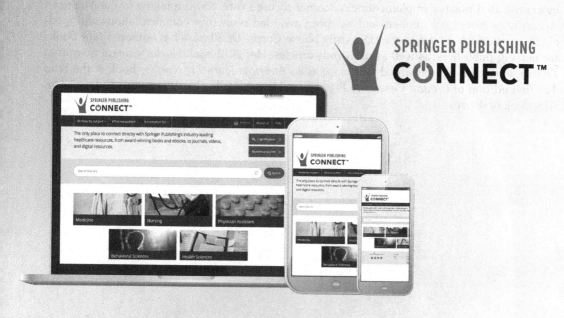

SPRINGER PUBLISHING
CONNECT™

Your print purchase of *Clinical Consult to Psychiatric Mental Health, Second Edition,* **includes online access to the contents of your book—** increasing accessibility, portability, and searchability!

Access today at:
http://connect.springerpub.com/content/book/978-0-8261-6184-0
or scan the QR code at the right with your smartphone
and enter the access code below.

Scan here for quick access.

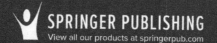

SPRINGER PUBLISHING
View all our products at springerpub.com

Jacqueline Rhoads, PhD, ACNP-BC, ANP-C, PMHNP-BE, CNL-C, FAANP, has held many faculty positions during her career and has taught in nurse practitioner programs since 1994. Dr. Rhoads has been awarded major research funding for a variety of research projects and continues to foster an evidence-based practice implementing outcomes-focused care. She is a fellow in the American Academy of Nurse Practitioners and has been awarded numerous commendations and medals for meritorious service in the U.S. Army Nurse Corps. Dr. Rhoads has authored four books for nursing publishers, as well as numerous articles. Her 2012 book *Nurses' Clinical Consult to Psychopharmacology* was awarded first place as an *American Journal of Nursing* Book of the Year. The first edition of *Clinical Consult to Psychiatric Mental Health Care* won second place as an AJN Book of the year.

Clinical Consult to Psychiatric Mental Health

Management for Nurse Practitioners

Second Edition

Jacqueline Rhoads, PhD, ACNP-BC, ANP-C, PMHNP-BE, CNL-C, FAANP

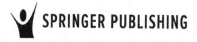
SPRINGER PUBLISHING

Copyright © 2021 Springer Publishing Company, LLC
All rights reserved.
First Springer Publishing Company edition 2014.

Springer Publishing Company, LLC
11 West 42nd Street
New York, NY 10036
www.springerpub.com
connect.springerpub.com/

Acquisitions Editor: Adrianne Brigido
Compositor: Transforma

ISBN: 978-0-8261-6183-3
E-book ISBN: 978-0-8261-6184-0
DOI: 10.1891/9780826161840

20 21 22 23 24 / 5 4 3 2 1

Medicine is an ever-changing science. Research and clinical experience are continually expanding our knowledge, in particular our understanding of proper treatment and drug therapy. The authors, editors, and publisher have made every effort to ensure that all information in this book is in accordance with the state of knowledge at the time of production of the book. Nevertheless, the authors, editors, and publisher are not responsible for any errors or omissions or for any consequence from application of the information in this book and make no warranty, expressed or implied, with respect to the content of this publication. Every reader should examine carefully the package inserts accompanying each drug and should carefully check whether the dosage schedules therein or the contraindications stated by the manufacturer differ from the statements made in this book. Such examination is particularly important with drugs that are either rarely used or have been newly released on the market.

Library of Congress Cataloging-in-Publication Data
Names: Rhoads, Jacqueline, 1948–author.
Title: Clinical consult to psychiatric mental health management for nurse
  practitioners / Jacqueline Rhoads.
Other titles: Clinical consult to psychiatric nursing for advanced practice
Description: Second edition. | New York, NY : Springer Publishing Company, LLC, [2021] | Preceded by
  Clinical consult to psychiatric nursing for advanced practice / Jacqueline Rhoads, Patrick J.M. Murphy.
  [2015]. | Includes bibliographical references and index. | Summary: "Provides "what to do next" guidelines
  when working with and beginning the treatment of a patient with a mental health disorder. Compiled by
  expert practitioners in psychiatric care, this work provides an overview of the management of the major
  Diagnostic and Statistical Manual of Mental Disorders, Fifth Edition (American Psychiatric Association, 2013)
  disorders across the life span and delivers complete clinical guidelines for their diagnosis, treatment options,
  and psychopharmacologic management"-- Provided by publisher.
Identifiers: LCCN 2020037433 (print) | LCCN 2020037434 (ebook) | ISBN
  9780826161833 (paperback) | ISBN 9780826161840 (ebook)
Subjects: MESH: Mental Disorders--nursing | Mental Disorders--therapy | Psychiatric Nursing--methods |
  Nurse Practitioners--standards | Psychopharmacology--methods
Classification: LCC RC440 (print) | LCC RC440 (ebook) | NLM WY 160 | DDC 616.89/0231--dc23
LC record available at https://lccn.loc.gov/2020037433
LC ebook record available at https://lccn.loc.gov/2020037434

Contact sales@springerpub.com to receive discount rates on bulk purchases. We can also customize our books to meet your needs.
For more information please contact: sales@springerpub.com

Publisher's Note: **New and used products purchased from third-party sellers are not guaranteed for quality, authenticity, or access to any included digital components.**

Printed in the United States of America.

This book is dedicated to all the healthcare workers out there—doctors, nurses, technicians, medical staff, administrators, food service workers, pharmacists, security guards, and our military deployed to set up hospitals and deliver aid. I, as a provider, understand the sacrifice, pain, and suffering you are exposed to every day. I understand the sleepless nights and difficulty concentrating especially when you get those precious days off. I'm so proud of you and feel a great deal of pride knowing I'm part of this special group of men and women.

Contents

Contributors   *ix*
Preface   *xi*
Abbreviations   *xiii*

PART ONE. Overview of Psychiatric Patient Disorders

SECTION I. PSYCHIATRIC PATIENT MANAGEMENT

1. The Psychiatric Interview and Diagnosis   *3*

2. Psychotherapeutic Management   *17*

3. Behavioral, Cognitive–Behavioral Therapy, and Psychoanalysis   *23*

SECTION II. PRINCIPLES OF CLINICAL PSYCHOPHARMACOLOGY

4. The Relationship of Psychopharmacology to Neurotransmitters, Receptors, Signal Transduction, and Second Messengers   *37*

5. Clinical Neuroanatomy of the Brain   *43*

6. Principles of Pharmacokinetics and Pharmacodynamics   *53*

7. Principles and Management of Psychiatric Emergencies   *63*

SECTION III. SYNDROMES AND TREATMENTS IN ADULT PSYCHIATRY

8. Behavioral and Psychological Disorders in Older Adults   *71*

9. Substance Use Disorders   *83*

10. Psychotic Disorders   *99*

11. Mood Disorders   *127*

12. Anxiety Disorders   *169*

13. Obsessive-Compulsive and Related Disorders   *197*

14. Dissociative Disorders   *221*

15. Sexual Dysfunction   *235*

16. Feeding and Eating Disorders   *255*

17. Sleep Disorders   *281*

18. Personality Disorders   *299*

19. Neurodevelopmental Disorders   *311*

PART TWO. Psychopharmacological Drug Monographs

20. Drug Monographs   *357*

   Index   *589*

Contributors

Angela Chia-Chen Chen, PhD, RN   Assistant Professor, College of Nursing and Health Innovation, Arizona State University, Phoenix, Arizona

Karen Crowley, DNP, APRN-BC, ANP, WHNP, CNE   Associate Dean, Graduate Online Nursing, Associate Professor, Regis College, Weston, Massachusetts

Shari Harding, DNP, PMHNP-BC, CARN-AP   Assistant Professor, University of Massachusetts Medical School, Worcester, Massachusetts

Rachael Hovermale, DNP, APRN   Coordinator and Associate Professor, Psychiatric-Mental Health Nurse Practitioner Program, Baccalaureate and Graduate Nursing, Eastern Kentucky University, Richmond, Kentucky

Jo-Ann Marrs, EdD, FNP, MSN, RN   Professor, College of Nursing, East Tennessee State University, Johnson City, Tennessee

Brenda Marshall, EdD, MSN, RN, APRN, ANEF   Professor, Department of Nursing, William Paterson University, Wayne, New Jersey

Anne M. Mingolelli, DNP, PMHNP-BC, APRN-BC   Assistant Professor, Nursing, Regis College, Weston, Massachusetts

Jacqueline Rhoads, PhD, ACNP-BC, ANP-C, PMHNP-BE, CNL-C, FAANP Professor of Nursing, Retired

CONTRIBUTORS TO THE FIRST EDITION

Athena J. Arthur, MS, LCDC

Renee R. Azzouz, ARNP

Sandra S. Bauman, PhD, ARNP, LMHC

Virginia Brooke, PhD, RN

Deonne J. Brown-Benedict, DNP, ARNP, FNP-BC

Lawrence S. Dilks, PhD

Susan O. Edionwe, MD

Elizabeth Hite Erwin, PhD, APRN-BC

Deborah Gilbert-Palmer, EdD, FNP-BC

Nnenna I. Igbo, MD

Jose Levy, MA, BCBA, CBIST

Patrick J. M. Murphy, PhD

Meena Patel, ARNP, DNP (Candidate)

Nancy Pierce, ARNP

Theresa Raphael-Grimm, PhD, RN, CS

Judy Rice, BSN, MSN FNPCS

Victoria Soltis-Jarrett, PhD, PMHCNS/NP-BC

Kimberly Swanson, PhD

Hisn-Yi (Jean) Tang, PhD, APRN

Kristen Vandenberg, MSN, ARNP, FNP-BC

Alma Vega, EdD, MSN, ARNP-BC

Lucinda Whitney, MSN, ARNP-BC

Elizabeth Willford

Preface

The devastation of the Gulf Coast after Hurricane Katrina and the recent pandemic of COVID-19 are imprinted in our memories not only by the sensational news coverage but also by the personal experiences of many healthcare providers who volunteered countless hours in helping the people affected by these crises. I was one of the providers who responded during Hurricane Katrina. From that experience came a realization of how many people were and are affected by mental illness and how little I knew of the protocols that could be used to provide mental healthcare to those I served. I went back to school for my post–master's degree in psychiatric mental health and saw the lack of published information that would lend assistance to those caring for people with mental disorders.

As a result of this realization, this text provides *what to do next* guidelines when working with and beginning the treatment of a patient with a mental health disorder. Compiled by expert practitioners in psychiatric care, this work provides an overview of the management of the major *Diagnostic and Statistical Manual of Mental Disorders, Fifth Edition* (American Psychiatric Association, 2013) disorders across the life span and delivers complete clinical guidelines for their diagnosis, treatment options, and psychopharmacological management.

We have constructed each chapter using a bulleted format for quick reference within a structured approach. This reference is organized into two major parts: The first is an overview of the principles of clinical psychiatry (interview, clinical decision-making, diagnostic evaluation, and treatment planning), psychotherapeutic management, behavioral therapy and cognitive-behavioral therapy, the principles of psychopharmacology (neurotransmitters, receptors, neuroanatomy, pharmacokinetics, and pharmacodynamics), syndromes and treatment in adult psychiatry, and syndromes and treatment in child and adolescent psychiatry. The second part presents monographs representing current major drug therapies for the major disorders that benefit from drug intervention.

A clinically useful drug selection table appears with each disorder for which psychopharmacology is an appropriate intervention and identifies the first- and second-line of drug therapy along with adjunctive therapies. It is important to note that the order in which drugs are listed within the drug classification on the drug table is significant in helping to guide drug choice. Additionally, it is important to note that not every drug within a classification is included for all disorders; rather, drugs that have been shown to have clinical efficacy are listed in a priority fashion to help guide the drug choice by the prescriber.

Essential drug information that is needed to safely prescribe and monitor the patient's response to those drugs includes the following: drug name, brand name, and generic name; drug class, usual and customary dosage, and administration of the drug; availability (e.g., as tablet, injection, intravenous, capsule); side effect, drug interaction, pharmacokinetics, precautions; patient education; and special populations. The Special Populations section includes management of those who are pregnant, breastfeeding, older adults, children, adolescents, and patients with impaired renal, hepatic, or cardiac function.

The book provides a concise, complete, easy-to-access clinical resource so the primary care provider can quickly access the following:

- Diagnostic criteria and differential diagnoses for each disorder
- The range of therapeutic interventions useful for managing disorders, including psychotherapeutic management, psychotherapy, and cognitive behavioral therapy
- The main psychotropic medications, when to prescribe, and how to select the most efficacious drug for each patient
- Special considerations for patient populations, including older adults, those who are pregnant, those who are breastfeeding, children, and adolescents
- Clinical considerations for prescribing in patients with impairment of renal, hepatic, and/or cardiac function
- Easy-to-read drug-selection tables for reliable clinical consultation

Pharmacology knowledge and applied clinical practices are constantly evolving due to new research and applied science, which expand our diagnostic capabilities and treatments. Therefore, it must be emphasized that practitioners carry an important responsibility to ensure that the treatment they select reflects current research and is appropriate according to manufacturer drug information for drugs selected; that dosages, route of administration, effects/precautions have been taken into consideration; and also that interactions and use in special populations are all accurate and appropriate for each patient. The practitioner is ultimately responsible to know each patient's history, to have conducted a thorough physical examination, and to consult appropriate diagnostic test results to ascertain best possible pharmacotherapeutic actions for optimal patient outcomes and appropriate safety procedures.

The contributors to this text have worked hard to present current and applicable content that is of therapeutic value in the understanding of specific mental health disorders. We are very grateful to the contributors of this text for their hard work and focused support.

Jacqueline Rhoads

Abbreviations

AA	Alcoholics Anonymous
AAIDD	American Association on Intellectual and Developmental Disabilities
ABA	applied behavioral analysis
ACG	anterior cingulate gyrus
ACh	acetylcholine
AD	Alzheimer's disease
ADAA	Anxiety Disorders Association of America
ADHD	attention deficit hyperactivity disorder
ADIS-C/P	Anxiety Disorder Interview Schedule for *DSM*-5-child/parent
ADLs	activities of daily living
AIMS	abnormal involuntary movement scale
ALP	alkaline phosphatase
ALT	alanine amino transferase
AMPA	alpha-amino-3-hydroxy-5-methyl-4-isoxazolepropionic acid receptor
AN	anorexia nervosa
ANA	antinuclear antibody
ANC	absolute neutrophil count
ANS	autonomic nervous system
APS	antipsychotics
ASAB	assigned sex at birth
ASD	autism spectrum disorder
ASPD	antisocial personality disorder
AST	aspartate amino transferase
AUD	alcohol use disorder
BBW	black box warning
BDD	body dysmorphic disorder
BDD-YBOCS	Body Dysmorphic Disorder-Yale Brown Obsessive Compulsive Scale

BDNF	brain-derived neurotrophic factor
BED	inge-eating disorder
BMI	body mass index
BN	bulimia nervosa
BP	blood pressure
BPD	borderline personality disorder
BPH	benign prostatic hypertrophy
BSDS	bipolar spectrum diagnostic scale
BUN	blood urea nitrogen
BZDs	benzodiazepines
BZPs	enzylpiperazines
CA	cocaine anonymous
CAD	coronary artery disease
CAGE	cut down, annoyed, guilty, and eye opener
CAM	complementary and alternative medicine
CAM-ICU	confusion assessment method for the intensive care unit
cAMP	cyclic adenosine monophosphate
CBC	complete blood count
CBT	cognitive behavioral therapy
CC	chief complaint
CHADD	Children and Adults with Attention Deficit/Hyperactivity Disorder
CHF	congestive heart failure
CIDI	Composite International Diagnostic Interview
CIR	clutter image rating
CIWA-Ar	clinical institute withdrawal assessment for alcohol
CMP	comprehensive metabolic panel
CNS	central nervous system
COPD	chronic obstructive pulmonary disease
COWS	Clinical Opiate Withdrawal Scale
CP/CPPS	chronic prostatitis/chronic pelvic pain syndrome
CPAP	continuous positive airway pressure
CR	controlled release
CrCl	creatinine clearance
CRH	corticotropin-releasing hormone
CRSD	circadian rhythm disorder
CSA	childhood sexual abuse
CT	cognitive therapy
CV	cardiovascular
CVA	cerebrovascular accident
CVLT	California Verbal Learning Test

CY-BOCS	Children's version of Y-BOCS
CYP	Cytochrome P450
DAN	Defeat Autism Now!
DATA	Drug Addiction Treatment Act
DBSA	depression and bipolar support alliance
DBT	dialectical behavior therapy
DD	depression disorder
DES	dissociative experiences scale
DEXA	dual emission x-ray absorptiometry
DHEA	dehydroepiandrosterone
DISCUS	Dyskinesia Identification System: Condensed User Scale
DM	diabetes mellitus
DXA	dual-energy x-ray absorptiometry
ECT	electroconvulsive therapy
ED	excoriation disorder
EDITS	Erectile Dysfunction Inventory of Treatment Satisfaction
EENT	eyes, ears, nose, throat
EIAED	enzyme-inducing antiepileptic drug
ELISA	enzyme-linked immunosorbent assay
EMDR	eye movement desensitization and reprocessing
EMG	electromyography
EOMs	xtraocular movements
EPS	extrapyramidal symptom
ERP	exposure and response prevention
FDA	food and drug administration
FGAs	first-generation antipsychotics
FH	family history
FSH	follicle stimulating hormone
GABA	gamma-aminobutyric acid
GAD	generalized anxiety disorder
GERD	gastroesophageal reflux disease
GGT	amma-glutamyl transferase
GI	gastrointestinal
GPCRs	G protein-coupled receptors
GTP	guanosine triphosphate
HCG	human chorionic gonadotrospin
5-HIAA	5-hydroxyindoleacetic acid
HIPAA	Health Insurance Portability and Accountability Act
HLA	human leukocyte antigen
H&P	history and physical

HPD	histrionic personality disorder
HPI	history of present illness
HRS	Hoarding Rating Scale
HTN	hypertension
IBS	irritable bowel syndrome
ICDSC	intensive care delirium screening checklist
IDEA	Individuals with Disabilities Education Act
IEP	individualized education program
IGF-1	insulin-like growth factor 1
IIEF	international index of erectile function
IM	intramuscular
INH	isoniazid
INR	international normalized ratio
IP$_3$	inositol trisphosphate
IV	intravenously
LFT	liver function test
LH	luteinizing hormone
LSD	lysergic acid diethylamide
M	muscarinic
MAOIs	monoamine oxidase inhibitors
MAT	medication assisted treatment
MCV	mean corpuscular volume
MDD	major depressive disorder
MDEs	major depressive episodes
MDMA	3,4-methylenedioxymethamphetamine
MDQ	mood disorder questionnaire
MET	motivational enhancement therapy
MGH-HPS	Massachusetts General Hospital Hairpulling Scale
MI	myocardial infarction
MR	mental retardation
MS	multiple sclerosis
MSE	mental status examination
MSLT	multiple sleep latency test
N	nicotinic
NA	Narcotics Anonymous
NAION	non-arteritic anterior ischemic optic neuropathy
NAMI	National Alliance on Mental Health
NaSSAs	noradrenergic and specific serotonergic antidepressants
NCD	neurocognitive disorder
NDRIs	norepinephrine/dopamine reuptake inhibitors

NE	neurotic excoriation
NE-Y-BOCS	Neurotic Excoriation Yale-Brown Obsessive-Compulsive scale
NIMH	National Institute of Mental Health
NIMH-TIS	NIMH Trichotillomania Impairment Scale
NIMH-TSS	NIMH Trichotillomania Severity Scale
NMDA	N-methyl-D-aspartate receptor
NMS	neuroleptic malignant syndrome
NOWS	neonatal opioid withdrawal syndrome
NPD	narcissistic personality disorder
NSAIDs	nonsteroidal antiinflammatory drugs
OCD	obsessive-compulsive disorder
OCPD	obsessive-compulsive personality disorder
ODD	oppositional defiant disorder
ODTs	orally disintegrating tablets
OTC	over-the-counter
PAIRS	psychological and interpersonal relationship scales
PANDAS	Autoimmune Neuropsychiatric Disorders Associated With Streptococcal Infections
PANSS	positive and negative symptoms scale
PCIT	parent–child interaction therapy
PCOS	polycystic ovary syndrome
PCPs	phencyclidines
PD	panic disorder
PDD	pervasive development disorder
PDE5	Phosphodiesterase Type 5
PHQ	Patient Health Questionnaire
PIAT-R	Peabody Individual Achievement Test-Revised
PI-WSUR	Pandua Inventory-Washington State University Revision
PKU	phenylketonuria
PLMS	periodic leg movements of sleep
PMDD	premenstrual dysphoric disorder
PMH	past medical history
PNS	peripheral nervous system
PSG	polysomnography
PSNS	parasympathetic nervous system
PT	prothrombin time
PTSD	posttraumatic stress disorder
QT	heart rhythm
QTc	corrected QT interval
RAD	reactive attachment disorder

RADQ	Randolph Attachment Disorder Questionnaire
RBC	red blood cell
RCTs	randomized controlled trials
RDAs	recommended daily allowances
REM	rapid eye movement
RLS	restless legs syndrome
ROS	review of systems
RPG	random plasma glucose
SAD	seasonal affective disorder
SARIs	serotonin-2 antagonist/reuptake inhibitors
SC	subcutaneous
SCAN	Schedules for Clinical Assessment in Neuropsychiatry
SCARED	screen for child anxiety-related emotional disorders
SCID	Structured Clinical Interview for *DSM-5* disorders
SCID-5	Structured Clinical Interview for *DSM-5* dissociative disorders
SEAR	self-esteem and relationship
SEP	sexual encounter profile
SGOT	serum glutamic oxaloacetic transaminase
SGPT	serum glutamic pyruvic transaminase
SH	ocial history
SIADH	syndrome of inappropriate antidiuretic hormone
SIR	Saving Inventory-Revised
SJS	Stevens-Johnson syndrome
SLD	specific learning disorder
SLP	speech/language pathologist
SM	selective mutism
SMAST	Short Michigan Alcoholism Screening Test
SNRIs	serotonin-norepinephrine reuptake inhibitors
SNS	sympathetic nervous system
SR	sustained-release
SSRIs	selective serotonin reuptake inhibitors
START	short-term assessment of risk and treatability
STDs	sexually transmitted diseases
SUD	substance use disorder
SWAN	Strengths and Weaknesses of ADHD Symptoms and Normal Behavior
TCAs	tricyclic antidepressants
TD	tardive dyskinesia
TEACCH	treatment and education of autistic and related communication-handicapped children
TEN	toxic epidermal necrolysis

TIA	transient ischemic attacks
TMJ	temporomandibular joint
TSH	thyroid-stimulating hormone
TTM	trichotillomania
UA	urinalysis
UCD	urea cycle disorder
VDRL	Venereal Disease Research Lab
VEGF	vascular endothelial growth factor
VSC	violence screening checklist
WBC	white blood cell
WISC	Wechsler Intelligence Scale for Children
XR	extended-release
Y-BOCS-II	Yale-Brown Obsessive-Compulsive Scale
Y-BOCS-TM	Yale-Brown Obsessive-Compulsive Scale-Trichotillomania

PART ONE

Overview of Psychiatric Patient Disorders

Section I. Psychiatric Patient Management

The Psychiatric Interview and Diagnosis

THE PSYCHIATRIC INTERVIEW

Introduction

- The psychiatric interview is the core of proper psychiatric evaluation. It plays an important role not only in clinical assessment but also in therapy. The interviewer should come to understand the patient's behaviors; emotions; experiences; psychological, social, and religious influences; and motivations through verbal and nonverbal communication with the patient.
- The psychiatric interview can be divided into the following stages: building an alliance with the patient, psychiatric history, diagnostic evaluation, and treatment plan formulation.
- As with all interviews, the patient–provider relationship is very important. An intact relationship between the interviewer and the patient increases the patient's confidence and willingness to disclose the personal or sensitive information necessary for diagnosis and facilitates patient compliance.
- The psychiatric interview depends on more than verbal communication; it requires that the physician be observant and listen. Nonverbal communication can provide insight necessary for the patient's clinical assessment and diagnosis, especially in patients significantly impaired by psychiatric disease.
- The extent of psychiatric impairment may necessitate that the interviews occur in multiple sessions or obtaining information from additional persons such as family members or friends.
- The interview should begin with an open-ended approach.
- A structured interview approach combines the psychiatric interview with diagnostic criteria in attempts to derive a thorough psychiatric history.

The Patient–Provider Relationship: Building an Alliance

- The patient–provider relationship is fundamental to providing excellent care and improving patient outcomes and the healing process. It has special significance in psychiatry, where the "stigma" of psychiatric treatment can make even seeking treatment difficult.
- A solid patient–clinician relationship requires optimization of the following seven components:

- Communication
- Office experience
- Hospital experience
- Patient education
- Integration (information sharing among all members of the treatment team)
- Shared decision-making
- Outcomes
- The patient–provider relationship involves a working or therapeutic alliance, which is an agreement between the provider and the patient, based on mutual rapport and trust, to undertake treatment together.
- The interviewer must be sensitive to the importance of empathy, respect, and trust to develop a good working alliance.
- Distrust is a common reason for noncompliance. In fact, most instances of noncompliance come from interruption of the patient–provider relationship.
- The interviewer should develop a rapport with the patient:
  - Remain attentive:
    - Maintain eye contact.
    - Minimize distractions such as excessive note taking or interrupting the patient while speaking.
  - Be empathic:
    - Show your understanding of and appreciation for their situation.
    - Reinforce what the patient is feeling. One way to do this is by making statements such as "I can see that was a very difficult time for you."
  - Listen! Listen! Listen!

The Interview: Nonverbal Communication

- Active observation of the patient should occur within the first few minutes of the interview, before names have been exchanged and the "formal" interview has begun.
- Actively process the patient's nonverbal communication, such as the following:
  - How does the patient first greet the interviewer?
  - Does the patient make eye contact?
  - What items (books or pictures, etc.) are present?
  - What is the patient wearing, and is their appearance disheveled or neat?
  - What (if any) unusual sounds or smells are in the room?
- Observation of the patient should continue throughout the interview. The interviewer should take note of the patient's body language and emotional expressions during responses to the questions.
- For example, a patient who becomes emotional when asked about a spouse may be depressed about a recent divorce or loss of a loved one.
- Certain kinds of nonverbal communication are included in the diagnostic criteria, and the interviewer should be cognizant of their presence.
- Active observation becomes increasingly important with increases in psychiatric impairments.

The Interview: Verbal Communication

- Open-ended questions
  - After formally introducing yourself and your role in the patient's care, start by asking open-ended questions.

- Examples of open-ended questions include the following:
  - Tell me what brings you here.
  - Tell me what kinds of problems you have had, lately.
- Three reasons why an open-ended manner of interviewing is important are as follows:
  - It strengthens the patient–provider relationship by showing that the interviewer is interested in the concerns of the patient.
  - It provides insight into the patient's condition.
  - It allows the interviewer to understand what is most important to the patient rather than making assumptions.
- The interviewer should engage in active listening as the patient responds to questions.
- Diagnosis-specific questions
  - As the history develops, specific questions such as "Do you see things that others cannot see?" (hallucinations) or "Have you ever tried to harm yourself?" (suicidal ideations) become necessary. Follow up on the responses.
  - These specific questions aim at gathering information necessary for diagnosis based on the *Diagnostic and Statistical Manual of Mental Disorders*, Fifth Edition (*DSM-5*; American Psychiatric Association, 2013) criteria.
  - The interviewer should be able to transition from open-ended questions to more specific ones.
    - For example, "Now I would like to ask you about several psychological symptoms that patients might experience."

Structured Interviews
- A structured interview uses a series of questions that couple the interview method with the *DSM-5* diagnostic criteria in attempts to explore the signs and symptoms necessary for diagnosis.
- Examples include the following:
  - The MINI-International Neuropsychiatric Interview (MINI[-Plus])
  - Structured Clinical Interview for *DSM-5* disorders (SCID)
  - Composite International Diagnostic Interview (CIDI)
  - Schedules for Clinical Assessment in Neuropsychiatry (SCAN)

Psychiatric Interview ICD-10
ICD-10 Code: **Z046 (Z04.6)**; Code Type: **Diagnosis**

THE DIAGNOSTIC ENCOUNTER

Phases of the Diagnostic Encounter
The diagnostic encounter is divided into three phases:
- Opening phase
- Body of the interview
- Closing phase

Opening Phase
- Initial 5 to 10 minutes
- Goals

- Introductions
- Preinterview preparation
  - For example, easing the patient's fears or concerns about the necessity for the interview
  - Building a therapeutic alliance
  - Keeping questions open ended and allowing the patient to speak uninterrupted for an appropriate amount of time

Body of the Interview
- 30 to 45 minutes
- Goals
  - Psychiatric history
  - Diagnosis-specific questions such as "Does this patient meet *DSM-5* criteria for diagnosis?"
  - Mental status examination (MSE)
  - Physical examination
  - Additional investigations

Closing Phase
- 5 to 10 minutes
- Goals
  - Reviewing your assessment with the patient
  - Collaborating with the patient on a treatment and follow-up plan

Psychiatric History

- *Identifying data*: Collect basic details about the patient, such as name, gender, age, religion, educational status, occupation, relationship status, and contact details.
- *Chief complaint* (CC): Document the reason for the patient's presentation.
- *History of present illness* (HPI): The interviewer attempts to gain a clear understanding of the full history of the patient's problems, such as when they started, what they entail, worsening symptoms, or associated symptoms. The HPI allows the interviewer to formulate preliminary hypotheses as to a diagnosis.
- *Past medical history* (PMH): The interviewer should explore the PMH to look for surgical or medical diseases or medications that cause, contribute to, or mimic psychiatric disease.
- *Past psychiatric history*: Explore previous diagnoses, treatments, and outcomes.
- *Family history* (FH): Explore familial psychiatric disorders or medical conditions as a cause of or contributing factors to psychiatric disorders.
- *Social history* (SH): Document the social circumstances of the patient, such as finances, housing, relationships, drug and alcohol use, and problems with the law, as these can contribute to the cause of psychiatric disease.
- *Development history*: Document the past, present, family, social, and cultural history of the patient.
- *Review of systems* (ROS): Explore pertinent systems associated with the onset of psychiatric disease.

Mental Status Examination

- *Appearance*: Physique, grooming, dress, habits, nutritional status, posture, nervousness, and eye contact.
- *Attitude/rapport*: Attitude toward the examiner. For example, is the patient friendly, cooperative, bored, or defensive?

- *Mood*: The patient's emotions. Elicit the mood by asking the patient questions such as "How have you been feeling on most days?" List the mood in the patient's own words. Moods include being depressed, angry, anxious, stressed, or elevated.
- *Affect*: Defined by the interviewer. Observable emotion: euthymic (normal), neutral, euphoric, dysphoric, or flat (no variation in emotion); the range: full, constricted, or blunted; appropriateness: appropriate or labile.
- *Speech*: Quality, quantity, rate, and volume.
- *Thought process*: The organization of the patient's thoughts:
  - *Logical*: Normal thought process.
  - *Loose associations*: The patient slips off the track from one idea to an unrelated one.
  - *Flight of ideas*: The patient verbally skips from one idea to another before the previous one has been concluded.
  - *Tangentiality*: The responses never approach the point of the questions.
  - *Thought blocking*: The patient stops abruptly in the middle of a thought.
  - *Circumstantiality*: Delay in getting to the point because of unnecessary details and irrelevant remarks.
  - *Neologism*: Patient creates new words.
- *Thought content*
  - *Suicidal ideation*: Assess the plan and previous attempts.
  - *Homicidal ideation*: Assess the plan and previous attempts.
  - Obsessions and compulsions.
  - Phobias.
  - Paranoia.
- Perceptual disturbances
- *Hallucinations*: Perception of a stimulus in the absence of a stimulus—auditory (hearing things), visual (seeing things), olfactory (smelling things), tactile (feeling things), and gustatory (tasting things).
- *Delusions*: Grandiosity, religious delusion, persecution, jealousy, thought insertion (belief that someone is putting ideas or thoughts into their mind), ideas of reference (belief that irrelevant, unrelated phenomena in the world refer to them directly or have special personal significance).
- *Illusions*: Erroneous interpretation of a present stimulus.
- *Insight*: The patient's understanding of their illness.
- *Judgment*: Estimate the patient's judgment on the basis of the history or on an imaginary scenario. Ask the following question: "What would you do if you smelled smoke in a crowded theater?" (An adequate response is "Call 911" or "Get help"; a poor response is "Do nothing" or "Watch the smoke rise.")
- *Impulsivity*: The degree of the patient's impulse control.
- *Reliability*: Determine if the patient seems reliable or unreliable or if it is difficult to determine.

Physical Examination

- Medical conditions (central nervous system [CNS] malignancy, hypothyroidism, or pancreatic cancer) can mimic a psychiatric illness. A thorough physical examination (usually with the exception of genitourinary examination), including full neurological examination, should be documented.

Additional Investigations

- Lab investigations

- Additional information from accompanying friend or family members
- Other forms of pertinent information

CLINICAL DECISION-MAKING

- The decision-making process has been broken down into a systematic and individualized process involving the following:
  - *State-mandated criteria*: Clinical practice guidelines, *DSM-5*, and so forth
  - *Investigation of alternatives*: For example, ruling out medical conditions that mimic psychiatric disease through lab investigations
  - *Shared decision-making*: Requires an adequate patient–clinician relationship
  - *Intuitive reasoning and experiences:* For example, years of experience or exposure to previous psychiatric disorders
  - Connection with the client, caution, and inability to control all contingencies
- Strategies for clinical reasoning and decision-making include the following:
  - Tolerate uncertainty, avoid premature closure, and consider alternatives.
  - Separate cue from inference; refer inferences to the salient cues from which they were derived.
  - Be aware of personal reactions to the patient.
  - Be alert for fresh evidence, particularly evidence that demands a revision or deletion of a hypothesis or diagnosis.
  - Value negative evidence above positive evidence.
  - Be prepared to commit to a diagnosis when enough evidence has been gathered.
- Historically, decision-making has shown variability among practitioners. As a result, efforts have been made to create practice guidelines, processes, and recommendations that will result in consistency in the diagnostic evaluation and, subsequently, in the treatment of psychiatric disease.
- Trend toward evidence-based clinical decision-making:
  - Use of *DSM-5* guidelines
  - Goals
    - More clinical research independent of pharmaceutical companies
    - An efficient means of making evidence-based data easily accessible to clinicians

DIAGNOSTIC FORMULATION, TREATMENT PLANNING, AND MODES OF TREATMENT

Putting It All Together: Diagnostic Formulation

- Diagnostic formulation has been traditionally described as a summary of the relevant genetic, constitutional, and personality factors and their interaction with the etiological factors, taking into account the patient's life situation, together with a provisional diagnosis.
- Essentially, the full encounter, including psychiatric history, MSE, labs, referral information, additional information from family members/friends, and physical examination, is assessed to yield a diagnosis.
- Currently, a diagnostic formulation is best accomplished using the *DSM-5* multiaxial system of assessment.

DSM-5 Disorders and ICD-10 Codes

- These disorders will be listed as Axis I or Axis II on the multiaxial system assessment.
- Adjustment disorders
  - Adjustment Disorder Unspecified (F43.20)
  - Adjustment Disorder with Anxiety (F43.22)
  - Adjustment Disorder with Depressed Mood (F43.21)
  - Adjustment Disorder with Disturbance of Conduct (F43.24)
  - Adjustment Disorder with Mixed Anxiety and Depressed Mood (F43.23)
  - Adjustment Disorder with Mixed Disturbance of Emotions and Conduct (F43.25)
- Anxiety disorders
  - Acute Stress Disorder (F43.0)
  - Agoraphobia (without a history of Panic Disorder) (F40.02)
  - Generalized Anxiety Disorder (GAD; [F41.1])
  - Obsessive-Compulsive Disorder (OCD; [F42])
  - Panic Disorder—with Agoraphobia (F40.01) or without Agoraphobia (F41.0)
  - Social Phobia (F40.10)
  - Posttraumatic Stress Disorder (PTSD; [F43.1])
- Dissociative disorders
  - Dissociative Amnesia (F44.0)
  - Dissociative Fugue (F44.1)
  - Dissociative Identity (Multiple Personality) Disorder (F44.81)
  - Depersonalization-Derealization Syndrome (F48.1)
- Eating disorders
  - Anorexia Nervosa (F50.0)
  - Bulimia Nervosa (F50.2)
- Impulse control disorders
  - Intermittent Explosive Disorder (F63.81)
  - Kleptomania (F63.2)
  - Pathological Gambling (F63.0)
- Mood disorders
  - Bipolar Disorder (F31.0)
  - Cyclothymic Disorder (F34.0)
  - Dysthymic Disorder (F34.1)
  - Major Depressive Disorder (MDD; [F32.0])
- Sexual disorders
  - Exhibitionism (F65.2)
  - Fetishism (F65.0)
  - Frotteurism (52.8)
  - Pedophilia (F65.4)
  - Sexual Masochism (F65.51)
  - Sexual Sadism (F65.52)
  - Transvestic Fetishism (F65.1)
  - Voyeurism (F65.3)
- Sleep disorders
  - Primary Insomnia (F51.01)
  - Primary Hypersomnia (F51.11)
  - Narcolepsy (G47.4)
  - Nightmare Disorder (F51.5)
  - Sleep Terror Disorder (F51.4)

- Sleepwalking Disorder (F51.3)
- Psychotic disorders
  - Brief Psychotic Disorder (F23)
  - Delusional Disorder (F22)
  - Schizoaffective Disorder (F29.5)
  - Schizophrenia
    - Schizophrenia, Catatonic Type (F20.2)
    - Schizophrenia, Disorganized Type (F20.1)
    - Schizophrenia, Paranoid Type (F20)
    - Schizophrenia, Residual Type (F20.5)
    - Schizophrenia, Undifferentiated Type (F20.5)
  - Schizophreniform (F20.81)
  - Shared Psychotic Disorder (F24)
- Sexual dysfunctions
  - Dyspareunia (F52.6)
  - Female Orgasmic Disorder (F52.31)
  - Female Sexual Arousal Disorder (F52.31)
  - Gender Identity Disorder (F52.22)
  - Hypoactive Sexual Desire Disorder (F64.2)
  - Male Erectile Disorder (F52.21)
  - Male Orgasmic Disorder (F52.8)
  - Premature Ejaculation (F52.4)
  - Sexual Aversion Disorder (F52.1)
  - Vaginismus (F52)
- Somatoform disorders
  - Body Dysmorphic Disorder (F45.22)
  - Conversion Disorder (F44.9)
  - Hypochondriasis Disorder (F45.21)
  - Pain Disorder (F45.19)
  - Somatization Disorder (F45.20)
- Substance disorders
  - Substance Abuse (F19.18)
  - Substance Dependence (F19.28)
- Personality disorders
  - Antisocial Personality Disorder (F60.2)
  - Borderline Personality Disorder (F60.3)
  - Narcissistic Personality Disorder (F60.81)
  - Dependent Personality Disorder (F60.7)
  - Histrionic Personality Disorder (F60.4)
  - Paranoid Personality Disorder (F60)

Treatment Planning

- Treatment planning is the next step after a diagnosis is evident.
- Selection of a therapeutic method depends on the mode, time, and setting of treatment.
- Patient involvement is necessary in formulating a treatment plan.
- The following are treatment plan goals:
  - To clarify treatment focus
    - What the treatment is meant to accomplish and through what means
  - To set realistic treatment expectations and goals

- Treatment goals should have criteria for achievement, be achievable, and be collaboratively developed and prioritized.
  - Expectations should adequately clarify to patients what they can realistically expect from a treatment course.
  - Patient and provider roles should be clarified, setting the ground rules for therapy and establishing realistic goals agreed by the patient.
- To establish a standard for measuring treatment progress
  - Include a plan for reevaluation or follow-up.
- To facilitate communication among professionals
- For the purposes of managed healthcare, treatment plans also serve to support treatment authorization, to document quality assurance efforts, and to facilitate communication with external reviewers.

Modes of Treatment

- Pharmacotherapy
  - *Antidepressants*: Used to treat depression, panic attacks, OCD, PTSD, social anxiety disorder, anxiety, premenstrual dysphoric disorder, nicotine withdrawal symptoms
  - *Mood stabilizers*: Used to treat bipolar disorder, dementia (anticonvulsants), severe agitation, aggression, severe impulsive behavior, mania, and disinhibition
  - *Neuroleptics*: Used to treat schizophrenia, mania, delusional disorder, symptoms of psychosis, Tourette's disease, Asperger's syndrome
  - *Anticholinergics*: Used for anxiety and stress reactions; also used to offset extra-pyramidal symptoms (EPS) for patients experiencing these symptoms while on antipsychotics
  - *Anxiolytics*: Used to treat anxiety disorders
  - *Sedative hypnotics*: Used to treat insomnia and sleep disorders
- Electroconvulsive therapy
  - Major depression with or without psychotic features
  - Bipolar illness (used to treat both depressed and manic phases)
  - Catatonic schizophrenia
  - Schizophrenia with strong affective components or schizophrenia highly resistant to treatment
- Behavior therapy and cognitive therapy
  - Used to help patients eliminate target behaviors; refer to additional texts for more information.
- Group psychotherapy
  - Used to treat the following disorders in a group setting:
    - Most personality disorders
    - Most anxiety disorders
    - Somatoform disorders
    - Substance-related disorders
    - Schizophrenia and related psychotic disorders
    - Stable bipolar disorders
    - PTSD
    - Eating disorders
    - Medical illness
    - Depressive disorders
    - Adjustment disorders
- Family/marital therapy

THE DIAGNOSTIC EVALUATION

The Process of Diagnostic Evaluation

- A complete diagnostic evaluation involves obtaining a complete psychiatric history, including the presence of specific symptoms, course, and duration, in addition to the MSE, physical examination, pertinent labs, and other additional information. Diagnosis-specific questions for *DSM* criteria during the diagnostic encounter are the key.

Diagnosis-Specific Questions

- As the interviewer develops hypotheses for a diagnosis, diagnosis-specific questions are asked to elicit *DSM-5* criteria for diagnosis as follows:
  - *How long have you felt depressed?*—The *DSM-5* diagnosis for a MDD requires at least 2 weeks of symptoms.
  - *Do you still derive pleasure from doing your favorite activities?*—The *DSM-5* diagnosis for MDD must include the presence of lack of pleasure (anhedonia) or a depressed mood.
  - *Are you able to function during the day on little to no sleep?*—A decreased need for sleep is one of the possible criteria for a diagnosis of bipolar disorder.
  - *Do you have flashbacks or nightmares of the traumatic event?*—Reexperiencing a trauma (via nightmares, flashbacks, obsessive thoughts) is part of the *DSM-5* criteria of diagnosis for PTSD.
- The interview may refer to additional diagnosis-specific screening questionnaires such as the following:
  - Mini-Cog—Instrument to assess dementia
  - Mini-Mental State Examination—Screening tool for cognitive function and impairment
  - Clock drawing test—Screening tool to assess executive function
  - Beck Depression Inventory
  - Hamilton Depression Scale
  - Other primary clinician instruments based on *DSM* criteria (intended for and sufficiently diagnostic in primary care settings)

The Diagnostic and Statistical Manual of Mental Disorders

Diagnostic Criteria

- Standard classification of mental health disorders used by mental health professionals in the United States.
- Designed for use across settings, such as inpatient, outpatient, partial hospital, clinic, private practice, and primary care; with community populations; and by psychiatrists, psychologists, nurses, occupational and rehabilitation therapists, counselors, social workers, medical students, and other health and mental health professionals.
- Necessary tool for collecting and communicating accurate public health data.
- Three major components: the diagnostic classification, the diagnostic criteria sets, and the descriptive text.
- For each disorder in the *DSM*, a set of diagnostic criteria indicates inclusion criteria (symptoms and length of presence) and exclusion criteria to qualify for a particular diagnosis.

PSYCHOLOGICAL TESTING IN PSYCHIATRY

What Is Psychological Testing?

Psychological testing offers objective data about mental functioning. It involves administration, scoring, and interpretation of specific tasks in a controlled fashion. Tests must be

- normed on a representative population,
- administered in a controlled environment,
- administered in a standard fashion,
- reliable and valid,
- culturally fair,
- scored according to standardized procedures, and
- interpreted according to acceptable professional practices by a trained professional.

What Information Does Psychological Testing Provide, and for Whom Is It Appropriate?

Psychological testing gives the practitioner the ability to provide useful diagnostic information regarding level of intellectual functioning, identify and describe the nature of a mental health disorder, and indicate underlying motivation, personality attributes, and other variables.

- The patient must be able to participate in the assessment. Grossly confused or psychotic patients are not good candidates for psychological testing.
- Psychological testing is useful in treatment planning and outcome evaluation.
- Psychological testing is useful when objective data are required to establish a suspected diagnosis (sanity boards, interdiction).

Types of Psychological Tests

Many types of psychological tests are available to qualified users, which include the following:

- Measures of intellectual functioning
- Personality questionnaires
- Projective techniques
- Neuropsychological tests
- Measures of cognitive impairment

Associated tests include the following:

- Psychodiagnostic screening tests
- Educational diagnostic tests
- Aptitude tests
- Interest inventories

How to Determine the Appropriate Types of Patients for Psychological Testing

- Almost anyone who possesses a reasonable reality orientation and is nonpsychotic is an appropriate candidate for psychological testing.
- Individuals with better mental statuses are capable of participating in more complex psychological testing procedures.
- Not all patients are capable of participating in all psychological tests. Physical handicaps, language barriers, and illiteracy may limit the available testing procedures.
- The willingness of the patient has an influence on the procedure. Angry or deceptive individuals may distort the outcome data. There are specific psychological tests to detect malingering and deception.

■ Very specific referral questions allow for the selection of instruments (measures) to specifically address the reason for referral for testing.

How Long Should Psychological Testing Take?

■ The time to complete psychological testing depends on the referral questions and the number of testing procedures performed. The time may be as short as 2 hours or as long as 8 hours.
■ Testing can be expedited by prearranging appointments, providing relevant records and history, clear referral questions, and, when necessary, preapproval by third-party payers.
■ Testing may be delayed when a third-party payer has questions as to the necessity of testing procedures, schedules are full, referral questions are vague, funding is unavailable, or the client is inappropriate for assessment.

Who Performs Psychological Tests?

■ A licensed psychologist or a technician under the supervision of a licensed clinical psychologist conducts psychological testing.
■ Not all psychologists provide psychological testing, and referrals are frequently made to specialists, especially in the case of neuropsychological assessment.
■ Some states allow psychological testing to be conducted by nonpsychologists for specific purposes or in limited environments.

Important Issues in Psychological Testing

■ Reliability
■ Validity
■ Cultural bias
■ Confidentiality
■ Qualified examiners and assistants
■ Explaining test results to referral sources

Psychological Tests and Procedures of Importance in Psychiatry

The Wechsler Adult Intelligence Scale, Fourth Edition (WAIS-IV)
■ The gold standard in the assessment of intellectual functioning
■ Cross-culturally normed and can be used with any member of the U.S. population above the age of 16 years
■ Requires 60 to 90 minutes to administer
■ Provides several IQ and index scores for different realms of intellectual ability

The Minnesota Multiphasic Personality Inventory (MMPI-2)
■ The most widely investigated and empirically validated personality questionnaire available.
■ The self-report format consists of 556 true-or-false questions requiring 1 to 2 hours for completion.
■ Has built-in validity scales to detect malingering and deception.
■ Consists of 10 basic clinical scales and supplemental scales to assess personality.
■ Has a number of presentation formats: paper, short form, and computer administration.
■ Optic scan options are available, which can then generate a written report for rapid review.

The Rorschach
■ The classic inkblot projective technique.
■ Patients are instructed to provide a description of what they see in an ambiguous picture.
■ The responses have been correlated with personality variables and psychopathology.
■ Requires specialized training and supervised practice to administer and interpret.
■ Computer programs are available to assist with scoring and interpretation.

Self-Report Instruments
■ Typically, self-report inventories are pencil-and-paper tests, wherein the patient endorses items either with a true/false or with a Likert-scale format.
■ These reports can also be done in an interview format.
■ They come in "short" and "long" versions, which take time to complete.
■ These have been empirically validated with various clinical populations and demographic groups.

Common Measures
■ The Beck Depression Inventory
■ The Beck Anxiety Inventory
■ The Hamilton Depression Scales
■ The Hamilton Anxiety Scale

Neuropsychological Test Batteries
■ A group of tests that describe brain–behavior relationships.
■ Some tests are preselected and referred to as structured batteries while others are selected by the neuropsychologist as per the referral question and are known as flexible batteries.
■ Individual tests assess psychological functions in different regions of the brain.
■ The test results can be assembled to draw conclusions about damaged and persevered cognitive realms and abilities.
■ Tests are useful in assessing the loss secondary to neurological insult and making predictions about recovery.
■ Neuropsychological testing requires up to 8 hours of testing time.
■ Specialized training is required to administer, score, and interpret measures used in neuropsychological assessment.

Questions for Referral Sources to Ask in Making a Referral
■ Will psychological testing answer the questions I have about my patient?
■ How soon will the psychologist see my patient?
■ How long will the testing take?
■ Is the procedure covered by my patient's insurance?
■ Does your office have a payment plan?
■ How long will it take to get the results?
■ Will the psychologist go over the results with my patient and me?
■ If my patient has difficulty in understanding the results, can they come and see the psychologist for further review?
■ Will the results include recommendations that I can implement?
■ How will my patient's confidentiality and privacy be protected?

BIBLIOGRAPHY

American Medical Association. (2019). *AMA physician ICD-10-CM 2019* (Vols. 1 and 2). American Medical Association Press.

American Psychiatric Association. (2013). *Diagnostic and statistical manual of mental disorders* (5th ed.). American Psychiatric Publishing.

Andronikof, A. (2008). Exneriana-II—The scientific legacy of John E. Exner, Jr. *Rorschachiana, 29,* 81–107.

Carlat, D. J. (2017). *The psychiatric interview: A practical guide to psychiatry* (2nd ed.). Lippincott Williams & Wilkins.

Ebert, M. H., Loosen, P. T., Nurcombe, B., & Leckman, J. F. (Eds.). (2018). *Current diagnosis & treatment: Psychiatry* (3rd ed.). McGraw-Hill.

Gillis, M. M., Haaga, D. A. F., & Ford, G. T. (1995). Normative values for the Beck Anxiety Inventory, Fear Questionnaire, Penn State Worry Questionnaire, and Social Phobia and Anxiety Inventory. *Psychological Assessment, 7,* 450–455.

LeBlond, R. F., DeGowin, R. L., & Brown, D. D. (Eds.). (2014). *DeGowin's diagnostic examination* (10th ed.). McGraw-Hill.

Meyer, G. J., Riethmiller, R. J., Brooks, R. D., Benoit, W. A., & Handler, L. (2000). A replication of Rorschach and MMPI-2 convergent validity. *Psychological Assessment, 74,* 175–215.

Moras, K., di Nardo, P. A., & Barlow, D. H. (1992). Distinguishing anxiety and depression: Reexamination of the reconstructed Hamilton scales. *Psychological Assessment, 42,* 224–227.

Scheiber, S. C. (2011). The psychiatric interview, psychiatric history, and mental status examination. In R. A. Hales, S. C. Yudofsky, & J. A. Talbott (Eds.), *The essentials of clinical psychiatry* (2nd ed., pp. 187–220). American Psychiatric Press.

Valenstin, M. et al. (1997). Screening for psychiatric illness with a combined screening and diagnostic instrument. *Journal of General and Internal Medicine, 12*(11), 679–685.

2

Psychotherapeutic Management

ESTABLISH A PHILOSOPHY OF MANAGEMENT

Management of the psychotherapeutic process is a multidimensional endeavor that requires the following:

- Staff management
- Patient well-being
- Coordination with other professionals
- Time management

A fundamental philosophy guiding both outpatient and inpatient treatment needs to be established as follows:

- What are the variables that influence service delivery?
- How can you ensure that services meet a level of excellence?
- How will staff teamwork be accomplished?
- Selection of the appropriate psychotherapy
- Risk management

The interactions of these factors with other relevant factors, such as those given in the following list specific to the patient's environment, will determine the ultimate process of intervention.

- How can patient outcome be made optimal?
- How can the service program become accountable?
- How can the treatment program become flexible and adaptable?
- How can the program achieve total fairness and mutual respect?

STANDARDS OF CARE IN PSYCHOTHERAPY MANAGEMENT

In the realm of psychotherapy, surrounding issues are not as well established as they are in other realms of medicine. This is changing as more becomes known about the process and utility of the different forms of intervention. Current influences on the standard of care include the following:

- Laws and current statutes
- Regulations passed by state licensing boards

- Precedent and case law
- Professional codes of ethics
- Opinions of consumers and other professionals

The three standards of care established in mental health are as follows:

- Duty to report abuse
- The case of *Tarasoff v. the Board of Regents of the University of California*
- Health Insurance Portability and Accountability Act (HIPAA) guidelines

PSYCHOTHERAPY: INITIAL INTERVIEW

Presentation by the patient includes the following:

- Attire
- Overall attitude
- Gross motor skills
- Speech
- Language
- Hygiene

Initial assessment includes the following:

- Presentation of the problem
- Secondary problems
- Medical history
- Working with the patient to determine whether there were any past "manic or hypomanic" episodes—drug and alcohol history
- Legal history
- Developmental history
- Educational history
- Employment history
- Marital status and history
- Abuse issues

Mental status examination includes the following:

- Alertness
- Coherence
- Mental organization
- Thought processing
- Delusions
- Obsessions
- Suicidal/homicidal ideation
- Affect and mood
- Illusions
- Hallucinations
- Orientation
- Memory
- Fund of information
- Abstraction

PSYCHOTHERAPY RECORD MANAGEMENT AND THE STANDARD OF CARE

At a minimum, a psychotherapy chart or file should include the history of severe adverse drug reactions and allergies.

- Diagnosis
- Presentation of problem
- Mental status examination
- History of past mental illness
- Background information
- Treatment goals
- Progress notes

If appropriate, the chart or notes should display the following:

- Psychological test results
- Psychiatric consultation
- Relevant medical tests or history
- Consultations
- Unscheduled communications with the patient

Special population notes should include the following:

- Nature of the condition
- Concurrent problems
- Potential for violence
- Crisis intervention procedures
- Detailed notes concerning abuse or neglect

PSYCHOTHERAPEUTIC MANAGEMENT OF DISORDERS

Personality Disorders

The management of personality disorders presents an unusual challenge because many of the maladaptive features that have caused the patient pain and suffering are fundamental components of the personality structure. Key features in management include the following:

- Maintaining strict boundaries between the patient and the psychotherapist
- Establishing a clear reimbursement plan
- In writing, establishing the responsibility of the patient and the responsibility of the psychotherapist
- Setting rules and consequences for tardiness in the outpatient setting
- Enacting a no-suicide contract
- Agreeing on a plan of action if the patient becomes suicidal
- Always promptly addressing the patient's stated need to discontinue treatment
- Always assessing secondary issues such as drug and alcohol use
- Becoming alert to issues of secondary gain and disruptive behavior
- Addressing self-destructive behaviors

- Working on enhancing adaptive behaviors and social skills
- Focusing on educating the patient on cause-and-effect relationships
- Helping establish personal, spiritual, and vocational goals of a long-term nature
- Minimizing self-disclosure
- Not accepting excuses

Substance Abuse

Substance abuse disorders require that clinicians wear many hats and address many different aspects of the patient's experiences.

- Treatment goals should be simple and clear.
- Patients should be actively involved in treatment.
- Therapists should structure a supportive environment.
- Patients must take responsibility for their behavior.
- Therapists should emphasize self-direction.
- Confrontation must be appropriate to the client's tolerance level.
- Empathy should be conditional and measured.
- Avoid arguing with patients.
- Involve the significant other whenever possible.
- Always emphasize the patient's motivation.
- Enhance awareness of problem behaviors.
- Focus on self-destructive cyclic behaviors.
- Educate about the physical destructiveness of substance abuse.
- Engage the family in the treatment.
- Help the patient identify feelings and express them appropriately.

Dementia

Management of dementia is achieved in both inpatient and outpatient settings. A multidisciplinary team approach is necessary to manage most cases effectively.

- Address physical safety issues.
- Gauge psychotherapy to the level of impairment.
- Address issues of incontinence in counseling.
- Enhance mobility.
- Educate as to the dangers of falling.
- Address depression in both individual and group sessions.
- Offer orientation counseling to low-functioning patients.
- Offer family consultation and counseling to all family members.
- Address end-of-life issues in group therapy.
- Carefully investigate drug and alcohol issues.
- Consult with family about driving privileges.
- Assess memory repeatedly.
- Stress a wellness model.
- Prepare to address sundowning problems.
- Establish smoking and obesity groups.
- Offer counseling for depression and loss.

Depression

Depression is the most common illness in the general population. There are numerous diagnostic categories for the depressive disorders, but some basic management principles apply to all forms of depression.

- Assess the depth of the depression.
- Establish the etiology, duration, and frequency of the depression.
- Assess vegetative signs.
- Assess suicide risk.
- Stabilize the affect and mood with medication management.
- Educate the patient as to the nature of the illness.
- Reduce guilt.
- Initiate a supportive therapy to stabilize.
- Look for cultural influences that maintain depression.
- Reduce stressors.
- Enhance self-esteem.
- Build problem-solving skills.
- Manage self-defeating thoughts.
- Help explore self-defeating behaviors.
- Engage family support.

Psychotic Disorders

A lack of a reality orientation and disorganized thinking are the hallmarks of psychosis. Psychotherapy is unproductive in the acute phase but profitable in the prodromal and residual phases, assisting the client in maintaining the medication management program and discovering a rewarding life.

- Establish the patient's current level of functioning.
- Encourage compliance with the medication management program.
- Reduce stressors.
- Assist with acquiring basic necessities.
- Investigate drug and alcohol use.
- Consistently encourage a balanced lifestyle.
- Discourage self-medication.
- Assist with enrollment in day hospital programs.
- Urge self-exploration of illness.
- Help establish boundaries.
- Assist with financial management.
- Build social skills.
- Teach patient to recognize psychotic features.
- Encourage personal hygiene.
- Teach listening skills.
- Always redirect when patient avoids.
- Enhance independent living skills.
- Prevent self-pity and despondency.
- Directly address noncompliance with treatment.

BIBLIOGRAPHY

American Psychotherapy Association. (2008). Psychotherapist's oath. http://www.americanpsychotherapy.com/about/oath/

Bruce, N. G., Manber, R., Shapiro, S. L., & Constantino, M. J. (2010). Psychotherapist mindfulness and the psychotherapy process. *Psychotherapy: Theory, Research, Practice, Training*, 47(1), 83–97.

Richmond, R. L. (2009). The psychotherapy process. http://www.guidetopsychology.com/questions/questions.htm#process

Richmond, R. L. (2009). Termination issues. http://www.guidetopsychology.com/questions/questions.htm#termin.

Richmond, R. L. (2009). Transference issues. http://www.guidetopsychology.com/questions/questions.htm#trans.

3

Behavioral, Cognitive–Behavioral Therapy, and Psychoanalysis

BEHAVIORAL THERAPY AND COGNITIVE-BEHAVIORAL THERAPY

Definitions

Behavioral Therapy

Behavioral therapy is any intervention or set of interventions that focuses on patient behaviors as the primary focus of change. Maladaptive, self-defeating, self-destructive, or otherwise problematic behaviors can be replaced with more effective ones. Learning these new behaviors is a matter of education and reinforcement. Progressive muscle relaxation training and social skills training are two examples.

Cognitive Therapy

Cognitive therapy (CT) includes interventions that target a patient's thinking process. The central principle guiding CT is that thoughts produce feelings. Simply put, sadness and anxiety are, in part, products of the thinking process. Faulty thinking often precedes emotional distress. The thinking process is often fraught with faulty assumptions and unexamined tenets that often render the patient unnecessarily constrained and distressed. Through identification and examination of the faulty or distorted thinking practices, patients are helped to consider themselves and their circumstances from an alternate perspective and thereby mitigate feelings of distress.

Cognitive-Behavioral Therapy

Cognitive-behavioral therapy (CBT) is a body of work in psychotherapy that draws from multiple theories and focuses on the thoughts and behaviors that shape problematic emotional reactions and consequences.

- In the CBT framework, emotional distress is believed to be the result of faulty habits of thinking that result in dysfunctional attitudes and behaviors.
- Maladaptive patterns of thinking create emotional distress.
- In order to alleviate that distress, new objective, evidence-based thought patterns have to be developed and new behavioral skills have to be adopted.
- Through a systematic process of examining, labeling, and analyzing these cognitive errors, patients learn to replace them with more reality-based, self-enhancing ones.

Behavioral and Cognitive-Behavioral Processes

Background

■ Behavioral therapy is based, in part, on the work of B. F. Skinner and others, who analyzed how operant conditioning determines behavioral responses and how these responses could be altered through effective environmental reinforcement.

■ Reward-based measures, such as token economies, are used to reinforce desired behaviors. Variations in specific theoretical frameworks and treatment techniques exist within behavioral therapy.

■ Thought leaders in CT include Albert Ellis (rational emotive therapy) and Aaron Beck (CT), who through the 1960s advanced the notion that feelings or emotions were strongly influenced by the habitual patterns people used to make sense of their experiences.

■ These thought patterns were considered "automatic" in that they are an innate part of the "self-talk" that seems to be a universal human phenomenon.

■ These automatic thoughts are often based on misconceptions, deeply embedded erroneous assumptions (schema), and learned principles that confine the manner in which people respond to all kinds of life problems.

■ Although psychodynamically oriented approaches look to the origin of feelings in sometimes deeply conflicted psychosocial, developmental, and cognitive aspects, theorists propose that feelings originate from learned patterns of thinking that create unnecessarily confined mental structures that affect how people learn, grow, and solve problems.

■ These false, fixed notions of reality often create mental prisons for those who live within them.

Terms and Methods

Fundamental Features

CBT is a relatively short-term psychotherapy process (approximately 6–18 sessions) that is structured and formalized. Attention to this structure is a hallmark of the approach. The steps of treatment usually include the following:

1. A thorough diagnostic interview
2. The partnering of the patient and the therapist leads to an active collaborative team.
3. The therapist–patient team works together to identify problematic areas in the patient's life, by identifying cognitive distortions or errors that commonly impose a negative interpretation on everyday events.
4. The therapist–patient team adopts a step-by-step process to examine the underlying assumptions, fundamental beliefs, or schemas, from which these self-defeating thought patterns and distortions originate. They are often outside the immediate conscious awareness of the patient.
5. The creating and maintaining of a written daily thought record includes the following:
   ■ Documenting specific events that evoke emotional distress
   ■ Identifying the specific cognitive distortions that are at work in many of these situations
   ■ Labeling and analyzing of cognitive distortions
   ■ Identifying alternative methods for thinking about these same events (cognitive correction process)
6. The assignment of carefully planned homework so that the patient remains actively engaged in the CBT process outside of the formal sessions.

7. The therapist actively engages in coaching the patient through a systematic examination of the antecedents and consequences of these errors in thinking.
8. The therapist–patient team designs strategies to examine evidence to determine the validity of these erroneous mental constructs.
9. Prioritization and processing of these problems from the standpoint of a CBT framework.
10. Recording the process of identification of goals in behavioral, measurable terminology.
11. Trying on new behaviors that are outside the patient's usual pattern to explore potential results and sources of reinforcement.
12. Ultimately, the patient becomes their own therapist, able to quickly identify erroneous thinking when it occurs and take steps to neutralize or counter it.
13. Coupled with the ability to initiate behavioral measures (relaxation and assertiveness), the patient can choose from a repertoire of skills to meet the demands of the emotionally charged situation and return to a state of emotional equilibrium.

Psychoeducation

- Psychoeducation is a major and ongoing component of the treatment and is usually woven into sessions throughout the course of treatment.
- Patients are introduced to a cognitive conceptualization of their problems and goals from the beginning.
- Psychoeducation teaches patients about the terms, strategies, and processes of CBT and is included in most of the sessions.

Cognitive Distortions

Cognitive distortions are automatic thoughts that are often irrational, illogical, or self-defeating. If occurring regularly, they can result in patterns of ineffective behavior. Despite different theorists developing somewhat idiosyncratic terminology to designate similar phenomena, the following are common in many of them:

- *Emotional reasoning*: The tendency to conclude that if a person feels awkward or uncomfortable after a social event, then the person must actually be socially awkward.
- *Dichotomous thinking (all-or-nothing thinking)*: Drawing absolute conclusions. A person whose marriage fails believes that they are a "complete loser."
- *Discounting the positive*: Disqualifying all positive experiences or traits as being trivial or unimportant, especially when compared to a seemingly glaring error or shortcoming.
- *Personalization*: Interpreting external data as being related to oneself without evidence for such a conclusion.
- *Arbitrary inference*: Drawing a conclusion without supporting evidence, or even in spite of contradictory evidence.
- *Minimization and magnification*: Overinflating the negative or underestimating the positive in the evaluation of the relative importance of events.
- *Catastrophizing*: Assuming that the worst possible outcome is the most likely.

Interactive Techniques

- *Setting an agenda*: The agenda for each session is actively negotiated with the patient at the onset.
- *Feedback*: The therapist deliberately requests feedback to ascertain the patient's understanding of—and success with—the process and methods. Eliciting and processing

patient reactions to—and concerns about—the impressions of both the therapy and the therapist are considered essential components of the CBT experience.

■ *Socratic method*: Through a series of questions, the therapist gradually advances the nature of a discussion to lead the patient to first uncovering the distorted perspective and then drawing more accurate, self-affirming conclusions.

■ *Guided discovery*: The therapist–patient team examines the evidence, weighs the value of alternatives, and explores the advantages and disadvantages of various options. This is done in an integrated and accepting manner through a discussion format.

■ *Focused attentiveness*: The therapist–patient team focuses on the central ideas, relevant thoughts, assumptions, behaviors, and so forth that are germane to the problem being discussed.

■ *Formulating a strategy for change*: The plan is actively negotiated with the patient, and it clearly outlines the CBT strategies to be employed in the change process.

Qualities of the Therapist

■ CBT is a methodology that requires its practitioners to be well grounded in the essential skills of psychotherapy.

■ CBT does not replace basic psychotherapeutic practice. Rather, it builds from it.

■ The cognitive-behavioral therapist must be well versed in conceptual and operational underpinnings of psychotherapeutic processes.

■ A therapist trained in CBT must also be able to demonstrate features of any other trained therapist as well as possess the following:

   ▪ Graduate education in a mental health field (psychology, psychiatry, social work, nursing, professional counseling, etc.)

   ▪ Deeply embedded commitment to and demonstration of basic therapist skills and attributes:

      ● Expression of empathy
      ● Professionalism
      ● Sound judgment, ethical practice
      ● Active listening
      ● Authenticity
      ● Understanding of complex psychological phenomena that influence human experiences
      ● Ability to understand the patient within the social, cultural, and environmental context of that patient's lived experience

Evidence-Based Applications

■ Among psychotherapy methods, to its credit, CBT has the largest body of empirical evidence to support its efficacy.

■ Because of the formalized and structured nature of its tenets and interventions, CBT can be operationalized in a reproducible manner, which creates sound reliability and validity.

■ Common evidence-based applications include the following:

   ▪ Anxiety disorders in adults and children
   ▪ Depression
   ▪ Addictions
   ▪ Posttraumatic stress disorder (PTSD)/trauma-informed care
   ▪ Personality disorders (especially in the expanded method of dialectical behavioral therapy [DBT])

■ Examples of newer applications (some still under investigation) include the following:

- Chronic pain
- Chronic illness
- Chronic fatigue syndrome
- Tinnitus
- Headache, especially with comorbid psychiatric symptoms
- Sleep disorders
- Schizophrenia
- Child sexual abuse
- Treatment of sex offenders
- Somatoform disorders
- Anxiety, depression, and insomnia in older adults
- Psychological adjustment to breast cancer
- Occupational stress

Related Approach: Dialectical Behavioral Therapy

- Mindfulness and radical acceptance are concepts that complement, draw from, or enhance a CBT.
- These concepts supplement or extend CBT methods and techniques to further target treatment-resistant emotional distress.
- DBT, for example, provides a systematic and programmed method for dealing with the intense emotional distress that sometimes occurs in patients who struggle with borderline personality disorder.
- Mindful strategies and meditation help to decrease the emotional reactivity that may be, in part, physiologically activated, especially after prolonged periods of intense stress.
- Computer-based, program-driven CBT is now available, and these programs claim to provide effective CBT in the absence of a psychotherapist.

PSYCHOANALYSIS

Sigmund Freud

Biographical Information

- Born in Moravia in 1856; died in London in 1939.
- Member of the Jewish faith, which had a significant influence on his worldview.
- Trained in neurology, he developed an interest in patients who exhibited neurological symptoms without any organic etiology.
- Studied with Jean Baptiste Charcot at the Salpetrière in Paris. This greatly affected his thinking about the influence of the unconscious on personality development and behavior.
- After returning to Vienna, he developed the first comprehensive theory of personality.
- His theory of personality led to the development of psychoanalysis.

Freud's Personality Theory

Freud's ideas can be reviewed in two broad sections:

The Topographic Model (1900)

- Saw personality as analogous to an iceberg with three distinct sections.
  - *Conscious level*: Consists of current thoughts and perceptions.

- *Preconscious level*: Involves memories and stored knowledge that can be retrieved on demand.
- *Unconscious level*: Inaccessible feelings, urges, drives, desires, and demands. These are driven by a basic biological–sexual need for fulfillment.
- The topographic model was represented in Freud's 1900 publication *The Interpretation of Dreams*, in which he proposed that humans were guided by unconscious sexual energies that lead to conflicts in everyday life.

The Structural Model (ca. 1920)

- As Freud's ideas matured, so did his conceptualization of personality structure.
- While the topographical model was rigid with its three sections, the structural model remained fluid and offered interaction between the realms of one's personality.
- The structural model has three semi-independent realms as follows:
  - The id
    - The id is the only part of personality present at birth.
    - The id operates on the pleasure principle.
    - Wants instant gratification—"It wants, what it wants, when it wants it."
    - No frustration tolerance.
    - No empathy or compassion for others; it is completely egocentric.
    - The goal of the id is to increase pleasure and decrease pain and anxiety.
    - Inappropriate or psychotic behavior results when needs are delayed or denied.
    - The id runs on libido energy (or life energy). The libido energy is a biological energy that drives an individual toward growth and development.
    - Initially, because the id is unconscious, the image of an object is just as rewarding as the object itself.
    - The id is forced by the biological necessity to acknowledge the outside world and thus makes arrangements for some libido energy to act as a go-between.
  - The ego
    - The ego begins as a fragile subsection of the id with the goal of satisfying id needs by any practical means.
    - To satisfy id needs, the ego is in communication with reality and guides behavior.
    - Gratifying the id's needs results in greater libido energy being shifted to the ego, which results in a stronger reality reorientation, socialization skills, and frustration tolerance.
    - Failure to meet the id's needs leads to deteriorating ego influence and an increase in primitive, infantile, or psychotic behavior.
    - The ego is in touch with reality and operates by the reality principle, which endorses delayed gratification.
    - For most people, the ego continues to develop and becomes the executor of personality, balancing the other forces.
  - The superego
    - The superego is the last portion of personality to develop a relationship with both the unconscious and the conscious.
    - The superego begins to develop as the attitudes of authority figures are integrated into the personality structure and a sense of right and wrong is established.
    - As the superego develops, it influences behavior by enhancing self-esteem for appropriate actions and punishing inappropriate behavior through guilt.

- In a healthy personality, there is a flow of energy among the three realms.
- If the libido energy becomes focused on the id, psychotic behaviors become prominent in the personality.
- If the libido energy becomes focused on the superego, anxiety disorders become prominent.

In sum, the id is driven by inborn instincts such as anger and sex, while the superego is at the other extreme, urging social values and altruism. The ego is the executor and arbitrator, directing and balancing the demands of the id and the superego.

The Psychosexual Stages of Development

Freud adopted a stage theory of psychosexual personality development in his 1905 work *Three Essays on the Theory of Sexuality* (see Table 3.1).

- The stages are invariant; they cannot be circumvented or skipped.
- The stages represent a shifting of libido energy to different areas of the body. These realms become the center of developmental psychosexual issues and attention.
- Each stage has a psychosexual crisis associated with it, which must be successfully resolved before moving on to the next stage of development.
- Failure in resolving the psychosexual crisis associated with the stage results in fixation. Psychosexual energy remains stagnant, and the individual (unconsciously) attempts to resolve the crisis. These attempts usually become socially inappropriate as the person ages.

The Oedipal Conflict

- In Greek mythology, Oedipus was the son of the king of Thebes, whose lover, unbeknownst to him, was his mother.
- When Oedipus became aware of the identity of his lover, he gouged out his eyes for violating a sexual taboo.
- The Oedipal conflict provides an explanation of gender orientation and operates unconsciously.
- During this phallic stage, libido energy builds, and the child begins to develop a sexual attraction for the opposite-sex parent.
- The course for boys and girls is different.
  - Boys
    - The boy develops affection for his mother and jealously wishes to displace his father as the man in her life. As his psychosexual tension grows, he becomes fearful of reprisal, which leads to a belief that his father may remove him as a contender by removing his genitals, that is, the castration complex.

TABLE 3.1 The Psychosexual Stages of Human Development

STAGE	AGE (YEAR[S])	EROGENOUS ZONE	PSYCHOSEXUAL CONFLICT
Oral	0–1	Mouth	Weaning, sucking, eating
Anal	1–3	Anus	Toilet training, feces
Phallic	3–5	Genitals	Oedipal conflict, sex
Latency	5–6	None	Period of calmness
Genital	Puberty	Mature sexual relationships	

- At this point, the anxiety is intolerable, and the boy engages two defense mechanisms to reduce anxiety and resolve the psychosexual conflict. He represses his affection for his mother and identifies with his father, leading to a psychological male orientation that matches his physiology.
- A small proportion of boys fail to resolve this crisis and fail to establish a male identity. This concludes the phallic period, and the child enters a period of psychosexual tranquility until puberty.
- Girls
  - A girl develops affection for her father and wishes to displace her mother, who is now viewed as a rival.
  - Eventually, the conflict between losing her mother's love and having her mother separate her from the family becomes intolerable.
  - Repressing her affection for her father and identifying with her mother successfully resolves the conflict.
  - Her psychology now matches her physiology, and she now identifies herself as female.
  - A small proportion of females fail to resolve the crisis and experience gender identity issues.

Defense Mechanisms

- Defense mechanisms serve as protective devices for the three mental structures (see Table 3.2).
- Their mission is to mitigate anxiety and stress and enhance stability in the personality structure.

TABLE 3.2   Defense Mechanisms

DEFENSE MECHANISM	ACTIVITY	EXAMPLE
Repression	Suppression of anxiety-laden material from consciousness	A sailor cannot remember the attack on his ship.
Projection	Attributing repulsive attitudes and traits to another	A student alleges that the faculty is out to get him.
Denial	Refusal to admit an obvious reality	Following a divorce, the husband still says he's married.
Rationalization	Substituting a concocted reason rather than the real reason for an event	Making an excuse using rationale. "If you had a wife like mine, you wouldn't go home either."
Reaction formation	Attesting to the opposite emotion of an impulse or desire	After breaking up with Mary, Bob says he never really loved her.
Regression	Reverting to a more primitive behavior of an earlier developmental stage	After losing an argument, Bob assaults his coworker.
Displacement	Substituting a less threatening object for the original object of hostility	After being fired, Bob returns home and kicks his cat.
Sublimation	Substituting forbidden impulses for socially acceptable activities	Bob plays tennis when he feels angry with his mother.
Humor	Humor is an expression of feelings or thoughts without discomfort	Bob tells friends "I am going to die alone" while laughing.

■ The defense mechanisms operate unconsciously.

■ The implementation of defense mechanisms to manage a stressor is based on efficiency. If unsuccessful, less efficient mechanisms will be implemented and may, unfortunately, lead to a demonstration of age-inappropriate or pathological behavior.

■ Psychotic individuals rely heavily on primitive defense mechanisms such as denial and projection.

■ Healthy individuals use the most appropriate defense mechanism and can quickly select another when necessary.

■ Individuals with personality disorders are unable to select appropriate mechanisms and rely heavily, even exclusively, on just one defense mechanism, such as paranoia.

The Process of Psychoanalysis

■ Freud believed that patients would structure their own emotional resolution if allowed to explore the repressed conflicts that were impeding growth and development.

■ The unconscious is both an asset and an impediment to conflict resolution and development. It is, by its nature, protective of the structure by holding an aberrant impulse in abeyance and thus managing anxiety and pain. Simultaneously, it prevents resolution because of this material being inaccessible.

■ One of Freud's goals was to develop a mechanism that would prevent overwhelming anxiety to the conscious mind and slowly allow the patient to develop an understanding of unconscious conflicts and developmental failures.

■ To address the unconscious, Freud developed psychoanalysis, a procedure by which the client could address repressed issues at their own pace in an environment free of ridicule and condemnation.

■ The client would recline on a couch and engage in a process of free association, in a spontaneous discourse of whatever came to mind.

■ The psychoanalyst would position themselves out of the patient's line of sight and record the process and topics of discourse. Commentary by the psychoanalyst was held to a minimum.

■ Occasionally, patients were requested to recount dreams. Dream material was given special attention, as Freud believed defense mechanisms were less vigilant during sleep and repressed conflicts and desires would work their way toward consciousness or at least preconsciousness. Even in the sleep state, the repressed material was too anxiety producing and had to be modified.

■ Freud explained the problem as follows:

   ■ The actual material and recollection of the dream consists of the manifest material. Thus, the content the patient remembers is a defensive modification of the repressed material. To the patient, the material may appear bizarre or nonsensical.

   ■ The latent content is the underlying repressed conflicting material that has been distorted by the manifest content so as to prevent anxiety.

■ Periodically, the psychoanalyst will interpret the latent content to the patient to facilitate resolution.

■ As analysis continues, the client experiences the anxiety of the repressed conflicts. As conflict intensifies, the client will have a catharsis, an outpouring of emotion that facilitates resolution. The analyst's task is to facilitate a controlled release of emotion so the client is not overwhelmed by anxiety and does not suffer a regressive experience.

- The psychoanalyst must refrain from addressing specific behaviors or superficial material. Resolving a specific symptom without addressing the underlying conflict might predispose the patient to have symptom substitution, that is, the development of a new symptom to replace the old.
- The process of analysis may be impeded by the patient's unconscious, as the process of investigation will increase anxiety and conflict.
- Patients will develop resistance. They may become dissatisfied with the psychoanalyst, skip or be late for appointments, become silent, or fail to report important material.
- The psychoanalyst must address resistance as it occurs or it may (will) become self-defeating and prevent deeper understanding of conflict-laden material.
- The patient may develop transference (a specific type of projection), that is, the unconscious association of the psychoanalyst with someone of significance in the patient's past. This allows the patient to ascribe to the psychoanalyst feelings once attributed to that person.
- Because of the nature of psychoanalysis, the psychoanalyst may engage in the same phenomenon, a process known as countertransference.
- Repressed conflicts affect an individual's life in an adverse manner by persistent utilization of inappropriate defense mechanisms. The psychoanalyst must interpret and educate the patient about the self-destructiveness of defense mechanisms.

Prominent Ideas of Freud

- The role of the unconscious is paramount in personality development and daily behavior.
- Sex, or the enhancement of pleasure, is the driving force in development and behavior.
- Freud possessed a dark view of human nature. He theorized humans as driven by fantasies, conflicts, and sexual urges that were controlled by socialization, training, and religion.
- Freud placed tremendous emphasis on early-life experiences. He proposed that most of our personality is formed by the age of 5.
- Freud outlined set stages of development. These were invariant and could not be circumvented. To obtain adequate psychological growth, the conflict at the end of each stage must be resolved so that libido energy can follow the appropriate developmental path.

The Freudians

Carl Jung, Analytical Psychology

- Jung was a Swiss colleague of Freud and a member of the inner circle until he developed his own theory of personality development.
- Jung believed that the personal unconscious could be understood by studying dreams, folklore, religion and mythology, and symbolism.
- As significant as the personal unconscious was the collective unconscious. He thought that there was a deeper level of the unconscious that was common to the entire species.
- Jung postulated the concept of archetype, a universal concept common to all humans. Many archetypes exist regarding behaviors such as motherhood and physical form. Archetypes are expressed in cultural and religious symbols.
- Mental health is the result of insight and self-realization. Mental illness is the consequence of conflicts that prevent self-exploration and self-realization.

Anna Freud, Ego Psychology

- The daughter of Sigmund Freud, Anna studied with her father and became a psychoanalyst in Vienna and London.
- Although a strong supporter of her father's theoretical positions, Anna came to believe that the ego should be the focus of attention.
- Anna Freud felt that the ego was the executor of personality and that analytical work should be directed at strengthening the ego to mitigate anxiety and stress.
- Anna Freud felt that the ego could become overwhelmed by conflicting demands of the id and the superego.
- Later in life, Anna Freud became a leader in child psychoanalysis and the psychological effects of depravation and poor nurturance.

Otto Rank, Humanistic Psychology

- Rank was Freud's closest associate for 20 years, until publication of a paper advocating a different process of development and questioning the importance of early-life psychosexual growth.
- Over time, Rank moved further away from the classic tenets and eventually focused on the "here and now" in psychotherapy, rather than interpreting early-life experiences and repressed conflicts.
- Rank emphasized active learning and continued psychological growth throughout life. Psychotherapy concentrates on discovering give and take, separating and coming together. A patient must find a balance regarding all the forces in their environment to achieve mental health. The passiveness of the analysis was changed to an active dialogue with the patient.
- Rank had a profound effect on the professional development of Carl Rogers, Rollo May, and Erik Erikson. His writings are considered the foundation of humanistic and client-centered therapy.

Erik Erikson, Developmental Psychology

- Following his graduation from the Vienna Psychoanalytic Institute, Erikson moved to the United States, where he taught at a number of universities and began to work with disadvantaged children and adolescents.
- Erikson revised Freud's five stages of psychosexual development into eight and said that human psychological development continues throughout life and that each stage has its individual challenges.
- Three stages were specific to adulthood and described challenges unique to that period.
- Like Anna Freud, Erikson was an ego psychologist who believed that the ego, not the id, was the focal point of personality.
- Erikson believed that social development, and not sexual development, was the underlying force behind growth.

Alfred Adler, Individual Psychology

- Along with Freud, Adler was one of the founders of psychoanalysis and the first colleague to break with Freud and establish his own school of thought.
- Adler believed in the unconscious and held that dream analysis was productive. However, he de-emphasized the role of psychosexual forces in favor of a conflict between inferiority and superiority.
- It was the work of the analyst to bring these two opposing forces into harmony.
- Central to Adler's technique was the concept of holistic treatment, which emphasized all psychological aspects of personal and social functioning of the patient.

- He abandoned the couch and had the psychoanalyst and the patient face each other in chairs. His therapeutic style utilized humor, historical incidents, and paradox.
- Adler's holistic approach led him to address how individuals integrate with society, and he became an advocate of prevention, democratic family structure, parent training, birth order, child psychology, organizational psychology, and women's rights.
- His work has been described as a precursor to modern CT.

Karen Horney, Feminine Psychology and Anxiety
- Psychoanalysis's first female practitioner, teacher, and theoretician, Horney broke with traditional Freudian teachings regarding psychosexual development and neurosis.
- Unlike Freud, who felt that neurotic (anxiety) disturbance in mental functioning was the result of conflict, Horney viewed neurosis as a continuous process of managing stressors. All persons possessed some degree of "basic anxiety," which formed the foundation for a lifelong struggle.
- Because of adverse early experiences, some patients were more susceptible to periods of anxiety.
- The management of anxiety was the foundation of development. Horney developed 10 basic neurotic needs that were expressed in three categories: moving toward people, moving away from people, and moving against people.
- Horney suggested that the "self" was at the core of personality. All persons possess a dual perception of the self: the real self, who we are, and the ideal self, who we wish to be.
- Anxiety is generated when the two selves are in conflict and disharmony.
- The job of the analyst is to resolve the conflict and enhance growth or self-actualization. This is a lifelong process.
- Horney felt Freud had overemphasized male sexual issues.
- She postulated that if women had "penis envy," then men must have "womb envy."
- As such, women had a psychological advantage as self-actualization could be achieved by bearing children.
- Men, unable to bear children, compensated for their feelings of inferiority by seeking self-actualization through external means, such as dominance and aggressiveness.
- Horney felt that cultural mores led women to be subservient to men, thereby preventing the attainment of self-actualization. She proposed that both genders had the ability to be productive and was an advocate for gender equality.

BIBLIOGRAPHY

Beck, A. T., Rush, A. J., Shaw, B. F., & Emery, G. (1979). *Cognitive therapy of depression*. Guilford Press.

Beck, J. (1995). *Cognitive therapy: Basics and beyond*. Guilford Press.

Burns, D. (1999). *Feeling good: The new mood therapy*. HarperCollins.

Choi, I., Zou, J., Titov, N. et al. (2012). Culturally attuned Internet treatment for depression amongst Chinese Australians: A randomised controlled trial. *Journal of Affective Disorders*, *136*(3), 459–468.

Dimeff, L. A., & Koerner, K. (Eds.). (2007). *Dialectical behavioral therapy in clinical practice*. Guilford Press.

Farrer, L., Christensen, H., & Griffiths, K. M., Mackinnon, A. (2011). Internet-based CBT for depression with and without telephone tracking in a national helpline: Randomised controlled trial. *PLoS One, 6*(11), e28099.

Gosch, E. A., Flannery-Schroeder, E., Mauro, C. F., & Compton, S. N. (2006). Principles of cognitive-behavioral therapy for anxiety disorders in children. *Journal of Cognitive Psychotherapy, 20*, 247–262.

Kenneth, H. K., Vessey, J., Lueger, R., & Schank, D. (1992). The psychotherapeutic delivery system. *Psychotherapy Research, 2*, 164–180.

Kuyken, W., Byford, S., Taylor, R. S., Watkins, E., Holden, E., White, K., Barrett, B., Byng, R., Evans, A., Mullan, E., & Teasdale, J. D. (2008). Mindfulness-based cognitive therapy to prevent relapse in recurrent depression. *Journal of Consulting and Clinical Psychology, 76*(6), 966–978.

Linehan, M. (1993). *Cognitive-behavioral treatment of borderline personality disorder.* Guilford Press.

Silfvernagel, K., Carlbring, P., Kabo, J., Edström, S., Eriksson, J., Månson, L., & Andersson, G. (2012). Individually tailored internet-based treatment for young adults and adults with panic attacks: Randomized controlled trial. *Journal of Medical Internet Research, 14*(3), e65.

Wheeler, K. (Ed.). (in press). *Psychotherapy for advanced practice nurses* (2nd ed.). Springer Publishing Company.

van der Zanden, R., Kramer, J., Gerrits, R., & Cuijpers, P. (2012). Effectiveness of an online group course for depression in adolescents and young adults: A randomized trial. *Journal of Medical Internet Research, 14*(3), e86.

Zur, O. (2009). *The standard of care in psychotherapy and counseling: Bringing clarity to an illusive standard.* http://www.zurinstitute.com/standardofcaretherapy.html

The Relationship of Psychopharmacology to Neurotransmitters, Receptors, Signal Transduction, and Second Messengers

The past 20 years have afforded scientists a greater understanding of the brain. Extreme changes in psychopharmacology have produced newer medicines with fewer side effects and greater benefits than ever before. These changes translate into improved wellness for patients with mental health disorders.

This chapter presents the following:

- A basic outline of the currently understood processes by which the brain communicates
- Information to support an improved understanding of the inner brain mechanisms from synaptic and cellular viewpoints in regard to psychopharmacology
- The signaling pathways associated with the six neurotransmitters most commonly altered in modern psychopharmacological therapy
- A strong scientific background on which to base psychopharmacological prescribing practices

Neurotransmitters

These are the molecules that mediate intracellular signaling of the brain.

- Neurotransmitters are chemicals that communicate their messages to the interior of the neurons. This process happens
  - through their release from the presynaptic terminal,
  - by their diffusing across the synaptic cleft, and
  - to further bind to receptors in the postsynaptic membrane.
- There are several dozen known or suspected neurotransmitters in the brain.
- Theoretically, there may be several hundred neurotransmitters, based on the amount of genetic materials in the neurons.
- Neurotransmitters are endogenous molecules; examples include various peptides and hormones (Table 4.1).
- Psychoactive drugs act by increasing, decreasing, or otherwise modulating the actions of neurotransmitters at their receptor sites.
- *Ligand* is a generic term referring to either endogenous or exogenous receptor binding partner proteins to which neurotransmitters bind, resulting in changes to downstream cellular processes.

TABLE 4.1 Major Neurotransmitters in the Central Nervous System

NEUROTRANSMITTER	EFFECTS
ACh	Cognition, learning, memory, alertness, muscle contraction
Dopamine	Pleasure, pain, movement control, emotional response
Gamma-aminobutyric acid	Psychomotor agitation/retardation, stress, anxiety
Glutamate	Memory, energy
Norepinephrine	Arousal, dreaming, depressed mood, suicide, apathy, psychomotor agitation/retardation, constricts blood vessels, increases heart rate and blood pressure, affects attention and the sleep–wake cycle
Serotonin	Mood control, temperature regulation, impulsiveness, aggression, cognitive problems, depressed mood, suicide, apathy, psychomotor agitation/retardation

ACh, acetylcholine.

- The following six neurotransmitter systems are the major targets for psychotropic drugs:
  - *Serotonergic neurons* (neurotransmitter = serotonin), originating primarily in the raphe nuclei of the reticular formation extending from the medulla to the midbrain
  - *Noradrenergic neurons* (neurotransmitter = norepinephrine), originating in the locus coeruleus
  - *Dopaminergic neurons* (neurotransmitter = dopamine), originating primarily in the ventral tegmental area
  - *Muscarinic cholinergic neurons* (neurotransmitter = acetylcholine), one of the principal neurotransmitters in the autonomic nervous system
  - *Glutamatergic neurons* (neurotransmitter = glutamate), an amino acid transmitter synthesized by the brain from glucose and other nutrients for motor activity
  - *GABAergic neurons* (neurotransmitter = gamma-aminobutyric acid [GABA]), an inhibitory amino acid neurotransmitter, which is synthesized from glutamate in the brain and decreases activity in nerve cells
- These six neurotransmitters are relatively low-molecular-weight amines or amino acids.
- Multiple neurons that release more than one neurotransmitter may converge at a single synapse.
- Cotransmission involves a monoamine coupled with a neuropeptide.
  - This natural combination of multiple signaling molecules at the synapse is the basis for the modern treatment rationale of prescribing drugs affecting multiple neuronal signaling pathways.

Six Neurotransmitters Most Commonly Affected by the Psychopharmacology-Treatment Regimens*

Communication within the brain happens in three ways: *anterograde, retrograde,* or *nonsynaptic.* Chemical neurotransmission is the foundation of psychopharmacology.

- **Anterograde neurotransmission**
  - Most predominant means of excitation coupling and synapses
  - Occurs in one direction (i.e., presynaptic to postsynaptic), from the cell body, down the axon, to the synaptic cleft

*Currently prescribed psychotropic medications are developed to target these neurotransmitter signaling pathways.

- Involves stimulation of a presynaptic neuron causing electrical impulses to be sent to its axon terminal (may be regarded as "classic" neurotransmission).
- Electrical impulses are converted into chemical messengers, known as neurotransmitters.
- Chemical messengers (neurotransmitters) are released to stimulate the receptors of the postsynaptic neuron.
- Communication *within* a neuron is mediated by electrical conduction of an action potential from the cell body down the axon of the neuron, where it ends at the synaptic cleft.
- Communication *between* neurons is chemical and mediated by one of the several neurotransmitters described earlier.
- Excitation–secretion coupling is the process by which an electrochemical signal in the first (i.e., presynaptic) neuron is converted from a chemical impulse into the release of a chemical signal at the synapse.
- Electrical impulses result from the opening of *ion channels* in the neuronal cell membrane along the axon, causing a change in net charge of the neuron. The difference in charge between the inside of the cell and the outside of the cell is referred to as an *action potential*.
  - Voltage-sensitive sodium channels
  - Voltage-sensitive potassium channels
- All this happens very quickly once the electrical impulse enters the presynaptic neuron.
- Occurs predominately in one direction (from the cell body, down the axon, to the synaptic cleft).
- **Retrograde neurotransmission**
  - Postsynaptic neurons can talk back directly and indirectly.
    - Indirectly through a long neuronal feedback loop
    - Directly through retrograde neurotransmission from postsynaptic to presynaptic
  - Examples of retrograde neurotransmitters synthesized in the postsynaptic neuron, released, and diffused into the presynaptic neuron are
    - endocannabinoids (endogenous compounds similar to marijuana, also known as cannabis), and
    - nitric oxide.
- **Non-synaptic neurotransmission**
  - No neurotransmission across a synaptic cleft.
  - Chemical messengers sent by one neuron diffuse to compatible receptor sites distant to the synapse.

Receptors

These are proteins to which neurotransmitters bind, resulting in changes to downstream cellular processes.

- Found within plasma membranes and the cytoplasm of a cell
- Affected by psychoactive drugs
- Located on cell membranes of neurons

Receptors Specific to Psychopharmacology

Psychotropic medications are developed to target these various receptor sites.

- *Serotonin* binds to 5-HT1A, 5-HT1B, 5-HT1D, 5-HT1E, 5-HT1F, 5-HT2, 5-HT2A, 5-HT2B, 5-HT2C, 5-HT3, 5-HT4, and 5-HT5A receptors (Table 4.2).
- *Norepinephrine* binds to alpha$_1$ and alpha$_2$, beta$_1$, beta$_2$, and beta$_3$ receptors (Table 4.3).

■ *Dopamine* binds to D1, D2, D3, D4, and D5 receptors (Table 4.4).
■ *Acetylcholine* binds to nicotinic (N) and muscarinic (M) receptors (Table 4.5).
■ *GABA* binds to $GABA_A$ and $GABA_B$ receptors (Table 4.6).
■ *Glutamate* binds to AMPA (alpha-amino-3-hydroxy-5-methyl-4-isoxazolepropionic acid receptor), kainate, and NMDA (*N*-methyl-D-aspartate) receptors (Table 4.7).

SIGNAL TRANSDUCTION

Signal transduction is the movement of signals from the outside of a cell to the inside.

■ Signal → receptor → change in cell function
■ Plays a very specific role through messaging and activation of an inactive molecule
  ■ Starts a reaction that cascades through chemical neurotransmission via numerous molecules
    ● Long-term effects of late gene products and many more messages.
    ● Can occur over the time course of minutes, hours, days, or weeks.
    ● Effects may be temporary or permanent.
■ Signal transduction translates into the following diverse biological responses:
  ■ Gene expression
  ■ Synaptogenesis

TABLE 4.2 Serotonin

RECEPTOR TYPE	DISTRIBUTION	EFFECTS
5-HT1, 5-HT1A, 5-HT1B, 5-HT1D, 5-HT1E, 5-HT1F	Brain, blood vessels, intestinal nerves	*Inhibitory*: neuronal inhibition, cerebral vasoconstriction *Behavioral effects*: addiction, aggression, anxiety, appetite, impulsivity, learning, memory, mood, sexual behavior, sleep
5-HT2, 5-HT2A, 5-HT2B, 5-HT2C	Brain, blood vessels, heart, lungs, smooth muscle control, GI system, blood vessels, platelets	*Excitatory*: neuronal excitation, vasoconstriction *Behavioral effects*: addiction, anxiety, appetite, mood, sexual behavior, sleep
5-HT3	Limbic system, CNS, PNS, GI system	*Excitatory*: nausea *Behavioral effects*: addiction, anxiety, learning, memory
5-HT4	CNS, smooth muscle, GI system	*Excitatory*: neuronal excitation, GI *Behavioral effects*: anxiety, appetite, learning, memory, mood
5-HT5, 5-HT5A, 5-HT6, 5-HT7	Brain	*Inhibitory*: may be linked to BDNF *Behavioral effects*: sleep
5-HT6	CNS	*Excitatory*: may be linked to BDNF *Behavioral effects*: anxiety, cognition, learning, memory, mood
5-HT7	CNS, blood vessels GI system	*Excitatory*: may be linked to BDNF *Behavioral effects*: anxiety, memory, sleep, mood

BDNF, brain-derived neurotrophic factor; CNS, central nervous system; GI, gastrointestinal; 5-HT, serotonin; PNS, peripheral nervous system.

TABLE 4.3   Norepinephrine

RECEPTOR TYPE	DISTRIBUTION	EFFECTS
Alpha$_1$	Brain, heart, smooth muscle	*Excitatory*: vasoconstriction, smooth muscle contraction
Alpha$_2$	Presynaptic neurons in brain, pancreas, smooth muscle	*Inhibitory*: vasoconstriction, gastrointestinal relaxation presynaptically
Beta$_1$	Heart, brain	*Excitatory*: increased heart rate
Beta$_2$	Lungs, brain, skeletal muscle	*Excitatory*: bronchial relaxation, vasodilation, smooth muscle relaxation
Beta$_3$	Adipose tissue	*Excitatory*: stimulation of effector cells

TABLE 4.4   Dopamine

RECEPTOR TYPE	DISTRIBUTION	EFFECTS
D1	Brain, smooth muscle	*Excitatory*: possible role in schizophrenia and Parkinson's
D2	Brain, cardiovascular system, presynaptic nerve terminals	*Inhibitory*: possible role in schizophrenia
D3	Brain, cardiovascular system, presynaptic nerve terminals	*Inhibitory*: possible role in schizophrenia
D4	Brain, cardiovascular system, presynaptic nerve terminals	*Inhibitory*: possible role in schizophrenia
D5	Brain, smooth muscle	*Excitatory*: possible role in schizophrenia and Parkinson's

TABLE 4.5   Acetylcholine

RECEPTOR TYPE	DISTRIBUTION	EFFECTS
M1	Ganglia, secretory glands	*Excitatory*: CNS excitation, gastric acid secretion
M2	Heart, nerves, smooth muscle	*Inhibitory*: cardiac inhibition, neural inhibition
M3	Glands, smooth muscle, endothelium, secretory glands	*Excitatory*: smooth muscle contraction, vasodilation
M4	CNS, PNS, smooth muscle, secretory glands	*Inhibitory*
M5	CNS	*Inhibitory*
N$_M$	Skeletal muscle, neuromuscular junction	*Excitatory*: neuromuscular transmission
N$_N$	Postganglionic cell body dendrites	*Excitatory*: ganglionic transmission

CNS, central nervous system; M, muscarinic; N, nicotinic; PNS, peripheral nervous system.

TABLE 4.6   GABA

RECEPTOR TYPE	DISTRIBUTION	EFFECTS
GABA$_A$	CNS	*Inhibitory*
GABA$_B$	ANS	*Excitatory*

ANS, autonomic nervous system; CNS, central nervous system; GABA, gamma-aminobutyric acid.

TABLE 4.7 Glutamate

RECEPTOR TYPE	DISTRIBUTION	EFFECTS
AMPA	CNS	Excitatory
Kainate	CNS	Excitatory
NMDA	CNS	Excitatory

AMPA, alpha-amino-3-hydroxy-5-methyl-4-isoxazolepropionic acid receptor; CNS, central nervous system; NMDA, N-methyl-D-aspartate receptor.

TABLE 4.8 Endogenous Neurotransmitters

NEUROTRANSMITTER	RECEPTOR	SIGNAL TRANSDUCTION	SECOND MESSENGER
Acetylcholine	Muscarinic Nicotinic	G-protein linked Ion channel linked	cAMP or IP_3 Calcium
Dopamine	D1, D2, D3, D4, D5 alpha$_1$, beta$_2$	G-protein linked G-protein linked	cAMP or IP_3 cAMP or IP_3
GABA	GABA$_A$ GABA$_B$	Ion channel linked and ligand-gated ion channels G-protein linked	Calcium cAMP or IP_3
Glutamate	AMPA, kainate, and NMDA metabotropic	Ion channel linked G-protein linked	Calcium cAMP or IP_3
Norepinephrine	Alpha$_1$, alpha$_2$ beta$_1$	G-protein linked G-protein linked	cAMP or IP_3 cAMP or IP_3
Epinephrine	Alpha$_1$, alpha$_2$ beta$_1$, beta$_2$	G-protein linked G-protein linked	cAMP or IP_3 cAMP or IP_3
Serotonin	5-HT1A, 5-HT1B, 5-HT1D, 5-HT1E, 5-HT1F 5-HT2, 5-HT2A, 5-HT2B, 5-HT2C 5-HT3 5-HT4 5-HT5A	G-protein linked G-protein linked Ion channel linked G-protein linked G-protein linked	cAMP or IP_3 cAMP or IP_3 Calcium cAMP or IP_3 cAMP or IP_3

cAMP, cyclic adenosine monophosphate; GABA, gamma-aminobutyric acid; 5-HT, serotonin; IP3, inositol trisphosphate.

Second Messengers

Second messengers are synthesized and activated by enzymes and help mediate intracellular signaling in response to a ligand binding to its receptor.

- Relay and amplify signals received by receptors such as cyclic adenosine monophosphate (cAMP) and inositol trisphosphate (IP_3) are used for signal transduction in biological cells and Ca^{2+}.

Endogenous Neurotransmitters

- See Table 4.8.

5

Clinical Neuroanatomy of the Brain

Clinical neuroanatomy is the method of studying lesions of the human nervous system as a tool to reinforce and amplify learning of the structure and organization of the central nervous system (CNS).

Clinical neuropharmacology is the study of drugs that alter processes controlled by the nervous system.

This chapter deals with the basic anatomy and physiology of the CNS, peripheral nervous system (PNS), somatic nervous system, blood–brain barrier, basal ganglia, hippocampus, hypothalamus, and neurotransmitters.

NERVOUS SYSTEM

The central nervous system is composed of the brain and spinal cord, which are covered by protective membranes (meninges) and have fluid-filled spaces; weighs less than most desktop computers; receives and interprets sensory information and controls simple/complex motor behaviors. The peripheral nervous system is composed of cranial and spinal nerves; the nerves contain nerve fibers, which conduct information to (afferent) and from (efferent) the CNS; efferent fibers are involved in motor function, such as contraction of muscles or activation of secretory glands; afferent fibers convey sensory stimuli from the skin, mucous membranes, and deeper structures.

- *Somatic nervous system*: part of PNS; innervates the structures of the body wall (muscles, skin, and mucous membranes).
- *Autonomic nervous system*: part of PNS; contains the sympathetic nervous system (SNS) ("fight or flight") and the parasympathetic nervous system (PSNS); controls activities of the smooth muscles, glands, and internal organs, including blood vessels, and returns sensory information to the brain.

Central Nervous System

Brain and Spinal Cord

- CNS drugs are used medically to treat psychiatric disorders, seizures, and pain and as anesthetics; nonmedically, they are used as stimulants, depressants, euphoriants, and mind-altering substances.

- The CNS drugs include at least 21 neurotransmitters:
  - *Monoamines*: norepinephrine, epinephrine, dopamine, serotonin
  - *Amino acids*: aspartate, glutamate, gamma-aminobutyric acid (GABA), glycine
  - *Purines*: adenosine, adenosine monophosphate, adenosine triphosphate
  - *Peptides*: dynorphins, endorphins, enkephalins, neurotensin, somatostatin, substance P, oxytocin, vasopressin
  - *Others*: acetylcholine (ACh), histamine

Blood–Brain Barrier

The blood–brain barrier blocks the entry of some drugs and substances into the brain.

- *Elements*: supporting cells (neuralgia), particularly the astrocytes, and tight junctions between endothelial cells.
- *Function*: selectively inhibits certain substances in the blood from entering the interstitial spaces of the brain or cerebrospinal fluid. Certain metabolites, electrolytes, and chemicals have differing abilities to cross the blood–brain barrier. This has substantial implications for drug therapy because some antibiotics and chemotherapeutic drugs show a greater ability than others for crossing the barrier.
- *P-glycoprotein*: a protective element of the blood–brain barrier and a transport molecule that pumps various types of drugs out of cells. In the capillaries of the CNS, P-glycoprotein pumps drugs back into the blood, thus limiting their access to the brain.
- Passage limited to lipid-soluble substances and drugs that cross by means of transport systems (protein-bound and highly ionized substances cannot cross).
- Protects brain from injury due to toxic substances but also acts as an obstacle to entry of therapeutic drugs.

The Brain

- The brain is able to adapt to prolonged drug exposure, which can alter the therapeutic effects and side effects of some drugs (adaptive changes are often beneficial but can be harmful).
  - Increased therapeutic effects, decreased side effects, tolerance, and physical dependences may occur.
  - Acts as a control center by receiving, interpreting, and directing sensory information throughout the body.
- Composed of cerebrum (*telencephalon*—cerebral cortex, subcortical white matter, commissures, basal ganglia; *diencephalon*—thalamus, hypothalamus, epithalamus, subthalamus), brain stem (midbrain, pons, medulla oblongata), and cerebellum (cerebellar cortex, cerebellar nuclei). The cerebrum and cerebellum are organized into the right and left hemispheres.
- There are *three major divisions* of the brain—the forebrain, the midbrain, and the hindbrain.
  - The forebrain is responsible for receiving and processing sensory information, thinking, perceiving, producing and understanding language, and controlling motor function.
  - The midbrain is responsible for auditory and visual responses and motor function.
  - The hindbrain is responsible for maintaining balance and equilibrium, movement coordination, and the conduction of sensory information.

- *The limbic system* is often called the "pleasure center."
  - It is the group of structures that govern emotions and behavior.
  - It connects to all areas of the brain, especially the frontal cortex, which is the learning center.

Peripheral Nervous System

The PNS is divided into the *somatic nervous system* (controls movement of skeletal muscles) and the *autonomic nervous system (ANS)*. The ANS is further divided into the PSNS and the SNS.

- *PSNS*—directs the housekeeping chores of the body; stimulation of these nerves slows heart rate, increases gastric secretions, empties bladder and bowel, focuses eye for near vision, constricts pupil, and contracts bronchial smooth muscle.
- *SNS*—has three main functions: regulates the cardiovascular system, regulates body temperature, and implements the fight-or-flight response.
- The PNS uses three neurotransmitters to exert its actions: ACh (released by all preganglionic neurons of the PSNS and SNS, all postganglionic neurons of the PSNS, all motor neurons of the skeletal muscles, and most postganglionic neurons of the SNS that supply the sweat glands), norepinephrine (released by almost all postganglionic neurons of SNS with the exception of postganglionic neurons that supply sweat glands), and epinephrine (released by adrenal medulla).
- Two basic categories of PNS receptors and their subtypes (receptor subtypes make it possible for drugs to act selectively) are as follows:
  - Cholinergic-mediated responses to ACh subtypes include the following:
    - $Nicotinic_N$ activation stimulates parasympathetic and sympathetic postganglionic nerves and causes release of epinephrine from adrenal medulla.
    - $Nicotinic_M$ activation causes contraction of the skeletal muscle.
    - Muscarinic activation causes focus of lens for near vision, miosis, decreased heart rate, constriction of bronchi, promotion of secretions, increase in bladder pressure, urination, salivation, increased gastric secretions, increased intestinal tone and motility, sweating, erection, and vasodilation.
  - Adrenergic-mediated responses to epinephrine and norepinephrine subtypes include the following:
    - $Alpha_1$ activation by epinephrine, norepinephrine, or dopamine causes mydriasis, vasoconstriction, ejaculation, and prostate contraction.
    - $Alpha_2$ activation by epinephrine or norepinephrine causes *inhibition* of subsequent neurotransmitter release.
    - $Beta_1$ activation by epinephrine, norepinephrine, or dopamine causes increased heart rate, force of contraction, atrioventricular conduction, and increased renin release from the kidney.
    - $Beta_2$ activation (only by epinephrine) causes vasodilation, bronchial dilation, uterine relaxation, glycogenolysis, and enhanced contraction of the skeletal muscle.
    - Dopamine (responds only to dopamine) activation causes dilation of kidney vasculature.

Somatic Nervous System

- *Elements:* motor neurons arising from the spinal cord and brain and the neuromuscular junction.
- *Neuromuscular junction:* formed by the terminal of the motor neuron and the motor end plates (special sites on the muscle's membrane). Motor neurons release

neurotransmitter ACh to the junction; subsequently, ACh activates its receptor (nicotinic$_M$ receptor) on the motor end plates and causes muscle contraction.

■ *Drugs that target the neuromuscular junction:* cholinesterase inhibitors, nondepolarizing neuromuscular blockers, and depolarizing neuromuscular blockers.

Basal Ganglia (or Basal Nuclei)

It is a group of nuclei situated at the base of the forebrain and strongly connected to the cerebral cortex, thalamus, and other areas.

■ *Elements:* striatum, pallidum, substantia nigra, and subthalamic nucleus.

■ *Function:* They are associated with motor control and learning functions. The substantia nigra provides dopaminergic input to the striatum. The basal ganglia play a central role in a number of neurological conditions, including several movement disorders. The most notable are Parkinson's disease, which involves degeneration of the dopamine-producing cells in the substantia nigra, and Huntington's disease, which primarily involves damage to the striatum.

■ Drugs are used for Parkinson's disease to increase the dopamine level at the striatum.

Hippocampus

The hippocampus belongs to the limbic system, which forms the inner border of the cortex.

■ *Function:* emotion, behavior, and long-term memory. Beta-amyloid, neuritic plaques and neurofibrillary tangles, and tau in the hippocampus and cerebral cortex are the prominent features of Alzheimer's disease (AD). Another characteristic of AD is that the level of ACh, an important neurotransmitter in the hippocampus and cerebral cortex, is significantly below normal.

■ Drugs used to treat AD include cholinesterase inhibitors and N-methyl-D-aspartate (NMDA) receptor antagonist.

Hypothalamus

The hypothalamus is located below the thalamus and above the brainstem.

■ The *pituitary gland* is located below the third ventricle of the brain and the hypothalamus, composed of anterior pituitary (adenohypophysis) and posterior pituitary (neurohypophysis). The pituitary stalk connects the hypothalamus to the pituitary gland.

■ *Function:* The hypothalamus controls the anterior pituitary by hypothalamic-releasing factors, while it synthesizes oxytocin and antidiuretic hormone and projects its neuronal axon to the posterior pituitary. The hypothalamus controls body temperature, hunger, thirst, fatigue, and circadian cycles.

■ Drugs that target the pituitary stimulate or inhibit the synthesis and release of hormones from the anterior pituitary gland. In addition, some drugs act as agonists or antagonists of pituitary gland hormone receptors.

Both in the PNS and the CNS, neurons regulate physiological processes in the same way through two steps:

■ *Axonal conduction*—An action potential is sent down the axon of a neuron.

　▪ Drugs that influence axonal conduction are not selective, so they stop transmission in the axon of any neuron they reach.

　▪ The only group of drugs that affect axonal conduction are local anesthetics.

■ *Synaptic transmission*—A transmitter is released from the neuron carrying information across a synapse, or gap, to a postsynaptic cell receptor causing a change in that cell.
  ▪ Most drugs work by affecting synaptic transmission.
  ▪ Drugs that work by affecting synaptic transmission are very selective due to the different types of transmitters and receptor sites.
  ▪ To work, drugs must have either a direct or an indirect effect on target cell receptors. Synaptic transmission includes five steps:
■ *Transmitter synthesis*—synthesis of the transmitter in the neuron
  ▪ Drugs work here by
    ○ increasing the amount of transmitter synthesized,
    ○ decreasing the amount of transmitter synthesized, and
    ○ synthesizing a "super" transmitter that is more potent than the naturally occurring transmitter.
■ *Transmitter storage*—The transmitter is stored in vesicles in the axon terminal for later use.
  ▪ Drugs work here by
    ○ reducing the amount of transmitter stored.
■ *Transmitter release*—Axonal conduction causes release of the transmitter into the synapse between the neuron and the target cell.
  ▪ Drugs work here by
    ○ increasing the amount of transmitter released, and
    ○ decreasing the amount of transmitter released.
■ *Receptor binding*—The transmitter binds to receptor sites on the postsynaptic, or target, cell causing a change in that cell.
  ▪ Drugs work here by
    ○ mimicking the natural transmitter and binding to additional target cell receptor sites to increase the effects on a target cell (agonist),
    ○ binding to target cell receptor sites to block the naturally occurring transmitter from binding to the target cell and decreasing the effect that the naturally occurring transmitter has on the target cell (antagonist), and
    ○ binding to the same target cell receptor sites together with the naturally occurring transmitter to increase the target cell's response to the transmitter.
■ *Termination of transmission*—The transmitter is depleted by reuptake, enzymatic degradation, or diffusion.
  ▪ Drugs work here by
    ○ stopping the reuptake of the transmitter, allowing more transmitter to be available to bind to the target cell receptor sites, and
    ○ stopping the enzymatic degradation of the transmitter, allowing more transmitter to be available to bind to the target cell receptor sites.

NEUROTRANSMITTERS

Neurotransmitters are chemicals that account for the transmission of signals from one neuron to the next across a synapse. They are also found at the axon endings of motor neurons, where they stimulate the muscle fibers to contract.

■ Chemical substances stored in the terminal end of a neuron, released when the storing neuron "fires," have the potential to influence the activity of a receiving cell (either increasing or decreasing likelihood of action).

- Present in the synaptic terminal.
- Action may be blocked by pharmacological agents.
- Examples of CNS neurotransmitters include the following; see Table 5.1.
    - *ACh*—widely distributed throughout the CNS and the primary transmitter at the neuromuscular junction
    - *Dopamine*—involved in a wide variety of behaviors and emotions associated with parkinsonism and, perhaps, schizophrenia
    - *Serotonin*—involved in sleep regulation, dreaming, mood, eating, pain, and aggression and associated with depression (i.e., selective serotonin reuptake inhibitor)
    - *Glutamate*—an excitatory transmitter, associated in memory, arousal, and pain
    - *GABA*—widely distributed; largely an inhibitory transmitter

NEUROPHARMACOLOGY

Neuropharmacology is the study of drugs that alter processes regulated by the nervous system. The nervous system regulates almost all bodily processes and, therefore, almost all bodily processes can be influenced by drugs that alter neuron regulation. By blocking (antagonist) or mimicking (agonist) neuron regulation, neuropharmacological drugs can modify skeletal muscle contraction, cardiac output, vascular tone, respiration, gastrointestinal function, uterine motility, glandular secretion, and functions of the CNS, such as pain perception, ideation, and mood.

- Neurons regulate physiological processes through a two-step process involving axonal conduction and synaptic transmission.
    - *Axonal conduction*—process of conducting an action potential down the axon of the neuron
        - Drugs (local anesthetics) that alter this conduction are not very selective, because the process of axonal conduction is almost the same in all neurons; therefore, a drug that alters conduction will alter conduction in all cells.
    - *Synaptic transmission*—the process of carrying information across the synapse between the neuron and the postsynaptic cell; requires release of neurotransmitters and binding of these transmitters to receptors on the postsynaptic cell
        - Most drugs act by altering this synaptic transmission because they are able to produce more selective effects by altering the following:
            - Transmitter synthesis and receptor activation can be increased; transmitter synthesis and receptor activation can be decreased; or transmitters that are more effective than the natural transmitter, which will cause receptor activation to increase, can be synthesized.
            - Transmitter storage can cause receptor activation to decrease by decreasing the amount of transmitter available.
            - Transmitter release can promote release and increase receptor activation or can inhibit release and reduce receptor activation.
            - Termination of transmitter action blocks transmitter reuptake or inhibition of transmitter degradation; both these actions will increase the concentration of transmitter and cause receptor activation to increase.
        - In order for a drug to exert its effect, it must be able to directly or indirectly influence the receptor activity on the target cell. Drugs act on receptors by
            - binding to them and causing activation (agonist),

TABLE 5.1   Neurotransmitters

NEUROTRANS-MITTER	FOCUSED AREAS
ACh	Neuromuscular junction, autonomic ganglia, parasympathetic neurons, motor nuclei of cranial nerves, caudate nucleus and putamen, basal nucleus of Meynert, portions of the limbic system *Receptor:* N, *action:* excitatory *Receptor:* M, *action:* excitatory or inhibitory *Action:* CNS—memory, sensory processing, motor coordination ■ Muscarinic—found at postganglionic parasympathetic endings (heart, smooth muscle, glands); five subtypes of muscarinic receptors: M_1 receptors found in ganglia and secretory glands M_2 receptors predominate in myocardium and in smooth muscle M_3 and M_4 receptors found in smooth muscle and secretory glands M_5 receptors have been identified in the CNS along with the other four types ■ Nicotinic receptors found in ganglia and at neuromuscular junction. Identified as the following: N_M receptors found at the neuromuscular junction in skeletal muscle N_G receptors found in autonomic ganglia, adrenal medulla, and CNS
Norepinephrine	SNS, locus coeruleus, lateral tegmentum *Action:* CNS—positive mood and reward, orienting and alerting responses, basic instincts (sex, eating, thirst) *C-receptors:* ■ $Alpha_1$ (postsynaptic) causes contraction of blood vessels, sphincters, radial muscle of eye. ■ $Alpha_2$ (presynaptic): negative feedback loop inhibiting subsequent release of neurotransmitter; upregulation and downregulation occur in response to decreased or increased activation of receptors; present at extrasynaptic sites in blood vessels and the CNS; stimulation in the brain stem decreases sympathetic outflow; stimulation in the pancreas inhibits insulin release. ■ $Beta_1$ (predominately cardiac) stimulation increases heart rate or strength of contraction. ■ $Beta_2$ (predominately noncardiac) found on smooth muscle (bronchi; large blood vessels) causes relaxation and promotes insulin release, liver and muscle gluconeogenesis and glycogenolysis, and lipolysis in fat cells. ■ $Beta_3$ receptors are expressed in visceral adipocytes.
Dopamine	Hypothalamus, midbrain nigrostriatal system *Receptors:* D1 and D2, action: inhibitory ■ D1 (postsynaptic) receptors responsible for vasodilation in splanchnic and renal circulations; stimulation in chemoreceptor trigger zone causes nausea and vomiting. ■ D2 (presynaptic) receptors initiate a negative feedback loop; five forms are found in the brain. *Action:* Regulation of hormonal balance, voluntary movement, reward
5-HT	Parasympathetic neurons in gut, pineal gland, nucleus raphe magnus of pons *Action:* CNS—sleep and emotional arousal, impulse control, cognition, pain processing, dreaming, homeostatic processes
GABA	Cerebellum, hippocampus, cerebral cortex, striatonigral system *Receptor:* GABAa, *action:* inhibitory (postsynaptic) *Receptor:* GABAb, *action:* inhibitory (presynaptic)
Glycine	Spinal cord *Action:* inhibitory
Glutamic acid	Spinal cord, brainstem, cerebellum, hippocampus, cerebral cortex

ACh, acetylcholine; CNS, central nervous system; GABA, gamma-aminobutyric acid; 5-HT, serotonin; M, muscarinic; N, nicotinic; SNS, sympathetic nervous system.

- binding to them and blocking their activation by other agents (antagonists), and
- binding to their components and indirectly enhancing their activation by the natural transmitter.

Clinical Neuroanatomy: Rationale for Understanding

■ Understanding neuroanatomy helps guide pharmacological approaches to treatment. A key goal of pharmacotherapy is to modify a patient's pathogenic nervous system activity.
  ▪ The nervous system (CNS and PNS) regulates our bodily processes. Therefore, our body processes can be affected by the drugs that regulate neuronal activity. Understanding clinical neuroanatomy helps in the development of neuropharmacological drugs and treatment selection to modify a patient's pathogenic nervous system activity.

Clinical Neuroanatomy: Association With Drug Action

■ Drug enters the body through various *routes of administration*—injection, oral, sublingual, inhalation, and transdermal.
■ What the body does to the drug (*pharmacokinetics*) is discussed in the following:
  ▪ *Absorption* (transfer of drug from the site of application to the blood stream)
    ● Affected by the rate of dissolution, surface area, blood flow, lipid solubility, and pH partitioning
    ● Bioavailability (the fraction of unchanged drug that reaches site of action), affected by anything that alters absorption, distribution, or metabolism
  ▪ *Distribution* (drug leaves blood stream → interstitial space of tissues → target cells responsible for therapeutic and adverse effects)
    ● Determined by the blood flow to tissues, ability to exit the vascular system (capillary beds, blood–brain barrier, placental drug transfer, and protein binding), and ability to enter cells (lipid solubility and presence of transport system)
  ▪ *Metabolism* (enzymatic alteration of drug structure or "bagging the trash," usually by liver)
    ● Hepatic drug-metabolizing enzymes
  ▪ *Excretion* (removal of drugs from the body)
■ What the drug does to the body (*pharmacodynamics*) is discussed in the following:
  ▪ Dose–response relationship
    ● Size of administered dose
    ● Intensity of the response produced
  ▪ *Drug–receptor interactions* (drugs interact with chemical)
    ● *Receptor* (chemicals in the body to which the drug binds to produce effects)
      - Regulated by endogenous compounds or macromolecules (body's own receptors for hormones, neurotransmitters, and other regulatory molecules).
      - Can be turned on or off.
      - Turned on by interaction with other molecules.
      - When the drug binds to receptors, it either mimics (*agonists*) or blocks (*antagonists*) the action of endogenous regulatory molecules such as neurotransmitters (supplied to receptors by neurons of the nervous system).
      - There are receptors for each neurotransmitter, each hormone, and all other regulatory molecules.
      - Drugs are selective to specific receptors (a receptor is analogous to a lock and a drug is analogous to a key for that lock), so only drugs with proper size, shape, and properties can bind to a receptor.

BIBLIOGRAPHY

Carter, R. (1999). *Mapping the mind*. University of California Press.

Haines, D. E. (1995). *Neuroanatomy: An atlas of structures, systems, sections, and systems* (4th ed.). Williams & Wilkins.

Kasschau, R. A. (2003). *Understanding psychology*. Glencoe McGraw-Hill.

Myers, D. G. (2004). *Psychology* (7th ed.). Worth Publishers.

Tortora, G. J., & Grabowski, S. R. (2003). *Principles of anatomy and physiology* (10th ed.). John Wiley & Sons.

6

Principles of Pharmacokinetics and Pharmacodynamics

Pharmacokinetics and pharmacodynamics comprise the collective interactions between a drug and a patient.

- *Pharmacokinetics* refers to the effects of the patient on the drug. The four primary pharmacokinetic processes are absorption, distribution, metabolism, and excretion.
- *Pharmacodynamics* refers to the effects of the drug on the patient.

PHARMACOKINETIC PRINCIPLES

- The four pharmacokinetic processes of absorption, distribution, metabolism, and excretion describe the effects the patient's organ systems have on the drug from the time it enters until the time it leaves the body.
- The extent to which a psychoactive drug will undergo each process is dependent on drug-specific and patient-specific variables.
  - Examples of drug-specific variables include the *chemical structure* and *route of administration*.
  - Examples of patient-specific variables include any *comorbidities*, overall *health*, the patient's *age*, and *concurrent pharmacotherapy*.

Absorption

- *Absorption* refers to the movement of a drug from its site of administration into the circulatory system.
- Drug absorption is affected by the chemical properties of the drug as well as the route of drug administration.
  - Movement of drugs into the circulatory system most commonly requires drugs to pass across and through cellular compartments.
  - This movement occurs by active transport, passive diffusion, or direct penetration through the cell membranes.
  - Chemical properties of the drug, drug concentration, presence of drug-transporter molecules, and pH affect intercellular drug movement.
  - The dosage requirements for a drug may be noticeably different based on its route of administration.
  - Dosing differences are often necessary to ensure that *bioequivalence* is achieved when two different routes of administration of the same drug are employed.

- Absorption following *oral administration*
  - Drugs enter the gastrointestinal (GI) tract and are absorbed through the stomach or small intestine. They travel via the portal vein first to the liver and then through the heart and into general circulation.
  - Oral administration results in more variable drug absorption and drug bioavailability than other administration routes.
  - *First-pass metabolism* (also known as the *first-pass effect*) refers to the inactivation of an orally administered drug by liver enzymes immediately following absorption from the GI tract and prior to the drug reaching general circulation. *Enterohepatic recirculation* refers to the cyclical movement of orally administered drugs from the GI tract to the liver, then packaged into bile and secreted into the small intestine, and then reabsorbed back into the liver.
  - Drug dissolution may be protracted up to approximately 8 hours by formulating sustained-release, extended-release, and controlled-release preparations. Sustained-release formulations (e.g., controlled-release paroxetine [*Paxil CR*]) may minimize GI distress, decrease the number of daily dosages, and provide more uniform drug absorption.
    - Many controlled-release (CR) formulations are available only as brand name medications at a substantially increased price over standard-release formulations. CR formulations cannot be crushed or chewed. Only formulations that are scored can be split.
  - Drugs that are inactivated by gastric acid or that cause gastric irritation may be prepared with an *enteric coating*, which permits drug absorption to be delayed until the drug passes through the stomach and enters the intestine. Care should be exercised not to coadminister antacids with enteric-coated products; if so done, the coating will dissolve in the higher pH.
  - Patients with GI distress may have impaired oral absorption.
- Absorption following *transdermal administration*
  - Suitable formulation and route of administration for drugs able to permeate intact skin.
  - Toxic effects may occur during transdermal absorption if drugs are highly lipid soluble, or when applied to irritated or damaged skin, or if transdermal application is a patch and the previous patch was not removed prior to the next dose (or if patch is cut or divided prior to a topical application). Exposure to heat can increase drug absorption and thus should be avoided (use of heating blankets, saunas, etc.).
  - Controlled-release transdermal formulations (e.g., nicotine patches) are becoming increasingly available for various medications.
- Absorption following *intramuscular (IM) administration* and *subcutaneous (SC) administration*
  - Many similarities exist between IM and SC injections. Both provide relatively rapid absorption of aqueous solutions and relatively slow absorption of lipophilic solutions.
  - The rate of absorption and drug bioavailability following an IM or SC injection are dependent on the lipophilicity of the drug, fat content, and blood flow at the injection site.
  - Injections may provide even, prolonged absorption. A drug may be prepared in a depot formulation that is gradually absorbed over time. Coadministration of a vasoconstricting medication may prolong absorption.
  - SC injections may result in pain if irritant is present.
- Administration via *intravenous (IV) injection*

- Absorption is essentially instantaneous, as the drug is delivered directly into the circulatory system.
- It is useful when rapid drug effect is needed and allows for administration of poorly lipid-soluble drugs and irritants.
- Continued and repeated IV administration requires accessibility to patent veins.
- Absorption may involve passive diffusion or active transport.
    - *Passive diffusion* is the movement of a drug across a cell membrane down its concentration gradient.
    - Drugs that are smaller, less protein bound, and more lipophilic can be more readily absorbed via passive diffusion. Most psychotherapeutic drugs are absorbed via passive diffusion.
    - *Active transport* is the facilitated movement of a drug across a cell membrane.
    - Drugs unable to be absorbed via passive diffusion—because of either their chemical properties or the drug concentration gradient—require active transport in order to be absorbed.
    - Active transport mechanisms include membrane-spanning proteins that facilitate the movement of drugs across cell membranes and into the circulatory system. Active transport of drugs is limited to those medications structurally related to endogenous compounds for which active transport mechanisms already exist (e.g., ions, amino acids, and simple carbohydrates).
- *Ion trapping* occurs when a drug classified as a weak acid transfers from a body compartment that is more acidic to one that is more alkaline (e.g., from the stomach to the plasma) or, conversely, when a weak base transfers from a more alkaline to a more basic compartment.
- Absorption-related *drug–drug* or *food–drug interactions* should be closely monitored. Antacids, for example, may impair the absorption of orally coadministered psychiatric drugs, leading to subtherapeutic concentrations of the coadministered drug.

Distribution

- *Distribution* refers to the movement of a drug from the circulatory system to its site(s) of action. Drugs are distributed to sites in the body responsible for producing both therapeutic effects and adverse effects.
- The variables affecting drug distribution—and delivery of the drug to its site of action—include blood flow to the target tissue, lipid solubility, and plasma protein binding.
    - Tissues of the body with *high blood flow* (e.g., the brain and muscle) will receive higher concentrations of a drug faster than tissues with low blood flow (e.g., adipose tissue).
    - Drugs with *high lipid solubility* (e.g., nonpolar molecules) will more readily cross cell membranes, including the blood–brain barrier and placenta. These drugs will more readily localize in tissues with high lipid content (e.g., brain and adipose tissue).
    - Drugs with a *low level of plasma protein binding* (e.g., lithium) have a less encumbered movement and have generally increased bioavailability than drugs with a high level of plasma protein binding (e.g., valproic acid). Table 6.1 identifies psychiatric drugs with high and low plasma protein binding.
    - The most abundant plasma protein is *albumin*; the terms *plasma protein binding* and *albumin binding* are often used interchangeably.
    - The biochemical properties that make a drug more readily absorbed into the circulatory system (e.g., high lipid solubility and low molecular weight) also make the drug more readily distributed throughout the body.

TABLE 6.1 Relative Plasma Protein Binding

HIGH PROTEIN-BINDING PSYCHIATRIC DRUGS	LOW PROTEIN-BINDING PSYCHIATRIC DRUGS
Aripiprazole (>99%)	Lithium (0%)
Ziprasidone (>99%)	Gabapentin (3%)
Atomoxetine (99%)	Levetiracetam (10%)
Diazepam (99%)	Topiramate (15%)
Sertraline (98%)	Methylphenidate (15%)
Buspirone (95%)	Clonidine (20%)
Valproic acid (93%)	Venlafaxine (28%)

- The total accumulation of lipid-soluble drugs in *adipose tissue* is dependent on the fat content of an individual. Adipose tissue may serve as a drug reservoir, which may result in redistribution during instances of profound weight loss. This increase in adipose tissue is significant for older adults—loss of muscle and increase in fat can put them at heightened risk.
- The *blood–brain barrier* results from brain capillary endothelial cells possessing continuous tight junctions, which impede drug movement from the circulatory system into the central nervous system (CNS). Drugs passing into the CNS require specific transporter proteins or high drug lipophilicity.
- Variables affecting *in utero drug distribution*
  - For women who are pregnant, special considerations should be given to the potential for maternal–fetal drug transfer via the *placenta*.
  - Similar properties dictate passive diffusion across the placenta as the blood–brain barrier. Often, drugs are able to cross the placenta first.
  - Drugs that have a high degree of lipid solubility, low molecular weight, and low serum protein binding cross the placenta more readily than drugs with a low degree of lipid solubility, high molecular weight, and high serum protein binding.
  - Because fetal plasma is slightly more acidic than maternal plasma, ion trapping of alkaline drugs may result in the increased accumulation of drug in the placenta.
- Patients suffering from malnutrition or acute or chronic inflammatory responses may present with *hypoalbuminemia*. The decrease in serum protein caused by hypoalbuminemia may result in greater drug bioavailability, particularly for drugs that are highly protein bound, leading to potentially toxic effects.
- Distribution-related drug–drug or food–drug interactions should be closely monitored. Warfarin, for example, may compete for albumin binding with other highly protein-bound psychiatric drugs, leading to an *increased* bioavailable plasma concentration of either the psychiatric drug or warfarin. These increased drug levels may be toxic and thus require dosage adjustments.

Metabolism

- *Metabolism* refers to the chemical modification of the administered drug by enzymes in the patient's body. Drug metabolism may take place before or after the drug reaches its site of action.
- Drugs may be metabolized (1) from active to inactive compounds, (2) from inactive to active compounds, or (3) from an active compound to a slightly less active compound (or vice versa).

- Most commonly, drug metabolism leads to the *biotransformation* of a more lipophilic parent drug to a more hydrophilic metabolite, which is often essential to increase the rate of excretion from the body.
- The chemically modified variant of the administered drug is referred to as a *metabolite*.
- Metabolites of several commonly administered drugs are therapeutically active at the same sites as their parent drug (e.g., s-desmethylcitalopram, the metabolite of escitalopram).
- Metabolites of other drugs produce effects different from their parent drug (e.g., desipramine, the metabolite of imipramine, blocks noradrenaline uptake, whereas imipramine itself inhibits serotonin reuptake).
- *Cytochrome P450 (CYP)* refers to the large family of enzymes, found primarily in the liver, responsible for facilitating the majority of drug metabolism in the body.
  - Each CYP family member has a unique collection of substrates (i.e., drugs and other exogenous compounds), which it metabolizes.
  - Metabolism of one psychotherapeutic drug may increase or decrease the metabolism of a second medication. This is often a consequence of alterations in CYP activity.
  - Identification of a drug's CYP metabolism is routinely established in preclinical and clinical testing. This information is generally included in the pharmacokinetics sections of printed drug guides or online/mobile device–based clinical management software (e.g., Lexi-Comp or Epocrates).
  - Individual drug effects on or by P450s may also be included as drug side effects or as drug–drug or food–drug interactions.
  - The standard nomenclature for specific CYP isozymes includes a three- to four-digit number–letter–number sequence, which identifies each isoform's sequence homologies.
  - The primary CYP isozymes present in humans and involved in metabolizing psychiatric drugs are CYP1A2, 2B6, 2C19, 2D6, and 3A4.
  - In addition to being substrates for specific CYPs, drugs may induce or inhibit P450 activity. Grapefruit juice, for example, specifically inhibits the drug metabolizing activity of CYP3A4. This leads to an increase in plasma concentration of other drugs that would have normally been metabolized by CYP3A4.
- The majority of drug metabolism occurs via P450s in the liver; however, in addition to hepatic P450s, notable amounts of drug metabolism also take place in the small intestine, kidney, and lungs.
- Patients with impaired liver function, such as those suffering from hepatitis or cirrhosis, are at risk of having impaired drug metabolizing activity. This may lead to an increase in bioactive drug concentrations and require a decrease in dosing in order to avoid drug toxicity.
- Metabolism-related drug–drug or food–drug interactions should be closely monitored. Grapefruit juice inhibits the metabolism of buspirone and other CYP 3A4 metabolites, leading to an *increased* plasma concentration of buspirone.
- *Therapeutic drug monitoring* improves the quality and safety of psychiatric drug therapy. Valid specimens must be collected during a specific time window; for example, many psychiatric medications such as lithium and valproic acid are drawn as "trough" concentrations just prior to the time the next dose is due. Appropriate pharmacokinetic interpretation of monitoring data can decrease costs and improve therapeutic outcomes.

TABLE 6.2 Comparison of Half-Lives of Commonly Administered Selective Serotonin Reuptake Inhibitors and Atypical Antipsychotics

SSRIs	ATYPICAL ANTIPSYCHOTICS
Paroxetine ($t_{1/2}$ = 17 hr)	Ziprasidone ($t_{1/2}$ = 3 hr)
Fluvoxamine ($t_{1/2}$ = 15 hr)	Risperidone ($t_{1/2}$ = 3 hr)
Sertraline ($t_{1/2}$ = 23 hr)	Quetiapine ($t_{1/2}$ = 6 hr)
Citalopram ($t_{1/2}$ = 33 hr)	Clozapine ($t_{1/2}$ = 23 hr)
Escitalopram ($t_{1/2}$ = 33 hr)	Olanzapine ($t_{1/2}$ = 33 hr)
Fluoxetine ($t_{1/2}$ = 53 hr)	Aripiprazole ($t_{1/2}$ = 47 hr)

SSRIs, selective serotonin reuptake inhibitors.

- The term *half-life* ($t_{1/2}$) refers to the amount of time necessary to decrease the concentration of the drug in the patient by 50%. The term *plateau* refers to the steady-state drug levels achieved in the body with continual drug administration.
  - Due to the unique pharmacodynamic properties of psychiatric drugs (e.g., antidepressants), it is possible for there to be a significant delay in therapeutic response even after a plateau drug level has been reached.
  - Since psychoactive drugs often have delayed neurochemical effects (e.g., receptor remodeling), it is possible that physiological changes will be observed even after most of the medication has been removed from the body.
  - Drugs of the same pharmacological class may have very different half-lives (Table 6.2).

Excretion

- *Excretion* refers to the removal of the drug and any drug metabolites from the patient's body. Of particular concern is the excretion of (1) a therapeutically active parent drug, (2) any bioactive metabolites, and (3) any toxic metabolites.
- The primary organs facilitating drug excretion are the kidneys. Renal excretion includes (1) glomerular filtration, (2) active tubular secretion, and (3) passive tubular reabsorption.
- Nonprotein-bound drug is filtered through the glomerulus. Transporter proteins facilitate active reabsorption.
- Drugs may also be excreted through the *GI tract* via sequestration in bile or directly into the intestines. Drugs may also be excreted through the skin (e.g., sweat), oral mucosa (e.g., saliva), breast (e.g., lactation), and lungs (e.g., expiration).
- Enterohepatic recirculation may impede excretion. Patients with impaired kidney function may have impaired drug excretion.
- Although most drugs undergo hepatic metabolism, some drugs (e.g., lithium) are excreted in their active form.

PHARMACODYNAMIC PRINCIPLES

Pharmacodynamics refers to the effects of the drug on the patient. Pharmacodynamic effects can be observed at the molecular and cellular levels, as well as at the tissue and organ system levels.

Mechanisms of Drug Action or Molecular Drug Targets

- Drugs most commonly produce their physiological effects through interactions with cellular drug targets, known as *receptors*. Receptors are most typically proteins and are expressed on a variety of tissues.
- The term *ligand* refers to drugs and endogenous molecules (e.g., neurohormones).
- Drug–receptor interactions account for the majority of *drug side effects* as well as *therapeutic effects*. A drug may interact with one or more receptors.
  - The drug–receptor interaction responsible for the therapeutic drug effect may be the same or different from the drug–receptor interaction responsible for specific drug side effects.
  - An example of therapeutic and adverse drug reactions being caused by the same drug–receptor interaction is illustrated by morphine: Both analgesia (therapeutic effect) and respiratory sedation (drug side effect) are caused by the binding of morphine to the mu opioid receptor.
  - An example of therapeutic and adverse drug reactions being caused by different drug–receptor interactions is illustrated by imipramine: The antidepressant effects result from interactions with serotonin and norepinephrine transporters and receptors; its side effects result from binding to cholinergic receptors (dry mouth, blurred vision, constipation) and histamine receptors (weight gain).
- Drug receptors can be classified into five classes based on their cellular location and general function. The five classes are G protein-coupled receptors (GPCRs), ligand-gated ion channels, cell membrane–embedded enzymes and transporters, intracellular enzymes and signaling proteins, and nuclear transcription factors.
- GPCRs comprise a superfamily of proteins, each containing seven membrane-spanning alpha helices and coupled to a guanosine triphosphate (GTP)–binding protein, which alters the activity of a cellular enzyme or ion channel.
- Examples of GPCRs include muscarinic acetylcholine receptors, histamine receptors, serotonin receptors, and dopamine receptors.
- *Ligand-gated ion channels* are located across cell membranes and permit a specific ion to cross into or out of a cell, down its concentration gradient.
  - Examples of ligand-gated ion channels include nicotinic acetylcholine receptors and gamma-aminobutyric acid receptors.
- *Cell membrane–embedded enzymes and transporters* span the cell membrane and have catalytic activity. Examples include the insulin receptor and neurotransmitter reuptake pumps.
- *Intracellular enzymes and signaling proteins*, such as monoamine oxidase, alter the cellular environment by catalyzing chemical reactions or conveying chemical messages.
- *Nuclear transcription factors*, such as the glucocorticoid receptor and thyroid hormone receptor, bind to DNA and alter the transcription rates of specific gene families.

Drug–Receptor Interactions

- A drug or endogenous chemical that activates a receptor is referred to as an *agonist*. Agonists may be classified as producing maximal receptor activation (full agonist) or less than that (partial agonist). A partial agonist may impede the actions of a full agonist, thus diminishing receptor activity.
- A drug or endogenous chemical that inhibits a receptor from being activated is referred to as an *antagonist*. Antagonists block the actions of both drugs and endogenous chemicals (e.g., neurotransmitters).

- While the effects of *competitive antagonists* can be overcome by the increased concentration of an agonist, the effects of other antagonists, referred to as *noncompetitive antagonists*, will persist even if more agonist is present.
- Drugs often act on more than one receptor, causing a multitude of both therapeutic and adverse drug effects.
- The description of a drug binding to a receptor simply indicates a physical interaction. This may lead to either receptor agonism or antagonism.
- Prolonged stimulation of a receptor may result in *desensitization*, in which the same concentration of a drug produces diminished therapeutic effects.
- The amount of observed therapeutic effect produced by a drug is a measure of *efficacy*. Maximal efficacy is the greatest response produced.
- The amount of effect a drug produces at a specific drug concentration is a measure of *potency*. High-potency drugs produce effects even when a small dose is given. Low-potency drugs may be nonetheless efficacious; however, they may require a greater dose to be administered.
- The difference between high-potency and low-potency psychiatric drugs are exemplified by first-generation antipsychotics (FGAs), where high-potency FGAs such as haloperidol produce their therapeutic effects at 1/10 to 1/100 the dose of low-potency FGAs (e.g., chlorpromazine).

Pharmacodynamic Drug–Drug Interactions and Side Effects

- Pharmacodynamic drug–drug interactions occur when one drug affects the physiological activity of another drug unrelated to a direct chemical interaction or pharmacokinetic process. Most pharmacodynamic drug–drug interactions occur at the cellular or receptor level.
  - An example of a pharmacodynamic drug–drug interaction is serotonin syndrome, which is produced by the coadministration of a monoamine oxidase inhibitor (e.g., phenelzine) and a selective serotonin reuptake inhibitor (e.g., fluoxetine). Both drugs contribute to a toxic accumulation of serotonin because of their actions on their respective drug targets.

INTERPATIENT VARIABILITY

Pharmacokinetic and Pharmacodynamic Changes Across the Life Span

- Life span considerations affect both pharmacokinetic and pharmacodynamic drug properties.
- In general, pediatric and geriatric patients are more at risk of experiencing increased sensitivity to therapeutic and adverse drug actions.
- Pregnancy causes alterations in the pharmacokinetic actions of certain drugs, primarily by altering the rates of drug absorption and excretion.

Pharmacogenetic Implications to Pharmacokinetics and Pharmacodynamics

- *Pharmacogenetics* refers to the effect a patient's genetic profile has on the patient's response to drug therapy.
- Slight changes in the genetic code, referred to as *polymorphisms*, have been identified in DNA that direct the production of proteins that affect drug metabolism, leading to pharmacokinetic variability. Polymorphisms that direct the production of drug receptors have also been identified in DNA, leading to pharmacodynamic drug variability.

- An example of a genetic alteration affecting psychiatric drug pharmacokinetics is a polymorphism in CYP 3A4, leading to the rapid or delayed metabolism of CYP substrates.
- An example of a genetic alteration affecting pharmacodynamics is referred to as the short allele polymorphism of the serotonin (5-HT) transporter. Patients with short allele 5-HT transporter-experienced insomnia and agitation at higher rates during treatment with fluoxetine.

BIBLIOGRAPHY

Azzaro, A. J., Ziemniak, J., Kemper, E., Campbell, B. J., & VanDenBerg, C. (2007). Selegiline transdermal system: An examination of the potential for CYP450-dependent pharmacokinetic interactions with 3 psychotropic medications. *Journal of Clinical Pharmacology, 47,* 146–158. https://doi.org/10.1177/0091270006296151

Birkett, D. J. (2002). *Pharmacokinetics made easy.* McGraw-Hill.

Clark, B., & Smith, D. A. (1986). *An introduction to pharmacokinetics.* Blackwell Science.

Gibson, G. G., & Skett, P. (2001). *Introduction to drug metabolism.* Nelson Thornes Ltd.

Jambhekar, S. S. (2012). *Basic pharmacokinetics.* Pharmaceutical Press.

Gupta, A., Hammarlund-Udenaes, M., Chatelain, P., Massingham, R., & Jonsson, E. N. (2006). Stereoselective pharmacokinetics of cetirizine in the guinea pig: Role of protein binding. *Biopharmaceutics & Drug Disposition, 27,* 291–297. https://doi.org/10.1002/bdd.509

Hisaka, A., Ohno, Y., Yamamoto, T., & Suzuki, H. (2010). Theoretical considerations on quantitative prediction of drug–drug interactions. *Drug Metabolism and Pharmacokinetics, 25*(1), 48–61.

Llorente Fernández, E., Parés, L., Ajuria, I., Bandres, F., Castanyer, B., Campos, F., Farré, C., Pou, L., Queraltó, J. M., & To-Figueras, J. (2010). State of the art in therapeutic drug monitoring. *Clinical Chemistry and Laboratory Medicine: CCLM/FESCC, 48*(4), 437–446.

MacDonald, L., Foster, B. C., & Akhtar, M. H. (2009). Food and therapeutic product interactions: A therapeutic perspective. *Journal of Pharmacy & Pharmaceutical Sciences, 12*(3), 367–377.

Perlis, R. H., Smoller, J. W., Mysore, J., Sun, M., Gillis, T., Purcell, S., Rietschel, M., Nöthen, M. M., Witt, S., Maier, W., Iosifescu, D. V., Sullivan, P., Rush, A. J., Fava, M., Breiter, H., Macdonald, M., & Gusella, J. (2010). Prevalence of incompletely penetrant Huntington's disease alleles among individuals with major depressive disorder. *American Journal of Psychiatry, 167*(5), 574–579.

WEB RESOURCE

- School of Biosciences & Medicine—University of Surrey, Guildford. https://www.surrey.ac.uk/library

7

Principles and Management of Psychiatric Emergencies

Definition

A psychiatric emergency is any disturbance in thoughts, feelings, or actions for which immediate therapeutic intervention is necessary.

- *Major emergencies:* suicidal patients, agitated and aggressive patients
- *Minor emergencies:* grief reaction, rape, disaster, panic attack
- *Medical emergencies:* delirium, neuroleptic malignant syndrome (NMS), serotonin syndrome, monoamine oxidase inhibitors (MAOI)/tyramine reactions, overdosages of common psychiatric medications, overdosages, withdrawal from addicting substances

Etiology/Background

- Approximately 29% to 30% of psychiatric emergency patients are suicidal, approximately 10% are violent, and approximately 40% require hospitalization.
- Psychiatric emergencies peak between 6 p.m. and 10 p.m., when family members are home together and conflicts arise; substance use increases and aggravates disruptive behavior. Family physicians, pastors, counselors, and other resources are difficult to reach.
- Patients present with severe changes in mood, thoughts, or behavior; those experiencing severe drug adverse effects need urgent psychiatric assessment and treatment.
- Psychiatric emergencies often erupt suddenly. A person may curse, hit, throw objects, or brandish a weapon.
- Patients may neglect self-care, stop eating, exhibit confusion, wander into traffic, or appear unclothed in public.
- Because psychiatric emergencies can be concomitant with medical illnesses, it is imperative that the ED physician establish whether the patient's symptoms are caused or exacerbated by a medical disease, such as infection, metabolic abnormality, seizure, or diabetic crisis.
- Emergency psychiatry includes specialized problems such as substance abuse, child abuse, and spousal abuse, as well as violence (suicide, homicide, and rape) and social issues (homelessness, aging, and competence). People with mental illness often lack a primary care physician and seek healthcare in crisis. Often uninsured, they have been denied coverage due to medical illness.

Incidence

- Psychiatric emergencies from acute psychotic disturbances, manic episodes, major depression, bipolar disorder, and substance abuse are responsible for approximately 6% of all ED admissions in the United States.
- In bipolar mania, agitation occurs with a frequency of approximately 90%; in schizophrenia, agitation accounts for approximately 20% of psychiatric emergency visits.
- Drug and alcohol intoxication or withdrawal is the most common diagnosis in combative patients.
- In 2006, there were 1,742,887 drug-related ED visits nationwide. Today, the number is much higher.
  - Thirty-one percent involved illicit drugs only.
  - Twenty-eight percent involved misuse or abuse of pharmaceuticals (i.e., prescription or over-the-counter medications, dietary supplements) only.
  - Thirteen percent involved illicit drugs with alcohol.

Suicidal State

Suicidal ideation and behavior are the most serious and common psychiatric emergencies.

- Each year, approximately 30,000 people in the United States and 1 million worldwide commit suicide; 650,000 receive emergency treatment after attempting suicide. It is the 10th leading cause of death worldwide.
- Suicide is highly prevalent in the adolescent population. Confounding comorbidities include depression, antisocial behavior, and alcohol abuse.
- A history of suicide attempts increases the odds of completing suicide more than any other risk factor.
- Most people who commit suicide reportedly never made a prior attempt and have never seen a mental health professional.
- People who attempt suicide more than once and later complete the act tend to be more anxious and socially withdrawn.
- In the United States, the majority of suicides are completed with firearms, followed by hanging among men and poisoning among women.
- Risk factors for suicide include the following:
  - Psychiatric illnesses
    - More than 90% of persons who attempt suicide have a major psychiatric disorder.
    - The most common mental health disorders leading to suicide include major depression, substance abuse, schizophrenia, and severe personality disorders.
  - Impulsivity and hopelessness
  - History of previous suicide attempts
  - Age, sex, and race
    - Risk increases with age.
    - Young adults attempt suicide more frequently but successfully complete less frequently than older adults.
    - Older White males (above 85 years) have the highest suicide rate.
    - Suicide rates have traditionally been higher among Whites compared with Blacks. The incidence of suicide attempts among young Blacks is rising.
  - Marital status
    - Whatever the family structure, living alone increases risk of suicide.
  - Occupation
    - Unemployed and unskilled persons are at higher risk.

- Health status
  - Risk increases with physical illness such as chronic or terminal illness, chronic pain, and recent surgery.

Violent Behavior

Certain features can serve as warning signs that a patient may be escalating toward physically violent behavior. The following list is not exhaustive:

- Facial expressions being tense and angry
- Increased or prolonged restlessness, body tension, pacing
- General overarousal of body systems (increased breathing and heart rate, muscle twitching, dilating pupils)
- Increased volume of speech, erratic movements
- Prolonged eye contact
- Discontentment, refusal to communicate, withdrawal, fear, irritation
- Thought processes unclear, poor concentration
- Delusions or hallucinations with violent content
- Verbal threats or gestures
- Reporting anger or violent feelings
- Blocking escape routes

Agitation and Aggression

- Aggressive, violent patients are often psychotic and diagnosed with schizophrenia, delusional disorder, delirium, acute mania, and dementia, but these behaviors can also result from intoxication with alcohol or other substances of abuse, such as cocaine, phencyclidine (PCP), and amphetamines.
- Medical disorders associated with violent behavior include (not all inclusive) the following:
  - *Neurological illnesses*—seizure disorders, hepatic encephalopathy, cerebral infarcts, encephalitis, Wilson's disease, Parkinson's disease, intracranial bleeds
  - *Endocrinopathies*—hypothyroidism, Cushing's syndrome, thyrotoxicosis, diabetic crisis
  - *Metabolic disorders*—hypoglycemia, hypoxia, electrolyte imbalance
  - *Infections*—AIDS, syphilis, tuberculosis
  - *Vitamin deficiencies*—folic acid, pyridoxine, vitamin B12
  - *Temperature disturbances*—hypothermia, hyperthermia, vitamin D
  - *Poisoning*
- Behavioral signs of agitation include excessive motor restlessness, irritability, jitteriness, and purposeless and repetitive motor or verbal activity.
- Precautions should be taken to modify the environment to maximize safety.
  - Ensure that the patient is physically comfortable and in an environment with low levels of stimulation.
  - Minimize waiting time.
  - Communicate in a safe, respectful manner.
  - Remove all dangerous objects.
- Aggressive behavior is usually managed with some combination of seclusion, physical restraints, monitoring with constant observation by a sitter, and drug therapy.
  - Seclusion offers a decrease in external stimuli that may be enough to reduce aggressiveness.
  - Restraints may be needed to obtain a thorough assessment.
- Drug therapy such as tranquilization should target control of specific symptoms.

■ Rapid calming or tranquilization of a patient is achieved with benzodiazepine or an antipsychotic given via the intramuscular (IM) or the intravenous (IV) route.
  ▪ Typical or atypical antipsychotics may be used.
  ▪ Benzodiazepines act more quickly but often have erratic IM absorption.
  ▪ A combination of both drugs can be very effective.
■ If oral medications are appropriate, orally disintegrating or liquid formulations are available for haloperidol, risperidone, olanzapine, and aripiprazole.

Drug Therapy for Agitation in Psychiatric Emergencies

■ It is better for a patient to take medication voluntarily and orally before the behavior escalates than to be involuntarily medicated after a crisis.
■ The decision on which medication to use is often based on the underlying diagnosis. If the patient is known to be schizophrenic or bipolar and most likely is in a psychotic or manic state, then an antipsychotic should be used. If the diagnosis is unclear or the result of intoxication with drugs or alcohol, then lorazepam, a benzodiazepine, is most often administered.
■ Medications discussed are those that have injectable dosage forms. There are other antipsychotics in liquids or disintegrating tablet forms that would work as well in the appropriate patient.

Diagnostic Workup

■ Mental status examination to rule out contributing mental illness to psychiatric emergency
■ Physical examination to rule out physical explanation for psychiatric emergency
■ Laboratory evaluation
  ▪ *White blood cell count (WBC)*—to look for infectious contribution
  ▪ *Serum electrolytes, creatinine, blood urea nitrogen (BUN)*—to rule out electrolyte abnormalities, such as hyponatremia, dehydration, and renal insufficiency, which can contribute to agitation
  ▪ *Liver function tests*—to screen for hepatic encephalopathy and hyperammonemia, which can present with agitation and aggression
  ▪ *Toxicological analysis of serum and urine*—to screen for substance abuse contribution to emergency
  ▪ *Neuroimaging (CT/MRI)*—rule out stroke and tumor
  ▪ *EEG*—if seizure disorder is suspected

Medical/Legal Pitfalls

■ Involuntary administration of psychotropic medications is allowed in emergencies that are considered life threatening. Wide variations exist in the legal definition of "life-threatening" and in the practice of administering involuntary medication.
■ Timely documentation of the need for restraint and involuntary medication is essential.
■ *Informed consent*: The most important element of informed consent is the assessment of decisional capacity, for example, through the use of the Mini-Mental State Examination.
■ If the patient is suffering from either an organic or a functional acute change in mental status and is a danger to self or others, then the patient should undergo emergency medical evaluation. If the patient will not voluntarily submit to this evaluation, then a request for an emergency medical evaluation from a judge, justice of the peace, or police officer is obtained.

TABLE 7.1 Drug Selection for Psychiatric Emergencies

CLASS	DRUG
BZDs	
	Lorazepam (Ativan)
	Midazolam (Versed)
First-generation (typical) antipsychotics	
	Haloperidol (Haldol)
	Fluphenazine HCl (Prolixin)
Second-generation (atypical) antipsychotics	
	Aripiprazole (Abilify)
	Olanzapine (Zyprexa)
	Ziprasidone (Geodon)
Antihistamine	
	Cyproheptadine (Periactin) for supportive use during serotonin syndrome. Other antihistamines that are useful are benadryl/hydroxyzine, which can be used for anxiolysis and severe EPS resolution)
Skeletal muscle relaxant	
	Dantrolene (Dantrium)
Dopamine agonist	
	Bromocriptine (Parlodel)

BZDs, benzodiazepines; EPS, extrapyramidal symptom.

- Chemical or physical restraints may be necessary in the combative patient. Chemical restraints typically include benzodiazepines and/or antipsychotics. Physical restraints are a last resort and are used mostly by security with close observation.
  - Protocols for restraints will vary by community.
  - Physical restraints should be used in the least restrictive manner and for the least amount of time possible.

Drug Selection Psychiatric Emergencies
- See Table 7.1.
  - As required by the Joint Commission, institutions must have policies in place that deal with the use of restraints.
- A person with capacity cannot be confined or restrained against their will. Doing so can lead to a legal charge of false imprisonment or battery.
- Duty to warn refers to the following:
  - Requires a clinician to warn a person who may be in danger from a combative patient
  - Failure to do so may make the clinician liable for injury to the third party

Expert Consensus Guidelines
Treatment of Behavioral Emergencies: Highlights of Treatment
- Support the use of oral formulations (liquid concentrate, rapidly dissolving tablets) of atypical antipsychotics as first-line therapy for the initial management of agitation or aggression in the emergency setting. Provide faster times-to-peak

concentration. Injection peaks faster; however, oral formulations are more legally preferred and patient centered whenever possible.

■ Reserve IM injections for patients unable to cooperate with oral therapy.

OTHER MEDICAL EMERGENCIES IN PSYCHIATRY

Delirium

Clinical **Presentation**: A condition of impaired attention, changes in behavior, and a clouded sensorium, which follows a waxing and waning course. The patient may be agitated, disoriented, and confused. Delirium is a disturbance of attention, not a disturbance of memory. It is acute in onset and may have concomitant neurological disturbances such as tremor, increased muscle tone, visual hallucinations, and impaired speech.

Etiology: Delirium is often caused by changes in acetylcholine balance. It can be caused by medications such as anticholinergics, narcotics, or steroids, or an underlying medical condition such as a urinary tract infection, liver failure, drug or alcohol abuse, or electrolyte/metabolic abnormalities. People with delirium need immediate medical attention.

Incidence: Delirium occurs in 30% of all older medical patients. The risk of delirium increases for people who are demented and dehydrated and taking drugs that affect the nervous system.

Treatment: Treatment depends on the condition causing the delirium. The underlying medical condition should be treated first. Eliminate or change medications that can worsen confusion or that are unnecessary. Medications may be needed to control aggressive or agitated behaviors. These are usually started at very low doses and adjusted as needed. Most often, antipsychotics and sedatives are selected but should be titrated slowly in older adults and selected to target the symptom. It should be kept in mind that benzodiazepine usage in older adults can worsen confusion and delirium.

Outcome: Delirium often lasts about 1 week, although it may take several weeks for mental function to return to normal levels. Full recovery is common.

Neuroleptic Malignant Syndrome

Clinical Presentation: Neuroleptic malignant syndrome (NMS) is a rare but life-threatening neurological emergency associated with the use of antipsychotic agents and characterized by a clinical syndrome of mental status change, rigidity, fever, and dysautonomia. Mortality results from systemic complications and dysautonomia. The cardinal features include muscular rigidity, hyperthermia, autonomic dysfunction, and altered consciousness. Rigidity and akinesia usually develop initially or concomitantly with a temperature elevation as high as 41°C. Autonomic dysfunction includes tachycardia, labile blood pressure, diaphoresis, dyspnea, and urinary incontinence. Creatine kinase, complete blood count, and liver function tests are usually increased. Symptoms develop over 24 to 72 hours.

Etiology: The cause of NMS is unknown but is thought to be related to central dopamine blockade. The risk appears to be lower for the atypical antipsychotics than for the typical.

Incidence: It occurs in 0.2% to 3.2% of patients. Most patients are young adults, but the disease has been described in all age groups. It can occur hours to months after initial drug exposure.

Treatment: Discontinue any neuroleptic agent or precipitating drug. Maintain cardio-respiratory and euvolemic stability. Benzodiazepines can be used for agitation. Lower fever using cooling blankets.

Serotonin Syndrome

Serotonin syndrome is a potential life-threatening syndrome associated with increased serotonergic activity in the central nervous system (CNS), such as from the combination of a selective serotonin reuptake inhibitor and a MAOI. It is associated with therapeutic use, drug interactions, or intentional self-poisoning. Classically, it is a triad of mental status changes, autonomic hyperactivity, and neuromuscular abnormalities. It is a clinical diagnosis; no laboratory test can confirm the diagnosis.

Clinical Presentation: Serotonin syndrome can manifest as a wide range of clinical symptoms, from mild tremor to life-threatening hyperthermia and shock. Examination findings can include hyperthermia, agitation, ocular clonus, tremor, akathisia, deep tendon hyperreflexia, inducible or spontaneous clonus, muscle rigidity, dilated pupils, dry mucous membranes, increased bowel sounds, flushed skin, diaphoresis and increased heart rate, and hypertension. Neuromuscular findings are typically more pronounced in the lower extremities.

Etiology: Serotonin syndrome occurs due to increased serotonin in the CNS. Postsynaptic 5-HT1A and 5-HT2A receptors are implicated. It occurs most commonly with the concomitant use of serotonergic drugs, with drugs that impair metabolism of serotonin, including MAOIs, or with antipsychotics or other dopamine antagonists.

Treatment: Discontinue serotonergic agents. Provide supportive care such as IV fluids for hydration and benzodiazepines for agitation, myoclonus, hyperreflexia, and hyperthermia.

Specific Agents: Periactin (cyproheptadine) is an antihistamine with serotonergic antagonist properties. It should be considered in moderate to severe cases.

BIBLIOGRAPHY

Bezchlibnyk-Butler, K. Z., & Jeffries, J. J. (Eds.). (2013). *Clinical handbook of psychotropic drugs* (13th rev. ed.). Hogrefe & Huber.

Charney, D. S., & Nestler, E. J. (Eds.). (2004). *Neurobiology of mental illness* (2nd ed.). Oxford University Press.

Cooper, J. R., Bloom, F. E., & Roth, R. H. (1996). *The biochemical basis of neuropharmacology* (7th ed.). Oxford University Press.

Curran, S., & Bullock, R. (Eds.). (2005). *Practical old age psychopharmacology: A multi-professional approach*. Radcliffe Publishing.

Dziegielewski, S. F. (2006). *Psychopharmacology handbook: For the non-medically trained*. W. W. Norton & Company.

Fisher, S., & Greenber, R. P. (Eds.). (1989). *The limits of biological treatments for psychological distress: Comparisons with psychotherapy and placebo*. Lawrence Erlbaum Associates.

Freeman, L. (2004). *Mosby's complementary & alternative medicine: A research-based approach*. Elsevier.

Hadad, P., Durson, S., & Deakin, B. (Eds.). (2004). *Adverse syndromes and psychiatric drugs: A clinical guide*. Oxford University Press.

Healey, D. (1997). *The antidepressant era*. Harvard University Press.

Healey, D. (2002). *The creation of psychopharmacology*. Harvard University Press.

Healey, D. (2004). *Let them eat Prosac: The unhealthy relationship between the pharmaceutical industry and depression*. New York University Press.

Hollander, E. (2001). *Professional's handbook of psychotropic drugs*. Springhouse.

Hyman, S. E., & Nestler, E. J. (1993). *The molecular foundations of psychiatry*. American Psychiatric Press.

Kelsey, J. E., Newport, D. J., & Nemeroff, C. B. (2006). *Principles of psychopharmacology for mental health professionals*. Wiley-Liss.

Keltner, N. L., & Folks, D. G. (2005). *Psychotropic drugs* (4th ed.). Elsevier Mosby.

Lewis, B. (2006). *Moving beyond Prozac, DSM, and the new psychiatry: The birth of postpsychiatry*. The University of Michigan Press.

Meyer, J. S., & Quenzer, L. F. (2005). *Psychopharmacology: Drugs, the brain, and behavior*. Sinauer Associates.

Nestler, E. J., Hyman, S. E., & Malenka, R. C. (2001). *Molecular neuropharmacology: A foundation for clinical neuroscience*. McGraw-Hill.

Preston, J. D., O'Neal, J. H., & Talaga, M. C. (2005). *Handbook of clinical psychopharmacology for therapists* (4th ed.). New Harbinger Publications.

Rose, S. (2005). *The future of the brain: The promise and perils of tomorrow's neuroscience*. Oxford University Press.

Schachter, M. (Ed.). (1993). *Psychotherapy and medication: A dynamic integration*. Jason Aronson.

Schatzberg, A., & Nemeroff, C. (Eds.). (2004). *Textbook of psychopharmacology* (3rd ed.). American Psychiatric Publishing.

Spiegel, R. (2003). *Psychopharmacology: An introduction*. Wiley.

Stahl, S. M. (2000). *Essential psychopharmacology: Neuroscientific basis and practical applications* (2nd ed.). Cambridge University Press.

Stahl, S. M. (2005). *Essential psychopharmacology: The prescriber's guide*. Cambridge University Press.

Stein, D., Lerer, B., & Stahl, S. (2005). *Evidence-based psychopharmacology*. Cambridge University Press.

Walsh, B. T. (Ed.). (1998). *Child psychopharmacology*. American Psychiatric Press.

Whitaker, R. (2002). *Mad in America: Bad science, bad medicine, and the enduring mistreatment of the mentally ill*. Perseus.

WEB RESOURCE

■ Inter-university Consortium for Political and Social Research (ICPSR): http://www.icpsr.umich.edu

8

SECTION III. SYNDROMES AND TREATMENTS IN ADULT PSYCHIATRY

Behavioral and Psychological Disorders in Older Adults

DELIRIUM

Background Information

Definition of Disorder

- Acute abnormality in cognitive processing affecting thinking, attention, awareness, memory, perception, and orientation to at times person but predominantly to place and time.
- Onset is fairly rapid.
- Delirium is the direct result of an underlying medical condition, substance intoxication or withdrawal, medication, toxin exposure, or combination of etiologies.
- Mimics dementia.

Symptoms can fluctuate throughout the day, often worsening in the evening.

- Often the first sign of illness in older adults
- Disturbed attention and lack of environmental awareness
- May involve visual illusions, hallucinations, and delusions

Etiology

- Medications—prescription or over-the-counter (OTC)—are the most common causes of delirium.
- Anticholinergic toxicity from prescribed medications (diphenhydramine [Benadryl]), tricyclic antidepressants (TCAs; amitriptyline [Elavil], imipramine [Tofranil]), and antipsychotics (chlorpromazine [Thorazine], thioridazine [Mellaril]).
- Benzodiazepines or alcohol.
- Antiinflammatory agents, including prednisone.
- Cardiovascular (antihypertensives, digitalis).
- Diuretics, if dehydrated.
- Gastrointestinal (cimetidine, ranitidine).
- Opioid analgesics (especially meperidine).
- Lithium.
- Antipsychotic, sedative, or hypnotic drugs often used to treat confusion, agitation, or insomnia may precipitate an episode of delirium.

- *Infections*: pneumonia, skin, urinary tract.
- *Metabolic* acute blood loss, malnutrition, dehydration, electrolyte imbalance, organ failure, hyper- or hypoglycemia, hypoxia.
- *Heart*: arrhythmia, congestive heart failure, myocardial infarction (MI), or shock.
- *Neurological*: central nervous system infection, head trauma, seizures, stroke subdural hematoma, transient ischemic accidents, tumors.
- Sleep deprivation or severe emotional distress
- *Other*: fever fugue, fecal impaction, postoperative recovery, sleep deprivation, urinary retention.

Demographic
- Thirty to 40 percent of hospitalized patients above the age of 65 years have experienced an episode of delirium.
- Forty to 50 percent of patients with delirium are recovering from surgery to repair a hip fracture.
- Thirty to 40 percent of patients with delirium have AIDS.
- Forty to 70 percent of patients with delirium have cardiac problems.

Risk Factors
- *Age*: The very old and the very young are at risk for delirium.
- Persons with brain trauma, dementia, cerebrovascular disease, tumor, alcohol dependence, diabetes mellitus, cancer, blindness, or poor hearing are at risk for delirium.
- Persons on multiple medications.
- Another mental health disorder, such as depression or substance abuse (alcoholism or drug abuse), increases the risk of developing delirium.
- *Another physical disorder*: infection, dehydration.
- Metabolic, electrolyte, and endocrine disturbances.

Diagnosis
Differential Diagnosis
- Whether the patient has another neurocognitive disorder (NCD) is the most common differential diagnosis.
- Rule out the following:
  - *Infection*: urinary, pneumonia, skin
  - Diabetic-, hyper-, or hypoglycemia
  - Cardiac arrhythmias
  - Cerebral lesions
- Alcohol or other substance intoxication or withdrawal
- Psychotic disorders such as brief psychosis, schizophrenia, bipolar/depression with psychotic features
- Acute stress disorder
- Malingering or a factitious disorder

ICD-10 Codes
- Unspecified dementia (28 index entries)
- Delirium due to known physiological condition or multiple etiologies (F05)
- Delirium not otherwise specified (NOS) (R41.0)
- Alcohol withdrawal (F10)
- Opioid (F11)

- Sedative, hypnotic, or anxiolytic (F13)
- Inhalant (F18)
- Cannabis (F12)
- Other or unknown substance/medication (F19)

Diagnostic Workup
- Assume reversibility
- Identify and correct underlying cause(s)
- Physical evaluation
- Blood sugar
- Urinalysis (UA) for culture and sensitivity
- Serum levels of medications
- O_2 saturation
- Arrhythmia
- Vitamin B12
- Electrolytes
- Complete blood count (CBC) with differential
- Brain imaging tests and measures of serum anticholinergic activity: experimental laboratory tests that show promise

Initial Assessment
- Delirium is often underrecognized by healthcare personnel, especially if the patient has hypoactive delirium, is 80 years of age or older, has vision impairment, or has dementia. Periodic application of simple cognitive tests, such as the Mini-Cog, the confusion assessment method for the intensive care unit (CAM-ICU), or the intensive care delirium screening checklist (ICDSC), may improve identification.
- The clock face test is also a simple test of mental status.
- White blood cell count, CBC, electrolytes (potassium, sodium, chloride, bicarbonate).
- Interview.
- Rule out infection and other medical or substance abuse causes.
- Review prescriptions, especially recent ones, and OTC medications for anticholinergic delirium.
- History if drug and alcohol use is noted.
- EKG—to identify any arrhythmias.

Clinical Presentation
- Hypervigilance or inattention to the environment
- Disorganized thinking or altered level of consciousness
- Sleep–wake cycle disturbance
- Progressing to anxiety, agitation, flight syndrome—tries to leave hospital
- Perceptual disturbances (visual illusions, hallucinations, delusions)
- Disorientation in regard to time, place, and person
- Concomitant physical condition
- Also may exhibit anxiety, fear, depression, irritability, and anger
- Symptom fluctuation over a 24-hour period

Diagnostic and Statistical Manual of Mental Disorders, Fifth Edition: Diagnostic Guidelines
- Delirium is a disturbance in consciousness and/or a change in neurocognition that cannot be accounted for by a preexisting dementia.

Treatment Overview

Acute Treatment

See the American Psychiatric Association's *Practice Guideline for Treatment of Patients With Delirium.*

- Identify the underlying cause.
- Initiate psychiatric management through therapeutic interaction with the patient to reduce fear.
- Educate the family and other clinicians regarding the illness.
- Establish therapeutic trust when the patient is stable.
- Provide supportive measures.
- Modify the environment; ensure that the patient is oriented to the environment.
- Provide objects to orient patient to day and night (e.g., calendar, clock).
- Provide quiet and well-lit surroundings that dampen noise made by machines, overhead pagers, and equipment.
- Use physical restraints only as a last resort.
- Hydrate the patient.
- Provide familiar faces of family members or sitters.
- Stimulate daytime activity; mobilize the patient.
- Correct sensory deficits with eyeglasses, hearing aids, and portable amplification devices.
- Promote normal sleep with warm milk, massage, and nighttime noise reduction.
- Prevent dehydration (blood urea nitrogen [BUN] to creatinine ratio >18) and fecal impaction.
- *Review risk factors*: use of physical restraints, dehydration, and bladder catheter.
- For acute agitation, use a high-potency low-anticholinergic, low-arrhythmo-genic antipsychotic medication. If on antipsychotic medication (i.e., risperidone [Risperdal], olanzapine [Zyprexa], and quetiapine [Seroquel, Seroquel XR]), patients should have their EKGs monitored. Corrected QT interval (QTc) greater than 450 ms or 25% over baseline warrants a cardiology consultation and reduction or discontinuation of the medication.
- Morphine (not meperidine) may be required if pain is a factor.

Chronic Treatment

- Most people respond well to treatment and can return to normal functioning in hours to days.
- Treatment can be complicated if the patient has another condition at the same time, such as substance abuse, depression, or other anxiety disorders.

Recurrence Rate

If the rate of recurrence is high, the patient needs to be monitored frequently.

Patient Education

- Information regarding delirium may be found in MD Consult: Delirium: Patient Education (www.mdconsult.com).
- Advise patients to avoid OTC medications for colds and sleep with high anticholinergic effect, including pseudoephedrine or cimetidine.

Medical/Legal Pitfalls

- Delirium is associated with significant morbidity and mortality. Estimated 3-month mortality rate of a patient with delirium ranges from 23% to 33%; 1-year mortality rate is as high as 50%.

- Persons with delirium are more likely to have a fall in the hospital or other events, which will delay discharge and result in costlier hospital stays.
- Persons with delirium are more susceptible to dehydration or malnutrition because the lack of orientation delays satisfying the urge to eat or drink.
- Pain can also contribute to delirium.
- Alcohol/drug use and withdrawal can cause delirium.

MAJOR AND MILD NEUROCOGNITIVE DISORDERS

Overview

- More than 6 million people in the United States suffer from major NCD; the disorder is underdiagnosed.
- Depression, anxiety, or other behavioral disturbances may accompany major NCD.
- The cost of treating dementia in older adults is estimated to be more than $148 billion annually.
- There are several types of major NCD, including vascular, frontal, Lewy body, HIV Huntington's, Parkinson's disease, and Alzheimer's disease (AD).
- Reversible causes of dementia should be explored before initiating pharmacological therapy.
- In the United States, a patient is diagnosed with AD, a form of major cognitive disorder/dementia, every 71 seconds.
- AD accounts for 70% of all major NCD dementias; the other 30% is due to other or multiple causes.

Background Information

Definition of Disorder

- Noticeable decline in memory beginning with short-term memory loss
- Decline in other cognitive functions, including ability to perform familiar tasks (activities of daily living [ADLs]), language, orientation to time and place, poor or declining judgment, abstract thinking, misplacing objects in unusual places, changes in mood or behavior, loss of initiative sufficient to affect ADL
- Insidious onset, progressive over months to years, and rarely reversible

Etiology

- A common denominator of all dementia disorders is that memory and cognitive function are impaired due to neuron death. Therefore, it is not reversible.

Demographic

- Approximately 1% of people aged 65 years or older and more than 50% of people aged 90 years or older have a major or minor cognitive dementia disorder.
- Worldwide, nearly half of the persons with cognitive disorders (46%) live in Asia, 30% in Europe, and 12% in North America; 52% live in less-developed regions.
- Approximately 59% of women with dementia have AD.

Risk Factors

- *Age*: Major NCD risk increases with age.
- *Genetic changes*: Apolipoprotein E (ApoE and E4) allele is a strong risk factor.
- *Probable risks*: head trauma and genetics.

- Evidence is moderate that low education has a moderate risk effect on NCDs.
- Evidence is moderate at midlife that controlling high cholesterol levels and high blood pressure has a protective effect against NCDs.
- Evidence is strong that antihypertensive drugs have a protective effect against NCDs.
- Evidence is moderate that leisure activities/active lives have a protective effect.
- Evidence is insufficient that social network or personality type has a protective effect.
- Evidence is insufficient that obesity, high homocysteine levels, diet, folate/vitamin B12 deficiency, aluminum, and depression are risk factors for NCDs.
- Evidence is insufficient that statins, hormone replacement therapy, and nonsteroidal antiinflammatory drugs (NSAIDs) have a protective effect.
- Evidence is limited that moderate alcohol use has a protective effect on the risk of NCDs.

Relationship to Other Diseases
- NCDs are unrelated to hypothyroidism or hyperthyroidism but need to be diagnosed and treated.
- Studies show variable results in regard to correlation between low vitamin B_{12} (cyanocobalamin) and NCDs or AD. There is a correlation between low folic acid levels and impaired cognitive function.

Diagnosis
Differential Diagnosis
- Delirium
- Depression
- Thyroid disorders
- *Diabetic*: hyper- or hypoglycemia
- Cardiac arrhythmias
- Cerebral lesions
- Posttraumatic stress disorder (PTSD)
- Drug interactions or adverse effects
- Schizophrenia

ICD-10 Codes
- Major neurocognitive disorder due to Alzheimer's disease (G30.9)
- Unspecified mild neurocognitive disorder (R41.9)
- Major neurocognitive disorder with Lewy bodies (F02.8)
- Progressive dementia (F03.90)
- Vascular neurocognitive disorder (F01.5)
- Unspecified neurocognitive disorder (R41.9)

Diagnostic Workup
- Currently, there is no simple, reliable test for diagnosing NCD at an early stage.
- A physical and neurological evaluation must be done.
- Mental status for short- and long-term memory, problem solving, and depression must be evaluated.
- CBC with differential is done.
- CT scan and MRI scan can identify people who have AD.

- Electroencephalography brain mapping and apolipoprotein levels are currently not recommended for identifying AD.

Initial Assessment

- History from the family, friends, or the caretaker close to the person will supplement the patient's account.
- Clock-drawing test or other simple exercises will allow selection for additional testing.
- Functional status needs to be assessed.
- People with dementia are sometimes stigmatized. Understanding can lead to more compassion among patient, family, and friends.

Clinical Presentation

Early (1–3 years)

- Disorientation as to date
- Recall problems in relation to recent events
- Naming problems
- Mild language or decision-making problems
- Mild problem in copying figures (e.g., face of a clock)
- Social withdrawal
- Mood change
- Problems managing finances

Middle (2–8 years)

- Disorientation about date and place
- Getting lost in familiar areas
- Impaired new learning
- Impaired calculating skills
- Agitation and aggression
- Problems with cooking, shopping, dressing, or grooming
- Restlessness, anxiety, or depression

Late (6–12 years)

- Disoriented to time, place, or person
- Increasingly nonverbal
- Long-term memory erased
- Unable to copy or write
- Unable to groom or dress
- Incontinent
- Motor or verbal agitation end stage
  - Nonverbal
  - Not eating or swallowing well
  - Not ambulatory
  - Incontinent of bowel and bladder
- Depression noted in 50% of the patients, which may cause rapid decline if not treated

Diagnostic and Statistical Manual of Mental Disorders, Fifth Edition: Diagnostic Guidelines

- Major and minor NCDs are a syndrome rather than an illness, with a set of signs and symptoms that include a progressive decline in cognitive function due to damage or disease in the body beyond what might be expected from normal aging.

Although NCDs are far more common in the geriatric population, it may occur at any stage of adulthood.

■ Symptoms of NCD can be classified as either reversible or irreversible, depending on the etiology of the disease. Fewer than 10% of cases of NCD are the result of causes that may presently be reversed with treatment. Without careful assessment of history, the short-term syndrome of delirium can easily be confused with NCD, because they have many symptoms in common. Some mental illnesses, including depression and psychosis, may also produce symptoms that mimic those of NCDs.

Treatment Overview

Chronic Treatment

The focus of treatment is to improve the quality of life of the individual and the care provider by maintaining functional ability and by supporting remaining intellectual abilities, mood, behavior, and social support networks such as the Swedish Council on Technology Assessment in Health Care (www.sbu.se/en/).

■ Treat comorbid physical illnesses, blood pressure, and diabetes.
■ Support the family in setting realistic goals.
■ Limit all medications, especially psychotropics or sedatives, to only essential medications.
■ Maintain functional ability.

Nonpharmacological Approaches

■ Care of the family member with NCD requires multilevel resources that increase the caregiver's burden over time.
■ Behavior modification, including scheduled activities (e.g., toileting in late stages) and prompted activities (e.g., dressing in middle stages).
■ Assistance provided only for what the patient cannot do.
■ Familiar music.
■ Walking or light exercise.
■ Pet therapy.
■ Calm and slow approaches.
■ Well-lighted lit areas without shadows.

Pharmacological Treatment

■ Cholinesterase inhibitors such as donepezil, razadyne, rivastigmine (benefit for 1–3 years).
■ Record functional status and cognitive status.
■ Treat agitation.

Support Caregiver

■ Caregiver burden includes isolation and anxiety.
■ Arrange respite care to provide caregiver relief.

Recurrence Rate

Long-term chronic decline occurs.

Patient Education

■ Alzheimer's Association: www.alz.org/index.asp
■ Family caregiver alliance: www.caregiver.org/caregiver/jsp/home.jsp
■ National caregiver alliance: www.caregiving.org/members/

Drug Selection Table for Neurocognitive Disorders and Alzheimer's Disease

CLASS	DRUG
Cholinesterase inhibitors	First-line drug therapy Donepezil hydrochloride (Aricept) Rivastigmine tartrate (Exelon and Exelon patch) Galantamine (Razadyne and Razadyne ER)
NMDA receptor antagonist	
	Memantine (Namenda)

NMDA, *N*-methyl-d-aspartate.

Medical/Legal Pitfalls

- NCDs affect all areas of life, including physical, social, and financial aspects. The issues are complicated and require careful reflection on the human condition and the value of various interventions.
- NCDs affect the lives of family members in a way that requires treatment resources to support the caregiver.
- Legal resources are involved in drawing up living wills and wills before the patient is no longer able to make their wishes known.
- Protective services may be involved to protect the patient against financial or physical abuse.
- Judges and attorneys have few guidelines for amnesic cases.

MAJOR DEPRESSIVE DISORDERS IN OLDER ADULTS

Overview

- Prevalence of depression increases with aging.
- More than 30% of adults above 65 years of age have symptoms of depression.
- Symptoms may include decreased energy, sleep disturbances, weight changes, loss of interest, guilt, poor concentration, and thoughts of suicide.
- The ICD-10 code is F33, depression, unspecified.
- *Diagnostic and Statistical Manual of Mental Disorders,* Fifth Edition *(DSM-5) Criteria*: Presence of 2 to 4 depressive symptoms of greater than 2 weeks duration.
- Risk factors include acute stress, anxiety, and illness.
- Differential diagnoses include grief reaction, metabolic disorder, substance abuse, or medication-induced depression.

Treatment Overview

Acute Treatment

- Selective serotonin reuptake inhibitors (SSRIs) are indicated as first-line treatment for major depressive disorders (MDDs).
- Serotonin-norepinephrine reuptake inhibitors (SNRIs) may be considered if SSRIs do not achieve optimal results.

Drug Selection Table for Major Depressive Disorders

CLASS	DRUG
SSRIs	First-line drug therapy Fluoxetine (Prozac) Paroxetine (Paxil)

Drug Selection Table for Major Depressive Disorders (*continued*)

CLASS	DRUG
	Citalopram (Celexa)
	Escitalopram (Lexapro)
	Sertraline (Zoloft)
SNRIs	
	Duloxetine (Cymbalta)
	Venlafaxine (Effexor)
	Desvenlafaxine (Pristiq)

SNRIs, serotonin-norepinephrine reuptake inhibitors; SSRIs, selective serotonin reuptake inhibitors.

Chronic Treatment
■ SSRIs and SNRIs are also first-line options for persistent MDDs.

Psychopharmacology of Major Depressive Disorders in Older Adults
General Considerations
■ Patients should avoid consuming alcohol while taking this medication.
■ Use with caution in patients with a history of seizure disorder and/or diabetes.
■ Avoid abrupt withdrawal of this class of drug. Dosage should be tapered down prior to discontinuation.
■ Monitor closely for clinical worsening and suicide risk.
■ Monitor closely for serotonin syndrome.
■ Monitor sodium levels.
■ Contraindicated if patient has been on a monoamine oxidase inhibitor (MAOI) within 14 days or has taken thioridazine within weeks.

GENERALIZED ANXIETY DISORDER IN OLDER ADULTS

Overview
■ Prevalence of anxiety is not as common in older adults with the diagnosis of amnestic disorder.
■ Anxiety may be associated with depression and/or NCDs.
■ Symptoms may include excessive worry, restlessness, poor concentration, irritability, or sleep disturbance typically for longer than 6 months. Typically, at least three symptoms are present.
■ ICD-10 code: F41.1.
■ *DSM-5 criteria*: 6 months of excessive worry/anxiety about issues causing distress or impairment.
■ Differential diagnoses include anxiety disorder due to another medical condition, social anxiety disorder, obsessive-compulsive disorder, adjustment disorders, grief reaction, PTSD, depression, metabolic disorder, cardiovascular disease, infection, or substance abuse.

Drug Selection Table for Generalized Anxiety Disorder

CLASS	DRUG
Serotonin 1A agonist	First-line drug therapy
	Buspirone (BuSpar)

Drug Selection Table for Generalized Anxiety Disorder (*continued*)

CLASS	DRUG
SSRIs	
	Paroxetine (Paxil)
	Escitalopram (Lexapro)
SNRIs	
	Duloxetine (Cymbalta)
Benzodiazepines	Second-line drug therapy
	Lorazepam (Ativan)

SNRIs, serotonin-norepinephrine reuptake inhibitors; SSRIs, selective serotonin reuptake inhibitors.

Treatment Overview

Acute Treatment
- First-line drugs of choice for generalized anxiety disorder (GAD) are the SSRI antidepressants.
- Typical anxiolytics may be considered if atypical anxiolytics are ineffective.

Chronic Treatment
- Atypical or typical anxiolytics are also options for treatment of persistent generalized anxiety disorder (GAD).

Psychopharmacology of Generalized Anxiety Disorder in Older Adults

General Considerations
- Atypical anxiolytics are the most commonly used medications for GAD in the older-adult population.
- Typical anxiolytics are used with caution with older adults.
- Patients should avoid consuming alcohol while taking any of these medications.
- Use with caution in patients with history of seizure disorders.
- Avoid abrupt withdrawal of this class of drug. Dosage should be tapered down prior to discontinuation.
- Should start low and go slow.
- Monitor closely for clinical worsening and suicide risk.

BIBLIOGRAPHY

American Medical Association. (2019). *AMA physician ICD-10-CM 2019* (Vols. 1 and 2). American Medical Association Press.

American Psychiatric Association. (2013). *Diagnostic and statistical manual of mental disorders* (5th ed.). American Psychiatric Publishing.

Bourne, R. S., Tahir, T. A., Borthwick, M., & Sampson, E. L. (2008). Drug treatment of delirium: Past, present and future. *Journal of Psychosomatic Research, 65*(3), 273–282.

Chu, J. A., Frey, L. M., Ganzel, B. L., & Matthews, J. A. (1999). Memories of childhood abuse: Dissociation, amnesia, and corroboration. *American Journal of Psychiatry, 156*, 749–755.

Greenaway, M. C., Hanna, S. M., Lepore, S. W., & Smith, G. E. (2008). A behavioral rehabilitation intervention for amnesic mild cognitive impairment. *American Journal of Alzheimer's Disease and Other Dementias, 23*(5), 451–461.

Harrison, M., & Williams, M. (2007). The diagnosis and management of transient global amnesia in the emergency department. *Emergency Medicine Journal, 24*(6), 444–445.

Inouye, S. K., Foreman, M. D., Mion, L. C., Katz, K. H., & Cooney, L. M. (2001). Nurses' recognition of delirium and its symptoms. *Archives of Internal Medicine, 161,* 2467–2473.

Litaker, D., Locala, J., Franco, K., Bronson, D. L., & Tannous, Z. (2001). Preoperative risk factors for postoperative delirium. *General Hospital Psychiatry, 23,* 84–89.

Michaud, M., Bula, C., Berney, A., Camus, V., Voellinger, R., Stiefel, F., Burnand, B., & The Delirium Guidelines Development Group. (2007). Delirium: Guidelines for general hospitals. *Journal of Psychosomatic Research, 62,* 371–383.

Owen, D., Paranandi, B., Sivakumar, R., & Seevaratnam, M. (2007). Classical diseases revisited: Transient global amnesia. *Postgraduate Medical Journal, 83*(978), 236–239.

Pantoni, L., Bertini, E., Lamassa, M., Pracucci, G., & Inzitari, D. (2005). Clinical features, risk factors, and prognosis in transient global amnesia: A follow-up study. *European Journal of Neurology, 12*(5), 350–356.

Simeon, D., Guralnik, O., Knuntelska, M., & Schmeidler, J. (2002). Personality factors associated with dissociation: Temperament, defenses, and cognitive schemata. *American Journal of Psychiatry, 159,* 489–491.

Swedish Council on Technology Assessment in Health Care. (2008). *Dementia—Etiology and epidemiology: A systematic review* (Vol. 1). Elanders Infologistics.

Wilmo, A., Winblad, B., Aguero-Torres, H., & von Stauss, E. (2003). *The magnitude of dementia occurrence in the world.* Aging Research Center.

WEB RESOURCES

- Alzheimer's Disease and Dementia/Alzheimer's Association: http://www.alz.org/index.asp/
- American Psychiatric Association: http://www.psych.org/
- Family Caregiver Alliance: http://www.caregiver.org/caregiver/jsp/home.jsp/
- Family Caregiver Alliance: http://www.caregiving.org/members/
- Freedom from Fear: http://www.freedomfromfear.org/

9

Substance Use Disorders

Background Information

Definition of Disorder

- Substance use disorder (SUD) is a maladaptive pattern of substance use.
- The substance used poses a hazard to health, employment status, school achievement and/or personal relationships.
- In the *Diagnostic and Statistical Manual of Mental Disorders*, Fifth Edition (*DSM-5*), Substance Abuse and Substance Dependence are combined under SUD.
- Abuse and dependence exist on a scale of measurement directed toward time and degree of use.

Four Classes of Substance Use Disorders

- *Stimulants*: caffeine, nicotine, amphetamines, cocaine, ecstasy
- *Depressants*: tranquilizers/benzodiazepines, alcohol
- *Narcotics*: opioids
- *Hallucinogens*: lysergic acid diethylamide (LSD), peyote, marijuana

Etiology and Risk factors

- The etiology of SUD is unknown; however, contributing factors have provided support for multiple theories.
- Genetics—inclusive of the impact of environment on gene development is thought to account for up to 60% of the risk for SUD/substance use addiction.
  - Environmental
    - Developmental influences
    - Personality traits
    - Posttraumatic stress disorder (PTSD), attention deficit hyperactivity disorder (ADHD)
  - Social learning
    - Parental, peer, and online/TV societal role modeling
    - Supportive cultural attitudes

Demographics

- Males are more likely to use illicit drugs than females.

- Males have higher rates of dependency than women, but women have equal likelihood to develop an SUD.
- Women have increased likelihood to experience craving and relapse in SUD.
- One in seven young adults (aged 18–25 years) or 14.8% have an SUD.
- Ten percent of young adults (aged 18–25 years) have an alcohol use disorder (AUD).
- A total of 7.3% of young adults have an illicit use disorder.
- Six percent of adults (aged 26–65 years) have an SUD.
- Over 1 million seniors (aged 65 years and older) have an SUD, most of whom had the disorder before the age of 65.
- The highest rates of SUD (12.8%) are found among American Indians and Native Alaskans, followed by Caucasians (7.7%).
- The lowest rates are among Asian Americans (3.7%).
- African Americans (6.8%), Hispanics (6.6%), and 4.6% of native Hawaiians/Pacific Islanders had SUD in 2017.
- Sixty-five percent of incarcerated Americans meet the criteria for SUD.
- Seventy-five percent of those Americans who are incarcerated in jails or prisons have comorbid psychiatric/SUD illnesses.

Diagnosis

Each SUD has its own diagnosis and differential diagnosis. Criteria for each SUD is included in the *DSM-5*. Two of 11 criteria reflective of an SUD are required in a 12-month period for diagnosis. Following are the general criteria for SUD: use of substance over a period of time; experiences tolerance; develops dependence on the substance, using more than intended; inability to quit over time; engages in seeking behaviors; continues to use despite negative consequences; time engaged in using; failure to keep responsibilities; giving up activities; and experiences withdrawal symptoms when not using.

Differential Diagnosis
- Hypoglycemia
- Medication-induced intoxication
- Electrolyte (sodium, potassium, chloride, and sodium bicarbonate) imbalance
- Head injury/trauma
- Stroke
- Psychosis
- Neurological disorder

ICD-10 Codes
Mental and behavioral disorders due to psychoactive substance use (F10–F19)

Other psychoactive substance (OPS) abuse, uncomplicated (F19.10)

Diagnostic Workup
- Diagnosis of SUD is typically made by detailed subjective history.
- Blood, saliva, breath, or urine screening for substance(s).

Initial Assessment
- Medical history and examination
- Psychiatric history and examination
- Family and social history

- Cultural history related to substance use
- Detailed history of past and present substance use, tolerance, and withdrawal
- How do the substances affect the patient mentally and physically
- How is the substance use affecting the patient's occupational, family, or social life
  - CAGE (cut down, annoyed, guilty, and eye opener) screening questionnaire to assess alcohol dependence
  - SMAST (Short Michigan Alcoholism Screening Test) screening tool for alcohol use
  - CIWA-Ar (Clinical Institute Withdrawal Assessment for Alcohol) is a validated 10-item assessment tool to evaluate alcohol withdrawal symptoms
  - COWS (Clinical Opiate Withdrawal Scale) assessment tool to evaluate opioid withdrawal symptoms

Clinical Presentation

Signs and symptoms will vary with individuals/substances used but may include the following:

- Sudden weight loss/gain
- Periods of excessive sleep or inability to sleep
- Periods of excessive energy
- Chronic nosebleeds
- Chronic sinusitis
- Chronic cough or bronchitis
- Increased periods of agitation, irritability, or anger
- Depressed mood
- Temporary psychosis
- Interpersonal difficulties
- Inability to fulfill roles at work, home, or school

Diagnostic and Statistical Manual of Mental Disorders, Fifth Edition: Diagnostic Guidelines

- Patient must meet 2+ criteria within a 12-month period. Classification: mild (2–3 symptoms), moderate (4–5 symptoms), or severe (6+ symptoms).
- *Hazardous use*: use of the substance in situations in which use is physically hazardous to self or others.
- *Social or interpersonal problems secondary to substance use*: continued use despite persistent or recurrent social or interpersonal problems that are caused or worsened by the substance use.
- Experiencing withdrawal symptoms when ceasing to use.
- *Tolerance*: more of the substance being required to achieve same effect.
- Substance used in larger amounts and/or for a longer period of time than intended.
- Repeated unsuccessful attempts at controlling or quitting.
- Much time is spent engaging in activities to obtain, use, or recover from the substance.
- Continued use despite persistent or recurrent social or interpersonal problems that are caused or worsened by the substance use.
- Major social, recreational, or occupational activities are relinquished or reduced due to the substance use.
- Presence of craving or a strong desire or urge to use the substance.
- *Common comorbidities*: other SUDs, adolescent conduct disorder, adult antisocial personality disorder.

Treatment Overview

Psychosocial Therapy
- Cognitive behavioral therapy (CBT)
- Motivational enhancement therapy (MET)
- Behavioral therapy
- Psychotherapy

Psychopharmacotherapy
- Treatment of withdrawal states.
- Alcohol withdrawal symptoms cause clinically significant distress resulting from autonomic hyperactivity, anxiety, and gastrointestinal symptoms. Alcohol withdrawal is a life-threatening condition that can result in alcohol withdrawal delirium, tonic–clonic seizures, and in some cases death.
- Medication to decrease reinforcing effects of substance(s).
- Maintenance medication management (agonist therapy).
- Medication for relapse prevention.
- Treatment of comorbid conditions.

Self-Help Groups
- Alcoholics Anonymous (AA)
- Narcotics Anonymous (NA)
- Cocaine Anonymous (CA)

Pharmacological Treatment for Use of Specific Substances
- Nicotine
  - *Nicotine replacement*: patch, gum, spray, lozenge, and inhaler
  - Bupropion (Wellbutrin/Zyban)
  - Varenicline (Chantix)
- Alcohol
  - Symptoms of withdrawal may occur within 4 to 12 hours after cessation or reduction.
  - Thiamine replacement and fluids are given.
  - Benzodiazepine (BZD) is initiated using either "symptom-triggered" dosing or "fixed dosing"—there are advantages to the first in that the dose is administered based on CIWA-Ar and patient receives an individualized dose. BZDs manage seizure risk and also minimize the withdrawal. Only specific BZDs are indicated—not all.
  - Clonidine (Catapres) may be given as needed for hypertensive episodes due to withdrawal.
  - Naltrexone (Revia, Vivitrol, oral or intramuscular [IM]) or acamprosate (Campral) is given to decrease craving.
  - Disulfiram (Antabuse) is a deterrent to drinking.
- Marijuana
  - No recommended pharmacological treatment
- Cocaine
  - Pharmacological treatment is not indicated.
- Opioids
  - *Opioid overdose*: Naloxone is given to reverse respiratory depression.
  - *Maintenance treatment*: Methadone (Dolophine Methadose) or buprenorphine (Subutex) is gradually tapered.
  - *Alternative maintenance*: naltrexone (Revia, Vivitrol).

Drug Selection Table for Managing Substance Use Disorder

CLASS	DRUG
Nicotinic receptor agonists	Nicotine, nicotine transdermal system, nicotine polacrilex (Nicotrol NS, Nicotrol Inhaler, Commit, Habitrol, Nicoderm, Nicotrol ProStep, Nicorette Gum, Nicorette DS), varenicline (Chantix)
Opioid antagonists	Naltrexone hydrochloride (Revia, Vivitrol)
Substance abuse deterrents	Disulfiram (Antabuse) acamprosate calcium (Campral)
Vitamins	B-Complex (Vitamin B1/Thiamine)
NDRIs	Bupropion (Wellbutrin, Zyban)

NDRIs, norepinephrine/dopamine reuptake inhibitors.

Drug Selection Table for Substance Dependence

CLASS	DRUG
Nicotine replacement therapy	Nicotine, nicotine transdermal system, nicotine polacrilex (Nicotrol NS, Nicotrol Inhaler, Commit, Habitrol, Nicoderm, Nicotrol ProStep, Nicorette Gum, Nicorette DS)
BZDs	Chlordiazepoxide (Librium) Diazepam (Valium) Lorazepam (Ativan)
Partial opioid agonists	Buprenorphine HO (Subutex) Buprenorphine HCl and naloxone HCl dihydrate (Suboxone) Methadone HCl (Methadose)
Alpha-agonists	Clonidine (Catapres, Catapres-TTS)
Anticholinergic drugs	Dicyclomine (Bentyl)
NSAIDs	Ibuprofen (Motrin)
Antidiarrheal drugs	Loperamide (Imodium)
Opioid antagonists	Naltrexone (Revia)
Alcohol antagonists	Disulfiram (Antabuse)
Substance abuse deterrents	Acamprosate calcium (Campral)
Vitamins	B-Complex (Vitamin B1/Thiamine Hydrochloride)
Antidepressants	Bupropion HCl (Wellbutrin, Zyban)
Nicotinic receptor agonists	Varenicline (Chantix)

BZDs, benzodiazepines; NSAIDs, nonsteroidal antiinflammatory drugs.

Patient Education

- Clinicians can impact outcomes with patient education related to treatments and medications.
- Educate on importance of joining a support group.
- Teach about relapse prevention. Encourage CBT to increase coping skills and individual therapy to enhance personal insight.
- Patients taking disulfiram (Antabuse) must be advised to avoid alcohol and any substances that contain alcohol. This includes mouthwash, colognes, cough syrups, and so forth.

Medical/Legal Pitfalls

- Abuse of alcohol or drugs comes in second to depression as the risk for suicide.
- Rates of suicide are two to three times more prevalent in those who abuse alcohol or drugs as compared to the general population.
- Individuals withdrawing from substances are at great risk for depression. When not properly treated, depression can lead to suicide.
- Individuals being treated for addiction may have a history of seeing multiple healthcare professionals to obtain medications ("doctor shopping"). Such practices may lead to accidental and/or intentional overdose.

ALCOHOL USE DISORDER

Background Information

Definition of Disorder
- AUD meets 2 of the 11 criteria over a 12-month period and is considered a relapsing brain disorder that is chronic in nature. Specifically, the person with an AUD has a loss of ability to control alcohol use, compulsivity to use alcohol, and an emotional state of negativity when not using alcohol.

Diagnosis

- Meets 2 or more of the 11 criteria, with alcohol the specific substance of use
- History and physical examination completed to rule out differential diagnosis and comorbid diagnosis
- EKG
- Routine blood, urine, and toxicology screens

Clinical Presentation
- Uncoordinated movements
- Ataxia
- Tremors
- Rapid pulse
- Sweating
- Slurred speech
- Reports lack of appetite
- Nausea and vomiting
- Involuntary eye movements
- Blemishes on skin and/or abnormal muscle tone
- Face and palm flushing
- Spider veins on skin (especially ion face or abdomen)
- Yellow sclera
- Abdominal bloating
- Ecchymosis

Signs and Symptoms of Alcohol Withdrawal
- Can progress quickly to medical emergency
- Three stages with timeline:
  - *Stage 1*: 1 to 8 hours after last drink; signs/symptoms—nausea, abdominal pain, anxiety, insomnia
  - *Stage 2*: 1 to 3 days after last drink; signs/symptoms—increased body temperature, hypertension (high blood pressure)

■ *Stage 3*: 1 week or more after last drink; signs/symptoms—agitation, fever, seizures, hallucinations

Acute and Chronic Complication of Alcohol Use and/or Alcohol Withdrawal
■ Alcohol poisoning
■ Delirium tremens (5% of alcohol withdrawals)
■ Alcohol seizures
■ Alcohol psychosis
■ Wernicke-Korsakoff syndrome

Detoxification and Stabilization for Alcohol Use Disorder
■ Treat presenting symptoms
■ CIWA-Ar Scale
■ Assess for treatment modality (inpatient/outpatient detoxification)

ICD-10 Codes
Mental and behavioral disorders due to use of alcohol (F10.1–F10.99)

Treatment Overview

Drug Selection Table for Managing Alcohol Use Disorder

DRUG CLASS	DRUG
Benzodiazepines	Treating withdrawal symptoms: Diazepam (Valium) Chlordiazepoxide (Librium)
	Lorazepam (Ativan) Oxazepam (Serax) Promoting abstinence: Naltrexone (Revia, Vivitrol) Acamprosate (Campral) Lorazepam (Ativan) Disulfiram (Antabuse)

NICOTINE/TOBACCO USE DISORDER

Background Information
Definition of Disorder
The person with nicotine/tobacco use disorder has a dependence on nicotine as a result of tobacco product use or other delivery systems; compulsivity to use tobacco products (e.g., hookahs, cigars, chewing tobacco, snuff, smokeless tobacco cigarettes, e-cigarettes); and an emotional state of negativity when not using nicotine delivering products. Tobacco use disorder presents a negative impact on almost all body organs and is considered the most common SUD with over 37 million Americans smoking.

Diagnosis
■ Meets 2 or more of the 11 criteria, with nicotine/tobacco the specific substance of use
■ History and physical examination completed to rule out differential diagnosis and comorbid diagnosis
■ EKG

Clinical Presentation
- Fatigue
- Dizziness
- Cravings
- Cough
- Change in appetite (usually increased)
- Constipation
- Insomnia
- Slowed speech patterns
- Depression
- Anxiety
- Inability to concentrate
- Nervousness
- Sense of hopelessness

Detoxification and Stabilization for Nicotine/Tobacco Use Disorder
- Treat presenting symptoms.

ICD-10 Codes
Mental and behavioral disorders due to use of tobacco (F17.200–F17.299)

Treatment Overview

Drug Selection Table for Managing Tobacco Use Disorder

DRUG CLASS	DRUG
Nicotine replacement therapy	Gums and lozenges Transdermal systems
Non-nicotine-containing products and antidepressants	Bupropion SR (Zyban) Varenicline (Chantix) Nortriptyline (Pamelor) Cytisine (Tabex)

Note: Special consideration should be taken when the patient is pregnant, is breastfeeding, or has a comorbid diagnosis that would make any of these medications contraindicated.

Patient Education
- Reassure patient that signs and symptoms of withdrawal will abate in about 2 weeks.

CANNABIS/HALLUCINOGENIC USE DISORDER

Background Information
Definition of Disorder
- Canabis or hallucinogenic use disorder meets 2 of the 11 criteria over a 12-month period and is considered a relapsing brain disorder that is chronic in nature. Specifically, the person with either or both of these disorders will experience psychoactive effects from the drugs resulting from excessive use. The person with these disorders will have delusions, hallucinations, and unspecified anxiety symptoms, often concurrent with other SUD.

Diagnosis
- Meets 2 or more of the 11 criteria, with alcohol the specific substance of use.
- Legal use of cannabis will not prevent the patient from developing a SUD. Legal uses of cannabis include recreational use in states where it is legal and medicinal use to treat pain, anorexia nervosa, antiemetic, asthma, autism spectrum disorder (ASD), chronic prostatitis (CP), epilepsy, glaucoma, and other medical conditions.
- History and physical examination completed to rule out differential diagnosis and comorbid diagnosis.
- EKG if abnormal cardiac rhythm is detected.
- Routine blood, urine, and toxicology screens.

Clinical Presentation
- Dilated pupils
- Uncoordinated movements
- Ataxia
- Slurred speech
- May have increase (cannabis) or decreased (hallucinogens) appetite
- Nausea and vomiting
- Flushing
- Agitation
- Hallucinations
- Paranoia
- Panic

Signs and Symptoms of Cannabis Withdrawal
- May not appear for 1 to 2 days and peaks at 4 days usually last up to 2 weeks
- *Emotional/behavioral*: aggression, anger, restlessness, anxiety
- *Physical*: diarrhea or loose stools, sweating, insomnia, flu-like symptoms, runny nose, loss of appetite

Presentation of Severe Intoxication
- Serious impairment to thought process and judgment
- Serious impairment to motor coordination
- Dyspnea, chills, tachycardia
- Unconsciousness

Treatment for Cannabis/Hallucinogen Overdose
- Treat presenting symptoms
- Hydrate
- Be prepared for rapid change in vital signs
- High risk for falls
- Pharmacological treatment for anxiety

Detoxification and Stabilization for Cannabis/Hallucinogenic Use Disorder
- Treat presenting symptoms
- Assess for treatment modality (inpatient/outpatient detoxification)

ICD-10 Codes
Mental and behavioral disorders due hallucinogen abuse (F16.10–F16.99)

Treatment Overview

- There are presently no Food and Drug Administration (FDA)-approved medications.
- Treatment must be symptom specific.
- Where legal, oral doses of tetrahydrocannabinol (THC) have been effective in reducing signs and symptoms of acute withdrawal.

COCAINE AND OTHER STIMULANT USE DISORDER

Background Information

Definition of Disorder

- Meets 2 of the 11 criteria over a 12-month period and is considered a relapsing brain disorder that is chronic in nature. Specifically, the person with a cocaine or stimulant use disorder has persistent use of stimulants/amphetamines (cocaine and other stimulants), increasing emotional and behavioral stress and impairment, and compulsivity to use a stimulant (e.g., cocaine, amphetamine, methamphetamine).

Diagnosis

- Meets 2 or more of the 11 criteria, with alcohol the specific substance of use.
- History and physical examination completed to rule out differential diagnosis and comorbid diagnosis.
- EKG.
- Routine blood, urine, and toxicology screens.
- Legal use of amphetamines will not prevent the patient from developing an SUD.
- Legal uses include treatment for ADHD, narcolepsy, obesity, and depression.

Clinical Presentation—Stimulant Intoxication

- Dilated pupils
- Talkative
- Insomnia
- Dry mouth
- Decreased of appetite
- Jaw clenching
- Tachypnea
- Tremors
- Rapid pulse
- Sweating
- Mania
- Nausea and vomiting
- Increased temperature
- Stroke and heart attack

Clinical Presentation—Long-Term Use

- Dilated pupils
- Chronic exhaustion alternating with energy, malnourishment, behavioral disorders, brain damage, cardiac problems, vitamin deficiencies, birth defects, chronic insomnia, dermatological problems, chronic anxiety and paranoia, psychosis, stroke, and death

- Insomnia
- Malnourishment
- Behavioral disorders
- Brain damage
- Cardiac problems
- Vitamin deficiencies
- Birth defects
- Chronic insomnia
- Dermatological problems
- Chronic anxiety and paranoia
- Psychosis
- Stroke
- Death

Signs and Symptoms of Withdrawal

- Can progress quickly to a medical emergency but is not usually life threatening. Begins after 12 hours and can last for days.
- Three stages:
  - *Immediate (within 24 hours of last use)*: increased cravings, lethargic, depressed
  - *Secondary*: fatigue progressing to exhaustion accompanied by insomnia and depression
  - *Crash*: exhaustion
- During the withdrawal phase, patients can experience muscle pains, anxiety, cravings, sleep alterations, depression, hallucinations, and unpredictable and possibly violent behaviors toward self and others (high risk for suicide). Patients withdrawing from methamphetamines are at higher risk for more serious symptoms including but not limited to paranoia, serious thought disturbances, hallucinations and psychosis.

Detoxification and Stabilization

- Treat presenting symptoms.
- Assess for treatment modality (inpatient/outpatient detoxification).

ICD-10 Codes

Mental and behavioral disorders due to cocaine abuse (F14.10–F15.99)

Treatment Overview

- There are no current FDA-approved medications. Treat symptoms utilizing sharp professional assessment of patient condition.

OPIOID USE DISORDER

Background Information

Definition of Disorder

- Meets two of the 11 criteria over a 12-month period and is considered a relapsing brain disorder that is chronic in nature. Specifically, the person with an opioid use disorder has a compulsive use of opioids in excess of prescribed amounts and compulsive use of opioids without prescription or for nonmedical purposes. Common opioids include opium, oxycodone, heroin, hydrocodone, fentanyl, methadone, codeine, meperidine, tramadol, oxymorphone, buprenorphine, carfentanil, meperidine and hydromorphone.

Diagnosis
- Meets 2 or more of the 11 criteria, with opioid being the specific substance of use
- History and physical examination completed to rule out differential diagnosis and comorbid diagnosis
- Evaluation with the COW scale
- EKG
- Routine blood, urine, and toxicology screens

Clinical Presentation
- Pinpoint/constricted pupils
- Sedation
- Yawning
- Drowsiness or sleepiness
- Decreased or shallow respirations
- Uncoordinated movements
- Ataxia
- Nausea and vomiting
- Slurred speech

Signs and Symptoms of Opioid Withdrawal
- Dysphoria
- Restlessness
- Respiratory depression
- Flu-like symptoms (runny nose)
- Sweating skin with goose bumps
- Joint pain, muscle aches
- Bradycardia
- Gastrointestinal (GI) problems: diarrhea, vomiting, nausea, abdominal cramping
- Pupillary dilation
- Nonresponsive

Reversal Agent for Overdose
- Naloxone (Narcan)

Detoxification and Stabilization
- Treat presenting symptoms
- COW scale
- Medically assisted opioid withdrawal using clonidine as well as other non-narcotics to reduce symptoms followed by use of a tapering approach with methadone or buprenorphine. This should be used with a long-term plan for stabilization.

ICD-10 Codes
Mental and behavioral disorders due opioid abuse (F11.1–F11.99)

Treatment Overview
- *Medication-assisted treatment* (MAT): combines psychotherapy and medications to increase the success of stabilization

Drug Selection Table for Opioid Withdrawal Management and Long-Term Stabilization

DRUG CLASS	DRUG
Non-opioids	Clonidine (Catapres)
Opioids	Buprenorphine (Suboxone)
	Methadone (Diskets, Methadone Intensol, Methadose, Dolophine)

INHALANT AND OTHER PSYCHOACTIVE SUBSTANCE USE DISORDERS

Background Information

Definition of Disorder
- Meets 2 of the 11 criteria over a 12-month period and is considered a relapsing brain disorder that is chronic in nature. Specifically, the person with an inhalant use disorder has a loss of ability to control the use of inhalants, compulsivity to use inhalants, and an emotional state of negativity when not sniffing/breathing inhalants; it is usually seen in younger people (teenagers). Volatile solvents, aerosols, gases, and nitrites are commonly used as inhalants.
- *Methods of inhaling*: sniffing, spraying into nose or mouth, bagging, huffing (breathing in from a rag soaked with the chemical), and inhalation from balloons.
- Intoxication is very brief, requiring multiple consecutive applications for sustained sense of intoxication.

Diagnosis
- Meets 2 or more of the 11 criteria, with inhalant and other psychoactive substances being the specific substance of use
- History and physical examination completed to rule out differential diagnosis and comorbid diagnosis
- EKG
- Routine blood, urine, and toxicology screens

Clinical Presentation
- Intoxication not caused by alcohol or other drugs
- Ataxia
- Uncoordination
- Smell of the chemicals on body or clothes
- Sores and scabs around the nose and mouth (Glue sniffer's rash)
- Slurred speech
- Change in personal hygiene
- Drowsiness
- Headache

Emergency Effects from Inhalants (Can Progress Quickly to a Medical Emergency)
- Agitation, fever, seizures, hallucinations
- Loss of sensation
- Confusion
- Loss of consciousness
- Coma
- Fatal accidental injury

Detoxification and Stabilization for Inhalant Use Disorder
■ Treat presenting symptoms.
■ Therapy.
■ Assess for treatment modality (inpatient/outpatient detoxification).
■ Keep solvents and sprays away from children and teens.

ICD-10 Codes
Mental and behavioral disorders due to inhalant abuse (F18.1–F18.99)

Mental and behavioral disorders due to OPS abuse (F19.1–F19.99)

Treatment Overview

Drug Selection Table for Managing Inhalant Use Disorder

DRUG CLASS	DRUG
Benzodiazepines	Treating withdrawal symptoms Diazepam (Valium)
	Chlordiazepoxide (Librium) Lorazepam (Ativan) Oxazepam (Serax) Promote abstinence Naltrexone (Revia, Vivitrol) Acamprosate (Campral) Lorazepam (Ativan) Disulfiram (Antabuse)

BIBLIOGRAPHY

American Psychiatric Association. (2006). *Practice guidelines for the treatment of patients with substance use disorders* (2nd ed.). http://www.Psychiatryonline.com/contenc.aspx?aID=14079 (accessed on February 10, 2009).

American Psychiatric Association. (2013). *Diagnostic and statistical manual of mental disorder* (5th ed.). Washington, DC: American Psychiatric Publishing.

Anthony, J. C., Warner, L. A., & Kessler, R. C. (1994). Comparative epidemiology of dependence on tobacco, alcohol, controlled substances, and inhalants: Basic findings from the National Comorbidity Survey. *Experimental and Clinical Psychopharmacology, 2*(3), 244–268. https://doi.org/10.1037/1064-1297.2.3.244

Bogunovic, O. (2012). Substance abuse in aging and elderly adults. *Psychiatric Times, 29*(8), 39.

Center for Behavioral Health Statistics and Quality. (2017). *Results from the 2016 National Survey on Drug Use and Health: Detailed Tables.* Substance Abuse and Mental Health Services Administration.

Centers for Disease Control and Prevention. (2015). *Today's heroin epidemic.* https://www.cdc.gov/vitalsigns/heroin/index.html (accesed on 10 May 2019).

Centers for Disease Control and Prevention. (2019). *HIV and women.* https://www.cdc.gov/hiv/group/gender/women/index.html (accessed on May 21, 2019).

Centers for Disease Control and Prevention. (2020). *HIV and women.* https://www.cdc.gov/hiv/group/gender/women/index.html (accessed on May 21, 2019).

Cleary, M., Hunt, G. E., Matheson, S. L., Siegfried, N., & Walter, G. (2008). Psychosocial interventions for people with both severe mental illness and substance misuse. *Cochrane Database of Systematic Reviews, 10*(1), CD001088. https://doi.org/10.1002/14651858.CD001088.pub2

Dragisic, T., Dickov, A., Dickov, V., & Mijatovic, V. (2015, June). *Drug addiction as risk for suicide attempts.* https://www.ncbi.nlm.nih.gov/pmc/articles/PMC4499285/#ref4 (accessed on May 20, 2019).

Ferri, M. M. F., Amato, L., & Davoli, M. (2006). Alcoholics Anonymous and other 12-step programmes for alcohol dependence. *Cochrane Database of Systematic Reviews, 3*(3), CD005032. https://doi.org/10.1002/14651858.CD005032.pub2

Gowing, L., Ali, R., & White, J. M. (2006). Buprenorphine for the management of opioid withdrawal. *Cochrane Database of Systematic Reviews, 2,* 3.

Kennedy, A. P., Epstein, D. H., Phillips, K. A., & Preston, K. L. (2013). Sex differences in cocaine/heroin users: drug-use triggers and craving in daily life. *Drug Alcohol Depend, 132*(1–2), 29-37. https://doi.org/10.1016/j.drugalcdep.2012.12.025

Kippin, T. E., Fuchs, R. A., Mehta, R. H. et al. (2005). Potentiation of cocaine-primed reinstatement of drug seeking in female rats during estrus. *Psychopharmacology, 182*(2), 245–252. https://doi.org/10.1007/s00213-005-0071-y

Marshall, B., & Spencer, J. (2018). *Fast facts about substance use disorders: What every nurse, APRN and PA needs to know.* Springer Publishing Company.

Naegle, M. (2008). Substance misuse and alcohol use disorders. In E. Capezuti, D. Zwicker, M. Mezey, & T. Fulmer (Eds.), *Evidence-based geriatric nursing protocols for best practice* (3rd ed., pp. 649–676). Springer Publishing Company.

National Institute on Drug Abuse. (2012). *Inhalants: What are the unique risks associated with nitrite abuse.* https://www.drugabuse.gov/publications/research-reports/inhalants/what-are-unique-risks-associated-nitrite-abuse (accessed on May 25, 2019).

National Institute on Drug Abuse. (2015). *Drug and alcohol use - a significant risk factor for HIV.* https://www.drugabuse.gov/related-topics/trends-statistics/infographics/drug-alcohol-use-significant-risk-factor-hiv (accessed on May 21, 2019).

National Institutes of Health. (2018). *Addiction and the criminal justice system.* https://report.nih.gov/nihfactsheets/ViewFactSheet.aspx?csid=22 (accessed on May 21, 2019).

Sack, D. (2014). We can't afford to ignore drug addiction in prison. *The Washington Post.* https://www.washingtonpost.com/news/to-your-health/wp/2014/08/14/we-cant-afford-to-ignore-drug-addiction-in-prison/ (accessed on May 21, 2019).

Substance Abuse and Mental Health Services Administration. (2007). *2007 National survey on drug use & health: National results.* http://www.oas.samhsa.gov/nsduh/2k7nsduh/2k7Results.cfm#TOC (accessed on February 13, 2009).

Substance Abuse and Mental Health Services Administration. (2018). *Key substance use and mental health indicators in the United States: Results from the 2017 National Survey on drug use and health.* https://www.samhsa.gov/data/sites/default/files/cbhsq-reports/NSDUHFFR2017/NSDUHFFR2017.pdf (accessed on May 18, 2019).

U.S. Library of Medicine, Medline Plus. (nd). *Substance use disorder.* https://medlineplus.gov/ency/article/001522.htm (accessed on May 7)

Vaz de Lima, F. B., da Silveira, D. X., & Andriolo, R. B. (2008). Effectiveness aned safety of topiramate for drug dependents (Protocol). *Cochrane Database of Systematic Reviews, 4*(4), 431–435.

Ziedonis, D., Das, S., & Larkin, C. (2017). Tobacco use disorder and treatment: New challenges and opportunities. *Dialogues in Clinical Neuroscience, 19*(3), 271–280.

WEB RESOURCES

- DSM-5 Diagnosis Guide: https://www.optumsandiego.com/content/dam/san-diego/documents/dmc-ods/toolbox/Quick_Guide_--DSM5-ICD10_Diagnosis_Guide.pdf
- The Substance Abuse and Mental Health Services Administration: http://www.samhsa.gov/

10

Psychotic Disorders

BRIEF PSYCHOTIC DISORDER

Background Information

Definition of Disorder

- Sudden onset of psychotic symptoms occurs.
- These include delusions, hallucinations, disorganized speech, or grossly disorganized or catatonic behavior.
- Episode lasts from 1 day to less than 1 month, with return to premorbid level of functioning.
- Symptoms may or may not meet the definition of schizophrenia.

Etiology

- It is often precipitated by extremely stressful life events.
- Cause is unknown.
- Patients with personality disorder may have predisposition toward development of psychotic symptoms.
- May have prevalence of mood disorders in family.
- May have poor coping skills along with secondary gains for psychotic symptoms.
- May have defense against a prohibited fantasy, fulfillment of unattained wish, or escape from a distasteful situation.

Demographics

- Brief psychotic disorder is generally considered uncommon.
- More likely to occur in young rather than older patients.
- It generally first occurs in early adulthood (20s and 30s) and is more common in women than in men.
- More frequent in lower socioeconomic classes.
- Patient may have prior personality disorder.
- May predispose to survivors of disasters or major cultural changes.

Risk Factors

- Major life events that cause significant emotional stress.
- Severity must be in relation to the patient's life.

Family History
More common in families with history of mood (bipolar) disorders. This suggests a genetic link.

Stressful Events in Susceptible People
- Usually follows life-altering stressor.
- May present after series of less overtly stressful events.
- Stressor could be unrelated to the psychotic episode.
- Paranoia is often predominant.

Diagnosis

Differential Diagnosis
- Factitious disorder with mainly psychological symptoms
- Malingering
- Psychotic disorder with medical causation
- Substance-induced psychotic disorder
- Seizure disorders
- Delirium
- Dissociative identity disorder
- Borderline personality disorder symptoms
- Schizotypal personality disorder symptoms

ICD-10 Codes
Brief psychotic disorder (F23)

Diagnostic Workup
- Always includes at least one major symptom of psychosis.
- Delusions with rapidly changing delusional topics.
- Abrupt onset occurs.
- Affective symptoms, confusion, and impaired attention are presented.
- Emotional lability is observed.
- Inappropriate dress or behavior is seen.
- Patient is screaming or mute.
- Impaired recent memory.
- Organic workup includes complete blood count (CBC) with differentials; complete serum chemistry; thyroid function studies; and thyroid stimulating hormone, serum alcohol, and illegal substance levels (including anabolic steroids, cannabis, alcohol, tobacco, temazepam, opium, heroine/morphine, and methamphetamines).
- No imaging studies are required to diagnose brief psychotic disorder.

Initial Assessment
- Medical history is obtained.
- Psychiatric history is obtained.
- In-depth mental status examination is done. A careful mental status examination can distinguish this disorder from delirium, dementia, or other organic brain syndromes, such as meningitis, transient ischemic attack, and epilepsy.
- Family history is obtained.
- History may need to be obtained from significant others in acutely ill patients.
- Symptoms are observed.

Clinical Presentation
- Psychotic symptoms seen, most likely paranoia
- Sudden onset
- May not include the entire spectrum of schizophrenia
- Mood variability
- Reactive confusion
- Reactive depression
- Impaired attention span
- Reactive excitation
- Screaming or silence
- Impaired short-term memory
- Changes in sleep or eating habits, energy level, or weight
- Inability to make decisions
- Garish style of dress

Diagnostic and Statistical Manual of Mental Disorders, Fifth Edition: Diagnostic Guidelines
- Sudden onset of at least one psychotic symptom occurs (i.e., delusions, hallucinations, disorganized speech, or grossly disorganized or catatonic behavior).
- Psychotic episodes *last less than 1 month and are followed by a full recovery*. This disorder can occur in the presence or absence of a major stressor.
- Diagnosis can only be made if other medical or psychiatric disorders have been excluded.

Treatment Overview

Acute Treatment
- In the acute phase, inpatient hospitalization may be necessary for safety and evaluation. This includes close monitoring of symptoms and assessment of danger to self and others.
- *Mental status examination*: Patients usually present with severe psychotic agitation that may be associated with strange or bizarre behavior, uncooperativeness, physical or verbal aggression, disorganized speech, screaming or muteness, labile or depressed mood, suicidal and/or homicidal thoughts or behaviors, restlessness, hallucinations, delusions, disorientation, impaired attention, impaired concentration, impaired memory, poor insight, and poor judgment.
- A quiet, structured hospital setting may assist in regaining reality.
- Administration of antipsychotic (AP) medication as indicated is most frequently a high-potency dopamine receptor antagonist. Conventional (typical) AP medications most commonly used in this disorder include haloperidol (Haldol) and chlorpromazine (Thorazine). Thorazine is used less frequently now due to corrected QT interval (QTc) risks.
- Newer medications, called atypical AP drugs, are used.
- Benzodiazepine medication may be given to patients who present or are at high risk for excitation, as they also are beneficial in the treatment of brief psychosis. Lorazepam (Ativan) or diazepam (Valium) may be used if the person has a very high level of anxiety or insomnia.
- If symptoms are only minimally impairing the patient's function and a specific stressor is identified, removing the stressor should suffice.
- Further inpatient care is unnecessary once the acute attack has ended.

Chronic Treatment

- Following the resolution of the episode, hypnotic medications may be useful.
- Long-term use of medications should be avoided. If maintenance medications are necessary, reevaluation of the diagnosis is indicated.
- Individual, family, and group psychotherapies are essential to integrate the experience psychologically into the lives of the patient and/or significant others.
- Therapies should include discussion of the precipitating stressors, the psychotic episode itself, and development of successful coping strategies. Sessions should be done at least weekly, once the patient is discharged from the hospital, and last 6 to 8 weeks or longer.
- The length of acute and residual symptoms is usually less than a week.
- Depressive symptoms may present following cessation of psychosis.
- Risk for suicide can escalate in the postpsychotic depressive stage.

Recurrence Rate

Good prognosis can be predicted if

- prior good adjustment occurs,
- few premorbid schizoid tendencies occur,
- the precipitating stressor is severe,
- onset of symptoms is sudden,
- affective symptoms are present,
- during acute phase, manifestation of confusion and bewilderment is seen,
- minimal affective blunting occurs,
- there is a short duration of symptoms, and
- there is an absence of schizophrenic relatives.
  In general, 50% to 80% of all patients have no further major psychiatric episodes.

Patient Education

- Information for patients and families is available in easy-to-understand language at www.webmd.com.
- Signs, symptoms, and treatment information can be obtained from www.healthline.com.
- Data on foundations and support groups are available at www.organizedwisdom.com.
- The National Alliance on Mental Illness—at www.nami.org—is a government-sponsored organization for information regarding mental illness.
- Specific information regarding this disorder is presented at www.medicinenet.com/brief psychotic disorder.

There is no known way to prevent brief psychotic disorder. However, early diagnosis and treatment can help decrease the disruption to the person's life, family, and friendships. Both the patient and the family must be educated about the illness and the potential adverse effects of the medications.

Medical/Legal Pitfalls

Risk of suicide or harm to others may occur if no immediate safety measures are taken:

- Misdiagnosis may be the result of symptoms similar to those of other psychiatric/medical disorders. General recommendations include serious consideration of medical causes in any acute-onset new psychosis. This does not necessarily mean ordering every possible test; but history and the physical examination often alert the clinician to the need for additional medical evaluation.

■ Physical or chemical restraints may be necessary in cases of severe uncontrolled agitation to provide safety to self and/or others.

DELUSIONAL DISORDER

Background Information
Definition of Disorder

■ Delusions can include paranoia, grandiosity, erotica, jealousy, somatic, and mixed responses.

■ Incorrect inference about external reality persists despite evidence to the contrary, and these beliefs are not ordinarily accepted by other members of the person's culture or subculture.

Etiology

■ Cause is unknown.

■ Distinction between schizophrenia and mood disorders is seen.

■ Onset occurs later in life.

■ Predominance varies depending on source reviewed.

■ Increased prevalence occurs with personality traits of suspiciousness, jealousy, and secretiveness.

■ Relatively stable diagnosis can be made, with less than a quarter of delusional patients rediagnosed as schizophrenic and less than 10% as mood disordered.

■ Delusional disorder may involve the limbic system or basal ganglia when intact cerebral cortical function is present.

Demographics

■ Prevalence in the United States is estimated to be 0.025% to 0.03%.

■ Annually, new cases account for 1 to 3 cases per 100,000 people.

■ Four percent of all first admissions to psychiatric hospitals are for psychoses not due to a general medical condition or substance.

■ Average age of onset is 40 years, with a range from 18 through the 90s.

■ Slightly more females than men are affected.

■ Many patients are married or employed.

■ Some association with recent immigration or low socioeconomic status, celibacy among men, and widowhood among women is noted.

■ Because of poor insight into their pathological experiences, patients with delusional disorder may rarely seek psychiatric help and often may present to internists, surgeons, dermatologists, police officers, and lawyers rather than to psychiatric professionals.

■ Men are more likely than women to develop paranoid delusions; women are more likely than men to develop delusions of erotomania.

■ Patients often do not present for treatment, and thus they do not commonly make themselves available for research studies.

Risk Factors
Age
■ Eighteen to 40 years

Family History
- A hostile family environment is observed, usually with an overcontrolling mother and a distant or sadistic father.

Stressful Events in Susceptible People
- Social isolation
- Less-than-expected levels of achievement
- Hypersensitivity
- Specific ego function, including reaction formation, projection, and denial
- Distrust in relationships evolving from hostility and abuse

Having Another Mental Health Disorder
- May have a mood component but not severe enough to be classified as a mood disorder

Diagnosis
Differential Diagnosis
- Delusions can transpire simultaneously, with many medical and neurological illnesses.
- Most common sites for lesions are the basal ganglia and limbic system.
- Toxicology screening and routine lab studies, including CBC with differential, serum chemistries, and thyroid function, are done.
- Differs from malingering and factitious disorder.
- Separated from schizophrenia by the absence of other schizophrenic symptoms and non-bizarre qualities of delusions and impairment of functioning.
- Differs from depressive disorders in that somatic features are not pervasive.
- In differentiating delusional disorder from paranoid personality disorder, it is necessary to determine the distinction between extreme suspiciousness and delusion. If in doubt that a symptom is a delusion, a diagnosis of delusional disorder should not be made.

ICD-10 Code
Delusional disorder (F22)

Diagnostic Workup
By psychiatric presentation

- Olfactory or tactile hallucinations may be prominent but only if they are related to the content of the delusion.
- This disorder is unlike schizophrenia in that (1) it has no prominent auditory or visual hallucinations, (2) it has no thought disorder, (3) it has no significant flattening of affect, (4) psychosocial functioning is not markedly impaired, and (5) behavior is not obviously odd or bizarre.
- The delusions have lasted longer than any associated depression or mania.
- *Laboratory studies*: toxicology screening, CBC with differential, serum chemistries, and thyroid function studies (triiodothyronine [T3], thyroxine [T4], thyroid-stimulating hormone [TSH]).
- CT scan of the brain can help rule out physical reasons.

Initial Assessment
- Psychiatric history and presentation are assessed to establish whether pathology is present.

- Determining the presence or absence of important characteristics often associated with delusions is important.
- Delusional disorder should be seen as a diagnosis of exclusion.
- Medical history is obtained.
- Veracity of symptoms should be checked before automatically considering the content to be delusional.
- Assessment of homicidal or suicidal ideation is extremely important in evaluating patients with delusional disorder. The presence of homicidal or suicidal thoughts related to delusions should be actively screened for and the risk of carrying out violent plans should be carefully assessed.

Clinical Presentation

Mental status examination reveals patients as usually well groomed and remarkably normal except for the specific delusional system:

- Patients may attempt to engage clinicians to agree with their delusions.
- Moods and affects are congruent with the delusions.
- No significant hallucinations occur unless strictly pertaining to the delusions presented.
- Disordered thought content is the primary symptom.
- Delusions are characterized as being possible and may be simple or complex.
- Sudden onset occurs.
- Below-average intelligence is seen.
- Intact memory and orientation.
- No insight.
- Poor impulse control.

Diagnostic and Statistical Manual of Mental Disorders, Fifth Edition: Diagnostic Guidelines

- No prominent auditory or visual hallucinations.
- No thought disorder.
- No significant flattening of affect.
- Psychosocial functioning is not markedly impaired.
- Behavior is not obviously odd or bizarre.
- Delusions have lasted longer than any associated depression or mania.

Treatment Overview

Acute Treatment

- Hospitalization should be considered if a potential for harm or violence exists.
- A complete neurological and medical workup may be indicated to determine an organic cause for the symptoms.
- Delusional disorder is challenging to treat for various reasons, including patients' frequent denial that they have any problem, especially of a psychological nature; difficulties in developing a therapeutic alliance; and social/interpersonal conflicts.
- Avoiding direct confrontation of the delusional symptoms enhances the possibility of treatment compliance and response.
- Treatment of delusional disorder often involves both psychopharmacology and psychotherapy.
- Polypharmacy is common, most often including a combination of AP and antidepressant medications. Atypical APs) are effective in treating the symptoms of delusional disorder with fewer movement-related side effects than typical APs.

■ Antidepressants, particularly the selective serotonin reuptake inhibitors (SSRIs), have been successfully used for the treatment of the somatic-type delusional disorder.
■ Establishing a therapeutic alliance, establishing acceptable symptomatic treatment goals, and educating the patient's family are of paramount importance.
■ Outpatient treatment is preferred.

Psychopharmacology of Delusional Disorder

Atypical AP drugs are used as a first-line treatment of delusional disorder with success.

Owing to their more tolerable side effect profile, atypical APs are prescribed more frequently than conventional or typical AP medications. However, recent studies have not confirmed atypical drugs to be better than conventional APs in the treatment of delusional disorder. Lower doses of AP medications are used with delusional disorder than with schizophrenia. Most commonly used atypical antipsychotic drugs are all labeled by the Food and Drug Administration (FDA) with similar indications. Begin treatment usually in low doses. Clozapine (Clozaril) has also been used for treatment-resistant cases with some success but requires close monitoring owing to the potential side effect of agranulocytosis.

■ *Typical (conventional) AP drugs that may be* used for the treatment of delusional disorder include the following:
  ▫ Haloperidol (Haldol) and pimozide (Orap). Until recently, pimozide was touted as the drug of choice for delusional disorder; more recent evidence suggests no difference in improvement with pimozide and other APs. Also, the evidence suggests no difference in improvement between atypical and conventional APs in the treatment of patients with delusional disorder.
■ If patients fail to respond to drug monotherapy, low-dose combination therapy using drugs from different pharmacological classes may be employed. Depressive symptoms, if present, may be treated with antidepressants. SSRIs have proven helpful with somatic-type delusions.
■ Delusional disorder is difficult to treat due to the individual's frequent denial of any existing problem, difficulties in establishing a therapeutic alliance, and social/interpersonal conflicts. Nonetheless, recent evidence suggests that 50% of individuals who are adequately treated recover and 90% demonstrate at least some improvement.
■ Somatic delusions seem to be more responsive to AP therapy than the other types of delusions, and persecutory delusions respond less well (50% improvement rates with no reports of complete recovery).
■ Psychotherapy or cognitive-behavioral therapy (CBT) may be helpful, either as monotherapy or in combination with an AP agent.
  ▫ Some form of supportive therapy is helpful with the goal of facilitating treatment adherence, providing education about the illness and treatment, providing social skills training, minimizing risk factors that increase symptoms, and providing realistic guidance in dealing with problems resulting from the illness.
  ▫ CBT may be helpful to individuals with delusional disorder of the persecutory type by helping them to identify maladaptive thoughts and replacing them with alternative, more adaptive attributions.
  ▫ Social skills training directed toward increasing the individual's control and promoting interpersonal competence has also been found to be helpful.

■ Insight-oriented therapy may be indicated rarely and even contraindicated, according to the literature. Nonetheless, there are reports of successful treatment with the goals of the development of a therapeutic alliance, containment of projected negative feelings, and development of creative doubt in the internal perception of the negative worldview.

Drug Selection Table for Delusional Disorders

CLASS	DRUG
Antipsychotic drugs, atypical (second generation)	First-line drug therapy: Aripiprazole (Abilify, Abilify Discmelt ODT, Abilify Liquid, Abilify IM injection, long-acting Abilify once monthly injection) Clozapine (Clozaril, FazaClo) Olanzapine (Zyprexa, Zyprexa Relprevv, Zyprexa Zydis) Risperidone (Risperdal, Risperdal Consta) Quetiapine (Seroquel, Seroquel XR) Ziprasidone (Geodon, Geodon IM injection) Paliperidone (Invega, Invega Sustenna and Invega Trinza IM injection) Asenapine (Saphris) Lurasidone (Latuda) Iloperidone (Fanapt) Cariprazine (Vraylar) Brexpiprazole (Rexulti)
Antipsychotic drugs, typical (first generation)	Second-line drug therapy: Haloperidol (Haldol) Pimozide (Orap)
SSRIs	First-line drugs sometimes helpful for somatic delusions: Fluoxetine (Prozac, Prozac Weekly, Sarafem) Sertraline (Zoloft) Escitalopram (Lexapro)

SSRIs, selective serotonin reuptake inhibitors.

Chronic Treatment
■ The chronic nature of delusional disorders suggests that treatment strategies should be tailored to the individual needs of the patients and focus on maintaining social function and improving quality of life.
■ For most patients with delusional disorder, some form of supportive therapy is helpful. The goals of supportive therapy include facilitating treatment adherence and providing education about the illness and its treatment.
■ Educational and social interventions can include social skills training (e.g., not discussing delusional beliefs in social settings) and minimizing risk factors.
■ Providing realistic guidance and assistance in coping with problems stemming from the delusional system may be very helpful.
■ Cognitive therapeutic approaches may be useful for some patients by identifying delusional thoughts and then replacing them with alternative, more adaptive ones.
■ It is important that goals be attainable, because a patient who feels pressured or repeatedly criticized by others will probably experience stress, which may lead to a worsening of symptoms.
■ Insight-oriented therapy is rarely indicated.

Recurrence Rate
- Delusional disorder has a relatively good prognosis when adequately treated: 52.6% of the patients recover, 28.2% achieve partial recovery, and 19.2% do not improve.
- Less than 25% of all cases are later diagnosed with schizophrenia.
- Less than 10% develop mood disorders.
- Good prognosis is predicted with high levels of occupational and social functioning, female gender, onset before age 30, sudden onset, and short duration of illness.

Patient Education
- Educating the family about the symptoms and course of the disorder is helpful. This is especially true as the family frequently feels the impact of the disorder the most.
- In addition to being involved with seeking help, family, friends, and peer groups can provide support and encourage the patient to regain their abilities.

Medical/Legal Pitfalls
- Patients with delusional disorder are more susceptible to becoming dependent on alcohol, tobacco, and drugs.
- It is not uncommon for people with delusional disorder to make repeated complaints to legal authorities.
- Patients with delusional disorder may encounter legal or relationship problems as a result of acting on their delusions.
- In patients with delusional disorder who may be dangerous, civil commitment focuses on preventing harm to self or others.

SCHIZOAFFECTIVE DISORDER

Definition of Disorder
- A diagnosis midway between the diagnosis of schizophrenia and bipolar I disorder.
- An individual has a mixture of psychotic and depressive/manic/mixed episode(s) that fail to meet the diagnostic criteria for either schizophrenia or bipolar I disorder.
- This disorder is not caused by a drug, medication, or general medical illness.
- The bipolar type of schizoaffective disorder is more common in younger patients, whereas the depressive type is more common in older patients.
- Individuals with this disorder have a better prognosis than individuals with schizophrenia but a worse prognosis than individuals with bipolar I disorder.

Etiology
- May either be a type of schizophrenia or a mood disorder, or both occurring at the same time or not related to either.
- May encompass bipolar and depressive types and may have a genetic component.
- Relatives of the persons with the depressed type of schizoaffective disorder have a higher incidence of also having schizoaffective disorder.

- Imbalance of dopamine and serotonin in the brain may contribute to development of the disease. Other theories consider that it may be due to in utero exposure to viruses, malnutrition, or even birth complications.
- Abnormalities of the neurotransmitters serotonin, norepinephrine, and/or dopamine could all contribute to this disorder.

Demographics
- There is a lifetime prevalence rate of less than 1%.
- Diagnosis may be used when the clinician is unsure of the classification of symptoms.
- The prognosis for patients with schizoaffective disorder is thought to be between that of patients with schizophrenia and that of patients with a mood disorder, with the prognosis better for schizoaffective disorder than for schizophrenic disorder but worse than for a mood disorder alone.
- The incidence of suicide is estimated to be 10%. Whites have a higher rate of suicide than African Americans.
- As in other psychiatric disorders, women attempt suicide more than men, but men complete suicide more often.
- Schizoaffective disorder affects more women than men, with more women in the depressive type as compared with the bipolar type.
- A poor prognosis in patients with schizoaffective disorder is generally associated with a poor premorbid history, an insidious onset, no precipitating factors, a predominant psychosis, negative symptoms, an early onset, an unremitting course, or having a family member with schizophrenia.

Risk Factors
Age
- Young people with schizoaffective disorder tend to have a diagnosis with the bipolar subtype, whereas older people tend to have the depressive subtype.
- Age of onset is later in women than in men.

Gender
- Prevalence is lower in men and occurs less often in married women.
- Men with schizoaffective disorder may exhibit antisocial behavior and flat or inappropriate affect.

Family History
- Patients may have a genetic predisposition.
- Results of studies are inconsistent, although relatives with the depressed type may be at higher risk of acquiring the disorder; stressful events in the lives of susceptible people may trigger the disorder.

Diagnosis
Differential Diagnosis
Evaluate Medical Medications
- All mood and schizophrenic disorders should be considered in the differential diagnosis of schizoaffective disorder.
- Testing is done for use of amphetamines, phencyclidines (PCPs), hallucinogens, cocaine, alcohol, and steroids, as these can present with similar symptoms.

- Seizure disorders of the temporal lobe can mimic schizoaffective signs, as can HIV/autoimmune deficiency syndrome, hyperthyroidism, neurosyphilis, delirium, metabolic syndrome, or narcolepsy.

ICD-10 Codes
Schizoaffective disorder (F29.9)

Diagnostic Workup
- Schizoaffective disorder must meet *Diagnostic and Statistical Manual of Mental Disorders*, Fifth Edition (*DSM-5*) criteria for components of schizophrenia and mood disorders (depressed) concurrently.
- Delusions or hallucinations for at least 2 weeks may be seen in the absence of mood symptoms. A major mood episode must be present for a majority of the disorder's total duration.
- Laboratory studies include sequential multiple analysis, CBC, rapid plasma reagent, thyroid function, drug and alcohol screens, lipid panel, enzyme-linked immunosorbent assay (ELISA) test results, and the Western blot test.
- If the patient's neurological findings are abnormal, CT or MRI may be ordered to rule out any suspected intracranial pathology. Findings include decreased amounts of cortical gray matter and increased fluid-filled spaces.

Initial Assessment
- Medical workup, including neurological history and evaluation of laboratory data.
- Psychiatric assessment, including mental status examination and history.
- Mental status examination may reveal appearances ranging from well groomed to disheveled; possible psychomotor agitation or retardation; euthymic, depressed, or manic mood; eye contact ranging from appropriate to flat affect; speech that ranges from poverty to flight of ideas or pressured; suicidal or homicidal ideation may or may not be present; presence of delusions and/or hallucinations.
- Psychological testing may assist with diagnosis and in rating the severity of the disease. The following scales may be useful in assessing the patient's progress: Positive and Negative Symptoms Scale (PANSS), Hamilton Depression Scale, and Young Mania Scale. The CAGE questionnaire (cut down, annoyed, guilty, and eye opener) is helpful in determining alcohol consumption in patients with schizoaffective disorder.

Clinical Presentation: Symptoms
- All the signs and symptoms of schizophrenia, manic episodes, and depressive disorders occur.
- Symptoms can appear in concert or alternating.
- May be mood incongruent, which has a poor prognosis.
- Suicidal ideation or attempt(s) may occur.

Diagnostic and Statistical Manual of Mental Disorders, Fifth Edition: Diagnostic Guidelines
- An uninterrupted period of illness occurs during which a major depressive episode, a manic episode, or a mixed episode occurs with symptoms that meet criteria for schizophrenia. The major depressive episode must include a depressed mood.
- Symptoms that meet the criteria for mood episodes are present for a substantial portion of the active and residual periods of the illness.

■ The disturbance is not the direct physiological effect of a substance (e.g., illicit drugs, medications) or a general medical condition.

■ The bipolar type is diagnosed if the disturbance includes a manic or a mixed episode (or a manic or mixed episode and a major depressive episode).

■ The depressive type is diagnosed if the disturbance includes only major depressive episodes.

Treatment Overview

Acute Treatment

■ The major treatments include inpatient psychiatric hospitalization, medication, and psychosocial therapies. Inpatient treatment is mandatory for patients who are dangerous to themselves or others and for patients who cannot take care of themselves.

■ Activity should be restricted if patients represent a danger to themselves or to others.

■ Psychopharmacological treatment involves use of APs to treat aggressive behavior and psychosis, along with antidepressants, and/or mood stabilizers. Agent selection depends on whether the depressive or manic subtype is present.

■ In the depressive subtype, combinations of antidepressants plus an AP are used.

■ In refractory cases, clozapine (Clozaril, FazaClo ODT) has been used as an AP agent. In the manic subtype, combinations of mood stabilizers and an AP are used.

■ Early treatment with medication along with good premorbid functioning often improves outcomes.

Psychopharmacology of Schizoaffective Disorder

Overview

■ *Second-generation (atypical)* APs are the first-line treatment for schizoaffective disorder.

■ Consistent evidence has demonstrated that risperidone (Risperdal), olanzapine (Zyprexa), quetiapine (*Seroquel*), ziprasidone (*Geodon*), aripiprazole (*Abilify*), paliperidone (Invega), asenapine (Saphris), lurasidone (Latuda), Iloperidone (Fanapt), cariprazine (Vraylar), brexpiprazole (Rexulti) are efficacious in the treatment of global psychopathology and the positive symptoms of the schizophrenic spectrum disorders, including schizoaffective disorder. Less consistent evidence has demonstrated that the negative symptoms improve as well.

■ *Second-line treatment:* first-generation (typical or conventional) APs; although haloperidol (Haldol) was previously regarded as a first-line treatment for patients with schizoaffective disorder, it is now regarded as a second- or third-line treatment since atypical APs generally have a more tolerable side effect profile.

■ In addition to an AP agent, antidepressant medications may be prescribed for the depressive symptoms. Mood stabilizers may be used to treat mixed symptoms occurring in schizoaffective disorder. Any of the SSRIs may be used for the depressive symptoms, but evidence available most is for fluoxetine (Prozac).

■ Lithium (Eskalith, Lithobid, lithium carbonate) has proven helpful as an adjunct to the AP agents. It has limited effectiveness as monotherapy in treating schizoaffective disorders. When combined with an AP agent, lithium augments the AP response in general and negative symptoms specifically.

■ Valproate (Depakote) studies have reported positive and negative results. The evidence base is limited because most studies have few patients.

■ CBT, modified for this population, focuses on symptom management, symptom recovery in acute psychosis, relapse prevention, and early intervention. Patients are taught coping strategies; attention switching or attention narrowing, especially useful for dealing with hallucinations; modified self-statements and internal dialog; reattribution; awareness training; de-arousing techniques; increased activity levels; social engagement and disengagement; and reality-testing techniques.

■ Electroconvulsive therapy (ECT) has been suggested as a treatment for resistant schizoaffective disorders; however, the evidence has been limited to case studies and uncontrolled studies. In general, AP treatment alone has produced better outcomes than ECT.

■ Emphasis is being placed on early identification of any of the schizophrenic spectrum disorders, including schizoaffective disorders. Earlier identification allows for earlier intervention and not requiring patients and/or families to reach a high threshold of risk, disruption, or deterioration before accessing treatment. There is evidence that if symptoms are treated prior to the onset of a psychotic episode, full-blown consequences (such as schizoaffective disorder or schizophrenia) may be delayed or even prevented.

Drug Selection Table for Schizoaffective Disorder

CLASS	DRUG
Antipsychotic drugs, atypical (second generation)	First-line drug therapy: Aripiprazole (Abilify, Abilify Discmelt ODT, Abilify Liquid, Abilify IM injection, long-acting Abilify once monthly injection) Clozapine (Clozaril, FazaClo) Olanzapine (Zyprexa, Zyprexa Relprevv, Zyprexa Zydis) Risperidone (Risperdal, Risperdal Consta) Quetiapine (Seroquel, Seroquel XR) Ziprasidone (Geodon, Geodon IM injection) Paliperidone (Invega, Invega Sustenna and Invega Trinza IM injection) Asenapine (Saphris) Lurasidone (Latuda) Iloperidone (Fanapt) Cariprazine (Vraylar) Brexpiprazole (Rexulti)
Antipsychotic drugs, typical (first generation)	Second-line drug therapy: Haloperidol (Haldol) Fluphenazine (Prolixin)
SSRIs	Adjunct treatment for mood or depression: Fluoxetine (Prozac, Prozac Weekly, Sarafem) Paroxetine (Paxil, Paxil CR, Pexeva, Brisdelle) Sertraline (Zoloft) Citalopram (Celexa) Escitalopram (Lexapro) Vilazodone (Viibryd) Fluvoxamine (Luvox, Luvox CR) Vortioxetine (Trintellix)
Mood stabilizers	Adjunct treatment for mood; also approved for bipolar/mania, includes carbamazepine, lamotrigine—same as depakote: Lithium (Eskalith, Lithobid, lithium carbonate) Valproate (Depakote: divalproex = depakote ER tablets and the regular delayed-release) tablet

IM, intramuscular; SSRIs, selective serotonin reuptake inhibitors.

Chronic Treatment
- Patients who have schizoaffective disorder can benefit greatly from psychotherapy as well as psychoeducational programs and regularly scheduled outpatient medication management.
- When making the transition to outpatient treatment, stressing the importance of medication compliance is crucial.
- If possible, select once-daily or long-acting medications to help with patient compliance.
- Therapy is most effective if it involves their families, develops their social skills, and focuses on cognitive rehabilitation.
- Psychotherapies should include supportive therapy and assertive community therapy in addition to individual and group forms of therapy and rehabilitation programs.
- Family involvement is needed in the treatment of this particular disorder.
- Treatment includes education about the disorder and its treatment, family assistance in compliance with medications and appointments, and maintenance of structured daily activities.
- Otherwise, patients who are schizoaffective should be encouraged to continue their normal routines and strengthen their social skills whenever possible.

Recurrence Rate
- A good outcome is predicted in the presence of a good premorbid history, acute onset, a specific precipitating factor, few psychotic symptoms, a short course, and no family history of schizophrenia.
- The prognosis for patients with schizoaffective disorder is thought to lie between that of patients with schizophrenia and that of patients with a mood disorder. Therefore, the prognosis is better with schizoaffective disorder than with a schizophrenic disorder but worse than with a mood disorder alone.
- Individuals with the bipolar subtype are thought to have a prognosis similar to those with bipolar type I, whereas the prognosis of people with the depressive subtype is thought to be similar to that of people with schizophrenia.
- Overall, determination of the prognosis is difficult.

Patient Education
- Discuss compliance with patients as well as with family members. Always discuss all the risks, benefits, adverse effects, and alternatives of each medication.
- Stress-reduction techniques are employed to prevent relapse and possible rehospitalization.
- Education should also include social skills training and cognitive rehabilitation.
- Family education should involve reducing of expressed emotions, criticism, hostility, or overprotection of the patient.

Medical/Legal Pitfalls
- Patients with schizoaffective disorder often lack judgment and insight into their illness. They commonly refuse to continue the medications started in the hospital after they are discharged. Noncompliance may also be the result of adverse effects of the medication, such as sedation and weight gain.
- Patients may begin to feel better as a result of their medications and believe that they no longer need to take them. This thinking leads to discontinuation of the medication and can result in rehospitalization.

- Be familiar with local mental health laws as patients with schizoaffective disorder, who represent a danger to self or others or are unwilling to seek help on a voluntary basis, may need to be committed for further evaluation and treatment.
- If nonadherence with medications is an issue, a court order may be necessary to to treat the patient over their objection.
- Physical restraints may also be indicated for protection of self and/or others.

SCHIZOPHRENIA

Background Information
Definition of Disorder
- This is a chronic, severe, and disabling brain disorder characterized by disordered thoughts, delusions, hallucinations, and bizarre or catatonic behavior.

Etiology
- Several genes are found to be strongly associated with schizophrenia. However, genes alone are not sufficient to cause this disorder.
- Imbalance of the neurotransmitters dopamine and glutamate (and possibly others) are found to play a role in schizophrenia.
- Scientists believe that interactions between genes and the environment are necessary to develop schizophrenia. Environmental risk factors (e.g., exposure to viruses or malnutrition in the womb, problems during birth) and psychosocial factors (e.g., stressful conditions) are found to increase the risk of schizophrenia.
- Research shows that schizophrenia is hereditary. People who have first-degree relatives (a parent, sibling) or second-degree relatives (grandparents, aunts, uncles, cousins) with this disorder develop schizophrenia more often than the general population. The identical twin of a person with schizophrenia has the highest risk (40%–65%) of developing this disorder.

Demographics
- Schizophrenia occurs in 1% of the general population.
- Schizophrenia affects men and women equally and occurs at similar rates in all ethnic groups worldwide.
  - Patients with schizophrenia are found to abuse alcohol and/or drugs more often than the general population. Abusing a substance can reduce the effectiveness of treatment.
  - Patients with schizophrenia are more likely to be addicted to nicotine as compared with the general population (75%–90% vs. 25%–30%).
  - Patients may need higher doses of psychotropic medication if they smoke and dose reductions for some APs on cessation of smoking. Nicotine replacement does not mitigate the metabolic consequences of cessation.
  - Patients with schizophrenia attempt suicide much more often than people in the general population; approximately 10% succeed, especially among young adult males.

Risk Factors
Age
- In men, onset of symptoms typically emerges in the late teens and early 20s and in women, in the mid-20s to early 30s.

■ Psychotic symptoms seldom occur after age 45 years and only rarely before puberty (although cases of schizophrenia in children as young as 5 years have been reported).

Gender
■ The prevalence of schizophrenia among men and women is about the same.
■ Pregnancy can worsen mental health in a subset of women with schizophrenia. Women are found to be especially susceptible for acute exacerbation of symptoms in the postpartum period.
■ Compared to men, women tend to experience more pronounced mood symptoms.
■ The gender differences in course and outcome are probably due to the effect of estrogen in women before menopause.

Family History
■ Patients with immediate family members diagnosed as schizophrenic have approximately a 10% risk of developing the disorder.

Factors Associated With Birth
■ Infants who experience a complication while in mothers' wombs or who experience trauma during delivery are at higher risk for developing schizophrenia.
■ Intrauterine viral infection may occur in the womb.

Environmental Stressors
■ Environmental stressors are found to be associated with the development of schizophrenia, including problems with interpersonal relationships, difficulties at school/work, and substance abuse.

Substance Abuse
■ Most researchers do not believe that substance abuse causes schizophrenia; however, patients with schizophrenia abuse alcohol and/or drugs more often than the general population.

Diagnosis
Differential Diagnosis
■ Psychotic disorder due to a general medical condition, delirium, or dementia
■ Substance-induced psychotic disorder, substance-induced delirium, substance-induced persisting dementia, and substance-related disorders may be seen
■ Brief psychotic disorder
■ Delusional disorder
■ Schizophreniform disorder
■ Psychotic disorder may not be otherwise specified
■ Schizoaffective disorder
■ Mood disorder with psychotic features
■ Mood disorder with catatonic features
■ Depressive disorder may not be otherwise specified
■ Bipolar disorder may not be otherwise specified
■ Pervasive developmental disorders (e.g., autistic disorder)
■ Childhood presentations combining disorganized speech (from a communication disorder) and disorganized behavior (from attention-deficit/hyperactivity disorder)

- Schizotypal personality disorder
- Schizoid personality disorder
- Paranoid personality disorder

ICD-10 Codes
Schizophrenia (F20)

Diagnostic Workup
Check for Drug Interactions
- Physical and mental status examination.
- CBC, including hemoglobin, hematocrit, red blood cell (RBC) count, white blood cell (WBC) count, WBC differential count, and platelet count.
- Hepatic and renal function tests, including alanine transaminase (ALT), aspartate transaminase (AST), alkaline phosphatase (ALP), blood urea nitrogen (BUN), and creatinine.
- Thyroid function tests (T3, T4, and TSH).
- Electrolytes (potassium, chloride, sodium, bicarbonate), glucose, B12, folate, and calcium level.
- For patients with a history of suspicion, check for HIV, syphilis, ceruloplasmin, antinuclear antibody test, urine for culture and sensitivity and/or drugs of abuse, and 24-hour urine collections for porphyrins, copper, or heavy metals.
- Alcohol and drug screening.
- Pregnancy test for female patients of childbearing age.

Initial Assessment
- Current physical status and physical history
- Current mental status and mental health history, including symptoms patient experiences, how long patient has been having symptoms, when the symptoms started, how often the symptoms occur, when and where symptoms tend to occur, how long symptoms last, and what effect symptoms have on patient's ability to function
- Drug history including prescribed and over-the-counter drugs
- Safety needs

Clinical Presentation
- Positive symptoms are extreme or exaggerated behaviors, including
  - delusions (somatic, ideas of reference, thought broadcasting, thought insertion, and thought withdrawal),
  - hallucinations (visual, auditory, tactile, olfactory, and gustatory), and
  - inappropriate or overreactive affect.
- Negative symptoms include
  - blunted or flat affect, unable to experience pleasure or express emotion (anhedonia),
  - inability to carry out goal-directed behavior (avolition),
  - limited speech (alogia),
  - lack of energy and initiative, and
  - poor coordination and self-care.
- Thought disorganization
  - Abnormal thoughts
  - Tangential, incoherent, or loosely associated speech

Diagnostic and Statistical Manual of Mental Disorders, Fifth Edition:
Diagnostic Guidelines

- The diagnosis is given if two of the following criterion A symptoms are present:
  - Delusions
  - Hallucinations
  - Disorganized speech
  - Grossly disorganized or catatonic behavior
  - Negative symptoms
    - The individual must have at least one of these three symptoms: delusions, hallucinations, and disorganized speech.
- Continuous signs of the disturbance are exhibited for at least 6 months.
- Schizoaffective disorder and mood disorder have been excluded.
- Substance abuse and other general medical conditions have been excluded.
- Schizophrenia subtypes are defined by the predominant symptomatology at the time of evaluation. The five subtypes of schizophrenia are paranoid type, disorganized type, catatonic type, undifferentiated type, and residual type.
- The first signs for the adolescent population may include drops in academic performance, changes of friends, sleep problems, or irritability. A diagnosis of schizophrenia can be difficult to make for members of this age group since many normal adolescents also exhibit these behaviors.

Treatment Overview

Acute Treatment

- Inpatient treatment is necessary for patients with a serious suicidal or homicidal ideation and plan, whose behavior can unintentionally be harmful to self or others, who are incapable of providing self-care, or who are at risk for behavior that may lead to long-term negative consequences.
- The goal of acute-phase treatment, usually lasting for 4 to 8 weeks, is to alleviate the most severe psychotic symptoms, such as agitation, frightening delusions, and hallucinations.
- Low-dose, high-potency APs have been found to be safe and effective in managing agitated psychiatric patients. Following are examples:
  - Haloperidol (Haldol) intramuscular (IM) is used to calm patients with moderately severe to very severe agitation. Subsequent doses may be needed within 1 hour depending on the responses.
  - Ziprasidone (Geodon) IM is recommended.
  - A low dose of a short-acting benzodiazepine (e.g., lorazepam [Ativan]) is also found to be effective in decreasing agitation during the acute phase and may reduce the amount of AP needed to control patients' psychotic symptoms.
  - Atypical (second generation) AP drugs are suggested to be used as a first-line treatment of schizophrenia because of their fewer side effects than conventional or typical AP medications.
  - ECT, in combination with AP medications, can be considered for patients with schizophrenia who do not respond to AP agents. The rate and number vary from patient to patient depending on clinical responses and side effects.
  - Substantial improvement of symptoms is seen in many patients by the 6th week of treatment. Providers may switch to other AP medications if patients are not responding to an adequate trial of a prescribed medication, are not able to tolerate a medication, or have poor medication adherence.

Psychopharmacology of Schizophrenia

- *Second-generation (atypical) antipsychotic drugs*: These are used as a first-line treatment of schizophrenia due to fewer side effects when compared to conventional or typical AP medications.
  - Commonly used *second-generation* atypical AP drugs include aripiprazole (Abilify), clozapine (Clozaril), olanzapine (Zyprexa), quetiapine (Seroquel), quetiapine fumarate (Seroquel XR), risperidone (Risperdal), long-acting risperidone (Risperdal Consta), ziprasidone (Geodon), and paliperidone (Invega). Newer atypical APs including asenapine (Saphris sublingual formulation), lurasidone (Latuda), Iloperidone (Fanapt), cariprazine (Vraylar), and brexpiprazole (Rexulti) have demonstrated positive effects for schizophrenia.
  - Clozapine (Clozaril) is the drug of choice for treatment-resistant schizophrenia (little or no symptomatic response to at least two AP trials of an adequate duration—at least 6 weeks—and at a therapeutic dose range), and it has a lower risk of tardive dyskinesia (TD). However, due to the potential side effect of agranulocytosis (loss of WBC), a blood test is required weekly for the first 6 months and biweekly for the next 6 months. Monitoring can be done monthly if no hematological problems are found after 1 year of clozapine treatment.
- *First-generation (typical or conventional) antipsychotic drugs*
  - Commonly used *first-generation* (typical or conventional) AP drugs include the following: haloperidol (Haldol), fluphenazine (Prolixin), thioridazine (Mellaril), trifluoperazine (Stelazine).
  - Low-dose, high-potency APs such as haloperidol IM 2 to 5 mg have been found to be safe and effective in managing agitated psychiatric patients. Subsequent doses may be needed within 1 hour depending on responses.
- *Short-acting benzodiazepine*: A low dose of a short-acting benzodiazepine (e.g., lorazepam 0.5 to 2 mg every 1 hour IM or intravenous [IV] as needed no more than 2 mg every minute—maximum daily doses vary with diagnosis and condition) is effective in decreasing agitation during the acute phase and may reduce the amount of AP needed to control patients' psychotic symptoms.
- ECT in combination with AP medications can be considered for patients with schizophrenia who do not respond to AP agents. The rate and number of ECT varies from patient to patient depending on their clinical responses and side effects.
- Social skills training aimed to improve the way patients with schizophrenia interact with others (e.g., poor eye contact, odd facial expressions, inaccurate or lack of perceptions of emotions in other people) has been found to be effective in reducing relapse rate.
- CBT helps patients with schizophrenia acquire some insight into their illness and appears to be effective in reducing the severity of symptoms and decreasing the risk of relapse.
- Dialectical behavior therapy (DBT) combines cognitive and behavioral theories. Patients with schizophrenia may benefit from DBT to improve interpersonal skills.
- Individual psychotherapy focuses on forming a therapeutic alliance between therapists and patients with schizophrenia. A good therapeutic alliance is likely to help patients with schizophrenia remain in therapy, increase adherence to treatments, and have positive outcomes at 2-year follow-up evaluations.
- Personal therapy, a recently developed form of individual treatment, uses social skills and relaxation exercises, self-reflection, self-awareness, exploration of vulnerability and stress, and psychoeducation to enhance personal and social adjustment of

patients with schizophrenia. Patients who receive personal therapy have shown better social adjustment and a lower rate of relapse after 3 years than those not receiving it.

- Many patients with schizophrenia benefit from art therapy because it helps them communicate with and share their inner world with others.
- Employment programs that include individualized job development, rapid placement, ongoing job supports, and integration of mental health and vocational services have been found to be effective in helping patients with schizophrenia to achieve employment.

Chronic Treatment

- The treatment goals are to prevent relapse and to improve patient's level of functioning.
- It is estimated that 40% to 50% of patients are not adherent to treatment within 1 to 2 years. Long-acting medications are found to increase treatment adherence as compared to oral medications.
- It is important to monitor and manage the side effects of AP medications, including extrapyramidal side effects (mostly common in patients treated with first-generation APs), TD, sedation, postural hypotension, weight gain metabolic syndrome— including shifts in lipids and blood glucose—along with increased central adiposity, and disturbances in sexual function.
- If patients develop extrapyramidal symptoms (EPS), benztropine or trihexyphenidyl or diphenhydramine should be given as directed.
- For drug-induced dystonic reaction (especially of head and neck), diphenhydramine (Benadryl) should be given for pseudoparkinsonism reaction due to drug use; trihexyphenidyl (Artane) or benztropine (Cogentin) should be used.

Drug Selection Table for Schizophrenia

CLASS	DRUG
Antipsychotic drugs, atypical (second generation)	First-line drug therapy: Aripiprazole (Abilify, Abilify Discmelt ODT, Abilify Liquid, Abilify IM injection, long-acting Abilify once monthly injection) Clozapine (Clozaril, FazaClo) Olanzapine (Zyprexa, Zyprexa Relprevv, Zyprexa Zydis) Risperidone (Risperdal, Risperdal Consta) Quetiapine (Seroquel, Seroquel XR) Ziprasidone (Geodon, Geodon IM injection) Paliperidone (Invega, Invega Sustenna & Invega Trinza IM injection) Asenapine (Saphris) Lurasidone (Latuda) Iloperidone (Fanapt) Cariprazine (Vraylar) Brexpiprazole (Rexulti)
Antipsychotic drugs, typical (first generation)	Second-line drug therapy: Haloperidol (Haldol) Fluphenazine (Prolixin) Thioridazine (Mellaril) Trifluoperazine (Stelazine)
BZDs	During acute phase: Lorazepam (Ativan)

BZDs, benzodiazepines; IM, intramuscular.

- The neuroleptic malignant syndrome (NMS), characterized by fever (hyperthermia), muscular rigidity, altered mental status, and autonomic dysfunction, is a rare but potentially fatal reaction to neuroleptic medications. If a parent has hyperthermia, or stops AP medications, give dantrolene and continue as needed until cumulative total dose is up to 10 mg/kg. After the acute phase, give dantrolene to prevent recurrence.
- Body mass index (BMI), fasting blood glucose, and lipid profiles are important health indicators to monitor since weight gain has occurred with most AP agents. It is recommended to weigh patients and check the BMI every visit for 6 months after a change in medications and abdominal girth.
- Clozapine (Clozaril, FazaClo ODT) is the drug of choice for patients with treatment-resistant schizophrenia (little or no symptomatic response to at least two AP trials of an adequate duration [at least 6 weeks] and at a therapeutic dose range), and it has a lower risk of TD. However, due to the potential side effect of agranulocytosis (loss of WBCs), a blood test is required weekly for the first 6 months and biweekly for the next 6 months. Monitoring can be done monthly if no hematological problems are found after 1 year of clozapine (Clozaril, FazaClo ODT) treatment.
- Social skills training, aimed at improving the way patients with schizophrenia interact with others (e.g., poor eye contact, odd facial expressions, inaccurate or lack of perceptions of emotions in other people), has been found to be effective in reducing the relapse rate.
- CBT helps patients with schizophrenia to gain some insight into their illness and appears to be effective in reducing the severity of symptoms and decreasing the risk of relapse.
- DBT combines cognitive and behavioral theories. Patients with schizophrenia may benefit from DBT to improve interpersonal skills.
- Individual psychotherapy focuses on forming a therapeutic alliance between therapists and patients with schizophrenia. A good therapeutic alliance is likely to help patients with schizophrenia remain in therapy, increase adherence to treatments, and have positive outcomes at 2-year follow-up evaluations.
- Personal therapy, a recently developed form of individual treatment, uses social skills and relaxation exercises, self-reflection, self-awareness, exploration of vulnerability and stress, and psychoeducation to enhance personal and social adjustment of patients with schizophrenia. Patients who receive personal therapy have shown better social adjustment and a lower rate of relapse after 3 years than those not receiving it.
- Many patients with schizophrenia benefit from art therapy because it helps them communicate with and share their inner world with others.
- Family-oriented therapies that help family and patients with schizophrenia understand the disorder and encourage discussions of psychotic episodes and events leading up to them may be effective in reducing relapses.
- Treat patients for co-occurring substance abuse. Substance abuse is the most common co-occurring disorder in patients with schizophrenia. Integrated treatment programs for schizophrenia and substance use produce better outcomes.
- Many studies show that integrating psychosocial and medication treatment produces the best results in patients with schizophrenia.

Recurrence Rate

The reported recurrence rates range from 10% to 60%; approximately 20% to 30% of patients with schizophrenia can have somewhat normal lives, 20% to 30% continue to experience moderate symptoms, and 40% to 60% of them remain significantly impaired for their entire lives.

Patient Education

- Information regarding schizophrenia is available from the National Institutes for Mental Health website at www.nimh.nih.gov/health/publications/schizophrenia/index.shtml.
- AP medications can produce dangerous side effects when taken with certain drugs. It is important for patients to tell healthcare providers about all medications, including over-the-counter medications, prescribed medications, vitamins, minerals, and herbal supplements that patients take.
  - *Note*: Medications should be used with particular caution in children, pregnant/breastfeeding women, and older adults.
  - *Note* black box warnings.
- It is important to teach patients about the importance of medication adherence and to avoid using alcohol and other substances.
- For excellent patient education resources, visit eMedicine's Mental Health and Behavior Center. See also eMedicine's patient education article on schizophrenia.

Medical/Legal Pitfalls

- Misdiagnosis.
- Patients with schizophrenia are addicted to nicotine at three times the rate of the general population (75%–90% vs. 25%–30%).
- Approximately 20% to 70% of patients with schizophrenia have a comorbid substance abuse problem, which is associated with increased violence, suicidality, nonadherence with treatment, hostility, crime, poor nutrition, and so forth.
- Mental health providers should inform patients being treated with conventional AP medications about the risk of TD. The Abnormal Involuntary Movement Scale (AIMS) is recommended for detecting TD early.
- Patients with schizophrenia are found to have a higher risk for acquiring obesity, diabetes, cardiovascular disease, HIV, lung diseases, and rheumatoid arthritis. It is important for mental healthcare providers to monitor their physical conditions regularly.

SCHIZOPHRENIFORM DISORDER

Background Information

Definition of Disorder

- This is characterized by the presence of the principal symptoms of schizophrenia, including delusions, hallucinations, disorganized speech, disorganized or catatonic behavior, and negative symptoms.
- An episode of the disorder (including prodromal, active, and residual phases) lasts at least 1 month but less than 6 months.

Etiology

- The cause of schizophreniform disorder remains unknown.

- Current biological and epidemiological data suggest that some of the patients with schizophreniform are similar to those with schizophrenia, whereas others have a disorder similar to mood disorder.

Demographics
- The lifetime prevalence rate of schizophreniform is 0.2%, and a 1-year prevalence rate is 0.1%.

Risk Factors
Age
- Schizophreniform disorder is most common in adolescents and young adults.

Gender
- The prevalence of schizophreniform disorder is equally distributed between men and women, with peak onset between the ages of 18 and 24 years in men and 24 and 35 years in women.

Family History
- Studies show that relatives of individuals with schizophreniform disorder are at higher risk of having mood disorders than are relatives of individuals with schizophrenia.
- Relatives of individuals with schizophreniform disorder are more likely to have a psychotic mood disorder than are relatives of individuals with bipolar disorders.

Diagnosis
Differential Diagnosis
- Schizophrenia
- Brief psychotic disorder
- Substance-induced psychotic disorder
- Bipolar disorder and major depression with mood-incongruent features

ICD-10 Codes
Sohizophreniform disorder (F20.81)

Diagnostic Workup
Medical Medications (i.e., steroids)
- Physical and mental status examination
- Electrolytes (potassium, chloride, and bicarbonate)
- Thyroid function tests (TSH, T3, and T4)
- Screening for alcohol and drugs, including amphetamines, methamphetamines, barbiturates, phenobarbital, benzodiazepines, cannabis, cocaine, codeine, cotinine, morphine, heroin, lysergic acid diethylamide (LSD), methadone, and PCP

Initial Assessment
- Current physical status and physical history
- Current mental status and mental health history, including symptoms patient experiences, how long patient has been having symptoms, when the symptoms started, how often the symptoms occur, when and where symptoms tend to occur, how long symptoms last, and what effect symptoms have on patient's ability to function

- Drug history, including prescribed and over-the-counter drugs
- Safety needs

Clinical Presentation: Symptoms

- Delusions (somatic, ideas of reference, thought broadcasting, thought insertion, and thought withdrawal)
- Hallucinations (visual, auditory, tactile, olfactory, and gustatory)
- Disorganized speech (e.g., frequent derailment or incoherence)
- Grossly disorganized or catatonic behavior
- Negative symptoms (e.g., flat affect, lack of energy and initiative)

Diagnostic and Statistical Manual of Mental Disorders, Fifth Edition: Diagnostic Guidelines

(1) Acute presentation of psychotic symptoms (2 weeks or less from a nonpsychotic to a clearly psychotic state); (2) symptoms present for the majority of the time since the establishment of an obviously psychotic clinical picture; and (3) acute polymorphic psychotic disorder ruled out.

Note: If the schizophrenic symptoms last for more than 1 month, the diagnosis should be changed to schizophrenia.

Treatment Overview

Acute Treatment

- Inpatient treatment is often necessary for patients with schizophreniform disorder for effective assessment and treatment. Patients who are at risk of harming themselves or others require hospitalization to allow comprehensive evaluation and to ensure their safety as well as others'.
- The pharmacotherapy for schizophreniform disorder is similar to that for schizophrenia. Atypical (second generation) APs are mostly used at this time. For details, see the schizophrenia discussion.
- Antidepressants may help reduce mood disturbances associated with schizophreniform disorder, but patients need to be monitored carefully for possible exacerbations of psychotic symptoms.

Chronic Treatment

- Long-acting medications are found to increase treatment adherence, including paliperidone (Invega Sustenna, Invega Trinza), a major active metabolite of risperidone (Risperdal Consta) and the first oral agent allowing once-daily dosing (6 mg PO in the morning).
- Ziprasidone (Geodon) and aripiprazole (Abilify) are available in injection form to help control acute psychotic symptoms. It is dose dependent; all second-generation APs are more likely to cause EPS for patients who are not AP-naive.
- Long-acting agents are made with aqueous vehicles—different from the typical injections that are sesame oil–based and can cause scarring and discomfort.
- It is critical to monitor and manage the side effects of AP medications (e.g., extrapyramidal side effects, TD, sedation, postural hypotension, weight gain, disturbances in sexual function). For details, see the schizophrenia section.
- Psychotherapeutic treatment modalities used in the treatment of patients with schizophrenia may be helpful in treating patients with schizophreniform disorder. However, patients with schizophreniform disorder can become frightened in groups in which they are mixed with patients who have chronic schizophrenia.

Drug Selection Table for Schizophreniform Disorders

CLASS	DRUG
Antipsychotic drugs, atypical (second generation)	First-line drug therapy: Aripiprazole (Abilify, Abilify Discmelt ODT, Abilify Liquid, Abilify IM injection, long-acting Abilify once monthly injection) Clozapine (Clozaril, FazaClo) Olanzapine (Zyprexa, Zyprexa Relprevv, Zyprexa Zydis) Risperidone (Risperdal, Risperdal Consta) Quetiapine (Seroquel, Seroquel XR) Ziprasidone (Geodon, Geodon IM injection) Paliperidone (Invega, Invega Sustenna and Invega Trinza IM injection) Asenapine (Saphris) Lurasidone (Latuda) Iloperidone (Fanapt) Cariprazine (Vraylar) Brexpiprazole (Rexulti)

IM, intramuscular.

- Family therapy is proven to be appropriate for patients with schizophreniform disorder and their families.
- In patients with schizophreniform disorder exhibiting impairments in social functioning, rehabilitative strategies similar to those described for patients with schizophrenia may be helpful.

It is estimated that 60% to 80% of patients with schizophreniform disorder will progress to full-blown schizophrenia despite treatment.

- Nonadherence to the medications is a common cause of treatment failure. It is critical to monitor and manage the side effects of AP medications.
- Psychotherapy (e.g., CBT) is recommended; individual therapy has been found to be more effective than group therapy.

Recurrence Rate
It is estimated that 50% of patients with shared psychotic disorder recover at long-term follow-up, 20% show improved symptoms, and 30% have no change in symptoms.

Patient Education

- AP medications can produce dangerous side effects when taken with certain drugs. It is important for patients to tell healthcare providers about all medications, including over-the-counter medications, prescribed medications, vitamins, minerals, and herbal supplements that patients take.
- It is important to teach patients about the importance of medication adherence and to avoid using alcohol and other substances.
- For excellent patient education resources, visit eMedicine's Mental Health and Behavior Center.

Medical/Legal Pitfalls

- Misdiagnosis.
- Mental healthcare providers should inform patients being treated with conventional AP medications about the risk of TD. AIMS is recommended for detecting TD early.
- Use medications with particular caution in children, pregnant/breastfeeding women, and older adults.

BIBLIOGRAPHY

American Psychiatric Association. (2006). *Practice guidelines for treatment: Compendium 2006.* Washington, DC: American Psychiatric Press.

American Psychiatric Association. (2013). *Diagnostic and statistical manual of mental disorders* (5th ed.). Washington, DC: American Psychiatric Press.

Azorin, J. M., Kaladjian, A., & Fakra, E. (2005). Current issues on schizoaffective disorder. *Encephale, 31*(3), 359–365.

Bond, G. R., & Drake, R. E. (2008). Predictors of competitive employment among patients with schizophrenia. *Current Opinions in Psychiatry, 21*(4), 362–369.

Cervini, P., Newman, D., Dorian, P., Edwards, J., Greene, M., & Bhalerao S. (2003). Folie a deux: An old diagnosis with a new technology. *Canadian Journal of Cardiology, 19*(13), 1539–1540.

Emsley, R., Oosthuizen, P., Koen, L., Niehaus, D. J., Medori, R., & Rabinowitz, J. (2008). Oral versus injectable antipsychotic treatment in early psychosis: Post hoc comparison of two studies. *Clinical Therapy, 30*(12), 2378–2386.

Etter, M., & Etter, J. F. (2004). Alcohol consumption and the CAGE test in outpatients with schizophrenia or schizoaffective disorder and in the general population. *Schizophrenia Bulletin, 30*(4), 947–956.

Fennig, S., Fochtmann, L. J., & Bromet, E. J. (2005). Delusional and shared psychotic disorder. In H. I. Kaplan & B. J. Sadock (Eds.), *Kaplan and Sadock's comprehensive textbook of psychiatry* (8th ed., pp. 1525–1533). Lippincott, Williams & Wilkins.

Fochtmann, L. J. (2005). Treatment of other psychotic disorders. In *Kaplan and Sadock's comprehensive textbook of psychiatry* (8th ed., pp. 1545–1550). Lippincott, Williams & Wilkins.

Harrow, M., Grossman, L. S., Herbener, E. S., & Davies, E. W. (2000). Ten-year outcome: Patients with schizoaffective disorders, schizophrenia, affective disorders and mood-incongruent psychotic symptoms. *British Psychiatry, 177*, 421–426.

Jones, R. T., & Benowitz, N. L. (2002). Therapeutics for nicotine addiction. In K. L. Davis, D. Charney, J. T. Coyle, & C. Nemeroff (Eds.), *Neuropsychopharmacology: The fifth generation of progress* (pp. 1533–1544). American College of Neuropsychopharmacology.

Jalali Roudsari, M., Chun, J., & Manschreck, T. C. (2015). Current treatments for delusional disorder. *Current Treatment Options in Psychiatry, 2*, 151–167. https://doi.org/10.1007/s40501-015-0044-7.

Kaplan, H. I., & Sadock, B. J. (Eds.). (2003). *Kaplan and Sadock's synopsis of psychiatry: Behavioral sciences/clinical psychiatry* (9th ed., pp. 508–511). Lippincott, Williams & Wilkins.

Kwon, J. S., Jang, J. H., Kang, D. H., Yoo, S. Y., Kim, Y. K., Cho, S. J. & APLUS Study Group. (2009). Long-term efficacy and safety of aripiprazole in patients with schizophrenia, schizophreniform disorder, or schizoaffective disorder: 26-week prospective study. *Psychiatry and Clinical Neuroscience, 63*(1), 73–81.

Marder, S. R. (2000). Integrating pharmacological and psychosocial treatments for schizophrenia. *Acta Psychiatrica Scandinavica Supplementum, 102*(407), 87–90.

Meltzer, H. Y., Alphs, L., Green, A. I., Altamura, A. C., Anand, R., Bertoldi, A., Bourgeois, M., Chouinard, G., Zahur Islam, M., Kane, J., Ranga Krishnan, Lindenmayer, J.-P., Potkin, S., & International Suicide Prevention Trial Study Group. (2003). Clozapine treatment for suicidality in schizophrenia: International Suicide Prevention Trial (InterSePT). *Archives of General Psychiatry, 60*(1), 82–91.

Meltzer, H. Y., & Baldessarini, R. J. (2003). Reducing the risk for suicide in schizophrenia and affective disorders. *Journal of Clinical Psychiatry, 64*(9), 1122–1129.

Möller, H. J. (2005). Occurrence and treatment of depressive comorbidity/cosyndromality in schizophrenic psychoses: Conceptual and treatment issues. *World Journal of Biology and Psychiatry, 6*(4), 247–263.

Morken, G., Widen, J. H., & Grawe, R. W. (2008). Nonadherence to antipsychotic medication, relapse and rehospitalisation in recent-onset schizophrenia. *BMC Psychiatry*, *8*, 32.

Mueser, K. T., & McGurk, S. R. (2004). Schizophrenia. *Lancet*, *363*(9426), 2063–2072.

Pharoah, F. M., Mari, J. J., & Streiner, D. (2003). Family intervention for schizophrenia. *Cochrane Database of Systemic Reviews*, *4*, CD000088.

Reif, A., & Pfuhlmann, B. (2004). Folie a deux versus genetically driven delusional disorder: Case reports and nosological considerations. *Comprehensive Psychiatry*, *45*(2), 155–160.

Sadock, B. J., & Sadock, V. A. (2008a). Delusional disorder and shared psychotic disorder. In B. J. Sadock & V. A. Sadock (Eds.), *Kaplan and Sadock's concise textbook of clinical psychiatry* (3rd ed., pp. 182–190). Wolters Kluwer/Lippincott Williams &Wilkins.

Sadock, B. J., & Sadock, V. A. (2008b). Schizophrenia. In B. J. Sadock & V. A. Sadock (Eds.), *Kaplan and Sadock's concise textbook of clinical psychiatry* (3rd ed., pp. 156–177). Wolters Kluwer/Lippincott, Williams & Wilkins.

Sadock, B. J., & Sadock, V. A. (2008c). Schizophreniform disorder. In B. J. Sadock & V. A. Sadock (Eds.), *Kaplan and Sadock's concise textbook of clinical psychiatry* (3rd ed., pp. 178–180). Wolters Kluwer/Lippincott Williams & Wilkins.

Shimizu, M., Kubota, Y., Toichi, M., & Baba, H. (2007). Folieà deux and shared psychotic disorder. *Current Psychiatry Report*, *9*(3), 200–205.

Silveira, J. M., & Seeman, M. V. (1995). Shared psychotic disorder: A critical review of the literature. *Canadian Journal of Psychiatry*, *40*(7), 389–395.

Solari, H., Dickson, K. E., & Miller, L. (2009). Understanding and treating women with schizophrenia during pregnancy and postpartum—Motherisk Update 2008. *Canadian Journal of Clinical Pharmacology*, *16*(1), e23–e32.

Suzuki, K., Awata, S., Takano, T., Ebina, Y., Takamatsu, K., Kajiwara, T., Ito, K., Shindo, T., Funakoshi, S., & Matsuoka, H. (2006). Improvement of psychiatric symptoms after electroconvulsive therapy in young adults with intractable first-episode schizophrenia and schizophreniform disorder. *Tohoku Journal of Experimental Medicine*, *210*(3), 213–220.

Wenning, M. T., Davy, L. E., Catalano, G., & Catalano, M. C. (2003). Atypical antipsychotics in the treatment of delusional parasitosis. *Annals of Clinical Psychiatry*, *15*(3–4), 233–239.

WEB RESOURCES

- American Psychiatric Association: http://www.psych.org/
- Cleveland Clinic: http://www.ClevelandClinic.org/
- National Alliance on Mental Illness (NAMI): http://www.nami.org/
- National Mental Health Information Center: http://mentalhealth.samhsa.gov/
- Psych Central: http://psychcentral.com/

11

Mood Disorders

Background Information

Definition of Disorder

- Feelings of overwhelming sadness or lack of enjoyment, sometimes with anxiety and irritability, are the primary indicators.
- Hopelessness and a sense of feeling overwhelmed or helpless are common.
- Sense of worthlessness or low self-esteem is a prominent feature.
- Fatigue or somatic symptoms are also usually present.
- Often follows chronic stress or significant acute stressor(s).
- May complicate the treatment of other medical conditions such as stroke and diabetes. For example, people with depression are four times more likely to develop a heart attack than those without a history of the illness. After a heart attack, they are at a significantly increased risk of death or a second heart attack.
- Negatively impacts social functioning, such as getting out of bed, going to work, and having positive relationships.
- Major depressive disorder (MDD) is a recurrent illness. Risk for relapse after one episode is 50%. After two episodes, risk for relapse is 80% to 90%. The average number of lifetime episodes is 4.

Etiology

- Although heterogeneous in nature and poorly understood, the chronic stress response and the subsequent continuous activation of the hypothalamic–pituitary–adrenal axis results in chronic brain changes, such as a smaller hippocampus and changes in neurotransmitters.
- Corticotropin-releasing hormone (CRH) is a neuropeptide released by the hypothalamus to activate the pituitary in response to acute stress but is hypersecreted in depression.
- Serotonin and norepinephrine are thought to be the primary neurotransmitters involved in depression, although dopamine can also be related to depression.
- Cognitive and personality factors, such as how people view their influence, their ability to change, and their interpretation of stressors, also play a role. The

person with an MDD thinks that good things are temporary, limited in scope, and the result of sheer luck. Bad things are considered permanent, pervasive in impact, and their fault.
- MDD has been found to run in families, and this may mean that inheritance (genes) plays a strong role in determining who will get it. However, people who have no family history of the disorder also develop it.
- Often, depression occurs in the context of chronic illness or major life stressors.

Demographics
- Affects approximately 17.3 million American adults, or about 7.1% of the U.S. adult population.
- The prevalence of MDE is higher among adult females (8.7%) compared to males (5.3%).
- In 2017, the prevalence of adults with a MDE was highest among individuals aged 18 to 25 (13.1%).
- MDD is the leading cause of disability in the United States for those aged 15 to 44 years and the leading cause of disability in the world for adolescents and adults.
- Suicide results in 47,000 deaths annually in the United States.
- Suicide is the second leading cause of death among individuals between the ages of 10 and 34 and the fourth leading cause of death among individuals between the ages of 35 and 54.
- Among females, the suicide rate is highest for those aged 45 to 54; among males, the suicide rate is highest for those aged 65 and older.
- The rate of substance abuse (especially of stimulants, cocaine, and hallucinogens) in persons with MDD is greater than that of the general population.
- Pregnant mothers with MDD are more likely to have infants of low birth weight for gestational age.

Risk Factors
Age
- First occurrence is often between the ages of 20 and 40 years.
- The prevalence of major depression is increasing in younger generations.

Gender
- Major depression is twice as common in women as in men.
- Pregnancy can either improve the condition or make it worse.
- The postpartum period is a time of especial susceptibility to major depression.

Family History
- Many studies have shown an increased incidence of major depression when there is a history of depression, alcoholism, or other psychiatric illnesses in first-degree relatives.
- The disorder is two times more common in first-degree relatives with MDD.

Past Medical History
- Comorbidities with chronic diseases are common, with conditions such as prior myocardial infarction, multiple sclerosis (MS), Parkinson's, and chronic pain having a >40% prevalence.
- Current alcohol or substance abuse incidence during an MDD episode may have occurred.

Stressful Events in Susceptible People
- The initial appearance of MDD may follow a highly stressful event, such as being the victim of a crime or the loss of a job, a loved one, or an important relationship.

Social History
- There is often a lack of social support.
- Frequent use of medical resources in the absence of serious illness may be seen.
- Past or current history of abuse (childhood, sexual, or domestic violence) increases the incidence of MDD.

Having Another Mental Health Disorder
- A previous episode of depression may increase the risk of subsequent episodes of depression by as much as 90%.
- A history of dysthymic disorder precedes MDD in 10% to 25% of individuals.
- Having another mental health disorder, such as substance abuse (alcoholism or drug abuse), or a sleep disorder may increase the risk of developing MDD.
- Past history of suicide attempt.

Risk Factors for Suicide
- Older adults
- Male gender
- Widows/widowers/unmarried people
- Unemployed
- People living alone
- History of previous psychiatric hospitalization
- Substance abuse
- Recent loss of significant relationship
- Recent loss of financial security
- Previous suicide attempt(s)

Diagnosis

Differential Diagnosis
- More common are as follows:
  - Thyroid disease
  - Anemia
  - Menopause
  - Chronic fatigue syndrome
  - If an underlying chronic health condition such as MS or stroke is the physiological *cause* of the depressed mood, the diagnosis is mood disorder due to a general medical condition
  - Bipolar disorder
  - Bereavement
  - Adjustment disorder with depressed mood
  - Anxiety disorders
  - Dementia
  - Drug interactions or adverse effects
  - Infectious disease, such as autoimmune disorder, mononucleosis, or hepatitis C
  - Fibromyalgia
  - Personality disorder

- Less common are as follows:
  - Amphetamine or cocaine withdrawal
  - Parathyroid disease
  - Adrenal disease
  - Cancer
  - Neurological disease, such as cerebrovascular accident (CVA), MS, subdural hematoma, normal pressure hydrocephalus, or Alzheimer's disease
  - Cardiovascular disease such as congestive heart failure (CHF) or cardiomyopathy
  - Nutritional deficiency, such as B vitamin, folate, or iron deficiency
  - Pulmonary disease, such as chronic obstructive pulmonary disorder (COPD)
  - Heavy metal poisoning

ICD-10 Codes
Major depressive disorder, single episode, unspecified degree (F32.9)

Major depressive disorder, single episode, severe with psychotic features (F32.3)

Major depressive disorder, recurrent episodes, unspecified degree (F33.0)

Diagnostic Workup
- Physical and mental evaluation
- Labs as needed to evaluate physical complaints
  - Thyroid function studies (triiodothyronine [T_3], thyroxine [T_4], thyroid-stimulating hormone [TSH])
  - Complete metabolic panel, including glucose, calcium, and albumin; total protein analysis; and levels of sodium, potassium, CO_2 (carbon dioxide, bicarbonate), chloride, blood urea nitrogen (BUN), creatinine, alkaline phosphatase (ALP), alanine aminotransferase (ALT, also called serum glutamic pyruvic transaminase [SGPT]), aspartate aminotransferase (AST, also called serum glutamic oxaloacetic transaminase [SGOT]), and bilirubin
  - *Complete blood count (CBC) with differentials*: hemoglobin, hematocrit, red blood cells, white blood cells, white blood cell differential count, and platelet count
  - Testing for infectious diseases, such as hepatitis C or HIV, if applicable

Initial Assessment
- *Screening question*: In the past month, have you felt down or depressed? In the past month, have you lost interest in the things you usually do?
- Use of a standard screening tool, such as the following:
  1. *SIG E CAPS* (Sleep, Interest, Guilt, Energy, Concentration, Appetite, Psychomotor, and Suicidal ideation)
     - Depressed mood
     - Decreased sleep (insomnia with 2 a.m. to 4 a.m. awakening)
     - Interest decreased in activities (anhedonia)
     - Guilt or worthlessness (not a major criterion)
     - Energy decreased
     - Concentration difficulties
     - Appetite disturbance or weight loss
     - Psychomotor retardation/agitation
     - Suicidal thoughts
  2. *Beck Depression Inventory*: 21-question survey completed by patient
  3. *Zung Self-Rating Scale*: 20-question survey completed by patient, in a Likert-type scale format
  4. *PHQ-9*: The Patient Health Questionnaire, a brief survey completed by patient

- Past medical history.
- Family medical history, with emphasis on psychiatric history.
- Social history, including safety of relationships, family support, recent or ongoing stressors.
- Past suicide attempts or past psychiatric hospitalizations.
- Any prior manic/hypomanic episodes (*any* history suggestive of bipolar or cyclothymia diagnosis): Mood Disorder Questionnaire (MDQ) is a helpful tool.
- What effect symptoms have had on ability to function (any missed work, etc.)?
- Assess for suicide ideation, suicide plan, and suicide intent.

Clinical Presentation

- *Somatization*: Often, presentation of depression is through complaints of (often multiple) physical symptoms that do not have clearly identifiable causes.
- Sadness
- Lack of enjoyment of usual activities (anhedonia)
- Fatigue
- Sleep problems (early-morning awakening with difficulty or inability to fall back asleep being typical)
- Feelings of guilt
- Feeling overwhelmed
- Difficulty concentrating, focusing, or remembering
- Appetite disturbances (lack of appetite or excessive eating)
- Irritability, agitation, or slowed movements
- Thoughts of suicide or wanting to "escape"
- Obsessive rumination about problems

Signs

- Flattened affect
- Slowed speech and movements, sighs, long pauses
- Tearfulness
- Lack of eye contact
- Memory loss, poor concentration, or poor abstract reasoning
- Sometimes, irritability, belligerence, or defiance (more common in adolescence)

Diagnostic and Statistical Manual of Mental Disorders, Fifth Edition: Diagnostic Guidelines

The Diagnostic and Statistical Manual of Mental Disorders, Fifth Edition (*DSM-5*) distinguishes between MDD—single episode and MDD—recurrent.

For MDD—single episode:

- At least five of the following symptoms have been present for at least 2 weeks: depressed mood, anhedonia, change in eating habits, sleep disturbance, psychomotor agitation or retardation, fatigue, excessive guilt or feelings of worthlessness, difficulty concentrating, and recurrent thoughts of death or suicide (at least one of the symptoms being depressed mood or anhedonia).
- Symptoms must cause a significant social or occupational dysfunction or subjective distress.
- Symptoms cannot be caused by a medical condition, medications, drugs, or bereavement.

For MDD—recurrent:

- Two or more major depressive episodes (MDEs) occur.
- Absence of manic, hypomanic, or "mixed" episodes.

Treatment Overview

Acute Treatment

- Psychotropic medication should be selected based on relative efficacy, tolerability and anticipated side effects, co-occurring psychiatric or general medical conditions, half-life, cost, potential drug interactions, and the patient's preference and prior response to medication.
- The onset of benefit from pharmacological treatment may be more gradual in MDD than the onset of benefit in nonchronic depression.
- Treatment of nonresponsive patients should be reevaluated for accuracy of diagnosis, unaddressed co-occurring medical or psychiatric disorders (such as substance abuse), the need for a change in treatment modalities, inadequate dose or duration of medical treatment, the need to augment medical treatment (with a second antidepressant from a different pharmacological class or use of an adjunctive such as a second-generation atypical antipsychotic, anticonvulsant or thyroid hormone), inadequate frequency of psychotherapy, complicating psychosocial factors, nonadherence to treatment, and poor "fit" between patient and therapist.
- Common combinations of medications include a selective serotonin reuptake inhibitor (SSRI) with the addition of bupropion or the combination of mirtazapine and an SSRI or venlafaxine.
- Pharmacotherapy may increase the potential of suicidal ideation, particularly in patients younger than 25 years of age. General guidelines include the following:
  - Patients initiated on any psychiatric medication intervention should be monitored carefully for changes in mood or suicidal behavior or ideation.
  - Depressed patients with suicidal ideation, plan, and intent should be hospitalized, especially if they have current psychosocial stressors and access to lethal means.
  - Depressed patients with suicidal ideation and a plan but without intent may be treated on an outpatient basis with close follow-up, especially when they have good social support and no access to lethal means.
  - Depressed patients who express suicidal ideation but deny a plan should be assessed carefully for psychosocial stressors. Weapons should be removed from the environment.
  - Careful attention should be paid in the first 1 to 4 weeks of treatment to a sudden lift of depression or to worsening mood as initial response to antidepressant therapy, as these could be signs of increased risk for suicide.
  - Pharmacotherapy for MDD should begin at the lowest dosage and gradually be increased, if needed, following a 4-week evaluation for therapeutic response. Patients should be observed for 1 to 2 weeks after initiation of therapy for evaluation of adverse drug effects. Frequency of monitoring should be determined based on symptom severity, co-occurring disorders, availability of social support, patient cooperation with treatment, and side effects of medication.
- The combination of pharmacological therapy and cognitive behavioral therapy (CBT), individually or in combination, is effective in more than 85% of cases.

Chronic Treatment

- Pharmacotherapy with or without individual counseling, particularly CBT, is the treatment of choice and should be considered for patients.
- Cognitive restructuring involves substituting positive perceptions for negative perceptions and assistance with problem solving and stress management.
- Once the patient has reached remission of symptoms, the patient is monitored for an additional 4 to 9 months prior to tapering the medication, or, in the case of three or more episodes, the patient is placed on maintenance treatment.

- In cases in which medication loses its effectiveness, alternative regimens and diagnoses should be explored.
- Electroconvulsive therapy (ECT) is recommended as the treatment of choice for patients with severe MDD that is not responsive to pharmacologic treatment and psychotherapy.
- Pharmacologic education should include the following:
  - Frequency of dosing
  - The likelihood that side effects will occur prior to improvement of symptoms
  - Expectations that it will take 2 to 4 weeks prior to beneficial effects and 4 to 8 weeks prior to full effects of the dosage
  - The importance of taking medication even after feeling better
  - Consulting with the healthcare provider before discontinuing medication
  - Correcting misconceptions about medication use and explaining what to do if side effects, questions, or worsening symptoms arise
- Nonpharmacologic recommendations should also be made, such as the following:
  - Proper sleep hygiene
  - Decreased use or elimination of caffeine, tobacco, and alcohol
  - Light therapy
  - Regular exercise
- Consider long-term treatment in patients with two or more episodes. A history of three or more episodes of depression indicates a very high risk for recurrence and the need for continuous treatment.
- Also may increase the risk of bleeding for patients on nonsteroidal antiinflammatory drugs (NSAIDs)/acetylsalicylic acid (ASA) and anticoagulation therapy.
- Stress management and lifestyle changes, such as regular exercise, which have been found to decrease depression, are essential for ongoing prevention.
- Behavioral therapy involves various relaxation techniques, self-care strategies, and cognitive and dialectical therapy, which may also be helpful. Studies suggest that augmentation of antidepressant effect occurs with adjunct use of omega-3 fish oil supplements, 1,000 mg BID daily. B vitamin supplementation has also been used in some studies, with equivocal results.
- Treatment can be complicated by having another condition at the same time, such as substance abuse, depression, or other anxiety disorders.

Notes on Selective Serotonin Reuptake Inhibitors as First Line of Drug Therapy

- SSRIs are one of the more commonly used medications for MDD.
- SSRI medications typically display fewer side effects than tricyclic antidepressants (TCAs) and monoamine oxidase inhibitors (MAOIs), with minimal risk of death in an intentional overdose. Treatment decisions should take into consideration patient symptoms and medication side effect profile.

Drug Selection Table for Major Depressive Disorder

CLASS	DRUG
SSRIs	First-line drug therapy
	Fluoxetine (Prozac)
	Sertraline (Zoloft)
	Paroxetine (Paxil, Paxil CR)
	Citalopram (Celexa)
	Escitalopram (Lexapro)
	Fluvoxamine (Luvox)
	Fluoxetine (Sarafem)

Drug Selection Table for Major Depressive Disorder (*continued*)

CLASS	DRUG
SNRIs	Venlafaxine (Effexor); Venlafaxine XR (Effexor XR) Duloxetine (Cymbalta) Desvenlafaxine (Pristiq)
SARIs	Second-line drug therapy Nefazodone (Serzone) Trazodone (Desyrel)
NaSSAs	Alternative therapy option Mirtazapine (Remeron)
NDRIs	Alternative therapy option Bupropion (Wellbutrin, Zyban), bupropion SR (Wellbutrin SR), and bupropion XL (Wellbutrin XL)
TCAs	Amitriptyline (Elavil) Clomipramine (Anafranil) Desipramine (Norpramin) Imipramine (Tofranil) Nortriptyline (Pamelor)
MAOIs	Phenelzine (Nardil) Isocarboxazid (Marplan) Tranylcypromine (Parnate) MAOIs, monoamine oxidase inhibitors; NaSSAs, noradrenergic and specific serotonergic antidepressants; NDRIs, norepinephrine/dopamine reuptake inhibitors; SARIs, serotonin-2 antagonist/reuptake inhibitors; SNRIs, Serotonin-norepinephrine reuptake inhibitors; SSRIs, selective serotonin reuptake inhibitors; TCAs, tricyclic antidepressants.

- They also may increase the risk of bleeding for patients on NSAIDs/ASA and anti-coagulation therapy.
- SSRI medications may not be preferred for patients with sexual dysfunction or who find sexual dysfunction as an intolerable side effect.
- Limited or no cholinergic, histaminergic, dopaminergic, or adrenergic receptor activity (i.e., they do not cause hypotension or anticholinergic response).
- May be of benefit to perimenopausal women experiencing hot flashes.
- Patients reporting intolerable side effects from one SSRI may benefit from switching to another SSRI.
- SSRIs inhibit serotonin 2A receptors and serotonin reuptake.
- Receptor inhibition produces a sedating effect.

Recurrence Rate
Rate of recurrence is 50% after one episode, 80% after two episodes, and >90% after three episodes.

Patient Education
- Information regarding MDD and support groups can be obtained from the National Institute for Mental Health (see further outpatient care).
- Advise patients with MDD to avoid nicotine and excess alcohol intake (no more than 1 svg/d for a woman, 2 svg/d for a man).

- Thirty minutes of daily exercise has been found to be beneficial for patients with MDD, and daily exposure to outdoor light may also be beneficial.

Medical/Legal Pitfalls

- Failure to monitor for suicide risk.
- Failure to screen for bipolar disorder (any history of mania/hypomania).
- Pay careful attention in the first 1 to 4 weeks of treatment to a sudden lift of depression or to worsening mood as initial response to antidepressant therapy, as these could be signs of increased risk for suicide.
- When initiating treatment, see patients on a more frequent basis until response to antidepressant is clear.
- Have a follow-up system to ensure that there are calls to patients who fail to schedule follow-up appointments or fail to show up for scheduled appointments.
- Patients with MDDs are more likely than the general population to use alternative therapies. Use of dietary supplements (e.g., herbs) should be discussed to avoid drug interactions.

BIPOLAR DISORDER

Background Information

Definition of Disorder

- Historically, it has been referred to as manic depression or manic-depressive illness.
- Neurobiological psychiatric disorder is characterized by sustained extreme mood swings from extremely low (depression) to extremely high (mania) and an abnormal increase in energy and activity.
- Both phases of this disorder are deleterious in that they adversely affect thoughts, behaviors, judgment, and relationships.
- Patients with bipolar I disorder have episodes of sustained mania and often experience depressive episodes.
- Patients with bipolar II disorder have one or more MDEs, with at least one hypomanic episode.
- Extreme mood swings that occur hourly or daily are very rarely associated with this disorder, and other medical and/or psychiatric diagnoses should be considered and ruled out first.
- An age of onset of mania after the age of 40 years alerts the practitioner that the symptoms are most likely due to a medical condition or substance use, and newly diagnosed mania is uncommon in children and adults older than 65 years.
- It is not uncommon for bipolar disorder to go undetected.
- Patients in the manic phase of the disorder often do not seek psychiatric or medical attention.
- Patients experiencing the depressive phase of the disorder often present initially to a primary care setting due to an increase in health issues, somatic complaints, or chronic pain that does not appear to have an objective or identifiable etiology. This is often erroneously diagnosed with unipolar depression, which can then be treated with unopposed antidepressant therapy (and may cause switch to mania).

Etiology

- The exact cause of bipolar disorder is not known.
- The *kindling theory* is the current predominant theory, meaning the disorder is likely caused by multiple factors that potentially interact and lower the threshold

at which mood changes occur. Eventually, a mood episode can start itself and thus become recurrent.

- Environmental factors
  - Sleep deprivation can trigger episodes of mania while hypersomnia can trigger MDEs.
  - Traumatic and/or abusive events in childhood.
  - Approximately one fifth of individuals with bipolar disorder, mostly those with bipolar II, have mood symptoms that wax and wane with the seasons. It is hypothesized that those with a diurnal pattern are affected mostly by both fluctuating light and temperature.
- Biological perspectives
  - Genetics
    - Twin studies consistently show that identical twins (40%–70%) are far more concordant for mood disorders than fraternal twins (0%–10%).
    - The overall heritability of bipolar spectrum disorders has been put at 0.71.
    - Between 4% and 24% of first-degree relatives of individuals with bipolar I disorder are also diagnosed with bipolar I disorder.
  - Neural processes
    - Hypersensitivity of melatonin receptors
    - Structural abnormalities in the amygdala, hippocampus, and prefrontal cortex
    - Larger lateral ventricles
- White matter hyperintensities
  - Endocrine models
    - Hypothyroidism can cause depression and/or mood instability.
    - Abnormalities have also been found in the hypothalamic–pituitary axis due to repeated stress.

Demographics
- True prevalence is not known due to misdiagnosis or undetected episodes of mania.
- Bipolar disorder affects approximately 2.8% of American adults annually.
- Lifetime prevalence is 1% for bipolar I and between 0.5% and 1% for bipolar II.
- First-degree biological relatives of individuals with bipolar I disorder are more likely to have an earlier onset of bipolar spectrum disorders.
- Forty percent or more of patients with this disorder experience mixed episodes (MDE + manic episode).
- The World Health Organization identified bipolar disorder as the sixth leading cause of disability-adjusted life years worldwide among people aged 15 to 44 years.
- Cardiovascular disease, obesity, type 2 diabetes mellitus, and other endocrine disorders occur more often in patients with bipolar spectrum disorders.
- Patients with bipolar disorder have higher rates of comorbid neurological disorders and migraine headaches.

Risk Factors
Age
- The average age of onset is 20 years.
- Late adolescence and early adulthood are peak years for the onset of bipolar disorder.
- Approximately 10% to 15% of adolescents with recurrent MDEs are more likely to develop bipolar I disorder.

- Mixed episodes appear more likely in adolescents and young adults than in older adults.
- Often, the cycling between depression and mania accelerates with age.

Gender
- Men and women are affected equally.
  - Men
    - The first episode in males is most likely to be a manic episode.
    - Early-onset bipolar disorder tends to occur more frequently in men and it is associated with a more severe condition.
    - Men with bipolar spectrum disorders tend to have higher rates of substance abuse (drugs, alcohol).
    - The number of manic episodes equals or exceeds the number of MDEs in men.
  - Women
    - The first episode in females is most likely to be an MDE.
    - There is a higher incidence of rapid cycling and mixed mood episodes among women.
    - Women have higher incidences of bipolar II disorder.
    - The number of MDEs exceeds the number of manic episodes in women.
    - Women with bipolar I disorder appear to have an increased risk for developing mood episodes in the immediate postpartum period.
    - Women in the premenstrual period may have worsening of ongoing major depressive, manic, mixed, or hypomanic episodes.

Family History
- Genetic factors account for 60% of the cases of bipolar disorder.
- The approximate lifetime risk in relatives of a bipolar proband is 40% to 70% for a monozygotic twin and 5% to 10% for a first-degree relative.
- Family members of patients with bipolar disorder also have a higher-than-average incidence of other psychiatric problems.
- Schizophrenia
- Schizoaffective disorder
- Anxiety disorders
- Attention deficit hyperactivity disorder
- Major depression
- Obsessive-compulsive disorder

Stressful Events in Susceptible People
- There have been repeated findings that about one third to one half of adults diagnosed with bipolar disorder report traumatic/abusive experiences in childhood, particularly events stemming from a harsh environment rather than from the child's own behavior. This is generally associated with earlier onset, a worse course, and more co-occurring mental health disorders such as posttraumatic stress disorder (PTSD) or other anxiety-related disorders.
- Ongoing psychosocial stressors have been shown to destabilize moods in patients with bipolar spectrum disorders.

Having Another Mental Health Disorder
- Anxiety disorders
  - There is a >50% lifetime comorbidity of anxiety disorders with bipolar illness and these patients appear to have a more difficult course of illness.

- Decreased likelihood of recovery.
- Poorer role functioning and quality of life.
- Greater likelihood of suicide attempts.
- Substance-use disorders
  - Sixty-one percent of patients diagnosed with bipolar I disorder and 48% of patients diagnosed with bipolar II disorder also have coexisting substance-use disorders.
  - The most common substance-use disorder appears to be alcohol abuse/dependence.
  - Lifetime prevalence of alcohol abuse/dependence is 49% for men and 29% for women diagnosed with bipolar spectrum disorders.
  - *Attention deficit hyperactivity disorder:* a diagnosis of attention deficit hyperactivity disorder as a child may be a marker for a bipolar spectrum diagnosis as an adult.
- Personality disorders
  - Approximately one third of patients with bipolar disorder also have a cluster B (borderline, narcissistic, antisocial, and histrionic) personality disorder.
  - Marked personality disorder symptoms negatively influence treatment-related outcomes in patients with bipolar disorder.

Risk Factors for Suicidal Behavior in Bipolar Spectrum Disorders
- Completed suicide occurs in 10% to 15% of individuals with bipolar I disorder.
- Personal or family history of suicidal behavior.
- Severity and number of depressive episodes or mixed mood states.
- Alcohol or substance abuse/dependence.
- Level of pessimism and hopelessness.
- Level of impulsivity and/or aggression.
- Younger age of onset of the disorder.
- A concomitant personality disorder diagnosis.
- Patients with remitting depressive symptoms are thought to be at increased risk for suicide.

Risk Factors for Harm to Others in Bipolar Spectrum Disorders
- A history of violent behavior has consistently been shown to be the best single predictor of future violence.
- The presence of symptoms that increase the risk of violence in the absence of overt threats includes being guarded and/or paranoid, psychosis, command hallucinations, cognitive disorders, and substance use. Child abuse, spouse abuse, or other violent behavior may occur during severe manic episodes or during mood episodes with psychotic features.
- Younger age.
- Gender is not a factor; the rates of violence among the genders are equal in patients who are acutely mentally ill.
- A history of victimization as a child or witnessing or experiencing violence after the age of 16 years.
- Level of impulsivity.
- More than half of victims of violence by persons with mental health disorders are family members.
- The availability of firearms and/or weapons.

Diagnosis

Differential Diagnosis

There is a broad differential diagnosis for bipolar spectrum disorders, which includes ruling out the following:

- Thyroid or other metabolic disorders
- Epilepsy (partial complex seizures)
- Diabetes mellitus
- Sleep apnea
- Brain lesions
- MS
- Systemic infection
- Tertiary syphilis
- Systemic lupus erythematosus
- Cerebral vascular accident
- HIV
- Steroid-induced mood symptoms
- Vitamin B12 deficiency
- Vitamin D deficiency
- PTSD
- Attention deficit hyperactivity disorder
- Cyclothymic disorder
- MDD
- Dysthymic disorder
- Schizoaffective disorder
- Schizophrenia
- Personality disorders
- Eating disorder
- Drug interactions or adverse effects that can cause mood symptoms (e.g., baclofen, bromide, bromocriptine, captopril, cimetidine, corticosteroids, cyclosporine, disulfiram [Antabuse], hydralazine, isoniazid, levodopa, methylphenidate [Ritalin], metrizamide, procarbazine, procyclidine [Kemadrin])
- Drug or alcohol intoxication or withdrawal

ICD-10 Codes

Bipolar disorder, unspecified (F31.9)

Bipolar disorder, current manic episode without psychotic features (F31.10)

Bipolar disorder, in partial remission, most recent episode manic (F31.73)

Bipolar disorder, in partial remission most recent episode depressed (F31.75)

Bipolar II disorder (specify if most recent episode is hypomanic/depressed) (F31.81)

Diagnostic Workup

- There are no biological tests that confirm bipolar disorder. Rather, tests are carried out to rule in/out medical issues that may be mimicking a mood disorder.
  - *Antinuclear antibody (ANA):* ANAs are found in patients whose immune systems may be predisposed to cause inflammation against their own body tissues. Antibodies that are directed against one's own tissues are referred to as autoantibodies.

- Thyroid and other metabolic function studies suggest hyperexcitability or hypo-excitability symptoms.
- Blood glucose level rules out diabetes.
- Serum proteins.
- Lithium levels are measured if patient has history of diagnosis and is taking this medication.
- CBC with differential is performed to rule out anemia or other blood dyscrasias.
- Urine toxicology screening for drugs and alcohol (see previous data).
- Urine copper level is measured.
- Venereal disease research lab (VDRL) test random plasma glucose (RPG) is performed.
- HIV testing (enzyme-linked immunosorbent assay [ELISA] and Western Blot test).
- EKG.
- Electroencephalography to exclude epilepsy.
- Sleep study.
- MRI.
- CT scan of head.
- Clinical history.
- Collateral information from close friends and family.

Initial Assessment

- It is important to gain a complete history and carefully assess for historical and/or current episodes of mania and/or hypomania as well as depression.
- Physical examination with a focus on neurological and endocrine systems and infectious diseases.
- Ask specific screening questions to assess for manic episodes, mixed episodes, or hypomanic episodes:
  - Have you ever experienced periods of feeling uncharacteristically energetic?
  - Have you had periods of not sleeping but not feeling tired?
  - Have you ever felt that your thoughts were racing and that there was nothing you could do to slow them down?
  - Have you ever experienced periods during which you were participating in risky activities, more interested in sex than usual, or spending more money than you usually would?
- Use standardized screening tools:
  - Bipolar Spectrum Diagnostic Scale (BSDS)
  - MDQ
  - *Violence Screening Checklist (VSC)*: reliably indicates the level of risk during the next 24-hour period
  - *Short-term assessment of risk and treatability (START)*: assesses risk and guides treatment for violence, suicide, self-neglect, substance use, and victimization
- Psychiatric assessment with a focus on current symptoms, date of onset, potential precipitating factors, perpetuating factors (e.g., drug or alcohol use), traumatic events in childhood, and substance use.
- Family history with an emphasis on psychiatric history and suicide attempts and completed suicides.
- Social history with an emphasis on current social support and safety issues in relationships, recent psychosocial stressors, ability to maintain employment, and financial concerns.

- Assessment of safety risk with an emphasis on history of harm to self or others, history of childhood abuse or victimization, plan and intent, and access to firearms and/or weapons.
- Level of functional impairment and need for hospitalization (e.g., assess ability to work, engage in self-care activities, ability to conduct activities of daily living, and ability to get along with others).

Clinical Presentation
- Manic episode
  - Affect/moods
    - Euphorically elevated, overly happy, outgoing
    - Irritable mood, agitation, jumpy, "wired"
    - Inappropriately joyous
  - Behaviors
    - Increased goal-directed activity
    - Excessive involvement in high-risk activities
    - Impulsivity
    - Restlessness
    - Energized behavior
    - Clothing may look disorganized or disheveled
    - Increased psychomotor changes
    - Religiosity
    - Decreased need for sleep
    - Behavior may become aggressive, intrusive, or combative
    - No patience or tolerance for others
    - Increased talkativeness or rapid, pressured speech
  - Thoughts
    - Inflated self-worth
    - Expansive and optimistic thinking
    - Flight of ideas and/or loose associations
    - Racing thoughts and feeling that their minds are active
  - Perceptions
    - Approximately three fourths have delusions.
    - Manic delusions reflect perceptions of power, prestige, position, self-worth, and glory.
    - Some have auditory hallucinations and delusions of persecution.
- Hypomanic episode
  - Affect/moods
    - Up
    - Expansive
    - Irritable
  - Behaviors
    - Busy
    - Active
    - Overinvolved
    - Increased energy
    - Increase in planning and doing things
    - Others notice the increase in their activity but the patient often denies that anything about their has changed

- Thoughts
  - Optimistic
  - Future focused
  - Positive attitude
- Perceptions
  - Patients with hypomania typically do not experience perceptual changes.
- MDE
  - Affect/moods
    - Sadness dominates affect and is often blunted or flattened
    - Feeling sad, depressed, empty, and isolated
    - Hopelessness
    - Helplessness
    - Worthlessness
    - Easily overwhelmed
  - Behaviors
    - Poor grooming
    - Increased tearfulness
    - Poor eye contact or no eye contact
    - *Psychomotor changes*: moves slowly or moves very little, with psychomotor retardation
    - Social withdrawal, shyness, or increase in social anxiety
    - Decreased interest in sexual activity and/or difficulty enjoying sexual activity
    - Somatization (e.g., increase in physical or somatic complaints without objective, identifiable cause)
    - Difficulty with attention and concentration
    - Appetite disturbances (increase or decrease)
    - Sleep disturbance
    - Decrease in energy and increase in fatigue regardless of amount of sleep
    - Attempts at suicide
  - Thoughts
    - Increased thoughts of death or morbid thoughts, and/or suicidal thoughts or specific plans for committing suicide
    - Thoughts that reflect their sadness (negative thoughts about self, world, and future)
    - Nihilistic concerns
    - Short-term memory deficits
    - Increase in worry and rumination; also referred to as brooding
    - Inappropriate guilt
  - Perceptions
    - In severe episodes, psychotic symptoms may be present (e.g., auditory hallucinations)
    - Delusions, for example, that they have sinned
- Mixed features (includes depressive signs and symptoms within manic or hypomanic phases of the illness)
  - Affect/moods
    - Marked irritability
    - Agitation
    - Anxiety
    - Rage
  - Behaviors
    - Aggressiveness
    - Belligerence

- Impulsiveness
- Sleep disturbance
- Rapid and pressured speech
- Psychomotor agitation
- Fatigue
- Thoughts
  - Confusion
  - Morbid thoughts and/or suicidal ideation
  - Paranoia and/or persecutory delusions
  - Racing thoughts
  - Increased worry and rumination
- Perceptions
  - Patients may exhibit hallucinations and/or delusions congruent with either depression or mania or both

Diagnostic and Statistical Manual of Mental Disorders, Fifth Edition: Diagnostic Guidelines
Manic Episode
- The patient's mood is disturbed and characterized as high, irritable, or expansive, with an increase in overall energy for at least 1 week.
- The patient exhibits three or more of the following:
  - Grandiose thinking
  - Diminished sleep
  - Volubility, or rapid and pressured speech
  - Racing thoughts
  - Distractibility, trouble concentrating
  - Increased goal-directed activity
  - Expanded pleasurable activities that have potential for adverse outcomes (e.g., spending sprees)
  - Psychomotor agitation
  - Psychotic features (e.g., delusions of grandeur, hallucinations)
- Symptom severity results in one or both of the following:
  - Reduced social functioning (social, marital, occupational)
  - Hospitalization (owing to the presence of safety risk)
- The symptoms are not more easily ascribed to other medical diagnoses, other medical conditions, substance use, or withdrawal from prescription medications.

Major Depressive Episode
- The patient has experienced five or more of the following in a 2-week period:
  - Depressed mood
  - Anhedonia
  - Change in eating habits, weight loss, or weight gain
  - Psychomotor agitation or retardation
  - Fatigue
  - Feelings of guilt; feelings of worthlessness
  - Problems with concentration; short-term memory deficits
  - Suicidal ideation
Note: Depressed mood or anhedonia must be one of the five.

- Symptom severity results in one or both of the following:
  - Reduced social functioning (social, marital, occupational)
  - Hospitalization (owing to the presence of safety risk)

- The symptoms cannot be more easily ascribed to other medical diagnoses, other medical conditions, substance use, or withdrawal from prescription medication.

Hypomanic Episode
- Elevated, expansive, or irritable mood for at least 4 days.
- During this same period, the patient has had three or more of the following:
  - Grandiose thinking, inflated self-esteem
  - Diminished sleep
  - Volubility
  - Racing thoughts
  - Problems with concentration
  - Psychomotor agitation
  - A focus on goal-directed activities
  - Poor judgment and increased engagement in activities that have potential for adverse consequences (e.g., spending sprees)
- Psychotic features are absent.
- Social functioning is not impeded.
- Hospitalization is not required.
- The symptoms are not more easily ascribed to other medical diagnoses, other medical conditions, substance use, or withdrawal from prescription medication.

Bipolar I
- Criteria for one manic episode have been met.
- If the patient is experiencing a hypomanic episode, they must have had at least one prior manic episode.
- Markedly reduced social or occupational functioning.
- For a majority of patients, depression is present more often than mania.
- The symptoms cannot be ascribed to other medical diagnoses, other medical conditions, substance use, or withdrawal from prescription medication.

Bipolar II
- The patient has had one or more MDEs.
- The patient has had one or more hypomanic episodes.
- A history of manic episodes is absent.
- The symptoms cause significant distress or significantly reduced functioning in the patient.
- The symptoms cannot be more easily ascribed to other medical diagnoses (including other psychiatric diagnoses), other medical conditions, substance abuse, or withdrawal from prescription medication.

Rapid Cycling (Can Be Applied to Both Bipolar I or Bipolar II Disorder)
- The patient has experienced four or more of the following: MDEs, manic episodes, or hypomanic episodes (any combination) within a 12-month period.
- Episodes are generally separated by periods of at least 2 months of full or partial remission, or there is a switch to an episode of the opposite polarity.

Treatment Overview
Acute Treatment
- The primary goal of the acute phase is to manage acute mania, hypomania, or depressive episodes and associated safety-risk issues.

- Diagnostic tests should be performed to rule out potential medical etiologies for mood symptoms, especially if this is the first episode of mania, hypomania, mixed mood symptoms, or depression.
- How to handle suicidal ideation?
  - A patient with suicidal ideation with plan and intent should be hospitalized (voluntarily or involuntarily) due to acute safety risk.
  - A patient with suicidal ideation with plan but no intent may be treated on an outpatient basis with close follow-up if they do not have access to the means to carry out the plan and do not have adequate social support.
  - A patient with suicidal ideation without plan and no intent requires careful assessment of current psychosocial stressors, access to weapons and other lethal means, substance use, and impulse-control issues. Any lethal means should be removed.
- How to handle aggression and potential harm to others?
  - If patients have access to firearms and or weapons, they should be removed.
  - Those with thoughts of harming others with plan and intent should be hospitalized (voluntarily or involuntarily).
  - Antipsychotics are often used for management in emergent situations, in which the patient presents as possibly psychotic, agitated, and making overt threats.
  - Those with thoughts of harming others with plan but no intent can be treated on an outpatient basis, with increased intensity of treatment with an established provider, depending on risk factors.
  - Those with thoughts of harming others without plan or intent do require increased intensity of treatment and perhaps increased dosages of medications.
- Acute manic episode with or without mixed features
  - Hospitalization is necessary in patients who present with significant suicide risk, increased aggressiveness, and significant risk of violence against others; who present with the potential for serious alcohol withdrawal symptoms; or when the differential includes other medical disorders that warrant admission.
  - Antidepressants, if they have been prescribed, should be discontinued if the patient is presenting with an acute manic episode with or without mixed features.
  - Patient should be advised to decrease alcohol, caffeine, and nicotine use.
  - Most patients are started on long-term mood stabilizers and also are given antipsychotic medications if agitated and/or experiencing psychotic symptoms.
  - Medications in the acute phase are commonly used to induce remission in acute mania or hypomania.
- Acute hypomanic episode
  - Treatment for hypomania, which can lead to either a manic or a depressive episode, may decrease symptom progression.
- Acute MDE
  - Hospitalization is necessary if patient presents with a significant suicide risk, if there is potential for serious withdrawal symptoms, or when the differential includes other medical disorders that warrant admission.
  - Antidepressant medications have not been shown to be an effective adjunctive therapy and, as a monotherapy, they can precipitate mania in individuals with bipolar disorder.
  - Be alert to sudden decreases of depressed mood or to worsening mood as initial response to antidepressant therapy, as these could be signs of increased risk for suicide.

- Medication noncompliance is common because mania and hypomania may be a desired state for many individuals with bipolar disorder, and many are reluctant to take medications to eliminate these states.
- Because bipolar disorder is a lifelong and recurrent illness, long-term treatment is needed to manage and control mood symptoms.
- Cardiovascular mortality is almost twice as high in patients with bipolar disorder. The risk of sudden death may also theoretically be increased due to reduced heart-rate variability.

Chronic Treatment

- The continuation phase of treatment lasts weeks to months and the primary goal is to reach full remission of symptoms and restoration of functioning.
- The primary goal of the maintenance phase of treatment is to achieve full and sustained symptom remission for at least 1 year after resolution of symptoms.
- Long-term life maintenance is recommended for patients who have suffered three or more manic episodes.
- Study results from a large-scale National Institute of Mental Health—funded clinical trial found patients treated with both medications and intensive psychotherapy (30 sessions over 9 months of therapy) demonstrated the following:
  - Fewer relapses
  - Lower hospitalization rates
  - Better ability to stick to treatment plans
  - More likely to get well faster and stay well longer
- Medications
  - Long-term management of bipolar disorder should be treated with a mood stabilizer.
  - Patients who fail to respond to one mood stabilizer may need to be switched to another or the addition of another mood stabilizer or an atypical antipsychotic may be required.
  - Risk of suicide is reduced 13-fold with long-term maintenance therapy with lithium.
  - There is limited research on all of the atypical antipsychotics in the maintenance phase of treatment; however, any of the atypical antipsychotics may be considered when other treatments are unsuccessful.
- ECT is used only as a last resort if the patient does not adequately respond to medications and/or psychotherapy.
  - Psychotherapy
  - *CBT*: helps individuals with bipolar disorder learn to change harmful and negative thought patterns and behaviors, as well as learn coping skills, such as stress management, identifying triggers for mood symptoms, and relaxation techniques.
  - *Family therapy*: This therapy includes family members. By doing so, it helps family members enhance coping strategies, such as recognizing new episodes and knowing how to help their loved one. Therapy also focuses on communication skills and problem solving.
  - *Interpersonal therapy*: helps people with bipolar disorder improve their relationships with others.
  - *Social rhythm therapy*: focuses on maintaining and managing daily routines, such as regular sleep–wake cycles, eating patterns, and social routines.

- *Psychoeducation*: focuses on teaching individuals with bipolar disorder about the illness and its treatment. This form of treatment helps people realize signs of relapse so that they can access treatment early before a full episode occurs. This usually occurs in a group format and may also be helpful for family members and caregivers.
- Follow-up care by a chemical dependence treatment specialist is recommended when indicated.
- Patients with cardiac comorbidity, abnormal findings on cardiac examination, or significant risk factors for heart disease should be referred to a cardiologist.
- Patients with endocrine dysfunction, such as hyperthyroidism or hypothyroidism, should be referred to an endocrinologist.
- Treatment can be complicated or have a poorer course by having another condition at the same time, such as substance abuse, depression, anxiety disorders, or a personality disorder.
- Concomitant substance abuse/dependence is correlated with increased hospitalizations and a worse illness course coupled with increased safety risk.

Psychopharmacology of Bipolar Disorder

Overview of Psychopharmacology of Bipolar Disorder

- *Mood stabilizers,* including mood-stabilizing anticonvulsants and lithium, are identified as first-line treatment approaches. Lithium is recommended for bipolar depression. Mood-stabilizing anticonvulsants (e.g., valproate) are preferred for rapid-cycling disorders.
- Hypomanic episodes and mild depressive episodes are generally managed with a single mood stabilizer. Acute manic and severe depressive episodes often require two or three medications.
- A benzodiazepine (e.g., diazepam or lorazepam) may be considered as an adjunct short-term treatment for reducing insomnia or agitation.
- Use of antidepressants by primary care providers for treating bipolar patients should be avoided. Antidepressant monotherapy may precipitate mania or induce rapid-cycling disorders between mania and depression.
- Dosage adjustments may be required if the patient experiences a partial response or breakthrough symptoms.

Drug Selection Table for Bipolar Disorders

CLASS	DRUG
Mood-stabilizing anticonvulsants	First-line drug therapy Valproate sodium, valproic acid, divalproex sodium (Depacon, Depakene, Depakote, Depakote ER, Depakote Sprinkle) Carbamazepine (Tegretol, Equetro, Tegretol XR) Topiramate (Topamax) Lamotrigine (Lamictal, Lamictal XR)
Nonanticonvulsant mood stabilizer	First-line drug therapy for bipolar depression: Lithium (Eskalith, Lithobid)
Atypical antipsychotics (second generation)	Aripiprazole (Abilify) Olanzapine (Zyprexa) Risperidone (Risperdal, Risperdal Consta) Quetiapine (Seroquel, Seroquel XR) Ziprasidone (Geodon)

■ ECT may be considered for treatment-resistant or severe mania. In general, mood-stabilizer treatment has produced better outcomes than ECT.

Recurrence Rate
■ Bipolar I disorder
  ▪ The course of bipolar I disorder is marked by relapses and remissions, often alternating manic with depressive episodes.
  ▪ Ninety percent of individuals who have a single manic episode go on to have future manic or hypomanic episodes within another 5 years.
  ▪ Approximately 60% to 70% of manic episodes occur immediately before or after an MDE.
  ▪ The majority of individuals with bipolar I disorder experience symptom reduction among episodes; however, between 20% and 30% continue to have mood lability and other symptoms.
  ▪ Sixty percent of sufferers experience chronic interpersonal and occupational difficulties among acute episodes.
  ▪ Patients with bipolar I fare worse than patients with a major depression. Within the first 2 years after the initial episode, 40% to 50% of patients experience another manic episode.
  ▪ Psychotic symptoms can develop days or weeks after a previous nonpsychotic manic or mixed episode.
  ▪ Individuals who have manic episodes with psychotic features are more likely to have subsequent manic episodes with psychotic features.
  ▪ Ninety percent of individuals with bipolar I disorder have at least one psychiatric hospitalization and two thirds have two or more hospitalizations in their lifetime.
■ Bipolar II disorder
  ▪ This disorder has been studied less and the course is less well understood.
■ Patient behaviors that can lead to a recurrence of depressive or manic symptoms are as follows:
  ▪ Discontinuing or lowering one's dose of medication.
  ▪ An inconsistent sleep schedule can destabilize the illness. Too much sleep can lead to depression, whereas too little sleep can lead to mixed states or mania.
  ▪ Inadequate stress management and poor lifestyle choices. Medication raises the stress threshold somewhat, but too much stress still causes relapse.
  ▪ Using drugs or alcohol can either trigger or prolong mood symptoms.

Patient Education
■ Advise patients that it is important to deal with mania early in the episode, and thus recognizing the early warning signs is the key so that more intensive treatment can be administered before symptoms escalate.
■ Advise patient to stay on all medications and to not decrease or stop any medications without medical supervision. This is especially important when experiencing mania or hypomania.
■ Also advise patients that sometimes several medication trials are needed to find ones that will be efficacious in controlling mood symptoms.
■ Advise patients that symptoms will improve gradually, not immediately, as they begin to remit.
■ In general, there is little research about herbal or natural supplements for bipolar spectrum disorders and not much is known about their efficacy; however, St. John's

wort may cause a switch to mania and can make other medications less effective (e.g., antidepressants and anticonvulsants). Additionally, the effects of Sam-E or omega-3 fatty acids are not known. All herbal and natural remedies for mood symptoms should be discussed with a medical provider.

- The best approach to treatment is a combination of psychotherapy and medications. This helps prevent relapses, reduces hospitalizations, and helps the patient get well faster and stay well longer.
- If patients plan extensive travel into other time zones, advise them to call their doctor before leaving to determine whether any changes in their medicines should be made and what to do if they have a manic or depressive episode while away.
- Women who are pregnant or would like to become pregnant and have been diagnosed with a bipolar spectrum disorder should speak with their doctor about the risks and benefits of all treatments during pregnancy. Mood-stabilizing medications used today can cause harm to the developing fetus or a nursing infant. Additionally, stopping or reducing medications during pregnancy can cause a recurrence of mood symptoms.
- Helping the individual identify and modify stressors provides a critical aspect of patient and family awareness.
- Changes in sleep patterns can sometimes trigger a manic or depressive episode. Advise patients to keep a regular routine such as eating meals at the same time every day and going to sleep at the same time nightly and waking up at the same time daily.
- Patients should be encouraged to keep a chart of daily mood symptoms, treatments, sleep patterns, and life events to both help themselves and their providers treat the illness most effectively. This is often referred to as a *life chart*.
- Advise patients with bipolar spectrum disorders to avoid nicotine, sympathomimetic or anticholinergic drugs, caffeine, alcohol, or illicit drugs.
- For excellent patient education resources, visit eMedicine's Mental Health and Behavior Center and Bipolar Center. See also eMedicine's patient education articles on bipolar disorder.

Medical/Legal Pitfalls

- Failure to assess, monitor, and treat safety risk issues.
- Failure to assess for history of manic or hypomanic episodes when patient presents with depressive symptoms.
- Failure to assess for coexisting substance-use disorders.
- Failure to discontinue antidepressants if individual presents with acute mania or mixed mood symptoms.
- Failure to monitor for toxicity or metabolic changes associated with prescribed lithium and atypical antipsychotics.
- Prescribing an antidepressant during a MDE and not also prescribing a mood-stabilizing agent in patients with known bipolar spectrum disorders is a mistake. Only taking an antidepressant increases the risk of switching one's mood to either mania or hypomania, or developing rapid-cycling symptoms.

CYCLOTHYMIC DISORDER

Background Information

Definition of Disorder

- Cyclothymia is considered a mild, subthreshold form of bipolar disorder and is often referred to as a "soft" bipolar spectrum disorder.

■ The main difference between cyclothymic disorder and bipolar I disorder is the severity of the mania in that the symptoms do not meet the criteria for a manic episode in cyclothymia.

■ The main difference between cyclothymic disorder and bipolar II disorder is the severity of the depressive symptoms in that the depressive symptoms do not meet the full criteria for an MDE.

■ Mood changes in cyclothymic disorder can be abrupt and unpredictable, of short duration, and with infrequent euthymic episodes.

■ Both phases of the disorder appear deleterious to psychosocial functioning; however, they can also have high levels of achievement and creativity, which can be socially advantageous due to hypomania.

■ Hypomania or subthreshold depressive symptoms can last for weeks or days. In between up and down moods, a person may have normal moods or may continue to cycle continuously from hypomanic to depressed with no normal periods in between.

■ The mood swings in this disorder appear to be biphasic.

■ Cyclothymia symptoms are typically chronic, often do not appear to be related to life events, and appear to an observer as a personality trait.

■ Although the mood symptoms are milder than those of bipolar I and bipolar II disorders, they can be disabling due to unstable moods, and the unpredictability of the mood pattern can cause significant distress.

■ Some patients with cyclothymic disorder were characterized as being interpersonally sensitive, hyperactive, or moody as young children.

■ Onset of cyclothymic disorder after the age of 65 years is rare and alerts the practitioner to rule out organic reasons for the mood fluctuations.

■ It is not uncommon for cyclothymic disorder to go undetected.

■ Patients rarely seek treatment during the periods of hypomania because it is often considered a desired state.

Etiology
■ The exact cause of cyclothymic disorder is not known.

■ The *kindling theory* is the current predominant theory, meaning that the disorder is likely to be caused by multiple factors that potentially interact and lower the threshold at which mood changes occur. Eventually, a mood episode can start itself and thus become recurrent.

  ▪ Environmental factors
    ● Irregular sleep–wake patterns have been shown to trigger mood symptoms.
  ▪ Biological perspectives
    ● Genetics
      – Cyclothymic disorder appears more common in first-degree biological relatives of individuals with bipolar disorder.
      – An individual appears two to three times more likely to have cyclothymic disorder if first-degree biological relatives also have the disorder.
    ● Neural processes
      – The disorder appears to have a circadian component. Some patients state, for example, that they can go to bed in a good mood and wake up with subthreshold depressive symptoms.
      – Declines in rapid eye movement (REM) period latency during the sleep cycle have been noted in patients with cyclothymia.
      – Reduced skin conductance has been found in patients with cyclothymic disorder.

- Endocrine models
  - Endocrine studies in cyclothymia are very limited.
  - Hypothyroidism can cause depression and/or mood instability.
  - Cortisol hypersecretion and poor regulation of cortisol have been noted in patients with cyclothymia when faced with an experimental stressor.

Demographics

- True prevalence is not known due to misdiagnosis or undetected episodes of hypomania.
- At this time, it does not appear that epidemiological studies have been specifically conducted for cyclothymic disorder; however, lifetime prevalence of cyclothymic disorder is estimated to range from 0.3% to 6%, depending on the criteria used.
- Women and men are affected equally, but women typically present for treatment more often than do men.
- Medically, research has shown the following related to dysthymia, the subthreshold depression associated with this disorder:
  - Due to the subthreshold depression, patients with this disorder are approximately 2.6 times more likely to suffer a cerebral vascular accident and are at greater risk for cardiovascular disorders.
    - The presence of depressive symptoms in the absence of MDEs is associated with greater risk for cardiac events.
    - The aspect of depression—hopelessness—has been linked to sudden death.
    - The presence of vital exhaustion (fatigue, irritability, and demoralized feelings) has been reported to predict progression of coronary artery disease and/or cardiac events.
    - Cardiovascular mortality is almost elevated for individuals who have dysthymia. The risk of sudden death may also theoretically be increased due to reduced heart-rate variability.
  - Overall, 28% of patients who have mild depressive symptoms suffer from incapacitating medical conditions.
    - Forty-five percent of patients have chronic insomnia.
    - Four percent to 18 percent have comorbid diabetes mellitus.
    - Fourteen percent to 20 percent have HIV infection.
    - Three percent to 31 percent have significant premenstrual syndrome.
    - Fourteen percent have Parkinson's disease.
    - Twenty-eight percent experience chronic pain.
  - Individuals with dysthymia use medical treatment to a higher degree than the general population.

Risk Factors
Age

- Cyclothymic disorder usually begins in adolescence or in early adulthood.
- True age of onset is typically difficult to ascertain due to the insidious nature of the mood symptoms and its chronic course.
- Incidence rates are rare before puberty, and hypomanic episodes are not known in children.
- Cyclothymia and dysthymia appear common in adolescents, when the depressive onsets outnumber the nondepressive onsets.
- Often, the cycling between moods accelerates with age.

Gender
- Some studies indicate that men and women are affected equally and others state that women are affected more than men.
- Women in the premenstrual period may have worsening of ongoing hypomanic episodes or depressive symptoms.

Family History
- Individuals who have first-degree relatives diagnosed with bipolar disorder are at greater risk of cyclothymic disorder.

Stressful Events in Susceptible People
- Often, patients with cyclothymic disorder cannot identify an environmental precipitant to their moods.
- Ongoing psychosocial stressors have been shown to destabilize moods.
- Major life changes have also been shown to destabilize moods.

Having Another Mental Health Disorder
- Substance-use disorders
  - Individuals with cyclothymia are at heightened risk for substance abuse issues due to the high frequency of their mood symptoms.
  - Substance abuse is common in cyclothymic disorder, and it has been hypothesized that the individual is attempting to self-medicate the dysthymic mood symptoms and/or sleep disturbance or to precipitate and sustain hypomania.
- Bipolar I or bipolar II disorder
  - This disorder has a 15% to 50% risk that the individual will eventually develop bipolar I or bipolar II disorder.
- A diagnosis of attention deficit hyperactivity disorder
  - The diagnosis for a child may be a marker for a bipolar spectrum diagnosis as an adult.
- Personality disorders
  - Differentiating between individuals with cyclothymic disorder and particularly cluster B personality disorders (borderline personality disorder, histrionic personality disorder, and antisocial personality disorder) is difficult because the affective instability is similar.
  - Mood symptoms from cyclothymic disorder can be so flagrant that a personality disorder may be erroneously diagnosed.
  - Marked personality disorder symptoms negatively influence treatment-related outcomes in patients with bipolar disorder.

Risk Factors for Suicidal Behavior in Bipolar Spectrum Disorders
- Patients with cyclothymic disorder are at higher risk for suicide due to frequently changing mood episodes.
- Personal or family history of suicidal behavior.
- Severity and number of depressive episodes.
- Alcohol or substance abuse/dependence.
- Level of pessimism and hopelessness.
- Level of impulsivity and/or aggression.
- Younger age of onset of the disorder.
- A concomitant personality disorder diagnosis.
- Patients with remitting depressive symptoms are thought to be at an increased risk for suicide.

Risk Factors for Harm to Others in Bipolar Spectrum Disorders

- A history of violent behavior has consistently been shown to be the best single predictor of future violence.
- The presence of symptoms that increase the risk of violence in the absence of overt threats includes presenting as guarded and suspicious.
- Younger age.
- Gender is not a factor and the rates of violence among genders are equal in patients who are acutely mentally ill.
- A history of victimization as a child or witnessing or experiencing violence after the age of 16 years.
- Level of impulsivity.
- More than a half of victims of violence by persons with mental health disorders are family members.
- The availability of firearms and/or weapons.

Diagnosis

Differential Diagnosis

There is a broad differential diagnosis for bipolar spectrum disorders, which includes the following:

- Thyroid or other metabolic disorders
- Epilepsy (partial complex seizures)
- MS
- Diabetes mellitus
- Sleep apnea
- Brain lesions
- Systemic infection
- Systemic lupus erythematosus
- Cerebral vascular accident
- HIV
- Steroid-induced mood symptoms
- Vitamin B12 deficiency
- Vitamin D deficiency
- PTSD
- Attention deficit hyperactivity disorder
- Bipolar I or II disorder with rapid cycling
- MDD
- Dysthymic disorder
- Borderline personality disorder
- Eating disorder
- Drug interactions or adverse effects that can cause mood symptoms (e.g., baclofen, bromide, bromocriptine, captopril, cimetidine, corticosteroids, cyclosporine, disulfiram [Antabuse], hydralazine, isoniazid, levodopa, methylphenidate [Ritalin], metrizamide, procarbazine, procyclidine [Kemadrin])
- Drug or alcohol intoxication or withdrawal

ICD-Code

Cyclothymic disorder (F34.0)

Diagnostic Workup

- There are no biological tests that confirm cyclothymic disorder. Rather, tests are carried out to rule in/out medical issues that may be mimicking a mood disorder.

- *ANA*: ANAs are found in patients whose immune system may be predisposed to cause inflammation against their own body tissues. Antibodies that are directed against one's own tissues are referred to as autoantibodies.
  - Thyroid and other metabolic function studies suggest hyperexcitability or hypo-excitability symptoms.
  - Blood glucose level to rule out diabetes.
  - Serum proteins.
  - Lithium levels should be measured if patient has a history of diagnosis and is taking this medication.
  - CBC with differential is used to rule out anemia or other blood dyscrasias.
  - Urine toxicology screening for drug and alcohol screening.
  - Urine copper level; high levels indicate toxic exposure.
  - VDRL test.
  - HIV testing (ELISA and Western Blot test).
  - EKG determines cardiac anomolities.
  - Electroencephalogram may exclude epilepsy.
  - *Sleep study*: sleep apnea.
  - MRI determines presence of aneurysms, past head trauma, brain tumors.
  - CT scan of head is used to rule out head injury.
- Clinical history.
- Diagnosis is difficult to establish without a prolonged period of observation or obtaining an account from others about their moods and functioning across their life span. Thus, collateral information from close friends and family is important.

Initial Assessment

- It is important to gain a complete history and carefully assess for historical and/or current episodes of mania and/or hypomania as well as major depression and episodes of subclinical depression.
- Physical examination with a focus on neurological and endocrine systems and infectious diseases.
- Differentiation of cyclothymic disorder from personality disorders:
  - Periods of elevation and depression that typify affective disorders tend to be endogenous in cyclothymic disorder. This means that the mood symptoms come out of the blue with little external provocation.
  - Diurnal variations with worsening symptoms in the morning are typical in cyclothymic disorder.
  - The disturbances in cyclothymia are biphasic.
- Specific screening questions to assess for and rule out manic episodes, mixed episodes, or hypomanic episodes are as follows:
  - Have you ever experienced periods of feeling uncharacteristically energetic?
  - Have you had periods of not sleeping but not feeling tired?
  - Have you ever felt that your thoughts were racing and that there was nothing you could do to slow them down?
  - Have you ever experienced periods during which you did riskier things, were more interested in sex than usual, or were spending more money than you usually would?
- Uses of standardized screening tools:
  - BSDS
  - MDQ

▪ *The START*: assesses risk and guides treatment for violence, suicide, self-neglect, substance use, and victimization.
▪ Psychiatric assessment with a focus on current symptoms, date of onset, potential precipitating factors, perpetuating factors (e.g., drug or alcohol use), traumatic events in childhood, and substance use.
▪ Family history with an emphasis on psychiatric history and suicide attempts and completed suicides.
▪ Social history with an emphasis on current social support and safety issues in relationships, recent psychosocial stressors, ability to maintain employment, and financial concerns.
▪ Assessment of safety risk with an emphasis on history of harm to self or others, history of childhood abuse or victimization, plan and intent, and access to firearms and/or weapons.
▪ Level of functional impairment and need for hospitalization (e.g., ability to work, engage in self-care activities, ability to conduct activities of daily living, and ability to get along with others).

Clinical Presentation
Hypomanic Episode
▪ Affect/moods
  ▪ Up
  ▪ Expansive
  ▪ Irritable
  ▪ Moody
▪ Behaviors
  ▪ Busy
  ▪ Active
  ▪ Overinvolved
  ▪ Increased energy
  ▪ Increase in planning and doing things
  ▪ Social warmth
  ▪ Increased creativity and productivity
  ▪ Can be hypersexual
  ▪ Others notice their increase in activity but the patient often denies anything about them has changed
▪ Thoughts
  ▪ Optimistic
  ▪ Future focused
  ▪ Positive attitude
▪ Perceptions
  ▪ Patients with hypomania typically do not experience perceptual changes.

Dysthymia
▪ Vegetative symptoms usually seen in MDEs are not as common.
▪ Affect/moods:
  ▪ Continuously feeling sad
  ▪ Gloomy
  ▪ Irritable
  ▪ Excessive anger
▪ Behavior:

- Poor appetite
- Sleep disturbance
- Apathy
- Lack of motivation
- Introversion
- Social withdrawal
- Quiet and less talkative
- Generalized loss of interest or pleasure and incapable of fun
- Passive
- Somatization (e.g., increase in physical or somatic complaints without objective, identifiable cause)
- Conscientious and self-disciplining
- Thoughts:
  - Self-critical, self-reproaching, and self-derogatory
  - Pessimistic
  - Poor concentration and indecisiveness
  - Worry and rumination (brooding)
  - Preoccupied with their inadequacy, failures, or negative life events
  - Hopelessness
  - Helplessness
- Perceptions:
  - Patients with dysthymia typically do not experience perceptual changes.
  - Biphasic characteristics of cyclothymic disorder.
- Lethargy alternates with good moods.
- Unexplained tearfulness alternates with excessive wit and humor.
- Introversion and self-absorption alternate with uninhibited seeking of people.
- Mental confusion alternates with sharpened thinking.
- Shaky self-esteem alternates between low self-confidence and overconfidence.

Diagnostic and Statistical Manual of Mental Disorders, Fifth Edition: Diagnostic Guidelines
Cyclothymic Disorder
- For at least 2 years, the patient has had multiple periods in which hypomanic symptoms have been present and multiple periods of low mood that have not fulfilled the criteria for a MDE or hypomanic episode.
- The longest period in which the patient has been free of mood swings is 2 months.
- During the first 2 years of the disorder, the patient had not had periods of mood disturbance in which the criteria for a manic episode, a mixed episode, or a MDE were also met.
- The symptoms are not more easily ascribed to other medical diagnoses, other medical conditions, substance use, or drug withdrawal.
- The disturbances in mood engender significant distress for the individual and/or a reduction in social or other important areas of functioning.

Hypomanic
- For at least 4 days, the patient manifests a mood that is elevated, expansive, or irritable, and representing a distinct departure from the patient's nondepressed baseline mood.
- During this period, the patient has three or more of the following:
  - Grandiose thoughts, inflated self-esteem
  - Diminished sleep

- Volubility
- Racing thoughts
- Increased levels of distractibility
- Psychomotor agitation
- A focus on goal-directed activities
- Poor judgment; activities that have potential for adverse outcomes (e.g., spending sprees)
- Psychotic features are absent.
- Appropriate social and occupational functioning are maintained.
- Hospitalization is not required.
- The symptoms are not more easily ascribed to other medical diagnoses, other medical conditions, substance use, or withdrawal from prescription medication.

Treatment Overview

Acute Treatment

- The primary goal of the acute phase is to manage acute hypomania episodes and subclinical depression and associated safety risk issues.
- Specific treatment studies for cyclothymic disorder separate from other bipolar spectrum disorders are minimal.
- Diagnostic tests should be performed to rule out potential medical etiologies for mood symptoms, especially if this is the first episode of mania, hypomania, mixed mood symptoms, or depression.
- How to handle suicidal ideation:
  - Patients with suicidal ideation with plan and intent should be hospitalized (voluntarily or involuntarily) due to acute safety risk.
  - Patients with suicidal ideation with plan but no intent may be treated on an outpatient basis with close follow-up if they do not have access to the means to carry out their plan and adequate social support.
  - Patients with suicidal ideation without plan and no intent require careful assessment of current psychosocial stressors, access to weapons, and other lethal means, substance use, and impulse control issues. Any lethal means should be removed.
- How to handle aggression and potential harm to others:
  - If patients have access to firearms and/or weapons, they should be removed.
  - Those with thoughts of harming others with plan and intent should be hospitalized (voluntarily or involuntarily).
  - Those with thoughts of harming others with plan but no intent can be treated on an outpatient basis, with increased intensity of treatment with an established provider, depending on risk factors.
  - Those with thoughts of harming others without plan or intent do require increased intensity of treatment and perhaps increased dosages of medications.
- Acute hypomanic episode:
  - Treatment for hypomania, which can lead to either a manic or a depressive episode, may decrease symptom progression.
- Medication noncompliance is common because hypomania may be a desired state for many individuals with cyclothymic disorder, and many are reluctant to take medications.
- Because this disorder is considered a chronic and lifelong illness, long-term treatment is needed to manage and control mood symptoms.

Chronic Treatment

- The primary goal of long-term treatment is to prevent cyclothymia from worsening and progressing to full-blown manic episodes.
- Specific treatment studies for cyclothymia as distinct from other bipolar spectrum disorders are minimal.
- Study results from a large-scale National Institute of Mental Health–funded clinical trial found patients treated with both medications and intensive psychotherapy (30 sessions over 9 months of therapy) for bipolar spectrum disorders demonstrated the following:
  - Fewer relapses
  - Lower hospitalization rates
  - Better ability to stick to treatment plans
  - More likely to get well faster and stay well longer
- Medications:
  - Long-term management of cyclothymic disorder should be treated with a mood stabilizer.
  - Antidepressant medications have not been shown to be an effective adjunctive therapy, and as a monotherapy they can precipitate mania, mixed mood symptoms, or hypomania.

Overview of Pharmacotherapy for Cyclothymic Disorder

- *Mood stabilizers*, including mood-stabilizing anticonvulsants, atypical antipsychotic agents, and lithium, are identified as first-line treatment approaches. Lithium and Lamictal are recommended for bipolar depression. Mood-stabilizing anticonvulsants (e.g., valproate and lamotrigine) are preferred for rapid-cycling disorders.
- For patients unresponsive to monotherapy, a combination of lithium and mood-stabilizing anticonvulsant or mood stabilizer plus atypical antipsychotic may be considered.
- Hypomanic episodes and mild depressive episodes are generally managed with a single mood stabilizer. Acute manic and severe depressive episodes often require two or three medications.
- A benzodiazepine (e.g., diazepam or lorazepam) may be considered as an adjunct short-term treatment for reducing insomnia or agitation.
- Use of antidepressants by primary care providers for treating bipolar patients should be avoided. Antidepressant monotherapy may precipitate mania or induce rapid-cycling disorders between mania and depression.
- Dosage adjustments may be required if the patient experiences a partial response or breakthrough symptoms.

Drug Selection Table for Cyclothymic Disorder

CLASS	DRUG
Mood-stabilizing anticonvulsants	First-line drug therapy Valproate sodium, valproic acid, divalproex sodium (Depacon, Depakene, Depakote, Depakote ER, Depakote Sprinkle) Carbamazepine (Tegretol, Carbatrol, Tegretol XR) Topiramate (Topamax) Lamotrigine (Lamictal, Lamictal XR)

Drug Selection Table for Cyclothymic Disorder (*continued*)

CLASS	DRUG
Nonanticonvulsant mood stabilizer	First-line drug therapy for bipolar depression Lithium (Eskalith, Lithobid)
Atypical antipsychotics (second generation)	Aripiprazole (Abilify) Olanzapine (Zyprexa) Risperidone (Risperdal, Risperdal Consta) Quetiapine (Seroquel, Seroquel XR) Ziprasidone (Geodon)

- ECT may be considered for treatment-resistant or severe mania. In general, mood-stabilizer treatment has produced better outcomes than ECT.
- ECT is used only as a last resort, if the patient does not adequately respond to medications and/or psychotherapy.
- Psychotherapy:
  - *CBT*: helps individuals with bipolar disorder learn to change harmful and negative thought patterns and behaviors, as well as learn coping skills such as stress management, identifying triggers for mood symptoms, and relaxation techniques.
  - *Family therapy*: includes family members. By doing so, it helps family members enhance coping strategies, such as recognizing new episodes and how to help their loved one. Therapy also focuses on communication skills and problem solving.
    - *Interpersonal therapy*: helps people with bipolar disorder improve their relationships with others.
  - *Social rhythm therapy*: focuses on maintaining and managing their daily routines such as regular sleep–wake cycles, eating patterns, and social routines.
  - *Psychoeducation*: focuses on teaching individuals with bipolar disorder about the illness and its treatment. This form of treatment helps people realize signs of relapse so that they can access treatment early before a full episode occurs. This is usually in a group format and it may also be helpful for family members and caregivers.
- Psychodynamic and psychoanalytic therapies do not appear to have an effect in patients with this disorder.
- Follow-up care by a chemical dependence treatment specialist is recommended when indicated.
- Patients with cardiac comorbidity, abnormal findings on cardiac examination, or significant risk factors for heart disease should be referred to a cardiologist.
- Patients with endocrine dysfunction, such as hyperthyroidism or hypothyroidism, should be referred to an endocrinologist.
- Treatment can be complicated or have a poorer course by having another condition at the same time, such as substance abuse, depression, anxiety disorders, or a personality disorder.
- Concomitant substance abuse/dependence is correlated with increased hospitalizations and a worse course of the illness and increases safety risk.

Recurrence Rate

- Approximately one third of all patients diagnosed with cyclothymic disorder will develop a major mood disorder during their lifetime, and it is usually bipolar II disorder.

- Retrospective studies of patients with cyclothymia, taking lithium over a 2-year period, indicated the following:
  - Only 26% to 36% were free of depression symptoms as compared to 42% to 55% for patients with bipolar II and 31% to 42% for patients with a unipolar designation.
  - The probability rate for hospitalization due to severity of depression symptoms was 69% for patients with cyclothymia versus 51% for patients with bipolar II and 64% for patients with a unipolar designation.
- Patients diagnosed with cyclothymia and treated with valproate required lower doses and serum concentrations to achieve mood stabilization as compared to patients with blood pressure (BP) disorder.
- Patient behaviors that can lead to a recurrence of depressive or manic symptoms are as follows:
  - Discontinuing or lowering one's dose of medication.
  - An inconsistent sleep schedule can destabilize the illness. Too much sleep can lead to depression, whereas too little sleep can trigger and sustain hypomania.
  - Inadequate stress management and poor lifestyle choices.
  - Medication raises the stress threshold somewhat, but too much stress still causes relapse.
  - Using drugs or alcohol can either trigger or prolong mood symptoms.

Patient Education

- Advise patients that it is important to deal with mania early in the episode, and thus recognizing the early-warning signs is the key so that more intensive treatment can be administered before symptoms escalate.
- Advise patient to stay on all medications and to not decrease or stop any medications without medical supervision. This is especially important when experiencing mania or hypomania.
- Also advise patients that sometimes several medication trials are needed to find ones that will be efficacious in controlling mood symptoms.
- Advise patients that symptoms will improve gradually, not immediately, as they begin to remit.
- In general, there is little research about herbal or natural supplements for bipolar spectrum disorders and not much is known about their efficacy; however, St. John's wort may cause a switch to mania and can make other medications less effective (e.g., antidepressants and anticonvulsants). May cause serious drug interactions and serotonin syndrome—as this is a natural SSRI and people don't realize that. Additionally, the effects of Sam-E or omega-3 fatty acids are not known. All herbal and natural remedies for mood symptoms should be discussed with a medical care provider.
- The best approach to treatment is a combination of psychotherapy and medications. This helps prevent relapses, reduces hospitalizations, and helps the patient get well faster and stay well longer.
- If patients plan extensive travel into other time zones, advise them to call their doctors before leaving to determine whether any changes in their medicines should be made and what to do if they have mood episode while away.
- Women who are pregnant or would like to become pregnant and have been diagnosed with a cyclothymic disorder should speak with their doctors about the risks and benefits of all treatments during pregnancy. Mood-stabilizing medications used today can cause harm to the developing fetus or a nursing infant.

Additionally, stopping or reducing medications during pregnancy can cause a recurrence of mood symptoms.

■ Helping the individual identify and modify stressors provides a critical aspect of patient and family awareness.

■ Changes in sleep patterns can sometimes trigger a manic or depressive episode. Advise patients to keep a regular routine such as eating meals at the same time every day and going to sleep at the same time nightly and waking up at the same time daily.

■ Patients should be encouraged to keep a chart of daily mood symptoms, treatments, sleep patterns, and life events to help both themselves and their providers treat the illness most effectively. This is often referred to as a *life chart*.

■ Advise patients with cyclothymia to avoid nicotine, sympathomimetic or anticholinergic drugs, caffeine, alcohol, or illicit drugs.

■ For excellent patient education resources, visit eMedicine's Mental Health and Behavior Center and Bipolar Center. See also eMedicine's patient education articles on bipolar disorder.

Medical/Legal Pitfalls

■ Failure to assess, monitor, and treat safety–risk issues.

■ Failure to assess for history of manic or hypomanic episodes when patient presents with depressive symptoms.

■ Failure to assess for coexisting substance-use disorders.

■ Failure to monitor for toxicity or metabolic changes associated with prescribed lithium.

■ Prescribing and not properly monitoring divalproex (Depakote) and valproic acid (Depakene) for women younger than 20 years is problematic. This medication may increase the levels of testosterone, which can lead to polycystic ovary syndrome (PCOS). Most PCOS symptoms begin after stopping treatment with valproic acid (Depakene).

■ Prescribing an antidepressant for depressive symptoms and not also prescribing a mood-stabilizing agent in patients with known bipolar spectrum disorders is risky. Only taking an antidepressant increased the risk of switching the patient's mood to either mania or hypomania, or developing rapid-cycling symptoms.

PERSISTENT DEPRESSIVE DISORDER (DYSTHYMIC DISORDER)

Background Information

Definition of Disorder

■ This is a chronic mood disorder characterized by depressed mood more days than not, indicated by the individual or by others.

■ Dysthymic disorder is associated with increased morbidity from physical disease.

■ Patients often possess a negative, gloomy outlook on life with ruminative coping strategies.

■ Tendency toward self-criticism and a sense of inadequacy.

■ Tend to spend limited time in leisure activities.

Persistent depressive disorder is characterized by long-term (2 years or longer) but less severe symptoms that may not disable a person but that prevent normal functioning or feeling well. People with dysthymia may also experience one or more episodes of major depression during their lifetimes.

Etiology

- It is thought to be a result of an interplay between genetic factors, chronic stress, and personality factors.
- Biological factors such as alterations in neurotransmitters, endocrine, and inflammatory mediators are also thought to play a role.
- Cognitive and personality factors, such as how people view their influence, their ability to change, and their interpretation of stressors, play a role.
- Cases are very likely to have a family history of mood disorders, particularly dysthymia and MDD.

Demographics

- Data suggest that the disorder affects 3% to 6% of the U.S. general population and 5% to 15% of the primary care population. It affects approximately 36% of patients in outpatient mental health treatment centers.
- Women are twice as likely to present with dysthymic disorder than men.
- It often starts at childhood or adolescence with an early sense of unhappiness without clear cause.
- One large study showed it to be more common in African Americans and Mexican Americans than in Whites (the opposite pattern from MDD).
- One study showed a 77% lifetime risk for developing MDD and a higher risk for suicide attempts among patients with dysthymic disorder than patients with MDD.
- The prevalence rate of dysthymic disorder is 0.6% to 1.7% in children and 1.6% to 8% in adolescents.
- Patients with dysthymic disorder should not be seen as simply having a "mild form of depression." They are at high risk for developing MDD and often have MDD, which is harder to treat.
- Patients with dysthymic disorder should be evaluated for suicide risk.

Risk Factors

Gender

- Like other depressive disorders, dysthymic disorder is approximately two times more common in women than men.

Family History

- Studies have shown an increased incidence of dysthymic disorder when there is a history of depression, bipolar disorder, or dysthymia in first-degree relatives.
- There are learned or genetic personality factors such as poor coping skills, particularly ruminative rather than problem-solving or cognitive-restructuring strategies.

Past Medical History

- Chronic medical illness
- History of MDD

Social History

- Lack of social support
- Multiple relationship losses

Having Another Mental Health Disorder

- Diagnosis with a personality disorder (antisocial, borderline, dependent, depressive, histrionic, or schizotypal), in particular, places a patient at higher risk for dysthymia.

■ Alcohol abuse or substance abuse places a patient at higher risk for dysthymic disorder. Approximately, 15% of patients with depressive disorder (DD) have comorbid substance dependence.

Diagnosis

Differential Diagnosis

■ Common:
  ▪ MDD
  ▪ Recurrent brief depressive disorder
  ▪ Alcoholism or substance abuse
  ▪ Thyroid disease
  ▪ Anemia
  ▪ Chronic fatigue syndrome
  ▪ If an underlying chronic health condition such as MS or stroke is the physiological *cause* of the depressed mood, the diagnosis is mood disorder due to a general medical condition
  ▪ Anxiety disorders, such as PTSD or obsessive-compulsive disorder
  ▪ Dementia
  ▪ Drug interactions or adverse effects
  ▪ Sleep apnea
  ▪ Personality disorder
■ Less common:
  ▪ Bipolar disorder
  ▪ Amphetamine or cocaine withdrawal
  ▪ Infectious disease, such as autoimmune disorder, mononucleosis, or hepatitis C
  ▪ Parathyroid disease
  ▪ Adrenal disease
  ▪ Fibromyalgia
  ▪ Cancer
  ▪ Neurological disease, such as cerebral vascular accident, MS, subdural hematoma, normal pressure hydrocephalus, or Alzheimer's disease
  ▪ Cardiovascular disease such as CHF or cardiomyopathy
  ▪ Nutritional deficiency, such as B vitamin, folate, or iron deficiency
  ▪ Pulmonary disease, such as COPD
  ▪ Heavy metal poisoning

ICD-10 Code

Persistent depressive disorder (dysthymia) (F34.1)

Diagnostic Workup

■ Physical and mental evaluation:
  ▪ Thyroid function studies (T3, T4, TSH levels)
  ▪ Complete metabolic panel
  ▪ CBC with differential
  ▪ Vitamin D level
  ▪ Testing for infectious diseases such as hepatitis C or HIV, if applicable

Initial Assessment

■ Mental status examination often shows slowed speech, decreased eye contact, diminished range of facial expression with self-doubt, sadness, guilt, hopelessness, and/or negative outlook. Thought will be organized without disruption of intellect, memory, abstraction, or significant abnormalities (such as delusions).

■ Use of a standard depression screening tool such as Beck Depression Inventory, or Zung Self-Rating Scale, to rule out MDD.

■ *Past medical history*: If any MDD has been diagnosed in the past 2 years, the patient does not have dysthymic disorder.

■ Family medical history, with emphasis on psychiatric history.

■ Social history, including safety of relationships, family support, and recent or ongoing stressors.

■ Past suicide attempts or past psychiatric hospitalizations.

■ Any prior manic/hypomanic episodes (any history suggests bipolar or cyclothymia diagnosis).

■ What effect have symptoms had on ability to function, particularly participation in nonoccupational activities?

■ Assess for suicide ideation, suicide plan, and suicide intent.

Clinical Presentation
■ Low self-esteem
■ Difficulties with sleep
■ Low energy or fatigue
■ Difficulty in decision-making
■ Feeling hopeless
■ Changes in eating habits; either decrease or increase in appetite
■ Decreased facial expression
■ Slowed speech or movements
■ Decreased eye contact
■ Poor concentration

Diagnostic and Statistical Manual of Mental Disorders, Fifth Edition: Diagnostic Guidelines
■ Persistent, long-term depressed mood and/or anhedonia (2 years or more in adults, 1 year or more in children and adolescents) in combination with at least two of the following:
  ■ Changes in eating habits
  ■ Changes in sleep habits
  ■ Fatigue, low energy
  ■ Lowered self-esteem
  ■ Distractibility, problems with concentration
  ■ Hopelessness
■ Periods of remission have not been >2 months.
■ There has been no MDE during the same period.
■ Psychotic features are absent.
■ Absence of manic or hypomanic episodes.
■ Evidence for cyclothymia is absent.
■ The symptoms engender distress in the individual and/or a reduction in social functioning.

Treatment Overview
Therapies
■ Studies support the pharmacological approach as the first-line treatment for dysthymic disorder. Approximately 55% of patients with DD will respond to pharmacologic therapy. Doses are the same as for major depression.

■ Both psychological and pharmacological therapies are effective in the treatment of dysthymic disorder and each has its own merits. The combination of antidepressants and psychotherapy, such as talk therapy, is recommended for dysthymic disorder patients for long-term treatment.

■ Pay careful attention in the first 1 to 4 weeks of antidepressant treatment to a sudden lift of depression or to worsening mood as initial response to antidepressant therapy, as these could be signs of increased risk for suicide.

■ Be aware of the Federal Drug Administration black box warning regarding antidepressant treatment in children and younger adults and use appropriate caution in these patients.

■ Regular follow-up for medication management, assistance for overcoming treatment resistance through augmentation therapy, and so forth; tracking patient progress in individual psychotherapy; monitoring for MDD; and reinforcement of patient self-efficacy are all important to care.

■ Stress management and lifestyle changes, such as regular exercise, are essential to ongoing care.

■ Studies suggest that augmentation of antidepressant effect occurs with adjunct use of omega-3 fish oil supplements, 1,000 mg BID daily. B vitamin supplementation has also been used in some studies, with equivocal results.

■ Psychodynamic therapy, addressing an understanding of maladaptive interpersonal responses, CBT, and interpersonal therapy—which involves addressing interpersonal conflicts through improved strategies—have all been found beneficial in the treatment of patients with dysthymic disorder. Group therapy may also be helpful.

■ Treatment may be complicated by having another condition at the same time, such as substance abuse, personality disorders, or other anxiety disorders, and these should also be addressed.

Drug Selection Table for Dysthymic Disorders

CLASS	DRUG
SSRIs	First-line drug therapy Fluoxetine (Prozac) Sertraline (Zoloft) Paroxetine (Paxil, Paxil CR) Citalopram (Celexa) Escitalopram (Lexapro) Fluvoxamine (Luvox)
SNRIs	Venlafaxine (Effexor) Venlafaxine XR (Effexor XR) Duloxetine (Cymbalta) Desvenlafaxine (Pristiq)
SARIs	Second-line drug therapy Nefazodone (Serzone) Trazodone (Desyrel)
NaSSAs	Alternative therapy option Mirtazapine (Remeron)
NDRIs	Alternative therapy option Bupropion (Wellbutrin, Zyban) Bupropion SR (Wellbutrin SR)

Drug Selection Table for Dysthymic Disorders (*continued*)

CLASS	DRUG
TCAs	Bupropion XL (Wellbutrin XL) Amitriptyline (Elavil) Clomipramine (Anafranil) Desipramine (Norpramin) Imipramine (Tofranil)
MAOIs	Nortriptyline (Pamelor) Phenelzine (Nardil) Isocarboxazid (Marplan) Tranylcypromine (Parnate)

MAOIs, monoamine oxidase inhibitors; NaSSAs, noradrenergic and specific serotonergic antidepressants; NDRIs, norepinephrine/dopamine reuptake inhibitors; SARIs, serotonin-2 antagonist/reuptake inhibitors; SNRIs, serotonin-norepinephrine reuptake inhibitors; SSRIs, selective serotonin reuptake inhibitors; TCAs, tricyclic antidepressants.

Recurrence Rate
- In one study, there was a 53% estimated 5-year recovery rate from dysthymic disorder but a very high risk of relapse.

Patient Education
- Advise patients with dysthymic disorder to avoid nicotine and to avoid alcohol.
- Thirty minutes of daily exercise have been found to be beneficial for patients with dysthymic disorder, and daily exposure to outdoor light may be beneficial.
- For excellent patient education resources, visit eMedicine's Mental Health and Behavior Center and Depression Center. See also eMedicine's patient education articles on Dysthymic Disorder.

Medical/Legal Pitfalls
- Failure to monitor for suicidal thoughts.
- Failure to screen for bipolar disorder (any history of mania/hypomania).
- Pay careful attention, in the first 1 to 4 weeks of treatment, to a sudden lift of depression or to worsening mood as an initial response to antidepressant therapy, as these could be signs of increased risk for suicide.
- It is important that patients with dysthymic disorder be viewed as having a severe and chronic condition, which must be monitored and managed.
- When initiating treatment, see patients on a more frequent basis until response to antidepressant is clear.
- Have a follow-up system to ensure that there are calls to patients who fail to schedule follow-up appointments or fail to show up for scheduled appointments.
- Patients with dysthymic disorder are more likely than the general population to use alternative therapies. Use of dietary supplements (e.g., herbs) should be discussed to avoid drug interactions.

BIBLIOGRAPHY

Akiskal, H. S. (2001). Dysthymia and cyclothymia in psychiatric practice a century after Kraepelin. *Journal of Affective Disorders, 62*(1–2), 17–31.

American Psychiatric Association. (2013). *Diagnostic and statistical manual of mental disorder* (5th ed.). Washington, DC: American Psychiatric Publishing.

Bauer, M., Beaulieu, S., Dunner, D. L., Lafer, B., & Kupka, R. (2008). Rapid cycling bipolar disorder–diagnostic concepts. *Bipolar Disorders, 10*(1 Pt. 2), 153–162.

Ghaemi, S. N., Hsu, D. J., Thase, M. E., Wisniewski, S. R., Nierenberg, A. A., Miyahara, S., & Sachs, G. (2006). Pharmacological treatment patterns at study entry for the first 500 STEP-BD participants. *Psychiatric Services, 57*(5), 660–665.

Goldberg, J. F., Allen, M. H., Miklowitz, D. A., Bowden, C. L., Endick, C. J., Chessick, C. A., Wisniewski, S. R., Miyahara, S., Sagduyu, K., Thase, M. E., Calabrese, J. R., & Sachs, G. S. (2005). Suicidal ideation and pharmacotherapy among STEP-BD patients. *Psychiatric Services, 56*(12), 1534–1540.

Goldberg, J. F., Perlis, R. H., Ghaemi, S. N., Calabrese, J. R., Bowden, C. L., Wisniewski, S., Miklowitz, D. J., Sachs, G. S., & Thase, M. E. (2007). Adjunctive antidepressant use and symptomatic recovery among bipolar depressed patients with concomitant manic symptoms: Findings from the STEP-BD. *American Journal of Psychiatry, 164*(9), 1348–1355.

Harel, E. V., & Levkovitz, Y. (2008). Effectiveness and safety of adjunctive antidepressants in the treatment of bipolar depression: a review. *Israel Journal of Psychiatry and Related Sciences, 45*(2), 121–128.

Hirshfeld, R. M. (2002). The mood disorder questionnaire: A simple, patient-related screening instrument for bipolar disorder. *Primary Care Companion for the Journal of Psychiatry, 4*(1), 9–11.

Manning, J. S., Ahmed, S., McGuire, H. C., & Hay, D. P. (2002). Mood disorders in family practice: Beyond unipolarity to bipolarity. *Primary Care Companion to the Journal of Clinical Psychiatry, 4*(4), 142–150.

Martinez, J. M., Marangell, L. B., Simon, N. M., Miyahara, S., Wisniewski, S. R., Harrington, J., Pollack, M. H., Sachs, G. S., & Thase, M. E. (2005). Baseline predictors of serious adverse events at one year among patients with bipolar disorder in STEP-BD. *Psychiatric Services, 56*(12), 1541–1548.

Miklowitz, D. J., Otto, M. W., Frank, E., Reilly-Harrington, N. A., Kogan, J. N., Sachs, G. S., Thase, M. E., Calabrese, J. R., Marangell, L. B., Ostacher, M. J., Patel, J., Thomas, M. R., Araga, M., Gonzalez, J. M., & Wisniewski, S. R. (2007). Intensive psychosocial intervention enhances functioning in patients with bipolar depression: Results from a 9-month randomized controlled trial. *American Journal of Psychiatry, 164*(9), 1340–1347.

Miklowitz, D. J., Otto, M. W., Wisniewski, S. R., Araga, M., Frank, E., Reilly-Harrington, N. A., Lembke, A., & Sachs, G. S. (2006). Psychotherapy, symptom outcomes, and role functioning over one year among patients with bipolar disorder. *Psychiatric Services, 57*(7), 959–965.

National Mental Health. (n.d.). *Bipolar disorder.* https://www.nimh.nih.gov/health/statistics/bipolar-disorder.shtml

National Mental Health. (n.d.). *Major depression.* https://www.nimh.nih.gov/health/statistics/major-depression.shtml

National Mental Health. (n.d.). *A report of the surgeon general.* http://www.surgeongeneral.gov/library/mentalhealth/home.html

National Mental Health. (n.d.). *Suicide.* https://www.nimh.nih.gov/health/statistics/suicide.shtml

Perlis, R. H., Ostacher, M. J., Patel, J. K., Marangell, L. B., Zhang, H., Wisniewski, S. R., Ketter, T. A., Miklowitz, D. J., Otto, M. W., Gyulai, L., Reilly-Harrington, N. A., Nierenberg, A. A., Sachs, G. S., & Thase, M. E. (2006). Predictors of recurrence in bipolar disorder: Primary outcomes from the Systematic Treatment Enhancement Program for Bipolar Disorder (STEP-BD). *American Journal of Psychiatry, 163*(2), 217–224.

President's New Freedom Commission on Mental Health. (2003). https://www.federalregister.gov/documents/2002/05/03/02-11166/presidents-new-freedom-commission-on-mental-health

Sadock, B., Sadock, V., & Ruiz, P. (2015). *Kaplan & Sadock's synopsis of psychiatry* (11th ed.). Wolters Kluwer.

Schneck, C. D., Miklowitz, D. J., Miyahara, S., Araga, M., Wisniewski, S., Gyulai, L., Allen, M. H., Thase, M. E., & Sachs, G. S. (2008). The prospective course of rapid-cycling bipolar disorder: Findings from the STEP-BD. *American Journal of Psychiatry, 165*(3), 370–377; quiz 410.

Tusaie, K., & Fitzpatrick, J. (2017). *Advanced practice psychiatric nursing* (2nd ed.). Springer Publishing Company.

Wheeler, K. (2014). *Psychotherapy for the advanced practice psychiatric nurse* (2nd ed.). Springer Publishing Company.

WEB RESOURCES

- American Psychiatric Association: http://www.psych.org/
- American Psychological Association: www.apa.org/
- Depression and Bipolar Support Alliance (DBSA): www.dbsalliance.org/
- MacArthur Initiative on Depression and Primary Care: http://www.depression-primarycare.org/
- National Alliance of the Mentally Ill (NAMI): http://www.nami.org/
- National Institute of Mental Health: nimh.nih.gov/
- National Suicide Prevention Lifeline: http://www.suicidepreventionlifeline.org/

12

Anxiety Disorders

OVERVIEW

- Anxiety disorders are the most common type of psychiatric disorders, with an incidence of 18.1% and a lifetime prevalence of 28.8%.
- They account for an annual cost of $42.3 billion in the United States, with more than 50% of the total sum directed toward nonpsychiatric medical treatment costs.
- Patients with anxiety disorders also have a high comorbidity with mood disorders.
- Following are the types of anxiety disorders: separation anxiety disorder, selective mutism, social anxiety disorder, panic disorder (PD), agoraphobia, generalized anxiety disorder (GAD), substance/medication-induced anxiety disorder, anxiety disorder due to another medical condition, other specified anxiety disorder, and unspecified anxiety disorder.

SEPARATION ANXIETY DISORDER

Background Information

Definition of Disorder

The primary trait of separation anxiety disorder is a disproportionate fear or anxiety pertaining to separation from home or an attachment figure. The anxiety level exceeds what would be considered expected in relation to the individual's developmental level. To meet the diagnostic criteria for separation anxiety disorder, symptoms must persist for a period of at least 4 weeks for children and adolescents younger than 18 years and persist for a period of 6 months or longer for adults. In relation to adult separation anxiety, there is some degree of flexibility regarding the time frame and thus the criterion of symptoms over a period of 6 months is provided as a general guide. A key feature is that the symptoms result in significant distress or impairment in important areas of social functioning.

Etiology

Anxiety and overprotection by a parent may be associated with separation anxiety disorder, as is an insecure parent–child attachment. Separation anxiety may also be heritable to some degree. Separation anxiety often develops in response to life stress, especially related to a significant loss. Changes in a child's environment, such as a move to a different neighborhood or a different school, may also cause separation anxiety in a child.

Demographics
In adults, in the United States, there is 0.9% to 1.9% prevalence for a 12-month period, whereas for children, a 6- to 12-month prevalence is 1.6%.

Risk Factors
Age
- It is more prevalent in children younger than 12 years but can occur at any age.

Gender
- Equally prevalent in males and females. Girls may exhibit more avoidance behavior than boys, such as reluctance to go to school. The expression of separation anxiety disorder in boys may be more indirect, such as a reluctance to be away from home.

Family History
- Parental overprotection and anxiety may be associated with separation anxiety disorder.

Stressful Events in Susceptible People
- Stressful life events and significant loss are often related to the development of separation anxiety disorder.

Diagnosis
Differential Diagnosis
- GAD
- PD
- Agoraphobia
- Conduct disorder
- Social anxiety disorder
- Posttraumatic stress disorder
- Illness anxiety disorder
- Bereavement
- Depressive and bipolar disorders
- Oppositional defiant disorder
- Psychotic disorders
- Personality disorders

ICD-10 Code
Separation anxiety disorder (F93.0)

Diagnostic Workup
- Physical and mental evaluation

Initial Assessment
- Full history and physical (H&P) examination
- Developmental history and family history
- Assessment of trauma or past event/stressor
- *Symptoms*: emotional, cognitive, and physical

- Labs as needed to evaluate anxiety symptoms and physical symptoms
- Thyroid function, complete metabolic panel, B12 level, and complete blood count (CBC)

Clinical Presentation

Excess worry and anxiety related to actual or potential separation from home or attachment figures and avoidance of activities that would require being away from home or attachment figures. Psychophysiological symptoms, such as headaches, nausea, vomiting, stomachaches, palpitations, and dizziness when anticipating separation, particularly in young children. Children may also exhibit clinging behavior.

Diagnostic and Statistical Manual of Mental Disorders, Fifth Edition: Diagnostic Guidelines

Diagnostic Criteria Include the Following:
A. Excessive fear or anxiety related to separation from an attachment figure that is developmentally excessive, which includes at least one of the following criteria:
1. The distress experienced is recurrent in nature related to experiencing a separation from home or from attachment figures.
2. Ongoing worry related to losing an attachment figure.
3. Excessive fears related to an anticipated event such as getting lost, being kidnapped, or other event that would result in a separation from the attachment figure.
4. Fear of separation leads to a reluctance to leave home.
5. Fear of being alone without the presence of the attachment figure.
6. Reluctance to sleep away from home or go to sleep without the presence of the attachment figure.
7. Recurrent nightmares with the theme of separation.
8. Physical complaints with anticipation of separation from the attachment figure.
B. Fear and anxiety lasting a period of 4 weeks in children and adolescents and at least 6 months for adults; symptoms are persistent in nature.
C. There is marked distress along with impairment in social functioning in areas that are significant to the individual.
D. The symptoms are not better explained by another mental disorder, health problem, or concerns about significant others.

Treatment Overview

- Cognitive-behavioral therapy (CBT)
- Relaxation exercises
- Family therapy when young children or adolescents are experiencing separation anxiety disorder
- Stress reduction techniques (systematic desensitization)

Psychopharmacology

- Selective serotonin reuptake inhibitors (SSRIs), such as sertraline (*Zoloft*), are considered first-line treatment for anxiety.
  - Serotonin-norepinephrine reuptake inhibitors (SNRIs), such as venlafaxine XR, have shown some efficacy in management of anxiety but are not considered a first line of treatment in children.
  - Benzodiazepines (BZDs) may have a limited, short-term role, particularly in children who are suffering from impairing physical symptoms. Such symptoms may result in significant lost school time and may keep the child from benefiting from psychotherapy due to preoccupation with somatic symptoms.

Patient Education

■ Education regarding the development of separation anxiety disorder related to a significant loss; individual therapy for adults and adolescents.

Medical/Legal Pitfalls

■ Screen for a medical condition that mimics anxiety disorders.

SELECTIVE MUTISM

Background Information

Definition of Disorder

Children with selective mutism demonstrate a lack of speech in social situations. In such situations, they do not initiate speech or respond with speech. Children with selective mutism will speak in their homes with immediate family members but tend not to speak with extended family or friends. They often refuse to speak at school, leading to academic problems. Shyness, anxiety, clinging behavior, withdrawal, and social isolation are common associated features. Some children may exhibit mild oppositional behavior or temper tantrums. Children with selective mutism generally have normal language skills; however, at times there may be a communication disorder.

Etiology

Selective mutism is a rare disorder with a prevalence between 0.03% and 1%.

Demographics

The prevalence of selective mutism does not vary by gender, race, or ethnicity.

Risk Factors

The disorder occurs in young children rather than adolescents and adults. Risk factors have not been well identified. Shyness and a parental history of shyness may play a significant role. Children with language difficulties may be more predisposed as compared to young children without language difficulties. There may be a genetic component given that there is a significant co-occurrence between social anxiety disorder and selective mutism.

Age

■ Onset of selective mutism is usually before the age of 5 years. Social mutism may be detected when the child begins school, when there is an increase in social interaction.

Gender

■ There has been no difference identified between girls and boys.

Family History

■ There may be a genetic component given that there is a significant co-occurrence between social anxiety and selective mutism. Parental history of shyness may also be a contributing factor.

Stressful Events in Susceptible People
- Environmental factors that may contribute to selective mutism in children may include parents who themselves demonstrate social inhibition and who also are overprotective.

Diagnosis
- Differential diagnosis
- Communication disorders
- Neurodevelopmental disorders
- Schizophrenia and other psychotic disorders
- Social anxiety disorder

ICD-10 Code
Selective mutism (F94.0)

Diagnostic Workup
- There are no particular laboratory tests.

Initial Assessment
- Assess for communication disorders
- Psychiatric assessment and developmental history
- Family history
- Comprehensive medical H&P examination

Clinical Presentation: Symptoms
Children are reluctant to speak in social situations outside their immediate family. Children with selective mutism exhibit anxiety in situations where they are expected to speak, such as in class.

Diagnostic and Statistical Manual of Mental Disorders, Fifth Edition: Diagnostic Guidelines
A. Failure to speak in social situations where there is an expectation for speaking despite the ability to speak.
B. The failure to speak significantly interferes with education and/or occupational development.
C. The disturbance lasts at least 1 month.
D. The failure to speak is not due to a lack of language development or inability to use spoken language that would be required in a social situation.
E. Failure to speak is not related to a communication disorder.

Treatment Overview
- CBT
- Family education and family therapy
- Stress reduction techniques such as relaxation exercises, imagery, role play, and progressive desensitization
- Consultation with the school and teachers

Psychopharmacology
Treatment of symptoms of anxiety related to selective mutism may include SSRIs. Fluoxetine has shown efficacy in treatment for childhood selective mutism.

Patient Education
- Family education
- Stress reduction techniques

Medical/Legal Pitfalls
- Rule out biological bases of selective mutism.
- Rule out neurodevelopmental disorders and psychotic disorder.

PHOBIAS AND SOCIAL ANXIETY

Other Names
- Simple phobia
- Specific phobia
- Social anxiety disorder

Background Information

Definition of Disorder
- There are two types of phobias: specific and social.
- To be diagnosed with a phobia, the person must have a marked, persistent fear of specific objects or situations, social situations, or performance situations.
- The fear may be manifested in a panic attack or resemble a panic attack.
- The phobic stimulus is avoided or dreaded.
- An immediate anxiety response is provoked by exposure to the phobic object or situation.
- Adults recognize that the fear is unreasonable or excessive.
- The avoidance, fear, and panic attacks must significantly interfere with the person's daily routine, occupation, or social life, or else the phobia causes marked distress to the person.
- The anxiety, panic attacks, and avoidance must not be caused by another mental condition, a general medical condition, or a drug.

Etiology
- Specific phobia
  - Phobias are usually objects or situations that may be threatening or have been threatening in the past.
  - Persons may be predisposed to phobia onset by the following:
    - Personal traumatic experiences or viewing others' traumatic experiences.
    - Being attacked by an animal or viewing another being attacked by an animal.
    - Observing others fearing an object or situation.
    - Informational transmission of things to be feared.
    - Unexpected panic attacks in a to-be-feared situation.
  - Phobias secondary to trauma or unexpected panic attacks tend to be acute and have no characteristic age of onset.
  - Phobias continuing into adulthood remit in about 20% of cases.
- Social anxiety disorder
  - May emerge in a child with social inhibition and shyness.

- Onset may be abrupt or secondary to stressful or humiliating experience.
- Onset may be insidious.
- Duration is frequently lifelong with remission or attenuation in adulthood.
- Social anxiety severity may wax and wane depending on stressors and life events.

Demographics

- Prevalence for specific phobia in the community is 4% to 8.8%.
- Lifetime prevalence for specific phobia is 7.2% to 11.3%, with a decline in older adults.
- Prevalence estimates for social anxiety varies depending on the threshold used to determine distress and impairment in each study.
- Prevalence estimates have been as high as 20% in those with anxiety disorders but as low as 2% in the general population.
- Lifetime prevalence for social anxiety is 3% to 13%.

Risk Factors

Age

- Specific phobia
  - Onset depends on type of phobia.
  - Usually occurs in childhood/early adolescence.
- Social anxiety
  - Usually occurs in the mid-teens.
  - Childhood onset may occur if a child has social inhibition and shyness.

Overprotective parenting may promote increased interpersonal sensitivity, resulting in an increased risk for social anxiety.

Gender

- Specific phobia
  - Women are affected more than men (2:1).
  - About 90% of animal and natural environment phobias and situational phobias affect women.
- Social anxiety
  - Women are affected more than men in the general population.
  - Men are affected more than women or are equally affected in the clinical setting.

Family History

- Family members of those with a specific phobia have increased risk for a specific phobia, especially if the phobia is animal type, situational type, or fear of blood or injury.
- Especially in the generalized type of social anxiety, first-degree biological relatives are more likely to have this form of anxiety than the general population.

Stressful Events in Susceptible People

- Specific phobia
  - Traumatic events may trigger phobias.
  - Stressful events may cause reemergence of a phobia.
- Social anxiety
  - May be caused by a stressful experience.
  - Stress may cause resurgence of anxiety after remission or attenuation.

Having Another Mental Health Disorder

- Having one specific phobia does not predispose a person to having another phobia unless the phobia developed in adolescence.
- Having any specific phobia does not predispose or increase risk for another mental health disorder.
- Those with social anxiety are more likely also to have other anxiety disorders, depression, substance abuse, and dependence.

Treatment Overview

Acute Treatment
Specific Phobia

- Cognitive-behavioral interventions are the most studied and most efficacious for this disorder.
- Multiple exposure treatments, in vivo or virtual reality, work very well in extinguishing the phobia.
- Applied relaxation and tension treatments have shown promise but need more studies to show efficacy.
- Cognitive restructuring treatments and psychodynamic psychotherapy may also be useful but more studies need to be done.

Social Anxiety

- CBTs
  - These therapies work on the belief that dysfunctional beliefs and biased information processing strategies are responsible for the social anxiety.
  - The therapies focus on the patient's beliefs and avoidance.
  - Therapies used include exposure treatments alone, exposure treatments plus cognitive restructuring treatments (either in a group session or in an individual session), social skills training, and relaxation strategies.
  - Exposure treatments with cognitive restructuring treatments are most effective.
  - Social skills training and relaxation strategies are less effective alone but have increased efficacy when either is combined with exposure treatments and cognitive restructuring treatments in a group setting.
- Various medications have been used to treat patients with social anxiety, including SSRIs, SNRIs, MAOs, and BZDs.
- SSRIs, such as sertraline (*Zoloft*) and paroxetine (*Paxil*) are the treatment of choice— although some SSRIs have been studied more extensively than others, there is no evidence of superiority of one SSRI over another.

Monoamines, such as phenelzine (*Nardil*), are reserved as the last line of treatment due to the dietary interactions and side effects. Drug therapy should be continued for 6 to 12 months.

  - Medication use alone was associated with a high relapse rate despite an earlier initial benefit.
  - Relapse rate was decreased when medication use was combined with cognitive-behavioral group therapy.
  - More studies need to be done to determine better treatment guidelines.
- Psychodynamic therapy, interpersonal psychotherapy, and acceptance and commitment therapy are used clinically but should be studied more to determine efficacy as compared to CBTs and medication use.

Chronic Treatment
Specific Phobia
- Long-term therapy may be needed if exposure therapy does not work.
- More research needs to be done on therapy for the specific phobia.

Drug Selection Table for Phobias

CLASS	DRUG
Beta-blockers	Drugs used for short-term treatment. Treatment of physical symptoms—does not treat the root of the problem. Helps control heart rate Propranolol (*Inderal*)
BZDs	Drugs used for short-term treatments Alprazolam (*Xanax/Xanax XR/Niravam*) Lorazepam (*Ativan*) Diazepam (*Valium*) Clonazepam (Klonopin) Chlordiazepoxide (*Librium*)
SSRIs	First-line drug therapy Sertraline (*Zoloft*) Fluoxetine (*Prozac*) Paroxetine (*Paxil*) Fluvoxamine (*Luvox*) Citalopram (*Celexa*) Escitalopram (*Lexapro*)
SNRIs	First-line drug therapy Venlafaxine (*Effexor, Effexor XR*)
TCAs	Considered second-line drug therapy: drugs for treatment-resistant cases Imipramine (*Tofranil*) Desipramine (*Norpramin*) Clomipramine (*Anafranil*)

BZDs, benzodiazepines; SNRIs, serotonin-norepinephrine reuptake inhibitors; SSRIs, selective serotonin reuptake inhibitors; TCAs, tricyclic antidepressants.

Social Anxiety

- Long-term therapy may be needed if the patient is refractory to acute treatment.
- Therapy may include cognitive-behavioral, or another type of, therapy, along with medication.

Recurrence Rate
- Rate of recurrence is variable. It depends on life stressors, attenuation, and remission of phobia.

Patient Education

- Both MD Consult and e-Medicine have patient education articles on phobias.
- Many support groups can be found online, including www.dailystrength.org.
- Advise patients to avoid self-medication with alcohol or other drugs.

Medical/Legal Pitfalls

- Patients with some phobias and/or social anxiety may abuse alcohol or illicit drugs as a coping mechanism. Healthcare workers should screen for this during the H&P examination.

Diagnosis

Differential Diagnosis
- Specific phobia
  - Social anxiety
  - PD with agoraphobia
  - PD without agoraphobia
  - Posttraumatic stress disorder symptoms
  - Separation anxiety disorder
  - Obsessive-compulsive disorder (OCD)
  - Hypochondriasis
  - Anorexia nervosa
  - Bulimia nervosa
  - Schizophrenia or another psychotic disorder
- Social anxiety
  - Specific phobia
  - PD without agoraphobia
  - Agoraphobia without history of PD
  - Separation anxiety disorder
  - GAD
  - Pervasive development disorder
  - Schizoid personality disorder
  - Avoidant personality disorder

ICD-10 Codes
Specific phobia (F40.298)
Social anxiety (F40.10)

Diagnostic Workup
- Physical and mental evaluations are done.

Initial Assessment
- Full H&P examinations are included.
- Past medical history including psychiatric history is done.
- Traumatic or past event/stressor is determined.
- Symptoms experienced are identified (emotional or physical symptoms).
- Physical and mental evaluations are included.
- Thyroid function studies (thyroid-stimulating hormone [TSH], triiodothyronine [T3], and thyroxine [T4]) are done.
- Complete metabolic panel includes glucose, calcium, albumin, total protein count, levels of sodium, potassium, CO_2 (carbon dioxide and bicarbonate), chloride, blood urea nitrogen (BUN), creatinine, alkaline phosphatase (ALP), alanine amino transferase (ALT, also called serum glutamic pyruvic transaminase [SGPT]), aspartate amino transferase (AST, also called serum glutamic oxaloacetic transaminase [SGOT]), and bilirubin.
- CBC with differentials: hemoglobin, hematocrit, red blood cell (RBC) count, white blood cell (WBC) count, WBC differential count, and platelet count.

Clinical Presentation
- Panic (or panic-like) attacks
- Extreme anxiety and/or fear

■ Extreme avoidance of social situations that involve exposure to unfamiliar people or possible scrutiny by others

SPECIFIC PHOBIA

Diagnosis

Differential Diagnosis
- Agoraphobia
- Social anxiety disorder
- Separation anxiety disorder
- PD
- OCD
- Trauma- and stressor-related disorders
- Eating disorders
- Schizophrenia spectrum and other psychotic disorders

Diagnostic and Statistical Manual of Mental Disorders, Fifth Edition: Diagnostic Guidelines

A. Extreme anxiety or worry that occurs for 6 months or more and creates impairment in school or work requirements. It may also cause problems with social relationships.

B. When the individual is exposed to the item or situation, fear or anxiety is triggered and the individual will actively seek to avoid the item or situation.

C. The fear or anxiety is in excess to the real danger presented by a situation or item.

D. The avoidant behavior or fear and anxiety lasts for at least 6 months and results in work and social impairment.

E. The symptoms are not related to another medical condition.

SOCIAL ANXIETY DISORDER

Background Information

Social anxiety disorder's key characteristic is an intense fear or anxiety in social situations when an individual believes they are being negatively evaluated by others. The anxiety and fear occurs in most social situations. Individuals who occasionally experience fear and anxiety in social situations would not meet the criteria of social anxiety disorder. The fear and anxiety is out of proportion to the actual risk of being negatively evaluated. To distinguish social anxiety from a transient social fear, the disturbance usually spans at least 6 months. The disturbance significantly interferes with social functioning or occupational functioning.

A specific subtype of social anxiety disorder deals with a fear-of-performance type of social anxiety disorder. Individuals with performance fears experience impairment in their professional lives but do not experience fear or avoidance in nonperformance social situations.

Diagnostic Criteria

A. The individual believes they are being viewed negatively. Examples of such situations include meeting unfamiliar people, being observed, or performing in front of others.

Note: To meet criteria, children with social anxiety disorder need to experience fear and anxiety in peer settings and not just in situations with adults.

B. The individual fears that they will exhibit symptoms of anxiety that will result in their being negatively evaluated. They experience feelings of being humiliated or embarrassed with the belief that they will be rejected and/or that their behavior has offended others.

C. *Note*: In children, behaviors such as crying, tantrums, freezing, clinging, shrinking, or failing to speak in social situations may occur reflective of social anxiety and fear.

D. Individuals attempt to avoid social situations. When they cannot avoid social situations, they experience significant anxiety and fear.

E. The fear or anxiety experienced by the individual is disproportionate to the actual threat.

F. Symptoms of fear, anxiety, and avoidance are persistent, lasting most times for 6 months or more.

G. The individual experiences significant impairment and/or distress in social, occupational, or other significant areas of functioning.

H. Symptoms of fear, anxiety, or avoidance are not attributable to the physiological effects of a substance (drugs or medications) or a medical condition.

I. Symptoms of fear, anxiety, or avoidance are not better explained by another mental disorder.

J. If there is a co-occurring medical condition (e.g., Parkinson's disease, obesity, disfigurement from burns or injury), the fear, anxiety, or avoidance is unrelated or is excessive.

Differential Diagnosis

- Normative shyness
- Agoraphobia
- PD
- GAD
- Separation anxiety disorder
- Specific phobias
- Selective mutism
- Major depressive disorder
- Body dysmorphic disorder
- Autism spectrum disorder
- Personality disorders
- Other mental disorders
- Other medical conditions
- Oppositional defiant disorder

ICD-10 Code
Social anxiety disorder (F40.10)

Etiology
It may emerge in a child with social inhibition and shyness.

- Onset may be abrupt or secondary to stressful or humiliating experience.
- Onset may be insidious.
- Duration is frequently lifelong with remission or attenuation in adulthood.
- Social anxiety severity may wax and wane depending on stressors and life events.

■ First onset of social anxiety disorder is rare but is more likely to occur following a stressful or humiliating event.

Demographics

In the United States, the 12-month prevalence rate is higher than in much of the world. The comparison based on the same diagnostic instrument is as follows: United States, approximately 7%; Europe, approximately 2.3%; and worldwide, approximately 0.5% to 2.0%.

Risk Factors

■ *Age*: The onset of social anxiety in the United States is between the ages of 8 and 15 years, with a median age of 13 years.
■ *Gender*: Higher rates of social anxiety disorder occur in females than in males, with ratios ranging from 1.5% to 2.2%.
■ *Family history*: There is a two to six times greater chance of developing social anxiety disorder among first-degree relatives. Genetic and environmental factors contribute to the increased predisposition.
■ *Stressful events in susceptible people*: Persons who exhibit traits such as behavioral inhibition and fears of being negatively evaluated may be at greater risk.
■ Environmental factors that contribute to increased risk include stressful events that lead to a feeling of being humiliated or significantly embarrassed.

Diagnostic Workup

■ There are no specific laboratory studies for social anxiety disorder.

Initial Assessment

■ Comprehensive physical examination
■ Comprehensive psychiatric evaluation

Clinical Presentation

The major presentation is extreme anxiety or fear related to social situations. The person has an intense fear of being evaluated negatively by others. Persons who occasionally experience anxiety or fear in social situations would not meet the criteria for social anxiety disorder.

Psychopharmacology

Treating symptoms of anxiety related to social anxiety disorder generally includes SSRIs and SNRIs. Other medications, such as gabapentin, and pregabalin (*Lyrica*) have shown efficacy with social anxiety management as well.

BZDs, such as clonazepam (*Klonopin*), has shown efficacy when used as augmentation for SSRI or SNRI treatment. Such medications must be used with caution and use must be avoided in individuals with a history of substance abuse.

PANIC DISORDER

Background Information

■ Sudden feelings of terror that strike without warning.
■ Can occur at any time, even during sleep.

- Mimics a heart attack or a feeling that death is imminent.
- PD is defined as recurrent, unexpected panic attacks followed by at least 1 month of persistent concern about having another attack, worry about the consequences of panic attacks, and a change in behavior as a result of the attacks.
- Diagnostic workup includes physical and mental evaluation.
- Often, the first attacks are triggered by physical illnesses, a major life stress, or medications that increase activity in the part of the brain involved in fear reactions.

Risk Factors
- *Age*: PD typically strikes in the late teen years or young adulthood.
- *Gender*: Women are twice as likely as men to develop PD.
- *Family history*: PD has been found to run in families; this may mean that inheritance (genes) plays a strong role in determining who will get it. However, many people who have no family history of the disorder develop it.

Diagnosis
Differential Diagnosis
- Thyroid disorders
- Diabetic hyper- or hypoglycemia
- Cardiac arrhythmias
- Cerebral lesions
- Substance-induced anxiety disorder
- Asthma
- Somatic symptom disorder

Psychopharmacology
Overview
- SSRIs are the most commonly used medications for PD.
  - They include fluoxetine (*Prozac*), sertraline (*Zoloft*), paroxetine (*Paxil*), fluvoxamine (*Luvox*), citalopram (*Celexa*), and escitalopram (*Lexapro*).
  - They take up to 8 to 12 weeks to reach maximum therapeutic efficacy.
  - If these do not help or if more immediate symptomatic relief is necessary, use of BZDs may be considered if the person does not have a history of drug dependence.
- SNRIs, such as venlafaxine XR, are also used as first-line therapy for PD. Tricyclic antidepressants (TCAs) such as imipramine and clomipramine can be effective for reducing the frequency of PD, but they have substantial side effects and poor tolerability compared with SSRIs.
- BZDs have been found to be efficacious for PD. However, they are associated with dependence and addiction.
  - They are used on a temporary basis and for immediate relief.
- Monoamine oxidase inhibitors (MAOIs), such as phenelzine (*Nardil*), tranylcypromine (*Parnate*), and isocarboxazid (*Marplan*), are only used when all other drugs do not work due to dietary restrictions and potential side effects.
  - MAOIs have been shown to be effective medications for PD, but they have serious side effects and interactions with other drugs and foods. (Initiation of this type of treatment is recommended to be conducted with a mental health provider.)
  - Behavioral therapies should be used together with drug therapy. These include CBT, exposure therapy, relaxation techniques, pleasant mental imagery, and cognitive restructuring (learning to recognize and replace panic-inducing thoughts). Behavioral treatment appears to have long-lasting benefits.

- Regular exercise, adequate sleep, and regularly scheduled meals may help reduce the frequency of the attacks. Caffeine and other stimulants should be reduced or eliminated.

Patient Education

- Individuals with PD have a suicide rate 18 times higher than the general population.
- The rate of substance abuse (especially stimulants, cocaine, and hallucinogens) in persons with PD is 7% to 28%, 4 to 14 times greater than that of the general population.

Drug Selection Table for Panic Disorder

CLASS	DRUG
SSRIs	First-line drug therapy Sertraline (*Zoloft*) Fluoxetine (*Prozac*) Paroxetine (*Paxil, Paxil CR*); paroxetine mesylate (*Pexeva*) Fluvoxamine (*Luvox CR*) Citalopram (*Celexa*) Escitalopram (*Lexapro*)
SNRIs	First-line drug therapy Venlafaxine (*Effexor, Effexor XR*) Desvenlafaxine (*Pristiq*) Duloxetine (*Cymbalta*)
TCAs	Drugs for treatment-resistant cases Imipramine (*Tofranil*) Clomipramine (*Anafranil*) Desipramine (*Norpramin*) Nortriptyline (*Pamelor*)
BZDs	Drugs used only in first weeks while establishing levels of SSRIs or SNRIs Alprazolam (*Xanax/Xanax XR/Niravam*) Lorazepam (*Ativan*) Clonazepam (*Klonopin*) Diazepam (Valium)
Serotonin 1A agonist	Drug for augmentation Buspirone (*BuSpar*)

BZDs, benzodiazepines; SNRIs, serotonin-norepinephrine reuptake inhibitors; SSRIs, selective serotonin reuptake inhibitors; TCAs, tricyclic antidepressants.

Medical/Legal Pitfalls

- Pregnant mothers with PD are more likely to have infants of smaller birth weight for gestational age.
- PD patients are nearly twice as likely to develop coronary artery disease, and those with known coronary disease can experience myocardial ischemia during their panic episodes.

AGORAPHOBIA

Background Information

Definition of Disorder

- The disorder is associated with significant anxiety or fear with an anticipated or actual exposure to a place or situation with concurrent fear that one cannot escape the place.

■ To meet the criteria for agoraphobia, two of the following situations need to cause the person significant anxiety or fear: (1) using public transportation, (2) being in open spaces, (3) being in enclosed spaces, (4) being in a crowd, or (5) being outside one's home alone.

■ The level of fear and anxiety may vary in relation to the anticipation or presence of the agoraphobic situation.

■ A key feature is that the fear or anxiety is persistent in relation to the situation and occurs consistently.

■ Individuals with agoraphobia experience fear, anxiety, and avoidance in relation to the situation that is disproportionate to the actual threat.

Etiology

■ Individuals who are behaviorally inhibited and are more anxious are more predisposed to agoraphobia but they are also more predisposed to a range of anxiety disorders (phobias, PD).

■ Individuals who have experienced a negative or stressful event may have an increased risk of developing agoraphobia.

Demographics

■ Initial onset for agoraphobia is typically before the age of 35 years in two-thirds of individuals with agoraphobia.

■ The mean age of onset for agoraphobia is 17 years.

■ Although the greatest risk for agoraphobia is during adolescence and early adulthood, there is also an increased risk phase after the age of 40 years.

■ Agoraphobia tends to present as chronic. The prevalence of agoraphobia does not vary in relation to culture or race.

Risk Factors

■ *Age*: Low prevalence in children. Although the initial onset is most often seen in adolescents and young adults, agoraphobia does present across the life span.

■ *Gender*: Males present with a higher rate of comorbid substance abuse disorders.

■ *Family history*: Of the phobias, agoraphobia has the strongest association with heritability.

■ *Stressful events in susceptible people*: Many individuals with agoraphobia have experienced anxiety symptoms in the past. Common comorbid diagnoses include specific phobias, PD, and social anxiety disorder.

Diagnosis

■ Extreme fear and anxiety in two or more of the following situations: (1) anxiety related to the use of public transportation; (2) fear of open spaces; (3) fear of being in enclosed spaces; (4) anxiety and fear related to being in a crowd; and (5) fear of being outside one's home alone.

■ Avoidance of situation when an individual fears that they cannot escape readily in the event of increased anxiety and potential panic-like symptoms.

■ The agoraphobic situations consistently result in fear and anxiety.

■ The agoraphobic situations are avoided or are not avoided if accompanied by another or if the person in the agoraphobic situation experiences extreme fear and/or anxiety.

- The fear or anxiety is disproportionate to the actual situation.
- Avoidance of the feared situation has existed for at least 6 months.
- The fear and anxiety related to the feared situation has caused significant impairment in the person's social functioning.
- If the fear, anxiety, and avoidance are related to a medical condition, the symptoms are considered extreme and excessive.
- The fear, anxiety, and avoidance are not better explained by another anxiety disorder, OCD or posttraumatic stress disorder.

Note: The diagnosis of agoraphobia need not be accompanied by symptoms of panic. If the individual experiences panic with agoraphobia, both diagnoses would be given.

ICD-10 Code
Agoraphobia (F40.0)

Diagnostic Workup
There are no specific laboratory studies for agoraphobias.

Initial Assessment
- Comprehensive physical examination
- Comprehensive psychiatric evaluation

Clinical Presentation: Symptoms
Apart from anxiety and fear, the individual may have panic-like symptoms when exposed or potentially exposed to feared situations, as described in the diagnostic criteria.

Treatment Overview
- CBT includes systematic desensitization
- Supportive therapy
- Stress reduction techniques
- Exposure therapy
- Thought stopping

Psychopharmacology
- Anxiety associated with agoraphobia may be treated with SSRIs, such as fluoxetine (*Prozac*) and sertraline (*Zoloft*).
- In the case of panic or panic-like symptoms, a BZD may help to reduce the intensity of the fear and/or anxiety; in the case of panic or panic-like attacks, BZD may decrease the number and intensity of the attacks.

Patient Education
- Coping skills training and stress reduction techniques may help decrease the severity of symptoms.

Medical/Legal Pitfalls
- Rule out potential medical conditions that may be an underlying cause of anxiety.

GENERALIZED ANXIETY DISORDER

Background Information
Definition of Disorder
- This is the most common anxiety disorder seen by primary care physicians.
- Patients have chronic anxiety, worry, and tension, which is without, or out of proportion to, any provocation or stimulus.
- Symptoms are not situational or limited to certain events.
- Patients are unable to assure themselves that their anxiety is greatly exaggerated in comparison to what the situation warrants.

Etiology
- Exact cause of GAD is unknown.
- Some research suggests that environmental and genetic factors may play a role.
- GAD may be caused by an imbalance between dopamine and serotonin.

Demographics
- Prevalence is 5.9% among adolescents and 2.9% among adults in the United States.
- Prevalence rates in other countries range from 0.4% to 3.6%
- Females are twice as likely as males to experience GAD.
- The diagnosis peaks during middle age and declines as the individual ages.

Family History
- There is some evidence that anxiety disorders, including GAD, tend to run in families.
- Studies of twins suggest that there may be a genetic factor.

Stressful Events in Susceptible People
- Stressful events can exacerbate symptoms in patients with GAD.
- Childhood abuse is considered a cause/risk factor for GAD.

Having Another Mental Health Disorder
- The comorbidities that accompany GAD include other anxiety disorders (PD, social anxiety), substance abuse, and mood disorders (dysthymic disorder, major depressive disorder). These comorbidities should be treated along with GAD.

Diagnosis
Differential Diagnosis
- Anxiety disorder due to another medical condition
- Substance- or medication-induced anxiety disorder
- Social anxiety disorder
- OCD
- Posttraumatic stress disorder and adjustment disorders
- Depressive, bipolar, and psychotic disorders

ICD-10 Code
Generalized anxiety disorder (F41.1)

Diagnostic Workup
- There are no particular laboratory tests that diagnose GAD, but tests can be done to rule out other organic causes (e.g., thyroid function test, CBCs, basic metabolic panels, urinalysis).
- Diagnosis of GAD can be difficult because several other physical and mental health disorders may be confused with GAD.
- Physical and mental evaluations are done.
- Two scales are used to evaluate for GAD (GAD 2 and GAD 7 scales).

Initial Assessment
- Medical history
- Symptoms
  - How long has the patient been having symptoms?
  - When did the symptoms start?
  - How often do they occur?
  - When and where do they tend to occur?
  - How long do they last?
  - What effect do they have on the patient's ability to function?

Clinical Presentation
- Worry being excessive and typically interfering with psychosocial functioning
- Worry being pervasive, pronounced, and distressing to the individual
- Restlessness
- Feeling keyed up
- Easily fatigued
- Difficulty in concentrating
- Irritability
- Muscle tension
- Sleep disturbances with difficulty falling or staying asleep or restless, unsatisfying sleep
- Trembling
- Twitching
- Feeling shaky
- Sweating
- Nausea
- Diarrhea
- Accelerated heart rate
- Shortness of breath
- Irritable bowel syndrome (IBS)
- Headaches

Diagnostic and Statistical Manual of Mental Disorders, Fifth Edition: Diagnostic Guidelines
A. Extreme anxiety or worry that occurs for 6 months or more and creates impairment in school or work requirements. It may also cause problems with social relationships.
B. The patient has difficulty controlling the worry or anxiety.
C. The anxiety or worry may also accompany restlessness, complaints of being tired, problems concentrating, irritability, and difficulty with sleep. Children may only have one of the previous symptoms.

Treatment Overview

In the treatment of GADs, the main focus of treatment is to reduce the agent that is causing the anxiety. In the event the anxiety cannot be controlled or eliminated and is considered acute, psychopharmacology is the standard of care. Once the anxiety is under control, psychotherapy is the next step in treatment.

Psychopharmacology

- SSRIs are the most common first-line agents used with GAD.
- TCAs can be effective in treating GADs; however, the initial side effects of the drugs when first initiated (jitteriness and insomnia) can reduce patient adherence to therapy. These medications are generally reserved for GAD resistant to treatment with SSRIs and SNRIs.
- SNRIs have Food and Drug Administration (FDA) approval for treatment of GAD and are considered the first-line treatment for GAD along with SSRIs.
- The non-BZD anxiolytic agent buspirone can be efficacious for the anxiety component, but it has no effect on depression and should not be used if concomitant depression is present.
- Pregabalin (*Lyrica*) may be used alone and for augmentation of SSRIs and SNRIs and has shown efficacy in treatment of anxiety symptoms.
- BZDs are generally the most efficacious in patients who only have anxiety symptoms; however, the healthcare provider needs to be cautious while using these agents for treating older adults. Additionally, patients may become physically dependent with long-term use. These drugs may be used as part of an initial treatment regimen and then discontinued when a long-term treatment plan has been developed.

Chronic Treatment

- Follow-up care by a chemical dependence treatment specialist is recommended when indicated.

Drug Selection Table for Generalized Anxiety Disorder

CLASS	DRUG
SSRIs	First-line drug therapy Citalopram (*Celexa*) Fluoxetine (*Prozac*) Escitalopram (*Lexapro*) Sertraline (*Zoloft*) Paroxetine (*Paxil, Paxil PR*) Paroxetine mesylate (*Pexeva*)
SNRIs	First-line drug therapy Venlafaxine (*Effexor, Effexor XR*) Duloxetine (*Cymbalta*)
Calcium channel moderator	Drug augmentation Pregabalin (*Lyrica*)
TCAs	Drugs for treatment-resistant cases Imipramine (*Tofranil, Tofranil PM*) Desipramine (*Norpramin*)

Drug Selection Table for Generalized Anxiety Disorder (*continued*)

CLASS	DRUG
BZDs	Drugs used only in first weeks while establishing levels of SSRI or SNRI Alprazolam (*Xanax/Xanax XR/Niravam*) Clonazepam (*Klonopin*) Lorazepam (*Ativan*) Diazepam (*Valium*)
Antihistamines	Drug augmentation Hydroxyzine (*Vistaril*)
Anxiolytics	Drug augmentation Buspirone (*BuSpar*)
SN-Ran	Mirtazapine (*Remeron*)—useful for refractory anxiety with insomnia (not FDA approved for GAD)
SPARI	Vilazodone (*Viibryd*)—has been shown in some studies to be as efficacious as SSRIs for GAD

The SNRI duloxetine (Cymbalta) is the only FDA-approved medication for treatment of GAD in children aged 7 to 17 years. Most SSRIs have been found to be effective for treating anxiety in children and adolescents but none have been approved by the FDA for use in treating non-OCD anxiety in young people.

BZDs, benzodiazepines; FDA, Food and Drug Administration; GAD, generalized anxiety disorder; SNRIs, serotonin-norepinephrine reuptake inhibitors; SPARI, serotonin partial agonist reuptake inhibitor; SSRIs, selective serotonin reuptake inhibitors; TCAs, tricyclic antidepressants.

- Psychiatric referral should be considered in patients who do not improve with medical treatment or those with suicidal ideations.

Psychotherapy
- Complementary and alternative medicine (CAM)
  - Acupuncture
  - Aromatherapy

Patient Education
- Patients should continue to take all medications as prescribed and never stop any medicines before discussing this with their physician.
- For excellent patient education resources, visit eMedicine's Mental Health and Behavior Center and Anxiety Center.

Medical/Legal Pitfalls
- Persons with GAD are more likely to have other anxiety disorders (e.g., PD).
- Anxiety disorders are more frequently seen in patients with chronic medical illness (chronic obstructive pulmonary disease [COPD], IBS, hypertension) than in the general population.
- Patients are more likely to present to their primary care physicians frequently with multiple complaints over time.
- Patients with GAD tend to smoke cigarettes and abuse other substances (alcohol, prescription or illicit drugs).

SUBSTANCE- OR MEDICATION-INDUCED ANXIETY DISORDER

Background Information

Definition of Disorder

The signs and symptoms of the anxiety are related to a specific substance the patient ingested. The substance creates the anxiety symptoms rather than an underlying disorder.

Etiology

Substances that may cause the anxiety disorder include alcohol, caffeine, cannabis, phencyclidine, inhalants, opioids, sedatives, hypnotics, anxiolytics, stimulants, cocaine, hallucinogens, or an unknown substance.

Demographics

The disorder is rare, with a 12-month prevalence of around 0.002% of the general population. In the clinical population, the numbers may be higher.

Risk Factors

- *Age*: unknown
- *Gender*: unknown
- *Family history*: unknown

Diagnosis

Differential Diagnosis

- Substance intoxication and substance withdrawal
- Anxiety disorder (i.e., not induced by a substance/medication)
- Delirium
- Anxiety disorder due to another medical condition

Diagnostic Workup

- Urine drug screen

Diagnostic and Statistical Manual of Mental Disorders, Fifth Edition: Diagnostic Guidelines

- Anxiety or panic attacks are the main feature of the disorder, as well as obsessions or compulsions.
- The symptoms occur right after the substance has been ingested or occur when the substance is discontinued.
- The anxiety or panic attacks are not exclusive to delirium.
- The anxiety or panic attacks affect personal relationships and/or school or work.

Treatment Overview

Once the identified substance that created the anxiety or panic attacks is discontinued, the symptoms should resolve within several days, weeks, or a month. If the symptoms were present prior to the ingestion or discontinuation of the substance, other causes should be explored.

Patient Education

Anxiety or panic attacks can occur from the discontinuation of alcohol, opioids, sedatives, or cocaine. Medications that could create anxiety or panic attacks include anesthesia, antihistamines, antiparkinsonian drugs, corticosteroids, antihypertensive medications, bronchodilators, or birth control pills. Carbon monoxide, gasoline, paint, and other heavy metals can cause anxiety or panic attacks.

ANXIETY DISORDER DUE TO ANOTHER MEDICAL CONDITION

Background Information
Definition of Disorder
- The individual who exhibits an anxiety disorder due to a medical condition presents with symptoms of anxiety and/or panic that are not related to another anxiety disorder.
- The symptoms are best explained as a physiological response to the medical condition, and there is supporting evidence from a comprehensive history/physical examination, psychiatric evaluation, and laboratory findings indicating that the symptoms are a consequence of a medical condition.
- Anxiety due to another medical condition is the appropriate diagnosis (1) when the medical condition is known to be associated with symptoms of anxiety and (2) when the medical condition precedes the onset of the anxiety and/or panic symptoms.

Etiology
- Symptoms of anxiety and/or panic coincide with the medical condition and have not been present previously.
- The emergence of the anxiety and/or panic symptoms demonstrates a clear temporal association with the occurrence of a medical condition.

Risk Factors
- There are several medical diagnoses that are associated with the development of anxiety symptoms, including endocrine disease, cardiac disease, respiratory disease, metabolic disturbances, neurological diseases, and various cancers.

Stressful Events in Susceptible People
- Individuals who have medical conditions that have been associated with the development of anxiety as a manifestation of the medical condition are at risk for this diagnosis.

Diagnosis
- Anxiety and/or panic symptom.
- Findings from the history, physical examination, and laboratory tests support that the symptoms have a direct physiological basis.
- The symptoms are not related to another mental disorder.
- Anxiety and/or panic are not due to delirium.
- There is significant distress and impairment in important areas of social functioning.

Differential Diagnosis
- Delirium
- Mixed presentation of symptoms such as mood symptoms and anxiety symptoms
- Substance- or medication-induced anxiety disorder

ICD-10 Code
Anxiety disorder due to another medical condition (F06.4)

Diagnostic Workup
- Comprehensive H&P examination
- Laboratory studies relevant to medical diagnosis
- Psychiatric history and psychiatric assessment

Initial Assessment
- Rule out psychiatric history and existing psychiatric diagnosis.

Clinical Presentation: Symptoms
- Anxiety and/or panic symptoms that emerge as a consequence of a medical condition.

Treatment Overview
- Treatment of the medication condition
  - Relaxation exercises
  - Supportive therapy

Psychopharmacology
- SSRIs may be helpful.
- SNRIs may be effective for anxiety and may also reduce neuropathic pain.
- BZDs can be helpful for acute anxiety reactions but should be used with caution in the medically ill.

Patient Education
- Patient education regarding anxiety symptoms and the relationship to the medical condition.

Medical/Legal Pitfalls
- Careful assessment regarding any co-occurring substance use or abuse.
- Assessment of comorbid psychiatric disorders.

OTHER SPECIFIED ANXIETY DISORDER

Background Information
- An individual would meet the criteria for "other specified anxiety disorder" when their symptoms do not meet the full criteria for an anxiety disorder but they are experiencing symptoms that cause significant distress.
- There may also be significant impairment in social functioning.
- When this diagnosis is used, there needs to be a rationale for how it does not meet the criteria for a specific anxiety disorder using the diagnostic criteria for the justification. For example, in a case when the individual experiences significant anxiety that occurs some days but not the majority of days in a week, the rationale would be listed as "General anxiety does not occur more days than not."

UNSPECIFIED ANXIETY DISORDER

- Individuals who meet the criteria for unspecified anxiety disorder experience significant anxiety symptoms and may also experience impairment in social functioning but do not meet the full criteria for any of the anxiety disorders.

■ The clinician does not specify the reason why the criteria are not met but rather may include that there is insufficient evidence to make a specific diagnosis.

BIBLIOGRAPHY

Ahmari, S. E., Spellman, T., Douglass, N. L., Kheirbek, M. A., Simpson, H. B., Deisseroth, K., & Hen, R. (2013). Repeated cortico-striatal stimulation generates persistent OCD-like behavior. *Science, 340*(6137), 1234–1239.

American Psychiatric Association. (2000). *Diagnostic and statistical manual of mental disorders* (4th ed., text rev.). Washington, DC: American Psychiatric Association.

American Psychiatric Association. (2007). *Practice guideline for the treatment of patients with obsessive-compulsive disorder*. American Psychiatric Press.

American Psychiatric Association. (2013). *Diagnostic and statistical manual of mental disorders* (5th ed.). Washington, DC: American Psychiatric Press.

Angoa-Perez, M., Kane, M. J., Briggs, D. I., Sykes, C. E., Shah, M. M., Francescutti, D. M., & Kuhn, D. M. (2012). Genetic depletion of brain 5HT reveals a common molecular pathway mediating compulsivity and impulsivity. *Journal of Neurochemistry, 121*(6), 974–984.

Bakker, A., van Balkom, A. J., & Spinhoven, P. (2002). SSRIs vs. TCAs in the treatment of panic disorder: A meta-analysis. *Acta Psychiatrica Scandinavica, 106*(3), 163–167.

Bergman, R. L., & Lee, J. C. (2009). Selective mutism. In B. J. Sadock, V. A. Sadock, & P. Ruiz (Eds.), *Kaplan and Sadock's comprehensive texbook of psychiatry* (9th ed., Vol. 2, p. 3694). Lippincott Williams & Wilkins.

Beucke, J. C., Sepulcre, J., Talukdar, T., Linnman, C., Zschenderlein, K., Endrass, T., Kaufmann, C., & Kathmann, N. (2013). Abnormally high degree connectivity of the orbitofrontal cortex in obsessive-compulsive disorder. *JAMA Psychiatry, 70*(6), 619–629. https://doi.org/10.1001/jamapsychiatry.2013.173.

Bjorgvinsson, T., Hart, J., & Heffelfinger, S. (2007). Obsessive-compulsive disorder: Update on assessment and treatment. *Journal of Psychiatric Practice, 13*, 362–372.

Bloch, M. H., Green, C., Kichuk, S. A., Dombrowski, P. A., Wasylink, S., Billingslea, E., & Pittenger, C. (2013). Long-term outcome in adults with obsessive-compulsive disorder. *Depress Anxiety, 30*(8), 716–722.

Bloch, M. H., Landeros-Weisenberger, A., Kelmendi, B., Coric, V., Bracken, M. B., & Leckman, J. F. (2006). A systematic review: Antipsychotic augmentation with treatment refractory obsessive-compulsive disorder. *Molecular Psychiatry, 11*(7), 622–632.

Bloch, M. H., Sukhodolsky, D. G., Dombrowski, P. A., Panza, K. E., Craiglow, B. G., Landeros-Weisenberger, A., & Schultz, R. T. (2011). Poor fine-motor and visuospatial skills predict persistence of pediatric-onset obsessive-compulsive disorder into adulthood. *Journal of Child Psychology and Psychiatry, and Allied Disciplines, 52*(9), 974–983.

Burns, G. L., Keortge, S. G., Formea, G. M., & Sternberger, L. G. (1996). Revision of the Padua inventory of obsessive compulsive disorder symptoms: Distinctions between worry, obsessions, and compulsions. *Behavior Research and Therapy, 24*, 163–173.

Clomipramine Collaborative Study Group. (1991). Clomipramine in the treatment of patient with obsessive-compulsive disorder. *Archives of General Psychiatry, 48*, 730–738.

Davidson, J. R., Bose, A., & Wang, Q. (2005). Safety and efficacy of escitalopram in the long-term treatment of generalized anxiety disorder. *Journal of Clinical Psychiatry, 66*(11), 1441–1446. https://doi.org/10.4088/JCP.v66n1115.

Dougherty, D. D., Rauch, S. L., & Jenike, M. A. (2004). Pharmacotherapy for obsessive-compulsive disorder. *Journal of Clinical Psychology, 60*, 1195–1202.

Fan, Q., Palaniyappan, L., Tan, L., Wang, J., Wang, X., Li, C., & Liddle, P. F. (2013). Surface anatomical profile of the cerebral cortex in obsessive-compulsive disorder: A study of cortical thickness, folding and surface area. *Psychology Medicine*, *43*(5), 1081–1091.

Geller, D. A., March, J., & The AACAP Committee on Quality Issues, (CQI). (2012). Practice parameter for the assessment and treatment of children and adolescents with obsessive-compulsive disorder. *Journal of the American Academy of Child and Adolescent Psychiatry*, *51*(1), 98–113. https:/doi.org/10.1016/j.jaac.2011.09.019.

Gibbons, R. D., Brown, C. H., Hur, K., Davis, J., & Mann, J. J. (2012). Suicidal thoughts and behavior with antidepressant treatment: Reanalysis of the randomized placebo-controlled studies of fluoxetine and venlafaxine. *Archives of General Psychiatry*, *69*(6), 580–587.

Gommoli, C., Durgam, S., Mathews, M., Forero, G., Nunez, R., Tang, X., & Thase, M. E. (2015). A double-blind, randomized, placebo-controlled, fixed-dose phase III study of vilazodone in patients with generalized anxiety disorder. *Depression and Anxiety*, *32*(6), 451–459.

Goodman, W. K., Price, L. H., Rasmussen, S. A., Mazure, C., Fleischmann, R. L., Hill, C. L., & Charney, D. S. (1989). The Yale-Brown obsessive compulsive scale: Pt. I. Development, use, and reliability. *Archives of General Psychiatry*, *46*, 1006–1011.

Hachiya, Y., Miyata, R., Tanuma, N., Hongou, K., Tanaka, K., Shimoda, K., & Hayashi, M. (2013). Autoimmune neurological disorders associated with group-A beta-hemolytic streptococcal infection. *Brain & Development*, *35*(7), 670–674. https:/doi.org/10.1016/j.braindev.2012.10.003.

Hellerstien, D. J., & Flaxer, J. (2015). Vilazadone for the treatment of major depressive disorder: An evidence-based review of its place in therapy. *Core Evidence*, *10*, 49–62.

Kasper, S., Herman, B., Nivoli, G., Van Ameringen, M., Petralia, A., Mandel, F. S., Baldinetti, F., & Bandelow, B. (2009). Efficacy of pregabalin and venlafaxine-XR in generalized anxiety disorder: Results of a double-blind, placebo-controlled 8 week trial. *International Clinical Pwsychopharmacology*, *24*(2), 87–96.

Mavrogiorgou, P., Nalato, F., Meves, S., Luksnat, S., Norra, C., Gold, R., & Krogias, C. (2013). Transcranial sonography in obsessive-compulsive disorder. *Journal of Psychiatric Research*, *47*(11), 1642–1648.

Pollack, M. H., Van Ameringen, M., Simon, N. M., Worthington, J. W., Hoge, E. A., Keshaviah, A., & Stein, M. B. (2014) A double-blind randomized controlled trial of augmentation and switch strategies for refractory social anxiety disorder. *American Journal of Psychiatry*, *171*(1), 44–53.

Ponniah, K., Magiati, I., & Hollon, S. D. (2013). An update on the efficacy of psychological therapies in the treatment of obsessive-compulsive disorder in adults. *Journal of Obsessive-Compulsive and Related Disorders*, *2*(2), 207–218.

Posner, J., Marsh, R., Maia, T. V., Peterson, B. S., Gruber, A., & Simpson, H. B. (2013). Reduced functional connectivity within the limbic cortico-striato-thalamo-cortical loop in unmedicated adults with obsessive compulsive disorder. *Human Brain Mapping* (e-pub ahead of print).

Rauch, S. L., & Carlezon, W. A. Jr. (2013). Neuroscience: Illuminating the neural circuitry of compulsive behaviors. *Science*, *340*(6137), 1174–1175.

Russell, E. J., Fawcett, J. M., & Mazmanian, D. (2013). Risk of obsessive-compulsive disorder in pregnant and postpartum women: A meta-analysis. *Journal of Clinical Psychiatry*, *74*(4), 377–385.

Schatzberg, A. F. (2000). New Indications for antidepressants. *Journal of Clinical Psychiatry*, *61*(Suppl. 11), 9–17.

Stein, D. J., Koen, N., Fineberg, N., Fontenelle, L. F., Matsunaga, H., Osser, D., & Simpson, H. B. (2012). A 2012 evidence-based algorithm for the pharmacotherapy for obsessive-compulsive disorder. *Current Psychiatry Reports*, *14*(3), 211–219. https:/doi.org/10.1007/s11920–012-0268-9.

Thordarson, D. S., Radomsky, A. S., Rachman, S., Shafran, R., Sawchuk, C. N., & Ralph Hakstian, A. (2004). The Vancouver obsessional compulsive inventory (VOCI). *Behavior Research and Therapy, 42*, 1289–1314.

Venkatasubramanian, G., Zutshi, A., Jindal, S., Srikanth, S. G., Kovoor, J. M., Kumar, J. K., & Janardhan Reddy, Y. C. (2012). Comprehensive evaluation of cortical structure abnormalities in drug-naive, adult patients with obsessive-compulsive disorder: A surface-based morphometry study. *Journal of Psychiatric Research, 46*(9), 1161–1168.

Weissman, M. M., Bland. R. C., Canino, G. J., Greenwald, S., Hwu, H. G., Lee, C. K., Newman, S. C., Oakley-Browne, M. A., Rubio-Stipec, M., & Wickramaratne, P. J. (1994). The cross national epidemiology of obsessive compulsive disorder (The Cross National Collaborative Group). *Journal of Clinical Psychiatry, 55*, 5–10.

World Health Organization. (2001). *The World Health report 2001—mental health: New understanding, new hope.* World Health Organization.

Wu, K., Hanna, G. L., Rosenberg, D. R., & Arnold, P. D. (2012). The role of glutamate signaling in the pathogenesis and treatment of obsessive-compulsive disorder. *Pharmacology, Biochemistry, and Behavior, 100*(4), 726–735. https://doi.org/10.1016/j.pbb.2011.10.007.

Zhang, T., Wang, J., Yang, Y., Wu, Q., Li, B., Chen, L., & Gong, Q. (2011). Abnormal small-world architecture of top-down control networks in obsessive-compulsive disorder. *Journal of Psychiatry Neuroscience, 36*(1), 23–31.

WEB RESOURCES

- American Anxiety Disorders Association: http://www.adaa.org/
- Obsessive Compulsive Foundation: http://www.ocfoundation.org/
- Peace of Mind Foundation: http://www.peaceofmind.co/

13

Obsessive-Compulsive and Related Disorders

Overview

- People with obsessive-compulsive disorder (OCD) and related disorders often have other comorbid mental disorders.
- OCD and related disorders are closely related to each other and to anxiety disorders.
- Differentiating between subclinical symptoms and an actual disorder requires clinical judgment and consideration of the person's level of distress and functional impairment.
- *Types of OCD and related disorders*: OCD, body dysmorphic disorder (BDD), hoarding disorder, trichotillomania (TTM), excoriation disorder, substance- or medication-induced OCD and related disorder, OCD and related disorder due to another medical condition, other specified OCD and related disorder, and unspecified OCD and related disorder.

OBSESSIVE-COMPULSIVE DISORDER

Definition of Disorder

- This disorder is characterized by obsessions and/or compulsions; most people have both.
- *Obsessions*: recurrent and persistent thoughts, urges, or images; experienced as intrusive and unwanted.
- *Compulsions*: repetitive behaviors or mental acts that an individual feels compelled to perform in response to obsessions or rules (American Psychiatric Association, 2013).
- Level of insight occurs on a continuum from good or fair to poor, to absent/delusional, and can vary throughout the course of the illness.
- The obsessions and/or compulsions are time consuming and/or cause clinically significant distress or impairment.

Etiology

- Neuropsychiatric disorder
- Multiple theories of causation
  - Structural and functional brain dysfunction
  - Hyperactivity of frontal–subcortical neuronal circuit
    - Hyperactivity in orbitofrontal cortex
    - Subcortical frontal gyrus

- Hyperactivity in anterior cingulate cortex
- Deficient volume, thickness, and surface area of right anterior cingulate gyrus (ACG)
- Hyperactivity in striatum
  - Decreased right lingual gyrus surface area
  - Significant increase in the right inferior parietal cortical thickness
  - Significant increases in gyrification in the left insula, left middle frontal, and left lateral occipital regions extending to the precuneus and right supramarginal gyrus
  - Dysfunction in caudate nucleus; decreased volume but increased neurotransmission
  - Dysfunction of thalamus
  - *Genetics*: specific markers have been identified
- Cognitive and behavioral factors

Demographics
- There is a 2.5% lifetime prevalence.
- There is a 1.2% 12-month prevalence of OCD in the United States.
- Mean age of onset is 19.5 years: 6 to 15 years of age for males and 20 to 29 years for females. Females are affected at a slightly higher rate than males in adulthood, but males are more commonly affected in childhood.
- Similar prevalence rates appear around the world.
- No difference exists across socioeconomic backgrounds.

Temperament
- Greater internalizing symptoms, higher negative emotionality, and behavioral inhibition in childhood are possible temperamental risk factors.

Environment
- Childhood trauma including physical or sexual abuse
- Infection or postinfection autoimmune syndrome, especially with sudden onset of symptoms in children

Genetics and Physiology
- Pregnancy and perinatal period symptoms may worsen
- Family members with OCD

Obsessive-Compulsive Disorder Prevalence With Other Disorders

Depressive disorders: 19% to 90%
Bipolar disorder: Varying rates depending on source: 15% to 35%
Schizophrenia: 10% to 60%
Anxiety disorders: 76%

22% for specific phobia
   18% for social anxiety disorder (social phobia)
   12% for PD
   30% for GAD

Tic disorders: 30%
Personality disorders: 23% to 32%

GAD, generalized anxiety disorder; PD, panic disorder.

Diagnosis

Differential Diagnosis

- Subclinical symptoms (e.g., normal checking without impairment)
- Anxiety disorders
- Major depressive disorder
- Other OCD and related disorder
- Eating disorders
- Tics
- Psychotic disorders
- Other compulsive-like behaviors
- Obsessive-compulsive personality disorder
- Autism spectrum disorder
- Posttraumatic stress disorder

ICD-10 Codes

Obsessive-compulsive disorder, predominantly obsessional thoughts or ruminations (F42.0)

Obsessive-compulsive disorder, predominantly compulsive acts (F42.1)

Obsessive-compulsive disorder, mixed obsessional thoughts and acts (F42.2)

Diagnostic Workup

- Careful assessment is essential as patients may be embarrassed by their symptoms or have difficulty articulating them.
- Screening can be accomplished with a brief instrument, such as the Zohar-Fineberg Obsessive-Compulsive Screen, which can be administered in less than 1 minute.
- Neuropsychological/psychological testing may be helpful for a differential diagnosis.
- Yale-Brown Obsessive-Compulsive Scale (Y-BOCS-II) is used to determine severity.
- Assess symptoms against the Y-BOCS-II symptom checklist.
- Children's version of Y-BOCS (CY-BOCS) is available for the pediatric population.
- Vancouver Obsessional Compulsive Inventory assesses symptoms.
- Padua Inventory-Washington State University Revision (PI-WSUR) assesses symptoms.
- For use in further clinical evaluation and research, use the *Diagnostic and Statistical Manual of Mental Disorders*, Fifth Edition (*DSM-5*) Level 1—Crosscutting Symptom Measures, Domain X; if positive, can administer Level 2: Repetitive Thoughts and Behaviors.
- Assess medical needs due to lack of medical care in severe cases.
- Assess for possible underlying strep infection in the pediatric population if Pediatric Autoimmune Neuropsychiatric Disorders Associated with Streptococcal Infections (PANDAS) suspected.

Initial Assessment

- Onset of symptoms.
- Severity of symptoms.
- Psychiatric review of symptoms to assess for comorbid conditions.
- Suicide risk; as many as half of patients with OCD may experience suicidal thoughts during the illness.
- Alcohol and substance use.
- Family psychiatric history.
- Functioning at home, school, and work and social functioning.
- Level of insight, for example, how firmly held is the belief that something bad will happen if the patient does not engage in the compulsion?

- Impact on person/family.
- How much time is the patient spending ritualizing/obsessing?
- How much time is the family spending accommodating (obliging/responding to, or otherwise engaging/coping with the ill relative's OCD symptoms)?

Clinical Presentation
- Severe anxiety, worry, or distress
- Avoidant behavior
- Excessive time spent on parts of daily routine, that is, showering, cleaning, preparing to leave the home
- Obsessions and compulsions
  - Common themes for obsessions include contamination fears, taboo thoughts involving sex, aggression, or religion, and symmetry/order
  - Common compulsions include excessive washing/cleaning, arranging, checking, counting, or praying
- Odd or excessive behaviors
- Significant impairment (i.e., patient is unable to work/attend school or participate in social activities)

DSM-5 Diagnostic Guidelines
- Either obsessions or compulsions.
- Obsessions are defined by the following:
  - Recurrent thoughts, urges, or images are experienced as intrusive and unwanted and in most people cause marked distress or anxiety. Obsessions are ego dystonic.
  - The individual makes attempts to ignore or suppress the offending thoughts, urges, or images or to neutralize them with other thoughts and/or activities.
- Compulsions are defined by the following:
  - Repetitive behaviors (e.g., hand washing or repeating an action until it "feels right") or repetitive mental activities (e.g., counting items, repeating words silently).
  - The individual feels driven to perform these repetitive behaviors or mental activities (often according to rules that, they believe, must be stringently adhered to).
- Children may or may not be able to explain their behaviors or mental activities.
- The obsessions or compulsions cause distress for the individual, are time consuming, or significantly interfere with their daily routine.
- The obsessive-compulsive symptoms are not characteristic of the physiological effects of a substance (e.g., a drug of abuse, a medication) or another medical condition.
- If another psychiatric disorder is present, the content of the obsessions or compulsions does not center on that disorder (e.g., preoccupation with food in the presence of an eating disorder or excessive worrying about everyday events as seen in generalized anxiety disorder [GAD]).
- Specify level of insight.
- Specify if tic-related.

Treatment Overview
- OCD is usually a chronic (persistent) condition; therefore, treatment and support are offered indefinitely.
- OCD treatment can help bring symptoms under control so that they do not control the person's life. The two main treatments for OCD are psychotherapy and medication.

- For mild to moderate cases of OCD, psychotherapy may be offered without medication, while severe cases warrant medications and psychotherapy treatments.
- The individual's preferences and abilities should be considered when planning treatment; for example, treatment with medication alone may be indicated if the person is not willing or able to engage in therapy; in severe cases, starting medication may help the person engage in therapy later by reducing symptom severity.
- Comorbid psychiatric and medical disorders should also be considered.
- For therapy, exposure and response prevention (ERP) and cognitive-behavioral therapy (CBT) offer the greatest benefits, or efficacy and specificity, in treating the symptoms.
- ERP involves gradually exposing the person to a feared object or obsession, such as something dirty, while teaching the person ways to cope with the resulting anxiety.
- CBT involves retraining thought patterns and routines so that compulsive behaviors are no longer needed to relieve anxiety.

Psychopharmacology Overview for Obsessive-Compulsive Disorder

- Selective serotonin reuptake inhibitor (SSRI) medications are the preferred first-line medication treatments. It is not unusual to try several medications before finding one that works.
- *Pediatric psychopharmacology*: Fluoxetine, fluvoxamine, sertraline, escitalopram, and clomipramine are Food and Drug Administration (FDA) approved for use in pediatric patients.
- Clomipramine is FDA approved for OCD; it is a tricyclic antidepressant (TCA) medication and is generally not as well tolerated as SSRIs and is therefore used as a second-line treatment.
- Remember to rule out a bipolar disorder before initiating medication treatment.
- Individuals with OCD may need higher doses of medications, toward or at the maximum approved doses, to achieve full response.
- SSRIs have a black box warning for their potential to increase suicidal thoughts in children, adolescents, and young adults, although new analysis of data reveal conflicting information about this risk.
- Medication treatment should be continued for at least 1 to 2 years after adequate response; medication may be gradually tapered but may also need to continue indefinitely.
- Augmentation with an antipsychotic (off-label use) may be warranted after weighing the risk and benefits.
- Behavioral therapies should be used together with drug therapy wherever possible. Behavioral treatment appears to have long-lasting benefits and may delay relapse of symptoms or reduce symptom severity after discontinuing medication.

Drug Selection Table for Obsessive-Compulsive Disorder

CLASS	DRUG
	First line
SSRIs	Fluoxetine (*Prozac*)
	Fluvoxamine (*Luvox, Luvox CR*)
	Paroxetine (*Paxil, Paxil CR*)
	Sertraline (*Zoloft*)
	Escitalopram (*Lexapro*)
	Citalopram (*Celexa*)
	Second line
TCAs	Clomipramine (*Anafranil*)

SSRIs, selective serotonin reuptake inhibitors; TCAs, tricyclic antidepressants.

Patient Education

- Available treatment is discussed, with side effects carefully explained.
- Shared decision-making regarding treatment options including if or when to try to taper medication is also discussed.

Medical/Legal Pitfalls

- Person may present with life-threatening medical conditions but refuse treatment.
- Provider may have to determine whether patient needs commitment, based on symptoms.

BODY DYSMORPHIC DISORDER

Definition of Disorder

- This disorder is characterized by preoccupation with perceived defects or flaws in physical appearance that are not observable by or appear insignificant to others.
- The person engages in repetitive physical or mental acts related to this preoccupation.
- "Muscle dysmorphia" occurs when the person is preoccupied with the belief that their body is too small or not muscular enough.
- Level of insight occurs on a continuum from good or fair to poor, to absent/delusional.

Etiology

- Multiple theories of causation are as follows:
  - Some cross-sectional evidence that individuals with BDD have abnormal visual processing with abnormal patterns of brain activation and other neurocognitive differences
  - Possible impairment of frontostriatal and temporoparietal occipital circuits
  - Possible smaller mean volumes of the orbitofrontal cortex and anterior cingulate cortex with larger mean white matter volume
  - *Genetics*: higher prevalence if a first-degree relative has OCD
- Cognitive and behavioral factors

Demographics

- There is a 2.4% point prevalence in the United States, with a slightly lower prevalence outside the United States (1.7–1.8%).
- It is slightly more common in females than males (2.5% vs. 2.2%).
- Higher prevalence is found in certain specialty settings, for example, 9% to 15% among dermatology patients and 7% to 8% among cosmetic surgery patients in the United States.
- Mean age of onset is 16 to 17 years; most common age of onset is 12 to 13 years; symptoms often start with subclinical concerns and gradually worsen over time.

Environment

- History of childhood neglect or abuse.
- Culture may affect the person's content of preoccupation.

Genetics and Physiology

- First-degree relative with OCD

Diagnosis

Differential Diagnosis
- Normal appearance concerns and/or clearly noticeable physical defects
- Eating disorders
- Major depressive disorder
- Anxiety disorders
- Other OCD and related disorders
- Illness anxiety disorder
- Psychotic disorders
- Other disorders or symptoms (e.g., body identity integrity symptoms, gender dysphoria, olfactory reference syndrome)

ICD-10 Codes
Body dysmorphic disorder (F45.22)

Diagnostic Workup
- The Body Dysmorphic Disorder Questionnaire is a brief (1–5 minutes) screening.
- The Body Dysmorphic Disorder-Yale-Brown Obsessive Compulsive Scale (BDD-Y-BOCS) is used to assess severity of BDD symptoms.
- Neuropsychological/psychological testing may be helpful for a differential diagnosis.
- Assess general medical history and needs; some people with BDD may avoid medical care due to concerns about others seeing their body.

Initial Assessment
- Onset of symptoms
- Severity of symptoms
- Psychiatric review of symptoms to assess for comorbid conditions
- *Suicide risk*: rates of suicidal ideation and attempts are high among people with BDD
- Alcohol and substance use
- Family psychiatric history
- Functioning at home, school, and work and social functioning
- Level of insight
- Medical and surgical history
- Behaviors (e.g., use of anabolic steroids, compulsive skin picking, tanning, or cosmetic procedures or surgeries)

Clinical Presentation
- Severe anxiety and/or dysphoric mood.
- Preoccupation with perceived physical defect (can be any part of the body but common ones are the hair, nose, skin, and/or overall body/build).
- Excessive time is spent on checking or attending to one's physical appearance.
- Excessive behaviors intended to improve the defect (e.g., skin picking, exercise, use of beauty products or anabolic steroids/supplements).
- Significant impairment (i.e., person has difficulty with work/school or social activities). Many individuals with BDD may be housebound.

DSM-5 Diagnostic Guidelines
- Preoccupation with one or more perceived physical defects or flaws that appear slight or are not observable to others.

- Repetitive behaviors or mental acts in response to the concern (e.g., mirror checking, excessive grooming, skin picking, reassurance seeking, comparing appearance to others).
- The preoccupation causes clinically significant distress or impairment.
- The preoccupation is not better explained by another disorder (e.g., body fat or weight concerns in an eating disorder).
- Specify level of insight.
- Specify if with muscle dysmorphia.

Treatment Overview

- BDD is usually a chronic (persistent) condition; therefore, treatment and support are offered indefinitely.
- Treatment is similar to OCD treatment; the two main treatments are psychotherapy and medication.
- CBT, especially CBT tailored to BDD, should be offered to all individuals with BDD.
- There are no medications with FDA approval for BDD. However, medication can help reduce BDD symptoms and should especially be offered to individuals with moderate to severe BDD.
- The person's individual preferences as well as comorbid psychiatric and medical conditions should be considered when selecting treatment.
- Cosmetic or other procedures to "correct" the perceived flaw are specifically not recommended as they do not improve and may worsen symptoms.

Psychopharmacology Overview for Body Dysmorphic Disorder

- SSRI medications are the preferred first-line medication treatments. It is not unusual to try several medications before finding one that works.
- There are no medications that are FDA approved specifically for BDD; however, similarities between OCD and BDD support similar treatment strategies.
- Remember to rule out a bipolar disorder before initiating medication treatment.
- Individuals with BDD may need higher doses of medications toward or at the maximum approved doses to achieve full response.
- SSRIs have a black box warning for their potential to increase suicidal thoughts in children, adolescents, and young adults, although new analysis of data reveal conflicting information about this risk.
- Medication treatment should be reevaluated periodically, but most people will experience relapse of symptoms if treatment is stopped.
- Augmentation with an atypical antipsychotic or buspirone (off-label use) may be warranted after weighing the risk and benefits.

Drug Selection Table for Body Dysmorphic Disorder

CLASS	DRUG
	First line
SSRIs	Fluoxetine (*Prozac*)
	Escitalopram (*Lexapro*)
	Sertraline (*Zoloft*)
	Fluvoxamine (*Luvox, Luvox CR*)
	Paroxetine (*Paxil, Paxil CR*)
	Citalopram (*Celexa*)
	Second line
TCAs	Clomipramine (*Anafranil*)

SSRIs, selective serotonin reuptake inhibitors; TCAs, tricyclic antidepressants.

Patient Education

- Diagnosis and prognosis are discussed—treatable but chronic course.
- Available treatment is discussed, with side effects carefully explained.
- Shared decision-making regarding treatment options including if or when to try to taper medication is also discussed.

Medical/Legal Pitfalls

- The person may seek cosmetic or related surgical treatments and then respond poorly or become angry or litigious afterward.
- People with BDD may have additional medical needs related to their behaviors (e.g., infection from skin picking).
- The provider may have to determine whether the patient needs commitment, based on symptoms.

HOARDING DISORDER

Definition of Disorder

- This disorder is characterized by excessive clutter caused by persistent difficulty with discarding items regardless of value.
- The clutter causes impairment in basic activities such as activities of daily living and the general use of living spaces for their intended purposes.
- Level of insight occurs on a continuum from good or fair to poor, to absent/delusional.

Etiology

- Neuropsychiatric disorder.
- Multiple theories of causation.
- Possible common neurobiology with other disorders including OCD and attention deficit hyperactivity disorder (ADHD).
- Some evidence of decreased glucose metabolism in the dorsal ACG.
- *Genetics*: Some genetic markers have been identified.
- Cognitive and behavioral factors.

Demographics

- The point prevalence in the United States and Europe is approximately 2% to 6%.
- Onset of symptoms may begin early in life (ages 11–15), but symptoms appear to worsen to the point of clinically significant impairment later in life.
- The highest prevalence is among individuals aged 55 to 94 years old.
- Approximately 75% of people with hoarding disorder also have a comorbid mood or anxiety disorder; approximately 20% have comorbid OCD.

Temperament

- Indecisiveness in the person and their first-degree relatives.

Environment

- Stressors or trauma may precede the onset or exacerbation of the hoarding.

Genetics and Physiology

- Family members with hoarding disorder

Diagnosis

Differential Diagnosis

- Normal collecting
- Other medical condition
- Neurodevelopmental disorders
- Neurocognitive disorders
- Major depressive disorder
- Other OCD and related disorders
- Psychotic disorders

ICD-10 Codes

Hoarding disorder (F42.3)

Diagnostic Workup

- The Hoarding Rating Scale (HRS) is a brief 5-item scale that can be used to screen for hoarding disorder.
- The Saving Inventory-Revised (SIR) is a 23-item questionnaire used to measure features of hoarding disorder.
- The Clutter Image Rating (CIR) is a visual tool used to help standardize definitions of clutter; pictures #4 or higher indicate probable hoarding.
- Rule out underlying neurological or other medical disorders.

Initial Assessment

- Onset of symptoms
- Severity of symptoms
- Psychiatric review of symptoms to assess for comorbid conditions
- Alcohol and substance use
- Family psychiatric history
- Functioning at home, school, and work and social functioning
- Level of insight
- Current living situation and any risk or legal issues

Clinical Presentation

- May or may not report distress, depending on level of insight.
- Family members or other third party (e.g., landlord or housing/health officials) may prompt treatment.
- Person may exhibit indecisiveness, procrastination, perfectionism, avoidance, distractibility, and/or difficulty planning/organizing tasks.
- Possible symptoms of depression or anxiety (high rate of comorbidity).
- Continued excessive acquisition (either buying items or obtaining free items).
- Odd or excessive behaviors.
- Significant impairment (i.e., patient is unable to work/attend school or participate in social activities).

DSM-5 Diagnostic Guidelines

- Persistent difficulty discarding/parting with possessions, regardless of actual value.
- This difficulty is due to a perceived need to save the items and distress related to discarding them.
- This difficulty results in cluttered active living areas and substantially compromises their intended use or if the living areas are uncluttered it is only because of third party intervention.

- The hoarding causes clinically significant distress or impairment (which may include maintenance of a safe environment).
- The hoarding symptoms are not attributable to another medical condition.
- The hoarding symptoms are not better explained by another mental disorder.
- Specify level of insight.
- Specify if with excessive acquisition.

Treatment Overview

- Hoarding disorder is usually a chronic condition that worsens over time if untreated.
- Treatments for hoarding disorder are still being studied, but current evidence suggests that some types of therapy and some types of medications may help manage symptoms.
- CBT is the therapy of choice for hoarding disorder.
- Motivational interviewing and skills training may also be helpful.
- There are no medications with FDA approval for hoarding disorder, but similarities between hoarding disorder and other conditions such as OCD support the use of medications such as selective serotonin reuptake inhibitors (SSRIs).
- Some evidence suggests that the serotonin-norepinephrine reuptake inhibitor (SNRI) venlafaxine can be effective in hoarding disorder.

Psychopharmacology Overview for Hoarding Disorder

- Behavioral therapy should be combined with medication wherever possible.
- Comorbid psychiatric conditions should be considered when selecting medication treatment.
- The limited available evidence suggests efficacy for SSRI medications, the SNRI venlafaxine, and the TCA clomipramine.

Drug Selection Table for Hoarding Disorder

CLASS	DRUG
	First line
SSRIs	Fluoxetine (*Prozac*)
	Sertraline (*Zoloft*)
	Paroxetine (*Paxil, Paxil CR*)
	Paroxetine mesylate (*Pexeva*)
	Fluvoxamine (*Luvox, Luvox CR*)
	Citalopram (*Celexa*)
Selective SNRIs	Venlafaxine (*Effexor, Effexor XR*)
	Second line
TCAs	Clomipramine (*Anafranil*)

SNRIs, serotonin-norepinephrine reuptake inhibitors; SSRIs, selective serotonin reuptake inhibitors; TCAs, tricyclic antidepressants.

Patient Education

- Diagnosis and prognosis are discussed—treatable but generally persistent and worsens without treatment.
- Available treatment is discussed, with side effects carefully explained.
- Shared decision-making regarding treatment options including if or when to try to taper medication is discussed.
- Development of a relapse prevention plan can help with self-management.

Medical/Legal Pitfalls

- People with hoarding disorder may experience a number of safety and risk issues, including risk of falls or other injuries, fire hazards, unsanitary living conditions, and legal issues such as eviction or animal welfare issues.
- People with hoarding disorder may not be ready to accept treatment but may have relatives or authorities who are prompting treatment.

TRICHOTILLOMANIA

Definition of Disorder

- This disorder is characterized by recurrent pulling out of one's hair, resulting in hair loss.

Etiology

- Multiple theories of causation
  - Several small studies have found some evidence of structural and functional brain dysfunction, often comparable to that found in OCD.
  - Very limited evidence on neurochemistry indicates possible role in monoaminergic systems (serotonin, dopamine, and possibly norepinephrine) as well as the glutamate system.
  - Some evidence exists that the pulling behavior can alleviate anxiety but also that the behavior may be reinforcing with involvement of the dopamine reward pathway.
- Cognitive and behavioral factors

Demographics

- There is a 1% to 2% 12-month prevalence among adolescents and adults.
- Females are affected more frequently (10:1 ratio).
- Onset often during or after the onset of puberty.

Genetics and Physiology

- There is evidence of familial tendencies.

Diagnosis

Differential Diagnosis

- Normal hair removal or manipulation
- Other OCD and related disorders
- Neurodevelopmental disorders
- Psychotic disorders
- Another medical condition
- Substance-related disorders

ICD-10 Codes
Trichotillomania (F63.3)

Diagnostic Workup

- The Massachusetts General Hospital Hairpulling Scale (MGH-HPS) is a self-report instrument to measure symptom severity and can be used to measure symptoms over time.

- The NIMH Trichotillomania Severity Scale (NIMH-TSS) and the NIMH Trichotillomania Impairment Scale (NIMH-TIS) are semi-structured interviews to determine severity and impairment.
- The Yale-Brown Obsessive-Compulsive Scale-Trichotillomania (Y-BOCS-TM) is used to determine severity of hair pulling.
- Assess medical needs due to associated behaviors such as biting or swallowing hair; may need referral to gastroenterologist.
- Most individuals admit to hair pulling, but dermatological evaluation may be needed in some cases to confirm cause of hair loss.

Initial Assessment
- Onset of symptoms
- Severity of symptoms
- Quality of symptoms (e.g., sites from which the hair is pulled and frequency and duration of hair-pulling episodes)
- Pre-pulling behaviors or rituals
- Environmental and affective context of hair-pulling episodes
- Level of awareness of hair pulling (e.g., focused versus more automatic)
- Attempts to conceal hair loss (e.g., wigs, scarves, hats, make-up)
- Psychiatric review of symptoms to assess for comorbid conditions
- Alcohol and substance use
- Family psychiatric history
- Functioning at home, school, and work and social functioning
- Medical and surgical history
- Behaviors (e.g., does the person bite or swallow the hair or does the person have other related behaviors such as skin picking or nail biting)

Clinical Presentation
- Hair loss; highly variable in terms of location and pattern of loss
- Shame or embarrassment; attempts to camouflage hair loss
- Possible associated body-focused repetitive behaviors (e.g., nail biting, cheek or lip chewing)
- Distress or impairment in school/work/social settings
- Anxiety, depression

Diagnostic and Statistical Manual of Mental Disorders, Fifth Edition: Diagnostic Guidelines
- Recurrent pulling out of one's hair, resulting in hair loss.
- Repeated attempts to decrease or stop hair pulling.
- Hair pulling causes clinically significant distress or impairment.
- Hair pulling is not related to another medical condition.
- Hair pulling is not better explained by another mental disorder.

Treatment Overview
- TTM is typically chronic, with symptoms waxing and waning over time.
- TTM treatment is individualized; the overall goal is to reduce or eliminate hair-pulling behavior to improve functioning and reduce distress.
- Therapy for TTM consists of stimulus control and habit reversal training:
  - Stimulus control includes awareness and reduction of triggers and sensory reinforcement through behavioral changes.

▪ Habit reversal training includes awareness training followed by competing response training, where the person is taught to perform an action that physically prevents hair pulling (e.g., making a fist). Habit reversal training also includes social support.

▪ There is very limited evidence for medications in TTM treatment; SSRI medications or clomipramine are sometimes used and may help comorbid psychiatric conditions.

Psychopharmacology Overview for Trichotillomania

▪ There are no medications FDA-approved for TTM. Limited evidence suggests some efficacy with SSRIs or clomipramine; SSRIs are generally better tolerated

▪ Limited studies show possible future treatment options including N-acetylcysteine

Drug Selection Table for Trichotillomania

CLASS	DRUG
	Firstline
SSRIs	Fluoxetine (*Prozac*)
	Sertraline (*Zoloft*)
	Paroxetine (*Paxil, Paxil CR*)
	Paroxetine mesylate (*Pexeva*)
	Fluvoxamine (*Luvox, Luvox CR*)
	Citalopram (*Celexa*)
	Second line
TCAs	Clomipramine (*Anafranil*)

SSRIs, selective serotonin reuptake inhibitors; TCAs, tricyclic antidepressants.

Patient Education

▪ Diagnosis and prognosis are discussed—treatable; symptoms may remit and relapse; generally chronic.

▪ Available treatment is discussed, with side effects carefully explained.

▪ Individualized goals for treatment focused on the specific context of behaviors and impairment are discussed.

Medical/Legal Pitfalls

▪ The person may present with medical needs related to the disorder, for example, worn or broken teeth, trichobezoars from swallowing hair, and possible complications including bowel obstruction.

▪ People with TTM frequently have other psychiatric comorbidities.

EXCORIATION DISORDER

Definition of Disorder

▪ This disorder is characterized by recurrent picking of one's own skin, leading to clinically significant distress or impairment.

Etiology

▪ Multiple theories of causation

  ▪ A small study has shown functional underactivation in a cluster encompassing the bilateral dorsal striatum (maximal in right caudate), bilateral anterior cingulate. and right medial frontal regions on fMRI.

- Very limited evidence on neurochemistry indicates possible role in monoaminergic systems (serotonin, dopamine, and possibly norepinephrine) as well as the glutamate system.
  - Some evidence exists that the picking behavior can alleviate anxiety but also that the behavior may be reinforcing with involvement of the dopamine reward pathway.
- Cognitive and behavioral factors

Demographics
- There is a 1.4% lifetime prevalence.
- Females are affected more than males (3:1).
- Onset may occur at any time but commonly occurs during puberty.

Genetics and Physiology
- Family members with an OCD.
- Onset of symptoms may start with a dermatological condition such as acne, and then skin picking continues independent of the medical condition.

Diagnosis
Differential Diagnosis
- Psychotic disorder
- Other OCD and related disorders
- Neurodevelopmental disorders
- Somatic symptom and related disorders
- Other disorders or behaviors such as non-suicidal self-injury
- Other medical conditions (e.g., underlying dermatological condition)
- Substance-related disorders

ICD-10 Code
Excoriation (F42.4)

Diagnostic Workup
- The Skin Picking Scale (Revised) is an 8-item instrument that can be administered quickly.
- The Modified Neurotic Excoriation Yale-Brown Obsessive-Compulsive scale (NE-Y-BOCS) is used to determine severity.
- Assess medical needs related to skin picking (e.g., infection).
- Rule out underlying medical cause.

Initial Assessment
- Onset of symptoms
- Severity of symptoms
- Quality of symptoms (e.g., sites of skin picking, picking healthy skin versus scabs or minor abnormalities)
- Environmental and affective context of skin-picking episodes
- Level of awareness during skin picking (e.g., focused versus more automatic)
- Attempts to conceal or camouflage skin picking
- Psychiatric review of symptoms to assess for comorbid conditions
- Alcohol and substance use
- Family psychiatric history
- Functioning at home, school, and work and social functioning
- Presence of other repetitive body-focused behaviors (e.g., TTM, nail biting)

■ Medical needs (e.g., skin infection, tissue damage, scarring); rule out underlying medical conditions (e.g., scabies)

Clinical Presentation
■ Areas of skin excoriation, scarring, or infection; sites of picking may vary over time
■ Excessive time spent on skin-picking behavior or thinking about skin picking
■ Shame or embarrassment; attempts to camouflage skin excoriation
■ Possible associated body-focused repetitive behaviors (e.g., nail biting, cheek or lip chewing)
■ Distress or impairment in school/work/social settings
■ Anxiety, depression

Diagnostic and Statistical Manual of Mental Disorders, Fifth Edition: Diagnostic Guidelines
■ Recurrent picking of one's own skin, resulting in skin lesions
■ Repeated attempts to decrease or stop skin picking
■ Skin picking causing clinically significant distress or impairment
■ Skin picking being not related to another medical condition
■ Skin picking not better explained by another mental disorder

Treatment Overview

■ Excoriation disorder is typically chronic, with symptoms waxing and waning over time.
■ Excoriation disorder treatment is individualized; the overall goal is to reduce or eliminate skin-picking behavior to improve functioning and reduce distress.
■ Therapy for excoriation disorder consists of CBT and habit reversal training.
■ There is limited evidence for medications in excoriation disorder treatment; there is some support for use of SSRI medications.

Psychopharmacology Overview for Excoriation Disorder

■ There are no medications with FDA approval for excoriation disorder.
■ There is some evidence for the efficacy of SSRI medications.
■ Limited studies show possible future treatment options including *N*-acetylcysteine.
■ Comorbid psychiatric conditions should be considered when selecting medication.

Drug Selection Table for Excoriation Disorder

CLASS	DRUG
SSRIs	Fluoxetine (*Prozac*) Escitalopram (*Lexapro*) Sertraline (*Zoloft*) Paroxetine (*Paxil, Paxil CR*) Fluvoxamine (*Luvox, Luvox CR*) Citalopram (*Celexa*)

SSRIs, selective serotonin reuptake inhibitors.

Patient Education

■ Diagnosis and prognosis are discussed—treatable; symptoms may remit and relapse; generally chronic.
■ Available treatment is discussed, with side effects carefully explained.
■ Individualized goals for treatment are focused on the specific context of behaviors and impairment.

Medical/Legal Pitfalls

■ The person may present with medical needs (e.g., infection).
■ People with excoriation disorder frequently have other psychiatric comorbidities.

SUBSTANCE- OR MEDICATION-INDUCED OBSESSIVE-COMPULSIVE DISORDER AND RELATED DISORDER

Definition of Disorder

■ This disorder is characterized by obsessions, compulsions, skin picking, hair pulling, other body-focused repetitive behaviors, or other OCD-characteristic symptoms.
■ The symptoms develop during or soon after exposure to, intoxication by, or withdrawal from a substance capable of producing the symptoms.

Etiology

■ Substance induced (exposure to, intoxication by, or withdrawal from), commonly stimulants such as amphetamine or cocaine

Demographics

■ Prevalence is rare.

Diagnosis

Differential Diagnosis

■ Substance intoxication
■ OCD and related disorder
■ OCD and related disorder due to another medical condition
■ Delirium

ICD-10 Codes

Substance- or medication-induced obsessive-compulsive disorder is coded based on the substance and presence or absence of comorbid substance use disorder.

ICD-10 Codes for Substance- or Medication-Induced Obsessive-Compulsive Disorder and Related Disorder

SUBSTANCE	WITH MILD USE DISORDER	WITH MODERATE OR SEVERE USE DISORDER	WITHOUT USE DISORDER
Amphetamine (or other stimulant)	F15.188	F15.288	F15.988
Cocaine	F14.188	F14.288	F14.988
Other (or unknown) substance	F19.188	F19.288	F19.988

Diagnostic Workup

■ Substance and medication history
■ Labs (e.g., urine toxicology screening, especially amphetamine, cocaine, other stimulants).
■ Neuropsychological/psychological testing may be helpful for a differential diagnosis.

Initial Assessment

■ Onset of symptoms
■ Severity of symptoms

- Level of insight
- Psychiatric review of symptoms to assess for comorbid conditions
- Substance and medication use and history
- Family psychiatric history
- Functioning at home, school, and work and social functioning
- Medical needs

Clinical Presentation
- Obsessions and/or compulsions and/or body-focused repetitive behaviors
- Significant distress or impairment

Diagnostic and Statistical Manual of Mental Disorders, Fifth Edition: Diagnostic Guidelines
- Presence of obsessions, compulsions, skin picking, hair pulling, other body-focused repetitive behaviors, or other OCD and related disorder symptoms.
- There is evidence from the history, physical exam, or labs of the following:
  - The symptoms developed during or soon after the substance intoxication or withdrawal or after exposure to a medication.
  - The involved substance/medication is capable of producing the symptoms.
- The symptoms are not better explained by another OCD and related disorder (e.g., independent of substance/medication use or withdrawal).
- The symptoms do not occur exclusively during the course of a delirium.
- The symptoms cause clinically significant distress or impairment.
- Specify with onset during intoxication, withdrawal, or after medication use.

Treatment Overview
- Identify the causative agent and discontinue use if applicable.
- Monitor symptoms; if symptoms do not resolve within days/weeks, consider other underlying causes.

Patient Education
- Discuss substance and state of use (e.g., use, intoxication, withdrawal) that led to symptoms.
- If present, comorbid substance use disorder should be treated accordingly.
- Discuss timeline for resolution of symptoms after removal of the causative agent or completion of detoxification from agent; typically days to weeks.
- If symptoms do not resolve as expected, the patient should present for reevaluation.

Medical/Legal Pitfalls
- Patient may present with life-threatening medical conditions depending on substance and state of use.
- Patient may present with psychiatric comorbidities including psychosis and/or substance use disorder.
- Provider may have to determine whether patient needs commitment, based on symptoms.

OBSESSIVE-COMPULSIVE DISORDER AND RELATED DISORDER DUE TO ANOTHER MEDICAL CONDITION

Definition of Disorder
- Symptoms of obsessions, compulsions, skin picking, hair pulling, or other body-focused repetitive behaviors or hoarding that are due to an underlying medical condition.

Etiology
- Underlying medical condition (e.g., cerebral infarction) with clear temporal association between the condition and the OCD and related disorder symptoms.

Demographics
- Rare; the course generally follows that of the underlying medical condition.

Diagnosis

Differential Diagnosis
- Delirium
- Substance- or medication-induced OCD and related disorder
- OCD and related disorder (primary)
- Mixed presentation of symptoms (e.g., predominant mood symptoms)
- Illness anxiety disorder
- Associated feature of another mental disorder
- Other specified or unspecified OCD and related disorder

ICD-10 Code
Obsessive-compulsive disorder and related disorder due to another medical condition (F06.4)

Diagnostic Workup
- Physical exam and/or labs required to substantiate diagnosis of another medical condition.
- Psychiatric comprehensive assessment is done.
- Neuropsychological/psychological testing may be helpful for a differential diagnosis.

Initial Assessment
- Onset of symptoms
- Severity of symptoms
- Level of insight
- Psychiatric review of symptoms to assess for comorbid conditions
- Substance and medication use and history
- Family psychiatric history
- Functioning at home, school, and work and social functioning
- Medical and surgical history
- Medical needs

Clinical Presentation
- Obsessions, compulsions, hoarding, preoccupation with appearance, hair pulling, skin picking, and/or other body-focused repetitive behaviors
- Possible anxiety
- Significant distress or impairment due to symptoms
- Onset temporally connected to a medical condition capable of producing OCD and related symptoms

Diagnostic and Statistical Manual of Mental Disorders, Fifth Edition: Diagnostic Guidelines
- Obsessions, compulsions, preoccupations with appearance, hoarding, skin picking, hair pulling, other body-focused repetitive behaviors, or other symptoms of OCD and related disorders are predominant.
- The physical examination, history, and/or lab findings support the symptoms being a direct consequence of another medical condition.

- The symptoms are not better explained by another mental disorder.
- The symptoms do not occur exclusively during the course of a delirium.
- There is clinically significant distress or impairment related to the symptoms.
- Specify if with
  - OCD-like symptoms,
  - appearance preoccupations,
  - hoarding symptoms,
  - hair-pulling symptoms, and
  - skin-picking symptoms.
- Include the name of the other medical condition in the name of the disorder (e.g., OCD and related disorder due to cerebral infarction).

Treatment Overview

- Treatment of the underlying medical condition.
- Supportive therapy may be indicated depending on the context.

Patient Education

- Discuss the treatment of the underlying medical condition that is thought to be causing the symptoms.
- Discuss the timeline for resolution of symptoms after treatment of the medical condition.
- If symptoms do not resolve as expected, the patient should present for reevaluation.

Medical/Legal Pitfalls

- The provider will likely need to coordinate care with other providers to manage the medical condition.
- If symptoms do not resolve as expected, the provider should reevaluate and consider other diagnoses or comorbid conditions.

OTHER SPECIFIED AND UNSPECIFIED OBSESSIVE-COMPULSIVE DISORDER AND RELATED DISORDER

Definition of Disorder

- Other specified and unspecified OCD and related disorder applies to clinical presentations with symptoms of OCD and related disorders that cause clinically significant distress or impairment but do not meet the full diagnostic criteria for any of the other disorders.
- Other specified OCD and related disorder is selected when the clinician documents the specific reason that the full criteria for another disorder are not met (e.g., "other specified obsessive compulsive and related disorder: body-focused repetitive behavior disorder").
- Unspecified OCD and related disorder is selected when the clinician is not able to document the specific reason that full criteria for another disorder are not met, for example, when there is insufficient information to make a more specific diagnosis.
- Some examples include the following:
  - Olfactory reference syndrome
  - Body-focused repetitive behavior disorder (e.g., lip or nail biting)
  - Shubo-kyofu (excessive fear of having a bodily deformity)

Diagnosis

Differential Diagnosis

- Other OCD and related disorder (e.g., OCD, BDD)

ICD-10 Codes
Other obsessive-compulsive and related disorder (F42.8)
Unspecified obsessive-compulsive and related disorder (F42.9)

Diagnostic Workup
- Comprehensive psychiatric and medical evaluation is done.
- Neuropsychological/psychological testing may be helpful for a differential diagnosis.

Initial Assessment
- Onset of symptoms
- Severity of symptoms
- Level of insight
- Psychiatric review of symptoms to assess for comorbid conditions
- Substance and medication use and history
- Family psychiatric history
- Functioning at home, school, and work and social functioning
- Medical and surgical history
- Medical needs
- Level of insight

Medical/Legal Pitfalls
- Often difficult to treat symptoms without further clarifying diagnosis.
- Consider psychiatric and/or medical comorbidities including substance use disorders.

BIBLIOGRAPHY

Ahmari, S. E., Spellman, T., Douglass, N. L., Kheirbek, M. A., Simpson, H. B., Deisseroth, K., & Hen, R. (2013). Repeated cortico-striatal stimulation generates persistent OCD-like behavior. *Science, 340*(6137), 1234–1239.

American Psychiatric Association. (2013). *Diagnostic and statistical manual of mental disorders* (5th ed.). Washington, DC: American Psychiatric Press.

American Psychiatric Association. (2007). *Practice guideline for the treatment of patients with obsessive-compulsive disorder*. American Psychiatric Press.

Angoa-Perez, M., Kane, M. J., Briggs, D. I., Sykes, C. E., Shah, M. M., Francescutti, D. M., & Kuhn, D. M. (2012). Genetic depletion of brain 5HT reveals a common molecular pathway mediating compulsivity and impulsivity. *Journal of Neurochemistry, 121*(6), 974–984.

Beilharz, F., Castle, D. J., Grace, S., & Rossell, S. L. (2017). A systematic review of visual processing and associated treatments in body dysmorphic disorder. *Acta Psychiatrica Scandinavica, 136*(1), 16–36. https:/doi.org/10.1111/acps.12705

Beucke, J. C., Sepulcre, J., Talukdar, T., Linnman, C., Zschenderlein, K., Endrass, T., Kaufmann, C., & Kathmann, N. (2013). Abnormally high degree connectivity of the orbitofrontal cortex in obsessive-compulsive disorder. *JAMA Psychiatry, 70*(6), 619–629. https:/doi.org/10.1001/jamapsychiatry.2013.173

Bjorgvinsson, T., Hart, J., & Heffelfinger, S. (2007). Obsessive-compulsive disorder: Update on assessment and treatment. *Journal of Psychiatric Practice, 13*, 362–372.

Bloch, M. H., Green, C., Kichuk, S. A., Dombrowski, P. A., Wasylink, S., Billingslea, E., & Pittenger, C. (2013). Long-term outcome in adults with obsessive-compulsive disorder. *Depress Anxiety, 30*(8), 716–722.

Bloch, M. H., Landeros-Weisenberger, A., Kelmendi, B., Coric, V., Bracken, M. B., & Leckman, J. F. (2006). A systematic review: Antipsychotic augmentation with treatment refractory obsessive-compulsive disorder. *Molecular Psychiatry, 11*(7), 622–632.

Bloch, M. H., Sukhodolsky, D. G., Dombrowski, P. A., Panza, K. E., Craiglow, B. G., Landeros-Weisenberger, A., & Schultz, R. T. (2011). Poor fine-motor and visuospatial skills predict persistence of pediatric-onset obsessive-compulsive disorder into adulthood. *Journal of Child Psychology and Psychiatry, and Allied Disciplines, 52*(9), 974–983.

Burki, T. (2018). Hoarding disorder: A medical condition. *Lancet, 392*(10148), 626. https://doi.org/10.1016/S0140-6736

Burns, G. L., Keortge, S. G., Formea, G. M., & Sternberger, L. G. (1996). Revision of the Padua inventory of obsessive compulsive disorder symptoms: Distinctions between worry, obsessions, and compulsions. *Behavior Research and Therapy, 24,* 163–173.

Castro-Rodrigues, P., Camacho, M., Almeida, S., Marinho, M., Soares, C., Barahona-Corrêa, J. B., & Oliveira-Maia, A. J. (2018). Criterion validity of the Yale-Brown Obsessive-Compulsive Scale Second Edition for diagnosis of obsessive-compulsive disorder in Adults. *Frontiers in Psychiatry, 9,* 431. https://doi.org/10.3389/fpsyt.2018.00431

Clomipramine Collaborative Study Group. (1991). Clomipramine in the treatment of patient with obsessive-compulsive disorder. *Archives of General Psychiatry, 48,* 730–738.

Department of Health and Human Services, Centers for Medicare and Medicaid. (2015). *Antidepressant medications: Use in pediatric patients.* https://www.cms.gov/Medicare-Medicaid-Coordination/Fraud-Prevention/Medicaid-Integrity-Education/Pharmacy-Education-Materials/Downloads/ad-pediatric-factsheet11-14.pdf

Dougherty, D. D., Rauch, S. L., & Jenike, M. A. (2004). Pharmacotherapy for obsessive-compulsive disorder. *Journal of Clinical Psychology, 60,* 1195–1202.

Fan, Q., Palaniyappan, L., Tan, L., Wang, J., Wang, X., Li, C., & Liddle, P. F. (2013). Surface anatomical profile of the cerebral cortex in obsessive-compulsive disorder: A study of cortical thickness, folding and surface area. *Psychology Medicine, 43*(5), 1081–1091.

Feusner, J. D., Neziroglu, F., Wilhelm, S., Mancusi, L., & Bohon, C. (2010). What causes BDD: Research findings and a proposed model. *Psychiatric Annals, 40*(7), 349–355.

Geller, D. A. & March, J. (2012). Practice parameter for the assessment and treatment of children and adolescents with obsessive-compulsive disorder. *Journal of the American Academy of Child and Adolescent Psychiatry, 51*(1), 98–113. https://doi.org/10.1016/j.jaac.2011.09.019

Gibbons, R. D., Brown, C. H., Hur, K., Davis, J., & Mann, J. J. (2012). Suicidal thoughts and behavior with antidepressant treatment: Reanalysis of the randomized placebo-controlled studies of fluoxetine and venlafaxine. *Archives of General Psychiatry, 69*(6), 580–587.

Goodman, W. K., Price, L. H., Rasmussen, S. A., Mazure, C., Fleischmann, R. L., Hill, C. L., Heninger, G. R., & Charney, D. S. (1989). The Yale-Brown obsessive compulsive scale: Pt. I. Development, use, and reliability. *Archives of General Psychiatry, 46,* 1006–1011.

Grant, J. E., & Chamberlain, S. R. (2016). Trichotillomania. *American Journal of Psychiatry, 173*(9), 868–874.

Grant, J. E., Chamberlain, S. R., Redden, S. A., Leppink, E. W., Odlaug, B. L., Suck Won Kim, & Kim, S. W. (2016). N-acetylcysteine in the treatment of excoriation disorder: A randomized clinical trial. *JAMA Psychiatry, 73*(5), 490–496. https://doi.org/10.1001/jamapsychiatry.2016.0060

Hachiya, Y., Miyata, R., Tanuma, N., Hongou, K., Tanaka, K., Shimoda, K., & Hayashi, M. (2013). Autoimmune neurological disorders associated with group-A beta-hemolytic streptococcal infection. *Brain & Development, 35*(7), 670–674. https://doi.org/10.1016/j.braindev.2012.10.003

International Obsessive Compulsive Disorder Foundation. (2019). *Clinical assessment.* https://hoarding.iocdf.org/professionals/clinical-assessment/

Lochner, C., Roos, A., & Stein, D. J. (2017). Excoriation (skin-picking) disorder: A systematic review of treatment options. *Neuropsychiatric Disease and Treatment, 13*, 1867–1872. https://doi.org/10.2147/NDT.S121138

Mavrogiorgou, P., Nalato, F., Meves, S., Luksnat, S., Norra, C., Gold, R., & Krogias, C. (2013). Transcranial sonography in obsessive-compulsive disorder. *Journal of Psychiatric Research, 47*(11), 1642–1648.

Mufaddel, A., Osman, O. T., Almugaddam, F., & Jafferany, M. (2013). A review of body dysmorphic disorder and its presentation in different clinical settings. *Primary Care Companion for CNS Disorders, 15*(4), PCC.12r01464. https://doi.org/10.4088/PCC.12r01464

National Institute of Mental Health. (2016). *PANDAS: Questions and answers*. https://www.nimh.nih.gov/health/publications/pandas/pandas-qa-508_01272017_154202.pdf

Odlaug, B. L., Hampshire, A., Chamberlain, S. R., & Grant, J. E. (2016). Abnormal brain activation in excoriation (skin-picking) disorder: Evidence from an executive planning fMRI study. *British Journal of Psychiatry, 208*(2), 168–174. https://doi.org/10.1192/bjp.bp.114.155192

Phillips, K. A., & Hollander, E. (2008). Treating body dysmorphic disorder with medication: Evidence, misconceptions, and a suggested approach. *Body Image, 5*(1), 13–27.

Phillips, K. A., Hollander, E., Rasmussen, S. A., Aronowitz, B. R., DeCaria, C., & Goodman, W. K. (1997). A severity rating scale for body dysmorphic disorder: Development, reliability, and validity of a modified version of the Yale-Brown Obsessive Compulsive Scale. *Psychopharmacology Bulletin, 33*(1), 17–22.

Piacentino, D., Pasquini, M., Sani, G., Chetoni, C., Cappelletti, S., & Kotzalidis, G. D. (2019). Pharmacotherapy for hoarding disorder: How did the picture change since its excision from OCD? *Current Neuropharmacology, 17*(1), e-pub ahead of print. https://doi.org/10.2174/1570159X17666190124153048

Ponniah, K., Magiati, I., & Hollon, S. D. (2013). An update on the efficacy of psychological therapies in the treatment of obsessive-compulsive disorder in adults. *Journal of Obsessive-Compulsive and Related Disorders, 2*(2), 207–218.

Posner, J., Marsh, R., Maia, T. V., Peterson, B. S., Gruber, A., & Simpson, H. B. (2013). Reduced functional connectivity within the limbic cortico-striato-thalamo-cortical loop in unmedicated adults with obsessive compulsive disorder. *Human Brain Mapping* (e-pub ahead of print).

Rauch, S. L., & Carlezon, W. A. Jr. (2013). Neuroscience: Illuminating the neural circuitry of compulsive behaviors. *Science, 340*(6137), 1174–1175.

Rubio-Aparicio, M., Núñez-Núñez, R. M., Sánchez-Meca, J., López-Pina, J. A., Marín-Martínez, F., & López-López, J. A. (2020). The padua inventory-Washington State University Revision of obsessions and compulsions: A reliability generalization meta-analysis. *Journal of Personality Assessment, 102*(1), 113–123. https://doi.org/10.1080/00223891.2018.1483378

Russell, E. J., Fawcett, J. M., & Mazmanian, D. (2013). Risk of obsessive-compulsive disorder in pregnant and postpartum women: A meta-analysis. *Journal of Clinical Psychiatry, 74*(4), 377–385.

Sadock, B. J., Sadock, V. A., & Ruiz, P. (2015). *Kaplan & Sadock's synopsis of psychiatry: Behavioral sciences/clinical psychiatry* (11th ed.). Wolters Kluwer.

Saxena, S., Brody, A. L., Maidment, K. M., Smith, E. C., Zohrabi, N., Katz, E., Baker, S. K., & Baxter, L. R. Jr. (2004). Cerebral glucose metabolism in obsessive-compulsive hoarding. *American Journal of Psychiatry, 161*(6), 1038–1048.

Stein, D. J., Koen, N., Fineberg, N., Fontenelle, L. F., Matsunaga, H., Osser, D., & Simpson, H. B. (2012). A 2012 evidence-based algorithm for the pharmacotherapy for obsessive-compulsive disorder. *Current Psychiatry Reports, 14*(3), 211–219. https://doi.org/10.1007/s11920-012-0268-9

Thordarson, D. S., Radomsky, A. S., Rachman, S., Shafran, R., Sawchuk, C. N., & Ralph Hakstian, A. (2004). The Vancouver obsessional compulsive inventory (VOCI). *Behavior Research and Therapy, 42*, 1289–1314.

Venkatasubramanian, G., Zutshi, A., Jindal, S., Srikanth, S. G., Kovoor, J. M., Kumar, J. K., & Janardhan Reddy, Y. C. (2012). Comprehensive evaluation of cortical structure abnormalities in drug-naive, adult patients with obsessive-compulsive disorder: A surface-based morphometry study. *Journal of Psychiatric Research, 46*(9), 1161–1168.

Weissman, M. M., Bland, R. C., Canino, G. J., Greenwald, S., Hwu, H. G., Lee, C. K., Newman, S. C., Oakley-Browne, M. A., Rubio-Stipec, M., & Wickramaratne, P. J. (1994). The cross national epidemiology of obsessive compulsive disorder (The Cross National Collaborative Group). *Journal of Clinical Psychiatry, 55*, 5–10.

Woods, D. W., & Houghton, D. C. (2014). Diagnosis, evaluation, and management of trichotillomania. *Psychiatric Clinics of North America, 37*(3), 301–317.

World Health Organization. (2001). *The World Health report 2001—Mental health: New understanding, new hope.* World Health Organization.

Wu, K., Hanna, G. L., Rosenberg, D. R., & Arnold, P. D. (2012). The role of glutamate signaling in the pathogenesis and treatment of obsessive-compulsive disorder. *Pharmacology, Biochemistry, and Behavior, 100*(4), 726–735. https://doi.org/10.1016/j.pbb.2011.10.007

Zhang, T., Wang, J., Yang, Y., Wu, Q., Li, B., Chen, L., & Gong, Q. (2011). Abnormal small-world architecture of top-down control networks in obsessive-compulsive disorder. *Journal of Psychiatry Neuroscience, 36*(1), 23–31.

WEB RESOURCES

- International OCD and Related Disorders Foundation, Body Dysmorphic Disorder: https://bdd.iocdf.org
- International OCD and Related Disorders Foundation, Hoarding: https://hoarding.iocdf.org
- National Alliance on Mental Illness (NAMI): https://www.nami.org/#
- National Institute of Mental Health, OCD: https://www.nimh.nih.gov/health/topics/obsessive-compulsive-disorder-ocd/index.shtml
- Obsessive Compulsive Foundation: http://www.ocfoundation.org/
- Peace of Mind Foundation: http://www.peaceofmind.com

14

Dissociative Disorders

OVERVIEW OF DISSOCIATIVE DISORDERS

- The normal integrations of consciousness, memory, identity, emotion, perception, body representation, motor control, and behavior are disrupted.
- Symptoms include unbidden intrusions into awareness and behavior.
- Inability to access information or to control mental functions.
- Positive symptoms include fragmentation of identity, depersonalization, and derealization.
- Negative symptoms include amnesia.
- Dissociative symptoms are frequently found after a traumatic event.
- Acute stress disorder and posttraumatic stress disorder (PTSD) contain dissociative symptoms.
- Symptoms can include depersonalization (experiences of unreality or detachment from one's mind, self, or body) and/or derealization (experiences of unreality and detachment from one's surroundings).

DISSOCIATIVE IDENTITY DISORDER

Background Information

Definition of Disorder

- Disruption of identity exemplified by two or more distinct personality states (in some cultures possession).
- Related alterations in affect, behavior, consciousness, memory, perception, cognition, and sensory-motor function.
- Gaps in the recall of everyday events, important personal information, and/or traumatic events.
- Significant decline in important areas of functioning.
- Children's imaginary playmates or fantasy play do not explain the symptoms.
- The symptoms are not the result of physiological substances or medical conditions.

Etiology
- Dissociative identity disorder is strongly linked to early childhood trauma (maltreatment).
- Between 85% and 97% of the patients have had severe childhood trauma, with physical and sexual abuse being the most frequently reported trauma.
- There is no genetic predisposition.

Demographics
- Female-to-male ratios between 5 to 1 and 9 to 1 for diagnosed cases
- Fewer than 200,000 cases per year in United States
- Rare in anyone 13 years of age or younger

Risk Factors
- Interpersonal/environmental stressors during early childhood years (prior to age 9)
- History of recurring, overpowering, and often life-threatening disturbances at a young age
- History of persistent neglect or emotional abuse and not necessarily physical or sexual abuse
- Parents being perceived by children as being frightening or unpredictable

Diagnosis

Differential Diagnosis
- Factitious, imitative, and malingered dissociative identity disorder
- Affective disorders
- Psychotic disorders
- Anxiety disorders
- PTSD
- Personality disorders
- Neurocognitive disorders
- Neurological and seizure disorders
- Somatic symptom disorders
- Other dissociative disorders
- Deep-trance phenomena
- Conversion disorder
- Major depressive disorder

ICD-10 Code
Dissociative identity disorder 300.14 (F44.81)

Diagnostic Workup
- Careful and detailed mental status exam
- Physical examination
- Labs as needed to evaluate physical complaints:
  Thyroid function studies (T3, T4, thyroid-stimulating hormone [TSH])
  Complete blood count (CBC) with differentials: hemoglobin, hematocrit, red blood cell (RBC) count, white blood cell (WBC) count, WBC differential count, and platelet count
    - Comprehensive metabolic panel (CMP) including glucose, calcium, albumin; total protein count; levels of sodium, potassium, CO_2 (carbon dioxide and bicarbonate), chloride, blood urea nitrogen (BUN), creatinine, alkaline

phosphatase (ALP), alanine amino transferase (ALT), aspartate amino trans-ferase (AST), and bilirubin
- Psychological examination to include possible screening:
  The Dissociative Experiences Scale (DES): self-report screen
  - The Structured Clinical Interview for *DSM-5* Dissociative Disorders (SCID-D)
    - A clinician-guided interview, it is the gold standard in the diagnosis of disso-ciative disorders but is time consuming.

Initial Assessment
- Mental Status Examination Questions could include asking the following questions:
  Do you act so differently in one situation compared to another situation that you feel almost like you were two people?
  Do you feel that there is more than one of you? More than one part of you? Side of you? Are the two sides in conflict?
  Does the other part of you have their own ways of thinking, perceiving, relating to yourself and the world? Do they have their own memories, thoughts, and feelings?
  Does more than one of these entities take control of you? Have you felt like your body does not belong to you? Have you ever done things that did not seem like yourself?
  Do you ever feel like you are outside, inside, or beside yourself?
  Do you feel disconnected from yourself? Can you name the sides of you? Do you ever struggle against yourself?
  - Have you ever heard voices, sounds, or conversations in your mind that seem to be discussing you and what you might need to do? Have you felt like your body was not yours?

Clinical Presentation
- Presence of two or more distinct personality states.
- Experience losing time.
- Blackout spells.
- Major gaps in the continuity of recall for personal information.
- Significant gaps in autobiographical memory, especially for childhood memories.
- Odd first-person plural or third-person singular or plural self-references.
- Children have the same core dissociative symptoms and secondary clinical phe-nomena as adults, only their imaginary companions take control of their behavior.
- Rapid mood swings or obsessive-compulsive personality traits may be present.

Diagnostic and Statistical Manual of Mental Disorders, Fifth Edition: Diagnostic Guidelines
- Disruption of identity is characterized by two or more distinct personality states.
- Recurrent gaps in the recall of everyday events, important personal information, and/or traumatic events.
- Symptoms cause clinically significant distress or impairment in social, occupa-tional, or other areas.
- Not part of accepted cultural or religious practice. In children, not better explained by imaginary playmates or fantasies.
- Not attributable to the effects of a substance or another medical condition.

Treatment
- *Psychotherapy*: Comfort with family treatment and systems theory are helpful in working with individuals who see themselves as a complex system of interactions with seen and unseen individuals. Expertise in addressing somatoform disorders

may also be helpful as they present with numerous somatic symptoms. Some patients are beyond help, other than supporting their symptoms and stabilizing them in their chronic states. Some types of therapy might include the following:

- Psychoanalytic psychotherapy
  Cognitive therapy: Many cognitive distortions are associated with this disorder and are slowly responsive in most cases.
  Behavioral therapy
  Hypnotherapy: may alleviate flashbacks, dissociative hallucinations, and passive-influence experiences. Enables negative events to be viewed without overwhelming anxiety.
  Electroconvulsive therapy: ameliorates refractory mood disorders but does not worsen dissociative memory problems.
- Adjunctive therapies
- Group therapy with patients with dissociative identity disorders are the most successful.
- Family therapy is used to address pathological family and marital processes, which are common among these patients. Interventions for education and support of family members have also been found to be helpful. Sex therapy may be necessary because these patients become intensely phobic of intimate contact for periods of time.
- Self-help groups have not been found to be helpful because they intensify PTSD symptoms, exploit these patients by predatory group members, contaminate recall by group discussions of trauma, and alienate them from other sufferers of trauma.
- Expressive therapy, such as art and movement therapy, gives safer avenues to express thoughts, feelings, mental images, and conflicts that they otherwise may have difficulty doing.
- Occupational therapy provides focused, structured activities that can be completed successfully, helping ground the patient.
- Eye movement desensitization and reprocessing (EMDR) has not been fully studied but might be helpful in those patients who have been stabilized but not in those in initial stages of the disorder.
- Pharmacotherapy
  - Antidepressants/anxiolytics such as selective serotonin reuptake inhibitors (SSRIs), nonselective reuptake inhibitors, tricyclic antidepressants (TCAs), and monoamine oxidase inhibitors:
    - Used to treat comorbid symptoms, stabilize mood, and reduce intrusive symptoms, hyperarousal, and anxiety
  - Benzodiazepines
    - Used with caution to decrease anxiety; this medication class may exacerbate dissociation.
  - Betablockers, clonidine
    - Can be used to stabilize mood and reduce intrusive symptoms, hyperarousal, and anxiety.
  - Atypical second-generation antipsychotics
    - Stabilize mood and reduce overwhelming anxiety and intrusive symptoms.
  - Prazosin
    - Reduces nightmares.
  - Carbamazepine and other mood stabilizers
    - Reduce aggression, intrusive symptoms, hyperarousal.
  - Naltrexone
    - *Reduces self-injurious behavior.*

Chronic Treatment

- Psychotherapy is used to strengthen the ego, identify new ways to cope, deconstruct different personalities and integrate them into one, improve relationships, and optimize functioning.

Prognosis/Recurrence Rate

- More than 70% of people with dissociative identity disorder have attempted suicide at least once, and self-injurious behavior is common.
- With proper treatment, many people who are impaired experience improvement in their ability to function in their work and personal lives.

Medical/Legal Pitfalls

- Persons with dissociative identity disorder often present in the court system instead of the mental health system. Defendants claim that they committed serious crimes while they were in their dissociated state, asserting that their alter personality did the crime. There have been pleas of not guilty by reason of insanity. Debate exists as to whether this should exculpate them for their criminal acts.

DEPERSONALIZATION/DEREALIZATION DISORDER

Background Information

Definition of Disorder

- Depersonalization exists when the person feels like they are an outside observer of their life.
- Derealization is when one feels detached from one's surroundings.
- Dissociation occurs when there are persistent feelings of being detached from one's body or environment.
- The depersonalization/derealization disorder occurs when there are either or both of these symptoms.

Etiology

- *Psychodynamic*: ego disintegration as an affective response to defend the ego.
- *Traumatic stress*: One-third to one half report history of significant trauma. After an accident that was life threatening, as many as 60% report transient depersonalization. In military studies, symptoms of depersonalization/derealization are evoked by stress and fatigue.
- *Neurobiological theories*: Depletion of L-tryptophan, a serotonin precursor, and the involvement of N-methyl-D-aspartate as responsible for the genesis of depersonalization symptoms indicate the presence of neurobiological explanations for this disorder.

Demographics

- Transient experiences of depersonalization/derealization are common in both normal and clinical populations.
- In general, one half of all adults have experienced at least one lifetime episode of depersonalization/derealization.
- The gender ratio is 1:1.
- Lifetime prevalence is 0.8% to 2.8% for the general population.
- Mean age for onset is 16 years, although it can start in early or middle childhood.

Risk Factors

■ If you have a harm-avoidant temperament, immature defenses, and both discon-nection and over-connection schemata, then you are more likely to have a dissocia-tive identity disorder.

■ Cognitive disconnection includes emotional inhibition and themes of abuse, neglect, and deprivation.

　■ Over-connection involves impaired autonomy with dependency, vulnerability, and incompetence.

■ History of emotional abuse and emotional neglect, physical abuse, witnessing domestic violence, growing up with seriously impaired mentally ill parent, or unexpected death or suicide of family member or close friend are risk factors.

■ Precipitant likely to be severe stress, depression, anxiety (panic attacks), and illicit drug use.

■ Symptoms can be elicited by hallucinogens, ketamine, 3,4-methylenedioxymetham-phetamine (MDMA), salvia, and tetrahydrocannabinol.

Diagnosis

Differential Diagnosis

■ Illness anxiety disorder
■ Major depressive disorder
■ Obsessive-compulsive disorder
■ Other dissociative disorders
■ Anxiety disorders
■ Psychotic disorders
■ Substance- or medication-induced disorders
■ Mental disorders due to another medical condition

ICD-10 Code

Depersonalization/derealization disorder 300.6 (F48.1)

Diagnostic Workup

■ Thorough medical and neurological examination is essential.
■ Labs as needed to evaluate physical complaints:
Thyroid function studies (T3, T4, TSH)
CBC with differentials: hemoglobin, hematocrit, RBC count, WBC count, WBC dif-ferential count, and platelet count
Drug screens for marijuana, cocaine, and other psychostimulants
EEG
　■ CMP, including glucose, calcium, albumin; total protein count; levels of sodium, potassium, CO_2 (carbon dioxide and bicarbonate), chloride, BUN, creatinine, ALP, ALT, AST, and bilirubin. Rule out seizure disorders, brain tumors, post-concus-sive syndrome, migraines, vertigo, Meniere's disease, and metabolic syndromes.

Initial Assessment

■ Mental status examination.
■ Individual may report persistent and/or recurrent feelings of detachment or estrangement from one's self.
■ Patients may report feeling like an automaton or seeing themselves in a movie.
■ They may feel detached from their environment as though feeling like they were dreaming or dead.

Clinical Presentation

- Depersonalization can include a sense of bodily changes, duality of self as observer/actor, being cut off from others, and/or being cut off from one's emotions.
- They may say, "I feel dead," "nothing is real," or "I'm standing outside myself" as if in an "out-of-body experience."
- They may feel as if they are going crazy or have irreversible brain damage.
- Time moves too fast or too slow for them.

Diagnostic and Statistical Manual of Mental Disorders, Fifth Edition: Diagnostic Guidelines

- The presence of persistent or recurrent experiences of depersonalization, derealization, or both.
- During depersonalization or derealization, the testing of reality remains intact.
- The symptoms cause significant distress or impairment in important areas of functioning.
- The disturbance is not due to the physiological effects of a substance or other medical conditions.
- The disturbance is not better explained by another mental disorder.

Treatment

- *Psychotherapy*: Comfort with family treatment and systems theory are helpful in working with individuals who see themselves as a complex system of interactions with seen and unseen individuals. Expertise in addressing somatoform disorders may also be helpful as they present with numerous somatic symptoms. Some patients are beyond help, other than supporting their symptoms and stabilizing them in their chronic states. Some types of therapy might include the following:
  - Psychoanalytic Psychotherapy
  Cognitive therapy: Many cognitive distortions are associated with this disorder and are slowly responsive in most cases.
  Behavioral therapy
  Hypnotherapy: may alleviate flashbacks, dissociative hallucinations, and passive-influence experiences. Enables negative events to be viewed without overwhelming anxiety.
    - *Electroconvulsive therapy*: ameliorates refractory mood disorders but does not worsen dissociative memory problems.
- Adjunctive therapies
- Group therapy with patients with dissociative identity disorders are the most successful.
- Family therapy is used to address pathological family and marital processes, which are common among these patients. Interventions for education and support of family members have also been found to be helpful. Sex therapy may be necessary because these patients become intensely phobic of intimate contact for periods of time.
- Self-help groups have not been found to be helpful because they intensify PTSD symptoms, exploit these patients by predatory group members, contaminate recall by group discussions of trauma, and alienate them from other sufferers of trauma.
- Expressive therapy, such as art and movement therapy, gives safer avenues to express thoughts, feelings, mental images, and conflicts that they otherwise may have difficulty doing.
- Occupational therapy provides focused, structured activities that can be completed successfully, helping ground the patient.

- EMDR has not been fully studied but might be helpful in those patients who have been stabilized but not in those in initial stages of the disorder.
- Pharmacotherapy
  - Typically, these patients are refractory in their response. SSRIs such as fluoxetine (*Prozac*) may be helpful to depersonalization disorder. However, fluvoxamine (*Luvox*) and lamotrigine (*Lamictal*) have not been effective. Some patients respond to the usual groups of psychiatric medications, either singly or in combination: antidepressants, mood stabilizers, typical and atypical antipsychotics, anticonvulsants, and so forth.
- Psychotherapy techniques have been used, but many patients do not have a robust response to these.
  Psychodynamic
  Cognitive
  Cognitive-behavioral
  Hypnotherapeutic
  - Supportive
- Other therapies that seem to help include the following: stress management strategies, distraction techniques, reduction of sensory stimulation, relaxation training, and physical exercise.

Chronic Treatment
- Psychotherapy with other strategies (listed previously) seems to be of utmost efficacy in reducing symptoms.

Prognosis/Recurrence Rate
- Complete recovery is possible for many of these patients. Some of the symptoms go away on their own or after treatment; however, with no treatment to work out the underlying issues, additional episodes of depersonalization/derealization may occur.
- Recurrences can be triggered by stress, worsening mood or anxiety symptoms, novel or over-stimulatory environments, and lack of sleep or lighting.
- One-third have discrete episodes, one-third continuous symptoms, and another one-third an initial episode that eventually becomes continuous.

Medical/Legal Pitfalls
- Depersonalization carries with it the risk of suicidal ideation to suicide completion.

DISSOCIATIVE AMNESIA

Background Information
Definition of Disorder
- Inability to remember personal information.
- Information lost is important and too extensive to be caused by forgetfulness.
- Gaps in recall occur usually about traumatic events or stressful information.
- Is not caused by illness, substance use, or injury to the brain.
- Memories are stored in the brain and not retrievable, but lack of recall is reversible.

Etiology
- Can occur at any age.
- Onset can be gradual or sudden.

- Time lost can be from minutes to years. One episode of lost time is most common, but multiple time periods may be lost.
- Different types of memory loss may occur.
- Localized amnesia—inability to remember specific events, such as an earthquake.
- Systematized amnesia—inability to remember categories of information, such as friends.
- General amnesia—inability to remember anything about their lives, including their own identity.
- Continuous amnesia—inability to remember events in the past and up to the current time.
- Frequency increases during wartime or natural disasters.

Demographics
- Occurs more frequently in women than in men.
- Can occur at any age past infancy.
- Occurs most frequently at ages 30 to 50 years.
- Approximately 2% to 7% of the population are affected.
- Controversial as a scientific diagnosis; difference exists between how American and Canadian psychiatrists view dissociative amnesia. Only 13% of Canadian psychiatrists think there is strong scientific validity to include it as a mental health diagnosis.

Risk Factors
- Victims of sexual abuse, domestic violence, trauma, or combat
- Difficult to diagnose prior to puberty because inability to remember events prior to age 4 years is normal
- Appears to occur also in other family members, suggesting a possible genetic link
- *Comorbidities*: conversion disorders, bulimia nervosa, alcohol abuse, depression, personality disorders (borderline, dependent, histrionic)

Diagnosis
Differential Diagnosis
- Seizure disorder
- Head injury
- Alcohol or substance intoxication
- Korsakoff's disease
- Medication side effect
- Sleep deprivation
- Brain disease
- Delirium or dementia
- Other dissociative disorders
- Malingering factitious disorder

ICD-10 Code
Dissociative amnesia (F44.0)

Diagnostic Workup
- Diagnosis of exclusion
- Medical and psychiatric history
- Labs as needed to evaluate physical complaints:

- Thyroid function studies (T3, T4, TSH)
- CMP, including glucose, calcium, albumin; total protein count; levels of sodium, potassium, CO_2 (carbon dioxide and bicarbonate), chloride, BUN, creatinine, ALP, ALT, AST, and bilirubin
- *CBC with differentials*: hemoglobin, hematocrit, RBC count, WBC count, WBC differential count, and platelet count
- Psychological examination to include possible screening:
  - *The DES*: This is a self-report screen.
  - The Structured Clinical Interview for *DSM-5* Dissociative Disorders (SCID-D): This is a guided interview; it is the gold standard in the diagnosis of dissociative disorders but is time consuming.

Initial Assessment
- Is the amnesia transient or persistent?
- Has there been a recent blow to the head?
- Is there fever?
- Is recent memory intact?
- Any recent medication or substance?
- Functional limitations?

Clinical Presentation
- Loss of memory of important life events is usually retrograde (traumatic event is prior to amnesia).
- The unconscious memories influence the conscious state:
  - A rape victim may not remember being raped but may act like a victim of a violent crime.
  - Demoralization and detachment.
  - Mild depression and/or anxiety.
  - Agitation at stimuli related to the un-recalled traumatic event.

Diagnostic and Statistical Manual of Mental Disorders, Fifth Edition: Diagnostic Guidelines
- One or more episodes of inability to recall important personal information (often though not necessarily of stressful or threatening import).
- The deficit is too extensive to be ascribed to ordinary forgetfulness.
- The disturbance does not occur concurrently with dissociative identity disorder, dissociative fugue, somatization disorder, or PTSD.
- The disturbance is not the direct physiological effect of substance use or a neurological or other condition.
- The symptoms engender distress in the individual and impairment of social functioning.

Treatment Overview
Acute Treatment
- Initially, supportive therapy and creation of a safe environment may restore past memories.
- Hypnosis
  - Age regression may help patients access previously unavailable memories.
  - Screen technique—The patient recalls the traumatic event on an imaginary movie screen, which allows the patient to separate the psychological from the somatic aspects of the memory, to make it more bearable. Assists with the cognitive restructuring of the trauma. Patients who are not highly hypnotizable may benefit from this technique.

- Medication, if there is depression and/or anxiety:
    - Usually SSRIs, serotonin-norepinephrine reuptake inhibitors (SNRIs), anxiolytics, or atypical antipsychotics are used; antipsychotics are not used as monotherapy for anxiety or depression; SSRI/SNRI can be used with augmentation with anxiolytics or atypical antipsychotics for severe symptoms.

Chronic Treatment
- Psychotherapy is used to strengthen the ego, find new ways to cope, improve relationships, and optimize functioning.

Drug Selection Table for Dissociative Amnesia

CLASS	DRUG
SSRIs	First-line drug therapy Escitalopram (*Lexapro*) Sertraline (*Zoloft*) Paroxetine (*Paxil, Paxil PR*) Paroxetine mesylate (*Pexeva*)
SNRIs	First-line drug therapy Venlafaxine (*Effexor, Effexor XR*) Duloxetine (*Cymbalta*)
Calcium channel moderator	Drug augmentation Pregabalin (*Lyrica*)
TCAs	Drugs for treatment-resistant cases Imipramine (*Tofranil, Tofranil PM*) Desipramine (*Norpramin*)
BZDs	Use BZDs during the first few weeks of initiating SSRI/SNRI until full therapeutic effects are observed/reported. Alprazolam (*Xanax/Xanax XR/Niravam*) Clonazepam (*Klonopin*) Lorazepam (*Ativan*) Diazepam (*Valium*)
Antihistamines	Drug augmentation Hydroxyzine (*Vistaril*)
Anxiolytics	Drug augmentation Buspirone (*BuSpar*)

BZDs, benzodiazepines; SNRIs, serotonin-norepinephrine reuptake inhibitors; SSRIs, selective serotonin reuptake inhibitors; TCAs, tricyclic antidepressants.

Recurrence Rate
- Rarely recurs

Patient Education

- Advise patients to avoid alcohol and drugs.
- Encourage a healthy lifestyle and treatment follow-up.
- *Online resources*: Cleveland Clinic, National Alliance on Mental Health (NAMI), Psychcentral.org (also include support group information).

Medical/Legal Pitfalls

- Criminal cases have involved the recall of previously "repressed" memories of abuse. It is not completely accepted that recovery of repressed memories exists. Some argue that false memories can occur through the power of suggestion during therapy. The position of the American Psychological Association is that a recovered memory cannot be distinguished from a false memory without corroborating information.

OTHER SPECIFIED DISSOCIATIVE DISORDER

This category applies to presentations in which the symptoms are characteristic of a dissociative disorder that causes clinically significant distress but that does not meet the full criteria for any of the disorders in the dissociative diagnostic class. It is used to communicate the specific reason based on which the person does not meet the criteria. Some reasons might include trances, brainwashing, thought reform, indoctrination while captive, torture, long-term political imprisonment, and recruitment by cults or terror organizations.

Other conditions might include constriction of consciousness; depersonalization; derealization; perceptual disturbances such as time slowing, micro-amnesias, macropsias; transient stupors; and/or alterations in sensory-motor functioning due to analgesia or paralysis.

UNSPECIFIED DISSOCIATIVE DISORDER

This category is used when the symptoms do not meet the full criteria for a dissociative disorder but cause significant impairment in important areas of functioning but the clinician chooses not to specify the reason based on which the criteria do not meet a specific dissociative disorder. Usually the cause is insufficient information.

BIBLIOGRAPHY

American Psychiatric Association. (2013). *Diagnostic and statistical manual of mental disorders* (5th ed.). Washington, DC: American Psychiatric Press.

Collins, R. D. (2003). *Algorithmic diagnosis of symptoms and signs.* Lippincott, Williams & Wilkins.

Farrell, H. (2011). Dissociative identity disorder: Medicolegal challenges. *Journal of the American Academy of Psychiatry and the Law Online, 39* (3), 402–406.

Gentile, J., Dillon, K., & Gillig, P. (2013). Psychotherapy and pharmacotherapy for patients with dissociative identity disorder. *Innovations in Clinical Neuroscience, 10*(2), 22–29.

Jones, R. (2002). Readmission rates for adjustment disorders: Comparison with other mood disorders. *Journal of Affective Disorders, 71*(1), 199–203.

Kay, J., & Tasman, A. (2006). *Essentials of psychiatry.* John Wiley & Sons.

Sadock, B., & Sadock, V. (2000). *Kaplan & Sadock's comprehensive textbook of psychiatry* (7th ed.). Lippincott, Williams &Wilkins.

Sadock, B., Sadock, V., & Ruiz, P. (2015). *Kaplan & Sadock's synopsis of psychiatry* (11th ed.). Wolters Kluwer.

Steinberg, M., Barr, D., Sholomskas, D., & Hall, P. (2005). SCL-90 symptom patterns: Indicators of dissociative disorders. *Bulletin of the Menninger Clinic, 69*(3), 237–249.

Tusaie, K., & Fitzpatrick, J. (2017). *Advanced practice psychiatric nursing* (2nd ed). Springer.

Wheeler, K. (2014). *Psychotherapy for the advanced practice psychiatric nurse* (2nd ed). Springer.

WEB RESOURCES

- Cleveland Clinic: www.ClevelandClinic.org
- Freedom from Fear: www.freedomfromfear.org/; information on anxiety and mental health treatment, not specifically adjustment disorders
- www.icd10data.com/
- International Society for the Study of Trauma and Dissociation: www.isst-d.org/
- The Journal of the American Academy of Psychiatry and Law: www.jaapl.org
- National Alliance on Mental Illness: www.nami.com
- National Institute of Mental Health: www.nimh.nih.gov/
- Psych Central: www.psychcentral.com/
- Psychology Today: www.psychologytoday.com
- WebMD: www.webmd.com/

15

Sexual Dysfunction

ERECTILE DISORDER

Background Information

Definition of Disorder

In the *Diagnostic and Statistical Manual of Mental Disorders*, Fifth Edition (*DSM-5*; American Psychiatric Association, 2013), erectile disorder is classified as belonging to a group of sexual dysfunction disorders typically characterized by a clinically significant inability to respond sexually or to experience sexual pleasure. Criteria are as follows:

- In approximately 75%–100% of sexual activity, the experience of at least one of the following symptoms: (a) pronounced difficulty in obtaining an erection when engaging in sexual activity, (b) pronounced difficulty in maintaining an erection until the completion of sexual activity, or (c) pronounced decrease in erectile rigidity.
- Symptoms have persisted for approximately 6 months.
- Symptoms cause significant distress in the individual.
- The dysfunction cannot be better explained by nonsexual mental disorder, a medical condition, the effects of a drug or medication, or severe relationship distress or other significant stressors.

The duration of the dysfunction is specified as lifelong (present since first sexual experience) or acquired (developing after a period of relative normal sexual functioning). The context in which the dysfunction occurs is specified as generalized (not limited to certain types of stimulation, situations, or partners) or situational (limited to specific types of stimulation, situations, or partners).

Etiology

- Penile erections are produced by an integration of physiological processes involving the central nervous, peripheral nervous, hormonal, and vascular systems. Any abnormality in these systems, whether from medication or disease, has a significant impact on the ability to develop and sustain an erection, ejaculate, and experience orgasm.
- Erectile disorder usually has a multifactorial etiology. Biological, physiological, endocrine, and psychological factors are involved in the ability to obtain and maintain erections. In general, erectile disorder is divided into two broad categories: biological and psychological.

■ Psychological factors that might play a role include the following: early sexual experiences, sexual abuse, poor body image, depression, worrying about obtaining or maintaining an erection, and guilty feelings about sex.

■ Many men with erectile disorder also have problems with anxiety—either specifically about sexual performance or related to other issues.

■ Relationship factors may contribute to erectile disorder.

■ Many men with erectile disorder have comorbid conditions such as hyperlipidemia, hypercholesterolemia, tobacco abuse, diabetes mellitus, or coronary artery disease (CAD). Erectile disorder may be the earliest presentation of atherosclerosis and vascular disease.

■ Other biological causes may include abnormal hormone levels, abnormal levels of neurotransmitters, inflammation and infection of the prostate or urethra, and inherited traits.

Demographics

■ Erectile disorder affects 50% of men older than 40 years, and 50% of all sexually active men will report some degree of erectile difficulty.

■ It is estimated that 18 to 30 million men in the United States are affected by erectile disorder.

■ All studies demonstrate a strong association with age, which suggests that vascular changes in the arteries and sinusoids of the corpora cavernosa, similar to those found elsewhere in the body, are contributing factors.

■ Long-term predictions based on an aging population and an increase in risk factors suggest a large increase in the number of men with erectile disorder.

■ The prevalence of erectile disorder is underestimated because physicians frequently do not question their patients about this disorder.

Risk Factors

■ Vascular conditions (e.g., atherosclerosis, peripheral vascular disease, myocardial infarction, arterial hypertension)

■ Systemic conditions (e.g., diabetes mellitus, hypertension, dyslipidemia, renal failure)

■ Neurological conditions (e.g., stroke, multiple sclerosis, epilepsy)

■ Respiratory conditions (e.g., chronic obstructive pulmonary disease, sleep apnea)

■ Endocrine conditions (e.g., hypo-/hyperthyroidism, hypogonadism, diabetes)

■ Penile conditions (e.g., Peyronie disease, epispadias, priapism)

■ Psychiatric conditions (e.g., depression, performance anxiety, post-traumatic stress disorder)

■ *Medications*: antihypertensives, antidepressants, antipsychotics, antiulcer agents, 5-alpha reductase inhibitors, cholesterol-lowering agents, methadone

■ Malnutrition; zinc deficiency

■ Smoking

■ Stress

■ Fear of causing pregnancy, contracting a sexually transmitted disease (STD), or poor sexual performance

Diagnosis

Differential Diagnosis

■ Depression

■ Abdominal vascular injuries

- Type 2 diabetes mellitus
- Hypertension
- Hypogonadism
- Peyronie disease
- Noncoronary atherosclerosis
- Scleroderma
- Hemochromatosis
- Sickle cell anemia

ICD-10 Codes
Male erectile dysfunction, unspecified (F52.9)

Drug-induced erectile dysfunction (F52.2)

Erectile dysfunction due to diseases classified elsewhere (F52.1)

Diagnostic Workup
- Complete medical and surgical, sexual, and medication/nonprescription drug history; physical examination; and psychiatric assessment or evaluation.
- Erectile disorder may require specialized testing and referral and a stepwise management approach with ranking of treatment options.
- Incorporation of patient and partner needs and preferences is key in the decision-making process.
- The following questionnaires assist in the gathering of objective data:
  - International Index of Erectile Function (IIEF)
  - Sexual Encounter Profile (SEP)
  - Psychological and Interpersonal Relationship Scales (PAIRS)
  - Self-Esteem and Relationship (SEAR) questionnaire
  - Erectile Dysfunction Inventory of Treatment Satisfaction (EDITS)
- Laboratories as needed:
  - Testosterone (free, total, bioavailable)
  - Luteinizing hormone
  - Prolactin
  - Thyroid-stimulating hormone (TSH)
  - Hemoglobin A1c
  - Serum chemistry panel
  - Lipid profile
  - Urinalysis

Other diagnostic studies as indicated:

  - Injection of prostaglandin EI
  - Ultrasonography
  - Nocturnal penile tumescence testing

Initial Assessment
- Complete medical and surgical, sexual, and medication/nonprescription drug history.
- Psychiatric history.
- Traumatic history (including any form of abuse).
- Sexual history.
- How long have you had trouble attaining or maintaining an erection?
- Are you ever able to obtain an erection suitable for penetration, even momentarily?

- Is your erectile disorder getting worse or stable?
- How hard is the erection, on a scale of 0 to 100?
- Have you ever had a traumatic sexual experience?
- Are you able to achieve orgasm and ejaculation?
- Approximately how long are you able to have intercourse before ejaculating?
- Do you use any type of contraceptives, such as condoms?
- Do you experience nocturnal or morning erections?
- Does pain or discomfort occur with ejaculation?
- Do you have premature (early) ejaculation?
- Is penile curvature (Peyronie disease) a problem?
- How frequently do you have sexual activity? Is it typically spontaneous or planned?
- If your erections were functional, what would be your preferred frequency of intercourse? Do you and your sexual partner agree on this issue?
- Is adequate foreplay occurring? Is your sexual partner satisfied with the sexual experience?
- Have you already tried any treatments? If so, what were they? Are you interested in trying a particular treatment first? Are you opposed to trying a particular type of therapy?
- What effect is this having in your relationship?
- To what degree do you wish to proceed in determining the cause of the erectile disorder? How important is this to you?
- Is there anything you do not like or do not feel comfortable with in your sexual encounters?
- Do you feel like your partner pushes you or is upset with your erectile disorder?
- Does this problem occur only in a certain situation or with a certain partner?
- Do you regard sex as dirty?
- What effect is this problem having on your daily functioning?

Clinical Presentation
- No specific physical symptoms.
- Patients may be in distress if treatment has not worked or if this disorder recurs after treatment.

Treatment Overview

Acute Treatment
- Interventions include psychological and biological interventions, external erection-facilitating devices, and surgical interventions. It is best to include the patient's partner in treatment as much as possible to enhance both treatment compliance and treatment efficacy.
- Psychological therapy consists of sex therapy, explorations of emotions from abuse, psychotherapy for trust and intimacy issues, and cognitive behavioral therapy (CBT).
- Biological therapy includes the following:
  - Phosphodiesterase type 5 (PDE5) inhibitors: sildenafil, vardenafil, tadalafil, and avanafil
  - Hormone replacement therapy (oral, injectable, gel, transdermal)
  - Intracavernosal injection of vasodilators or intraurethral prostaglandin E1 pellets (agent: alprostadil)
  - Vascular endothelial growth factor (VEGF)

Drug Selection Table for Erectile Disorder

CLASS	DRUG
Phosphodiesterase type 5 inhibitors	First-line drug therapy Sildenafil citrate (*Viagra*) Tadalafil (*Cialis*) Vardenafil (*Levitra*) Vardenafil (as HCl; *Staxyn*) Avanafil (*Stendra*)
Prostaglandin E1	Alprostadil (injection; *Caverject, Caverject Impulse, Edex*) Alprostadil (urethral suppository; *Muse*)

- External erection-facilitating devices include the following:
  - Constriction devices
  - Vacuum devices
- Surgical interventions include the following:
  - Surgical revascularization
  - Surgical elimination of venous outflow
  - Placement of penile implant

Chronic Treatment
- Continue psychological therapy to completion.
- Continue medication with regular follow-up.
- Patients should be aware that this condition may recur and treatment may not be permanent.

Patient Education
- For patient education resources, visit WebMD's Erectile Dysfunction Health Center: www.webmd.com/erectile-dysfunction/default.htm

Medical/Legal Pitfalls
- Laboratory results should be discussed with the patient and, if possible, with his sexual partner. This educational process allows a review of the basic aspects of the anatomy and physiology of the sexual response and an explanation of the possible etiology and associated risk factors.
- Patient should be counseled on the side effects of medications.

FEMALE SEXUAL INTEREST/AROUSAL DISORDER

Background Information
Definition of Disorder
In the *DSM-5* (American Psychiatric Association, 2013), disorders of sexual desire and sexual arousal were combined into female sexual interest/arousal disorder.

- The disorder is defined as a lack of, or significantly decreased, sexual interest/arousal characterized by at least three of the following: (1) decreased or absent interest in sexual activity; (2) decreased or absent erotic or sexual thoughts or fantasies; (3) decreased or absent initiation of sexual activity along with a lack of receptivity to initiation by a partner; (4) decreased or absent

sexual excitement or pleasure during sexual activity in almost all or all sexual encounters either in identified situational or all contexts; (5) decreased or absent sexual interest/arousal in response to any external or internal written, verbal, or visual sexual cues; and (6) decreased or absent genital or nongenital sensations during sexual activity in almost all or all identified situations or all contexts.
- Symptoms have persisted for at least 6 months.
- Symptoms cause clinically significant distress in the individual.
- Symptoms cannot be attributed to a nonsexual mental disorder, to a consequence of severe relational distress or other stressors, or the effects of a substance or medication or a medical condition.

The disorder is specified as lifelong or acquired and generalized or situational. The severity of the symptoms are specified as mild, moderate, or severe.

Etiology
- Sexual response is not necessarily a linear process. Rather, phases of the sexual response cycle may occur in a variety of patterns. For example, some women have reported that desire precedes arousal, whereas others have experienced arousal prior to desire.
- Problems related to sexual response may be due to psychological factors, organic factors, or a combination of both. An understanding of interpersonal contexts is important.
- Examples of psychological factors include relationship issues/discord, cognitive and affective factors, and cultural and societal factors. For example, communication difficulties between partners, both inside and outside of the bedroom, can be the sole causative factor behind arousal dysfunction.
- Depression and anxiety often affect arousal. In fact, women who experience anxiety just prior to erotic stimuli often experience decreased subjective arousal.
- Other psychological factors include worry, stress, low self-esteem, negative attitudes toward sex, and unhappiness with one's body.
- Relationship factors such as longer relationship duration, low partner attractiveness, having a partner with a sexual dysfunction, and low outcome expectancy may decrease sexual desire. A history of sexual abuse can also impact arousal.
- Low sexual desire has not been linked with illicit drug or alcohol use.
- Organic causes include endocrine dysfunction, autonomic nervous system (ANS) dysfunction, and cardiovascular/medical issues.
- As women age, production of androgens, hormones linked to sexual desire, decreases. This occurs independent of menopause.
- Oral contraceptives may increase the sex hormone binding globulin, leading to a decrease in free testosterone.
- Low sexual desire has been correlated with hyperprolactinemia, however, not all patients with chronic hyperprolactinemia have low sexual desire.
- For sexual arousal to occur in women, normal amounts of estrogens and androgens must be present along with a normal, functioning sympathetic nervous system.
- Women with decreased or absent estrogen production have reduced tissue sensitivity of the vagina and vulva and decreased or absent vaginal lubrication.
- ANS dysfunction includes spinal cord lesions.
- Cardiovascular issues include vascular disease and hypertension.
- Female sexual arousal disorder may be lifelong or acquired and situational or generalized.

Demographics

- Consistently higher rates of sexual dysfunction have been reported in women with commonly identified decreased or absent desire.
- Although sexual desire may decrease with age, some older women report less distress about low sexual desire compared to their younger counterparts.
- Prevalence statistics differ depending on the population sampled, sample size, and the instruments used in the study.
- Literature reports vary on prevalence statistics due to nonstandardized approaches in studying female sexual disorders.
- It is fairly uncommon for a premenopausal woman to have an arousal problem without a decreased libido.
- Antidepressants and antipsychotics are two common classes of drugs that may interfere with orgasm.

Risk Factors

- *Age*: Symptoms can develop at any age and may be present for the woman's entire sexual life.
- *Family history*: There is no evidence that this disorder is familial.
- *Stressful events in susceptible people*: Stressful events in one's life and stressful situations between couples may be the sole cause of this disorder.
- Having another mental health problem, such as a mood or an anxiety disorder.
- The presence of another sexual function disorder.
- Negative thoughts and/or attitudes about sexuality.
- Environmental factors, such as developmental difficulties, childhood relationships, and stressors.
- Medical conditions, such as diabetes or thyroid dysfunction.
- It has been suggested that genetic factors may increase vulnerability to sexual problems in women.

Diagnosis

Differential Diagnosis

- Sexual dysfunction due to a general medical disorder
- Substance-induced sexual disorder
- Another Axis I disorder (major depressive disorder, etc.)
- Occasional problems with sexual arousal
- History of rape, physical, and/or sexual abuse
- Current rape, physical, and/or sexual abuse
- Relationship conflict
- Significant stress
- Other interpersonal factors
- Menopause

ICD-10 Code

Female sexual arousal disorder (F52.22)

Diagnostic Workup

- Complete history, physical examination, and psychiatric assessment or evaluation.
- This sexual dysfunction may be due to a general medical condition (female androgen insufficiency, chronic renal failure, hyperprolactinemia, pregnancy, and lactation).

- The patient should complete one of the following to aid in diagnosis and treatment: the Sexual Interest and Desire Inventory—Female, Hurlbert Index of Sexual Desire, or Sexual Desire Inventory Questionnaire.
- Laboratories as needed to evaluate physical complaints:
  - Thyroid function studies (triiodothyronine [T3], thyroxine [T4], TSH)
  - Comprehensive metabolic panel (CMP), including glucose, calcium, albumin; total protein count; levels of sodium, potassium, CO_2 (carbon dioxide and bicarbonate), chloride, blood urea nitrogen (BUN), creatinine, alkaline phosphatase (ALP), alanine amino transferase (ALT, also called serum glutamic pyruvic transaminase [SGPT]), aspartate amino transferase (AST, also called serum glutamic oxaloacetic transaminase [SGOT]), and bilirubin
  - *Complete blood count (CBC) with differentials*: hemoglobin, hematocrit, red blood cell (RBC) count, white blood cell (WBC) count, WBC differential count, and platelet count

Initial Assessment

There may be different symptom profiles in how the disorder is expressed. It is important to note that a woman who has a lower desire for sexual activity than her partner does not meet the criteria for this disorder.

In addition to the listed subtypes, the following five areas must be considered in assessing and diagnosing the disorder: (1) partner factors, (2) relationship factors, (3) individual vulnerability factors, (4) cultural/religious factors, and (5) medical factors.

- Medical history with detailed social history.
- Psychiatric history.
- Traumatic history (including any form of abuse).
- Sexual history.
- Current medication use.
- Any recent changes in medication?
- Have you ever had problems with low or absent sexual desire?
- For how long have you had low or absent sexual desire?
- Does this problem only occur in a certain situation or with a certain partner?
- Do you have decreased desire to masturbate or use a vibrator?
- What effect is this having in your relationship?
- Did any emotional or other stressful life event occur when you began to have decreased or absent sexual desire?
- What effect is this decreased/absent sexual desire having on your daily functioning?
- Is there anything you do not like or do not feel comfortable with in your sexual encounters?
- Do you feel like your partner pushes you or is upset with your decreased desire?
- Have you ever had problems with attaining arousal? If so, for how long?
- Have you ever had a problem with lubrication? If so, for how long?
- Do you ever have problems attaining orgasm?
- Do you have pain during sex?
- Do you have difficulty with arousal only while masturbating or using a vibrator?
- How long does it take to become aroused now, compared with the past?
- What effect is this having in your relationship?
- Did any emotional or other life stress occur when the problems with arousal began?
- When did you undergo menopause?

- Have you ever had your ovaries removed?
- Have you ever taken hormone replacement therapy?
- What brought you to seek treatment now?
- What effect is this problem having on your daily functioning?
- Do you feel safe with your partner?
- Have you ever been threatened or harmed by your partner in any way?

Clinical Presentation
- No specific physical symptoms.
- Patients may be in distress if treatment has not worked or if this disorder recurs after treatment.

Treatment Overview

Acute Treatment
- Interventions include psychological and biological interventions.
- Psychological therapy consists of marital therapy, explorations of emotions from abuse, psychotherapy for trust and intimacy issues, and CBT.
  - There is limited evidence of effectiveness of CBT therapy for this disorder.
  - CBT consists of identifying and correcting dysfunctional attitudes toward sexual pleasure, masturbation, and sensate focus.
  - Emphasis is also on couple communication.
- Biological therapy includes the following:
  - For decreased lubrication, there are lubricants and estrogen-related products.
    - In postmenopausal patients, be cautious using estrogen-related products.
    - Estrogen-related products may increase risk of breast cancer as well as endometrial cancer in women with an intact uterus.
  - Eros.
    - Clitoral vacuum device approved by Food and Drug Administration (FDA).
  - Zestra.
    - Botanical massage; oil is applied to vulva.
    - Investigation for efficacy is ongoing.
  - Phosphodiesterase inhibitors and alprostadil.
    - Only one study with un-replicated results showed any promise of these medications helping women with sexual arousal disorder and subnormal libido.
    - Sildenafil and nitric oxide do increase the physical arousal stage but do not affect the subjective arousal feelings in women with this disorder.
  - Flibanserin, a novel multifunctional serotonin agonist, has been shown to be efficacious in treating female hypoactive sexual disorder but has a significant side-effect profile.

Chronic Treatment
- Continue psychological therapy to completion.
- Continue medication with regular follow-up, with exception of flibanserin, which should be discontinued if no improvement is seen within 8 weeks.
- Patients should be aware that this condition may recur and treatment may not be permanent.

Recurrence Rate
More research needs to be done on this subject with more studies using standardized instruments.

Patient Education

Information regarding this disorder can be found at the Merck website under the subject of sexual dysfunction in women.

- For more patient education resources, visit eMedicine's website under the topic of female sexual problems and visit familydoctor.org under "Sexual dysfunction in women" (https://familydoctor.org/condition/sexual-dysfunction/)
- Patient education on disease process is needed.

Medical/Legal Pitfalls

- Patients may become very frustrated if treatments do not work.
- In some cases, therapy will not work unless the patient's partner agrees with the therapy.
- Patients may try herbal supplements in attempts to increase arousal.
- Patient should be counseled on side effects and interactions of supplements with other medications.
- Arousal difficulties may be due to cardiovascular issues; patients should be screened for hypertension and vascular disease.

GENDER DYSPHORIA

Background Information

Definition of Disorder

The diagnosis of gender dysphoria replaces the prior diagnosis of "gender identity disorder," which emphasized cross-gender identification. Gender dysphoria is not considered to be a sexual dysfunction or a paraphilia but rather a condition resulting from experienced gender incongruence with resulting gender dysphoria. Separate criteria are provided for children, adolescents, and adults.

Gender Dysphoria in Children

- In children, there is a marked incongruence between assigned gender and experienced/expressed gender manifested by at least six of the following: (1) a desire to be the other gender or insistence that one is the other gender; (2) a strong preference for cross-dressing as the opposite gender of one's assigned gender; (3) a strong preference for cross-gender roles; (4) a strong preference for toys, games, or activities typically engaged in by the opposite gender; (5) a strong preference for playmates of the opposite gender; (6) a strong rejection of typically masculine games and activities when the assigned gender is male and a strong rejection of typically feminine games and activities when the assigned gender is female; (7) a strong dislike of one's sexual anatomy; and (8) a strong desire for the primary or secondary sex characteristics matching the experienced gender.
- Associated with clinically significant distress or impairment in social, school, or other important areas of functioning.
- Must specify whether this occurs with a disorder of sex development.

Gender Dysphoria in Adults and Adolescents

- A marked incongruence between one's expressed/experienced gender and assigned gender of at least 6 months' duration and characterized by at least two of the following: (1) a marked incongruence between one's experienced/expressed gender and actual or anticipated primary and/or secondary sexual characteristics; (2) a strong desire to be rid of one's actual or anticipated primary and/or secondary sexual characteristics; (3) a strong preference for the primary or secondary sexual characteristics of the other gender; (4) a strong desire to be the other gender or an alternative gender from the assigned gender; (5) a strong desire to be treated as the other gender or an alternative gender from the assigned gender; and (6) a strong conviction that one has the typical feelings and reactions of the other gender or an alternative gender from assigned gender.

- Associated with clinically significant distress or impairment in social, school, occupational, or other important areas of functioning.
- Must specify whether this occurs with a disorder of sex development.
- Must specify whether the individual has transitioned to full-time living in the desired gender with or without a legal change and either has undergone or is preparing to have at least one cross-sex medical procedure or treatment regimen (post-transition).
- *Early onset*: starts in childhood and continues into adolescence and adulthood; may have a period where dysphoria remits and individual identifies self as gay.
- *Late onset*: starts near puberty or later.

Gender Dysphoria Associated With a Disorder of Sex Development
- For many, issues of gender assignment have already been raised by healthcare providers or parents.
- Frequently associated with early-onset gender atypical behavior.
- Individuals with a disorder of sex development may not develop gender dysphoria but may experience uncertainty about their gender.
- For females, there may be associated infertility.

Other Specified Gender Dysphoria
- Applies to individuals who present with symptoms characteristic of gender dysphoria that (1) cause clinically significant distress or impairment in social, occupational, or other important areas but who do not meet the full criteria for gender dysphoria or (2) the individual meets the criteria for gender dysphoria but the duration of symptoms is less than 6 months.
- The specified category is used in situations in which the reasons based on which the individual does not meet the criteria for gender dysphoria are specified.

Unspecified Gender Dysphoria
- Applies to individuals who present with symptoms characteristic of gender dysphoria that cause clinically significant distress or impairment in social, occupational, or other important areas but do not meet the full criteria for gender dysphoria.
- The unspecified category is used in situations in which the reasons based on which the individual does not meet the criteria for gender dysphoria are unspecified and/or in which there is insufficient information available.

Etiology
- Unknown etiology.
- One theory involves structure formation of the uncinate nucleus.
- In gender dysphoria without a disorder of sex development, twin studies suggest an increased concordance for transsexualism among monozygotic twin pairs and some degree of heritability.

- Possible androgen increase in some women.
- In gender dysphoria with a disorder of sex development, a prenatal androgen imbalance may increase vulnerability to gender dysphoria.
- For individuals with gender dysphoria without a disorder of sex development, gender dysphoria may develop as early as preschool, with increased likelihood of persistence into adolescence and adulthood.
- Males with gender dysphoria without a disorder of sex development are more likely to have older brothers.

Demographics
- In the United States, 0.6% of adults (approximately 1.4 million adults) and 1:137 13- to 17-year-old adolescents are estimated to experience incongruence between their assigned sex at birth (ASAB) and gender identity. (Note that prevalence is likely underreported.)
- Sixty percent (60%) of transgender adults were aware of their gender being different than their ASAB before puberty, while 81% knew before age 16.
- Male to female transexualism has a 1% to 6% prevalence.
- Female to male transsexuals and the homosexual MtF usually apply for gender reassignment surgery in their 20s.
- Heterosexual MtF patients usually apply for gender reassignment surgery much later.
- Heterosexual MtF patients usually have married and fathered children before applying.
- Those with this disorder will continue to have unresolved issues with gender, will accept their birth gender, will have part-time cross-gender behavior, or will have gender reassignment surgery.
- Individuals with gender dysphoria have been reported across many countries and cultures.

Risk Factors
Age
- Age of development varies.
- Most common ages of onset of gender dysphoria reported are from younger than 3 years old to middle childhood.

Gender
- This disorder is found in both genders.
- Men are affected two to three times more often than women.

Stressful Events in Susceptible People
- Significant crisis or loss may worsen this disorder.

Having Another Mental Health Disorder
- Higher likelihood of having schizophrenia, affective psychosis, or adjustment disorder.
- Patients with gender dysphoria are more likely to have substance abuse problems, although statistics vary on prevalence.
- Patients with gender dysphoria are more likely to have a personality disorder, have attempted suicide in the past, have engaged in self-harm behavior, have an increased risk for violence (assault, rape, attempted rape), HIV infection, and other STDs.

Diagnosis

Differential Diagnosis

- Nonconformity to gender roles
- Transvestic disorder
- Body dysmorphic disorder
- Schizophrenia and other psychotic conditions
- Other clinical presentations

ICD-10 Codes

Gender identity disorder of childhood (F64.2)

Gender identity disorder, unspecified (F64.9)

Other gender identity disorders (F64.8)

Transsexualism (F64.0)

Diagnostic Workup

- The diagnostic workup includes a comprehensive medical history, including a sexual history, a history of prior and current medications, a physical examination, and pertinent laboratory work.
- Psychiatric assessment should account for family, school, and occupational settings and relationships with peers.

Initial Assessment

- Complete medical history.
- Sexual history.
- Psychiatric history.
- Psychosexual development.
- For how long have you felt you are of the opposite sex?
- What brought you to seek help now?
- What is your sexual orientation?
- How do you feel about your body?
- Are you currently in a relationship?
- Tell me your feelings related to your birth gender.
- How were you raised?
- Did your family raise you in your birth gender?
- Do you have a social support system?
- What is your occupation?
- What outcome are you looking for? (counseling, gender reassignment surgery, etc.)

Laboratory Tests

None is relevant to diagnosis of this disorder.

Treatment Overview

Acute Treatment

- Psychodynamic psychotherapy focused toward acceptance of birth gender has been the accepted therapy for years.
    - Multiple studies have been unable to determine the exact efficacy of psychodynamic psychotherapy.
    - Patients with any of the following characteristics are most likely to respond to this therapy:
        - Patient treated and controlled for comorbid psychological problems

- Religious beliefs inconsistent with gender reassignment surgery
- Anatomic features prevent passing as the opposite gender despite sex reassignment surgery (extremely tall stature or very large size)
- Fear of losing spouse, children, and alienating other family members
- Individual psychotherapy can also help the patient.
  - It provides a safe setting for the patient to discuss feelings and concerns.
  - This is recommended but not required during real-life experience.
- Group psychotherapy is also helpful for patients.
  - It provides a supportive environment.
- Hormone therapy
  - This is used in those who decide not to undergo gender reassignment surgery but still want to be the opposite gender part-time.
  - These patients will undergo either masculinizing or feminizing hormonal therapy.
  - Episodically, they will live as the opposite sex.
  - This occurs more often in cross-dressing adult males and less often in adult females with this disorder.
- Real-life experience
  - Homosexual MtF transsexuals usually will undergo this "test."
  - Heterosexual MtF transsexuals are least likely to undergo this "test."
  - FtM transsexuals usually have an easier time with this "test" than the other two groups.
  - There are irreversible social consequences to living as the opposite sex without surgery.
  - This is usually done while taking hormone therapy.
- Gender reassignment surgery
  - This is a permanent solution.
  - The patient must have a thorough evaluation before being allowed to undergo surgery.
  - Patients must also have completed either at least 1 year of cross-sex hormone therapy or at least 1 year of real-life experience in their gender role.
  - The process to completely become the opposite sex takes years to decades.

Chronic Treatment
- Psychotherapy
  - About 50% of those undergoing evaluation or psychotherapy for this disorder will stop treatment.
  - Some, but not all, return to treatment at a later time.
  - Reasons for not continuing therapy include impatience, seeing the therapist as unempathetic, expensiveness of therapy, or decision not to resolve the gender identity problem.
- Hormone therapy
- Gender reassignment surgery
  - This is apermanent solution.
  - The surgery takes place in stages.
  - The physical transition may take place over years but the complete emotional, psychological, and identity changes may take decades.

Recurrence Rate
- Rate depends on the patient, the outcome decided by the patient, and other factors.

Clinical Presentation
- No specific physical symptoms are related to this disorder.
- Patients may have symptoms related to hormonal therapy or surgical procedures.

Patient Education

- Information on gender dysphoria disorder can be found at www.merck.com under the *Merck Manual of Diagnosis and Therapy* (psychiatric disorders, then sexuality and sexual disorders, then gender identity disorder).
- E-medicine (emedicine.medscape.com) also has a good website with information under the topic of psychiatry and sexual and gender identity disorders.

Medical/Legal Pitfalls

- During acute psychotic episodes, those with bipolar disorder, schizophrenia, and other psychotic disorders may have delusions of becoming the opposite sex.
- Care should be taken to diagnose and treat these conditions before jumping ahead toward treatment.
- Treatment of psychotic disorders will resolve the desire to become the opposite sex.
- Those with antisocial or borderline personality disorders will also seek gender reassignment surgery for unrelated reasons.
- Sex hormone therapy often leads to permanent sterilization, so patients should be counseled on sperm/egg preservation.
- Estrogen therapy can cause thrombosis and pulmonary embolism; patients should also be monitored for insulin resistance.
- Testosterone therapy may predispose the patient for cardiovascular disease; regular screening should be done, including lipid profiles and tests for insulin resistance.
- Patients undergoing sex hormone therapy should be monitored for cancer.
- Ovarian malignant changes and endometrial hyperplasia with testosterone therapy must also be monitored.

PREMATURE EJACULATION

Background Information

Definition of Disorder

In the *DSM-5* (American Psychiatric Association, 2013), premature (early) ejaculation is defined as a recurring or persisting pattern of ejaculation that occurs during partnered sexual activity before the individual wishes to ejaculate. Although the diagnosis may be applied to individuals who engage in non-vaginal sexual intercourse, specific duration criteria for such activities have not been established. Criteria are as follows:

- In 75%–100% of sexual activity, the individual experiences a pattern of ejaculation that occurs within 1 minute after vaginal penetration during partnered sexual activity and before the individual wishes it.
- Symptoms have persisted for at least 6 months.
- Symptoms cause significant distress in the individual.
- The dysfunction cannot be better explained by nonsexual mental disorder, a medical condition, the effects of a drug or medication, or severe relationship distress or other significant stressors.

The severity of premature (early) ejaculation is specified as follows:

- Mild (occurring within approximately 30 seconds to 1 minute of vaginal penetration)
- Moderate (occurring within approximately 15 to 30 seconds of vaginal penetration)

■ Severe (occurring before sexual activity, at the start of sexual activity, or within approximately 15 seconds of vaginal penetration)

The duration of the dysfunction is specified as lifelong (present since first sexual experience) or acquired (developing after a period of relative normal sexual functioning). The context in which the dysfunction occurs is specified as generalized (not limited to certain types of stimulation, situations, or partners) or situational (limited to specific types of stimulation, situations, or partners).

Etiology

■ Ejaculation is controlled by the central nervous system. When men are sexually stimulated, signals are sent to the spinal cord and brain. When men reach a certain level of excitement, signals are then sent from the brain to your reproductive organs. This causes semen to be released through the penis (ejaculation).

■ The exact cause of premature ejaculation is not known. It involves a complex interaction of psychological and biological factors.

■ Psychological factors that might play a role include the following: early sexual experiences, sexual abuse, poor body image, depression, worrying about premature ejaculation, and guilty feelings that increase the tendency to rush through sexual encounters.

■ Erectile dysfunction may play a role. Men who are anxious about obtaining or maintaining an erection during sexual intercourse might form a pattern of rushing to ejaculate, which can be difficult to change.

■ Many men with premature ejaculation also have problems with anxiety—either specifically about sexual performance or related to other issues.

■ Relationship factors may contribute to premature ejaculation.

■ Biological causes include abnormal hormone levels, abnormal levels of neurotransmitters, inflammation and infection of the prostate or urethra, and inherited traits.

Demographics

■ An estimated 30% to 70% of males in the United States experience premature ejaculation.

■ The prevalence is likely underreported as many men do not report premature ejaculation to their clinician, possibly because of embarrassment or a feeling that no treatment is available for the problem. Some men might not even perceive premature ejaculation as a psychological or medical problem.

■ Although more than 20% to 30% of men aged 18 to 70 years report being concerned about the rapidity of their ejaculation, only 1% to 3% would be classified as having premature (early) ejaculation according to the current *DSM-5* criteria.

■ It is most common in men aged 18 to 30 years but may also occur in conjunction with secondary impotence in men aged 45 to 65 years.

■ Antidepressants and antipsychotics are two common classes of drugs that may interfere with orgasm.

Risk Factors

■ Erectile dysfunction
■ Stress
■ Lack of sexual experience
■ Lack of knowledge about male and female sexual responses
■ Fear of causing pregnancy, contracting an STD, or poor sexual performance

Diagnosis

Differential Diagnosis
- Erectile dysfunction
- Side effect of pharmacological treatment
- Delayed orgasm in female partner
- Preejaculation

ICD-10 Code
Premature ejaculation (F52.4)

Diagnostic Workup
- Complete history, physical examination, and psychiatric assessment or evaluation.
- Patient should measure length of time from penetration to ejaculation (ejaculation latency), subjective feelings of control over ejaculation, and personal and relational distress caused by the condition.
- Screening for chronic prostatitis/chronic pelvic pain syndrome (CP/CPPS).
- Laboratories as needed to evaluate physical complaints:
    - Testosterone (free and total)
    - Prolactin

Initial Assessment
In addition to the listed subtypes, the following four areas must be considered in assessing and diagnosing the disorder: (1) partner factors, (2) relationship factors, (3) individual vulnerability factors, and (4) medical factors.
- Medical history with detailed social history.
- Psychiatric history.
- Traumatic history (including any form of abuse).
- Sexual history.
- Current medication use.
- Any recent changes in medication?
- For how long have you experienced premature ejaculation?
- What is the time between penetration and ejaculation?
- Can you delay ejaculation?
- Do you feel bothered, annoyed, and/or frustrated by your premature ejaculation?
- What effect is this having in your relationship?
- Did you experience a traumatic sexual episode as a child or teenager?
- Does your family have a history of incest or sexual assault?
- Is there anything you do not like or do not feel comfortable with in your sexual encounters?
- Do you feel like your partner pushes you or is upset with your premature ejaculation?
- Have you ever had problems with attaining arousal? If so, for how long?
- Does this problem occur only in a certain situation or with a certain partner?
- Do you regard sex as dirty?
- How long does it take to become aroused now, compared with the past?
- Did any emotional or other life stress occur when the premature ejaculation began?
- What brought you to seek treatment now?
- What effect is this problem having on your daily functioning?

Clinical Presentation
- No specific physical symptoms.
- Patients may be in distress if treatment has not worked or if this disorder recurs after treatment.

Treatment Overview

Acute Treatment
- Interventions include psychological and biological interventions. Premature ejaculation is often viewed as a "couple's problem"; it is recommended to include the partner in treatment as much as possible to enhance both treatment compliance and treatment efficacy.
- Psychological therapy consists of sex therapy, explorations of emotions from abuse, psychotherapy for trust and intimacy issues, and CBT.
  - There is limited evidence of the effectiveness of CBT therapy for this disorder.
  - CBT consists of addressing unhelpful thoughts (cognitions) in the male that get in the way; establishing a cooperative partner relationship; and teaching the patient behaviors for delaying ejaculation.
  - Sex therapy includes techniques such as the stop–start or squeeze–pause technique popularized by Masters and Johnson.
- Biological therapy includes the following:
  - Desensitizing agents such as prilocaine/lidocaine cream or related topical anesthetic agents
  - Selective serotonin reuptake inhibitors, such as sertraline, fluoxetine, and paroxetine, because of their known side effects of delaying or inhibiting orgasm

Chronic Treatment
- Continue psychological therapy to completion.
- Continue medication with regular follow-up.
- Patients should be aware that this condition may recur and treatment may not be permanent.

Recurrence Rate
- Relapse rates may range from 20% to 50%; more research needs to be done on this subject with studies using standardized instruments.

Patient Education
- Referral to licensed sex therapist.
- Sex education during adolescence may decrease incidence of premature ejaculation in young men.
- Early treatment of erectile disorder may help prevent acquired premature ejaculation in older men.
- For patient education resources, visit WebMD's Premature Ejaculation Directory: www.webmd.com/men/premature-ejaculation-directory

Medical/Legal Pitfalls
- Patients may become very frustrated if treatments do not work.
- In some cases, therapy will not work unless the patient's partner agrees with the therapy.
- Patient should be counseled on the side effects of medications.

REFERENCE

American Psychiatric Association. (2013). *Diagnostic and statistical manual of mental disorders* (5th ed.). Washington, DC: American Psychiatric Press.

BIBLIOGRAPHY

Baid, R., & Agarwal, R. (2018). Flibanserin: A controversial drug for female hypoactive sexual desire disorder. *Industrial Psychiatry Journal, 27*(1), 154–157.

Basson, R. (2002). A model of women's sexual arousal. *Journal of Sex and Marital Therapy, 28*, 1–10.

Basson, R., Leiblum, S., Brotto, L., Derogatis, L., Fourcroy, J., Fugl-Meyer, K., Graziottin, A., Heiman, J. R., Laan, E., Meston, C., Schover, L., van Lankveld, J., & Schultz, W. W. (2003). Definitions of women's sexual dysfunction reconsidered: Advocating expansion and revision. *Journal of Psychosomatic Obstetrics and Gynecology, 24*(4), 221–229.

Covington, S. (1991). *Awakening your sexuality*. Harper.

Deem, S., & Kim, D. E. (2019). *Premature ejaculation*. https://emedicine.medscape.com/article/435884-overview

Dennerstein, L., & Lehert, P. (2004). Confronting the challenges: Epidemiological study of female sexual dysfunction and menopause. *Journal of Sexual Medicine, 2*(3), 118–132.

Flores, A. R., Herman, J. L., Gates, G. J., & Brown, T.N.T. (2016). *How many adults identify as transgender in the United States?* The Williams Institute.

Graham, C. A., Sanders, S. A., Milhausen, R. R., & McBride, K. R. (2004). Turning on and turning off: A focus group study of the factors that affect women's sexual arousal. *Archives of Sexual Behavior, 33*(6), 527–538.

Herman, J. L., Flores, A. R., Brown, T. N. T., Wilson, B. D. M., & Conron, K. J. (2017). *Age of individuals Who identify as transgender in the United States*. The Williams Institute.

James, S. E., Herman, J. L., Rankin, S., Kesiling, M., Mottel, L., Anafi, M. (2016). *The report of the 2015 U.S. transgender survey*. Washington, DC: National Center for Transgender Equality.

Kim, E. D. (2018). *Erectile dysfunction*. https://emedicine.medscape.com/article/444220-overview#a1

Latini, D. M., Penson, D. F., Lubeck, D. P., Wallace, K. L., Henning, J. M., & Lue, T. F. (2003). Longitudinal differences in disease specific quality of life in men with erectile dysfunction: results from the Exploratory Comprehensive Evaluation of Erectile Dysfunction study. *Journal of Urology, 169*(4), 1437–1442. https://doi.org/10.1097/01.ju.0000049203.33463.9e

Masters, W. H., & Johnson, V. E. (1970). *Human sexual inadequacy*. Churchill.

Mathers, N., Bramley, M., Draper, K., Snead, S., & Tobert, A. (1994). Assessment of training in psychosexual medicine. *British Medical Journal, 308*, 969–972.

Nelson, S. (2005). Women's sexuality. In G. Andrews (Ed.), *Women's sexual health* (pp. 3–13). Elsevier.

Pollack, M. H., Reiter, S., & Hammerness, P. (1992). Genitourinary and sexual adverse effects of psychotropic medication. *International Journal of Psychiatry in Medicine, 22*(4), 305–327.

Sadock, B., Sadock, V., & Ruiz, P. (2015). *Kaplan & Sadock's synopsis of psychiatry* (11th ed.). Wolters Kluwer.

Sobczak, J. A. (2009). Female sexual dysfunction: Knowledge development and practice implications. *Perspectives in Psychiatric Care, 45*(3), 161–173.

Tusaie, K., & Fitzpatrick, J. (2017). *Advanced practice psychiatric nursing* (2nd ed.). Springer Publishing Company.

Wheeler, K. (2014). *Psychotherapy for the advanced practice psychiatric nurse* (2nd ed.). Springer Publishing Company.

16

Feeding and Eating Disorders

ANOREXIA NERVOSA

Background Information

Definition of Disorder and Diagnostic Criteria

- Anorexia nervosa (AN), as defined in the *Diagnostic and Statistical Manual of Mental Disorders*, Fifth Edition (*DSM-5*; American Psychiatric Association, 2013), is the purposeful and persistent energy intake restriction, an intense fear of becoming fat or gaining weight or persistently engaging in behaviors that interfere with weight gain, and a disturbance in self-perceived weight or shape. The *DSM-5* criteria for the diagnosis of AN include the following:
  - A restriction of energy intake relative to energy requirements, leading to the patient being significantly below weight (i.e., less than minimally normal or minimally expected weight) in the context of patient norms.
  - An intense fear of becoming fat, gaining weight, and/or persistent behaviors that preclude normal weight gain, such as excessive exercise and/or purging.
  - A disturbance in the way the patient experiences their body weight, undue influence of body weight or shape on the evaluation of self, or persistent nonrecognition of the graveness of their current low body weight.
  - In addition, specification in three areas is required. The areas are (1) subtype of AN, whether restricting or binge eating/purging; (2) remission status, partial or full; and (3) current level of severity, using body mass index (BMI) scoring. Severity levels are as follows: BMIs of 17 kg/m² or greater are mild, BMIs of 16 to 16.99 kg/m² are moderate, BMIs of 15 to 15.99 kg/m² are severe, and BMIs of 15 kg/m² or less are extreme.

Associated Features

- AN is not just a desire to be thin but an overwhelming desire to be thin and to reduce weight to meet lower and lower weight targets. The individual, in lowering their weight, may thereby reduce stress and improve their sense of empowerment.
- Individuals are most often brought to medical attention by family members who are concerned with marked weight loss or failure to gain expected weight. Individuals with AN lack insight into, or deny, a problem, making it important

for the practitioner to obtain information from family members or other legitimate sources.

■ Nutritional compromise seen in AN can affect most major organ systems and produce a wide range of disturbances. Depending on the specific behaviors the individual is engaging in, laboratory values may or may not reflect the disturbances.

■ Depressive symptoms, such as a depressed mood, social withdrawal, irritability, insomnia, and diminished interest in sex, may be present. These features may be secondary to starvation or severe enough to warrant an additional diagnosis of clinical depression. Suicide risk is elevated in AN. A complete suicide assessment, including suicide-related ideation, behaviors, other risk factors, and history of attempts should be conducted.

■ Obsessive-compulsive tendencies both related and unrelated to food are often present. As with depressive symptoms, food, body shape, and weight preoccupation are often secondary to starvation. Preoccupations commonly noted are rigid calorie counting, eating only low-calorie foods, cutting food into very small pieces, using only toothpicks to eat, recipe collecting, meal preparation without consumption, chewing food and spitting it out, repeated weighing of self, and frequent comments about feeling fat.

■ When individuals with AN exhibit obsessions and compulsions not related to food, body shape, or weight, an additional diagnosis of obsessive-compulsive disorder may be warranted.

■ Individuals with AN who use excessive exercise to control weight are at risk during treatment due to the difficulty in controlling physical activity.

■ Medications may be misused by the individual with AN to avoid weight gain or achieve weight loss. Medications may include (1) diet pills containing caffeine, ephedrine, or phenylpropanolamine and (2) medications that induce purging, such as laxatives and emetics. Withholding or reducing insulin to minimize carbohydrate metabolism is seen in individuals with both AN and insulin-dependent diabetes mellitus (DM).

■ Other features that may be associated with AN include feelings of ineffectiveness, a strong desire to control the environment, concerns about eating in public, inflexible thinking, limited social spontaneity, and overly restrained emotional expression.

■ Individuals with binge-eating/purging type of AN have higher rates of impulsivity and are more likely to abuse alcohol and other drugs than those with the restricting type.

■ The individual denies their weight problem and feels better as a result of continued weight loss.

■ Younger individuals (preadolescent) may not lose weight but may fail to gain weight and to achieve their ideal weights. Younger children very often have a poor ability to express inner turmoil and may refuse to eat certain foods or to increase exercise activity.

■ Approximately half of the individuals with AN have experienced a phase of bingeing/purging. During bingeing, the amounts of food ingested may not be large, and the foods themselves are often "forbidden foods," high in calories or fat.

Prevalence and Etiology

■ The lifetime prevalence rate for women is 0.9% and 0.3% in men for diagnosis in developed countries. The gender difference in the development of this disorder is a 10:1 female-to-male ratio. The disorder commonly begins during adolescence or young adulthood. Rarely does it begin before puberty or after the age of 40 years, though both can occur. Hospitalization may be required to restore weight and stabilize medical complications. Most individuals with AN experience remission within 5 years of presentation. Mortality rate is approximately 5% per decade, with the cause of death being medical complications associated with the disorder or suicide. The development of AN is associated with combinations of biological, psychological, and societal factors.

- Any individual who participates in restrictive diets can trigger obsessive focus on food and feelings of loss of control, often seen with repeated weight loss and weight gains: "yo-yo dieting." Modern Western culture cultivates and reinforces a desire for thinness, compounded by the influence of the media of very thin models and actors and the emphasis on elite athletes. Individuals in this society may view thinness as "successful." AN, however, did exist prior to the sociocultural values of the modern Western culture.
- Although social, economic, and cultural factors may be influencing factors, eating disorders have not been found among the majority of people in society.
- Individuals with AN may have low self-worth and an obsessive–compulsive personality trait for perfectionism. In these cases, the individuals will never be the "perfect weight."
- AN can be influenced by transitions in life experiences; requirements of sports, work, or artistic activity; and the media and society.
- Studies have indicated the interplay of an imbalance of neurotransmitters, such as serotonin (5-HT), as a factor in AN. Whether changes in the brain are a causative factor or caused by the disorder is not yet clear.

Demographics
- Eating disorders occur more in female patients (90%) and Whites (95%); it first develops in adolescence in 75% of cases.
- Although most patients are from middle- or upper-socioeconomic status families, the disorders can be found among any gender, race, age, or socioeconomic group. In fact, recent studies suggested that the disorder among minority females and adolescents of color is higher than suspected.

Complications
- *Death*: AN has the highest incidence of death related to starvation than any other mental illness.
- *Hematological*: Anemia, leukopenia, and thrombocytopenia.
- Cardiovascular
  - *Structural complications*: mitral valve prolapse, arrhythmias, decrease cardiac mass, myocardial fibrosis, and heart failure
  - *Functional complications*: hypotension, bradycardia, decreased diastolic function, and prolonged heart rhythm (QT) interval
- *Respiratory*: wasting of respiratory muscles and decrease in pulmonary capacity
- *Gastrointestinal*: gastroparesis, constipation, elevated liver enzymes, and occasionally acute pancreatitis
- *Genitourinary*: Electrolyte imbalance, renal insufficiency, and/or renal failure
- *Reproductive*: amenorrhea and infertility
- *Muscular-skeletal*: Osteoporosis
- *Neurological*: Wernicke encephalopathy, Korsakoff syndrome, and brain atrophy
- *Dermatologic*: alopecia, presence of lanugo, petechiae and carotenoderma

Risk Factors
Age
■ AN first occurs in middle school and then continues throughout adolescence.
    ▪ Onset usually occurs in young girls of middle-school age. Dieting, either for legitimate reasons or as a result of a body image distortion, is in itself a risk factor for the development of AN.
    ▪ Children who refuse to eat.
    ▪ Young children who do not gain weight as expected.
■ Children who develop anxiety disorders or display obsessional traits are at risk for developing AN.

Gender
■ Young girls of the White race, most often adolescents

Family History
■ In a study on risky eating disorders of mothers and sisters who had AN, the incidence of occurrence was eight times more often.
■ Genetic studies also have indicated an underlying biological influence on eating disorders, especially in twins. AN and other anxiety disorders tend to run in the family.
■ History of perfectionism coupled with compulsive behaviors
■ There is an increased risk for AN and bulimia nervosa (BN) among first-degree relatives of individuals with the disorder.

Stressful Events in Susceptible People
■ Females in late childhood and adolescence who feel a need to diet or lose weight are at risk for harmful weight-loss habits.
■ Transitioning events in childhood or adolescence, such as when entering high school or college.
Individuals who engage in low-weight-oriented sports or occupations, such as gymnasts, jockeys, runners, and wrestlers.

Having Another Mental Health Disorder
Those with other mental health disorders have a higher risk for developing AN. Individuals with a comorbidity of mood disorders; anxiety disorders; substance abuse disorders; disruptive, impulse control, and conduct disorders; attention-deficit/hyperactivity disorders; obsessive compulsive disorders; and posttraumatic stress disorder have an increased lifetime prevalence of a co-diagnosis of AN. Fifty-six percent of patients diagnosed with AN had a lifetime history of at least one mental health disorder, and 34% had three or more mental health diagnoses.

Diagnosis
Differential Diagnosis
■ Hyperthyroidism
■ Cardiac insufficiency or arrhythmias
■ Gastrointestinal disease
■ Malignancy, central nervous system (CNS) neoplasm
■ Pregnancy
■ AIDS/acute onset
■ Depression

- Substance abuse
- Schizophrenia
- Social anxiety disorder
- Obsessive-compulsive disorder
- Body dysmorphic disorder
- Avoidant/restrictive food intake disorder

ICD-10 Codes
Restricting type (F50.01 1)

Binge eating/purging type (F50.02)

Diagnostic Workup
- Low white blood cell count, increased margination of the leukocytes not related to an infection.
- Complete blood count (CBC) with differential; elevated hemoglobulin levels may be related to dehydration. Low hemoglobin and hematocrit seen with anemia; low platelets seen in thrombocytopenia. Low mean corpuscular volume (MCV) indices indicate iron deficiency anemia or active bleed; high MCV indices indicate macrocytic anemia from low B12 or folate.
- Transferrin and iron levels may be low.
- Blood plasma protein levels and prealbumin (determine malnourishment).
- Erythrocyte sedimentation rate is usually normal and may be elevated with organic illness, such as inflammatory bowel disease.
- Thyroid function studies—may be depressed.
- CMP-14—biochemical profiles, especially for presence of electrolyte imbalance such as hypoglycemia, hypomagnesemia, and hypokalemia.
- Liver function studies—may be elevated with severe dehydration as much as two times the normal level.
- Cholesterol levels may be elevated, with starvation due to depressed triiodothyronine (T3); cholesterol binding with globulin is low and fatty infiltration and leakage of cholesterol into the hepatic system is possible.
- Blood urea nitrogen (BUN) and creatinine to assess for renal function, urinalysis high specific gravity.
- EKG may reveal presence of bradycardia and prolonged QT interval.
- Echocardiogram to assess cardiomyopathy.
- Dual-energy x-ray absorptiometry (DXA) bone mineral density and 25-hydroxyvitamin D (25[OH]D).
- Human chorionic gonadotrospin (HCG), follicle stimulating hormone (FSH), luteinizing hormone (LH), prolactin, estradiol, thyroid stimulating hormone (TSH), and testosterone in males.
- X-rays to rule out fracture, pneumonia, respiratory, or infectious process.

Initial Assessment
- Medical history
- Symptoms experienced
- Assess vital signs, especially for hypothermia and for presence of orthostatic hypotension
- Assess for hypovolemia
- Dental assessment for presence of dental enamel erosion

- Assess for Russell sign—abrasion or callus of metacarpophalangeal joint of the index of middle finger of dominant hand
- Assess for alopecia
- Assess for edema, especially peripheral, which is indicative of poor capillary integrity due to malnutrition
- Assessment of weight and height is done by using standard growth charts for children or for those younger than 10 years of age; calculate BMI. Children, especially boys, have an increase of BMI with age; it is best to use standard growth charts
  - BMI = (weight in kg)/(height in m^2)
- Physical, mental, and psychosocial evaluation; use of screening tools for depression and mood
- Nutritional intake history and assessments for weight loss or weight cycling
- Diet recall
  - How does the patient feel about their weight?
  - Is the patient satisfied with their eating patterns?
  - Has the patient tried to control or lose weight by vomiting, diet pills, laxative, or starving?
  - Exercise practices of the patient.
- Family history or sibling eating disorder patterns
- History of mental illness/affective disorders, inpatient, and/or of family members
- Physical symptoms
  - Amenorrhea
  - Cold hands and feet
  - Constipation
  - Dry skin and hair
  - Headaches
  - Fainting or dizziness
  - Lethargy or lack of energy
  - Anorexia
  - Lanugo (body's attempt to maintain body heat)
  - Cutting, picking, or burn scars
  - Low blood pressure for the age
- Emotional and behavioral symptoms
  - Refusal to eat
  - Denial of hunger
  - Excessive exercise
  - Flat mood or lack of emotion
- Social withdrawal
  - Difficulty concentrating
  - Preoccupation with food
  - Black-and-white thinking (resistant to change)

Diagnostic and Statistical Manual of Mental Disorders, Fifth Edition: *Diagnostic Guidelines*
- Difficult disorder to diagnose because individuals with anorexia often attempt to hide the disorder.
- Denial and secrecy.
- It is unusual for an individual with anorexia to seek professional help because the individual typically does not accept that they have a problem (denial).
- In many cases, the actual diagnosis is not made until medical complications have developed.

- The individual is often brought to the attention of a professional by family members only after marked weight loss has occurred.
- Warning signs of developing anorexia or one of the other eating disorders include excessive interest in dieting or thinness.
- Restriction of energy intake relative to requirements, leading to a significantly low body weight.
- Weight in the context of age, sex, developmental trajectory, and physical health.
- Significantly low weight is defined as a weight that is less than minimally normal or, for children and adolescents, less than that minimally expected.
- Intense fear of gaining weight or becoming fat, or persistent behavior that interferes with weight gain even though the individual is already at a significantly low weight.
- Disturbance in the way body weight or shape is experienced, undue influence of body weight or shape on self-evaluation, or persistent lack of recognition of the seriousness of the current low body weight.

Treatment Overview

- The psychiatrist may assume the leadership role within a program or team that includes other physicians, psychologists, registered dietitians, and social workers or may work collaboratively on a team led by others. Additionally, these same practice guidelines require that communication among all disciplines is essential (Recommendation I).
- A team approach is recommended by the American Psychiatric Association (APA) Practice Guidelines (Recommendation III) as well as using various resources for treatment: inpatient, outpatient, psychological therapy, and pharmacotherapy, including patient education (Recommendation I).
- Obtain a history; schedule a physical that is comprehensive, with a review of the patient's height and weight history; restrictive and binge eating and exercise patterns and their changes; purging and other compensatory behaviors; core attitudes regarding weight, shape, and eating; and associated psychiatric conditions (Recommendation I).
- Obtain a family history of eating disorders or other psychiatric disorders, including alcohol and other substance-use disorders; a family history of obesity; the family's reactions or interactions in relation to the eating disorder; and family attitudes toward eating, exercise, and appearance (Recommendation I).
- It is important to determine stressors that may trigger the eating disorders in order to facilitate amelioration of the eating disorder.
- When assessing children and adolescents, it is essential to involve parents, significant others, and, when appropriate, school personnel and health professionals who routinely work with the patient (Recommendation I).
- With older adults, although spouses and significant others should be part of the treatment program, the clinician should consider whether others should be involved (Recommendations II and III).

Acute Treatment

- Treatment is multifaceted and interprofessional.
- The goal is to stop weight loss and gain weight. The ultimate goal is to establish a structured pattern of three meals and one to three snacks daily.
- Breakfast is essential as this is the meal most often missed by dieters, anorexics, and adolescents. Patients who eat breakfast often have less chance of binge eating later in the day, are less hungry, and thus may avoid bingeing.

- In severe situations, acute treatment may be indicated for life-threatening conditions, such as cardiac arrhythmias, severe dehydration, or electrolyte imbalance. Intensive care has been instituted for life-threatening situations.
  - Total parenteral nutrition may be indicated along with intravenous replacement of electrolytes.
  - Albumin may be given to prevent sudden refeeding syndrome—a potentially fatal condition resulting from rapid changes in fluids and electrolytes in malnourished individuals given oral, enteral, or parenteral feeding. Monitor for hypophosphatemia occurring as a result of glycolysis.
  - Hypophosphatemia can result in impairment of myocardial contractility.
  - Heart failure can occur in the presence of fluid retention with an inadequate cardiac status.
  - Hypokalemia may result as well from insulin secretion in response to an increase in calories, which shifts the potassium into the cells.
  - A daily multivitamin with thiamine should be used to prevent Wernicke's encephalopathy.
  - Nasogastric feeding may be necessary to replenish caloric requirements once the acute phase for refeeding occurs.
- Supervise and monitor weight daily; some patients with AN have learned how to increase weight by drinking fluids.
- Monitor vital signs for hypothermia and fluid and electrolytes, especially urine-specific gravity. Patients may try to falsify weight by wearing increased underclothing garments; however, urine-specific gravity can indicate dehydration or starvation.
- A dietitian should be an integral part of the inpatient treatment to evaluate and treat specific deficiencies or excesses.
- Food should be balanced, with a flexible exchange system to allow for variety. All food consumption should be monitored. Diet must be balanced; "fat-free foods" should be limited and healthy foods emphasized. Adolescents may perceive "fat-free foods" as "good" food, not realizing the increase in sugar and calories. The patient should be educated on a balanced diet and nutritional concepts.
- The patient can maintain a journal of eating patterns and identify dysfunctional eating patterns (purging) that occur during the inpatient episode. Provide feedback and encouragement for adherence to health; try not to stress the increase in food intake.
- Individuals with AN may not think that they have a problem but rather that they have chosen a lifestyle.
- Inpatient treatment in a mental health setting is necessary in patients with a suicidal ideation and plan and serious alcohol or sedative withdrawal symptoms or when the differential includes other medical disorders that warrant admission (e.g., unstable angina, acute myocardial ischemia).
- Cognitive-behavioral therapy (CBT), including dialectical behavior therapy, allows patients to monitor progress and identify triggers for dieting, binge eating, and purging as well as refusal to eat. CBT focuses on restructuring thoughts that lead to distorted eating.
- Psychotherapy that establishes trust is essential, as individuals with AN may not be willing to relinquish their coping mechanism or eating patterns. AN must be explained in terms of the patient's stage of psychosocial development. Reassure the patient that others need to be incorporated in care to assist with improving health and that the clinician is not abandoning the patient.

- Family therapy can help resolve family conflicts or elicit support from concerned family members; this is especially important for children who live at home.
- Group therapy can help persons with AN to connect with others facing similar complications, stressors, and coping behaviors. Group therapy must be carefully monitored as persons with AN may use it as a means to compete as to who is thinnest.

Chronic Treatment

- A multidisciplinary approach with a psychologist, primary care provider, and a dietitian is essential. Any therapy can last for over 1 year while the individual attempts to gain insight into triggers that can induce the eating-disordered behavior.
- Interpersonal therapy and family therapy have proven to be more effective than CBT, with or without pharmacotherapy, for AN.
- A meta-analysis revealed that intervention was more successful if it was interactive and had multiple sessions.
- Measurement of bone density should be evaluated initially and every 6 months. Findings demonstrate that depressive symptoms and anxiety are associated with low bone density.
- Menses resumption occurs with return to at least 86% of ideal body weight; therefore, the goal should be to assist adolescents in acquiring a healthy habit of eating nourishing foods and exercising.

Pharmacotherapy Overview for Anorexia Nervosa

- Selective serotonin reuptake inhibitors (SSRIs) may be useful with AN to maintain weight gain and prevent relapse, such as fluoxetine (Prozac, Sarafem, with the initial dose of 20 mg once daily increased to 40 to 60 mg for maintenance).
- SSRIs are not useful in AN when patients are at low weights due to decreased protein levels, including tryptophan, which is needed for serotonin production.
- Although tricyclic antidepressants, such as clomipramine (Anafranil) and amitriptyline (Elavil), have been prescribed to individuals with AN, cardiac toxicity due to electrolyte abnormality, as seen in AN patients, can occur. This category of drugs can also cause sedation, tachycardia, constipation, dry mouth, and confusion.
- Cyproheptadine (Periactin), an antihistamine, and serotonin antagonists have proven beneficial in increasing food intake. Serotonin in the hypothalamus is responsible for decreased food consumption; therefore, it is hypothesized that a serotonin antagonist would have the opposite effects. Cyproheptadine has been successful in treatment of patients with inappropriate caloric intake, such as patients with HIV, cancer, and other chronic illnesses.
- Dronabinol (Marinol), a cannabinoid, has been used with patients to increase appetite (see the Web Resources section).
- In some patients with AN, anxiolytic agents such as olanzapine (Zyprexa, Zyprexa Zydis), prior to eating, have been effective.
- Because gastric motility is impaired with AN, drugs such as metoclopramide (Reglan) and cisapride (Propulsid) help to accelerate gastric emptying and enhance gastric motor activity. Osmotic agents such as Gl-Lytely or Glycolax can help with constipation and bloating.
- Zinc supplementation, alone or along with a multivitamin, has been associated with weight gain.

- Rate, growth factors (insulin-like growth factor 1 [IGF-1]), and dehydroepiandrosterone (DHEA), a naturally occurring adrenal hormone, may be of some benefit in patients with severe bone loss.
- The Society for Adolescent Medicine has suggested 1,200 to 1,500 mg of elemental calcium, a multivitamin with 400 units of vitamin D, along with dual emission x-ray absorptiometry (DEXA) scans on baseline and to monitor bone regrowth.
- Natural herbs may improve appetite and have a placebo effect on weight gain; Kiddie Florish™, an herbal supplement, has been used by some parents with younger school-age children to improve appetite.

Note: The Food and Drug Administration (FDA) has not approved natural remedies as pharmacological treatments for eating disorders.

- Appropriate pharmacological therapy and CBT, individually or in combination, are effective in more than 85% of cases.
- In general, pharmacotherapy has limited usefulness in the treatment of AN.

Recurrence Rate

- Rate of recurrence is approximately 15% to 25%. Individuals with AN who are hospitalized have a 75% to 85% chance of full recovery.

Patient Education

- Advise patients with AN to avoid nicotine, sympathomimetic or anticholinergic drugs, caffeine, and alcohol.

Drug Selection Table for Anorexia Nervosa

CLASS	DRUG
SSRIs	Drugs sometimes useful to treat symptomatology Citalopram (Celexa) Fluoxetine (Prozac) Sertraline (Zoloft)
Tricyclic antidepressants	Drugs sometimes useful to treat symptomatology Amitriptyline (Apo-Amitriptyline, Elavil) Clomipramine (Anafranil)
Antipsychotics, atypical (second-generation)	Drugs sometimes useful to treat symptomatology: Quetiapine (Seroquel) Olanzapine (Zyprexa, Zyprexa Zydis) SSRIs, selective serotonin reuptake inhibitors.

- Avoid weighing self; resist urge to isolate self from caring individuals.
- Provide information on healthy lifestyles, such as supplements and vitamins.
- Avoid pro-anorexia websites, chat rooms, or media that emphasize thinness.
- Avoid contact with friends who also have AN. Stick to your healthy lifestyle plan and use of cognitive-behavioral interventions, such as participating in appropriate student organizations, journaling, and identifying feelings and thoughts and linking to an internet support program.
- Information regarding AN and support groups can be obtained from the National Institute of Mental Health (NIMH).

Medical/Legal Pitfalls

- A common finding in those who commit suicide is the presence of more than one mental health disorder, such as mood disorder (i.e., depression), personality disorder, and other psychiatric disorders (WHO, 2000). Individuals with AN are at risk for depression due to their distorted body image and perfectionist psychological profile (Wattula, 2008).

- As of May 2, 2007, the National Clearing House labeled all antidepressant drugs with a black box warning on the prescribing information to include warnings about the increased risks of suicidal thinking and behavior in young adults aged 18 to 24 years during the first months of treatment.
- In 2006, the antidepressant Paxil received the first warning—to be followed by others in 2007, that is, a Clinical Worsening and Suicide Risk label in the prescribing information related to adult patients, especially younger adults.
- Individuals with an eating disorder display symptoms as a result of psychological problems; failure to recognize the relationship may result in inappropriate care.

BULIMIA NERVOSA

Background Information

Definition of Disorder

- BN occur when a large amount of food is eaten in a short time period. The essential features of BN include recurrent episodes of binge eating, recurrent inappropriate compensatory behaviors to prevent weight gain, and self-evaluation that is unduly influenced by body shape and weight. A diagnosis of BN can be made when the binge eating and inappropriate compensatory behaviors occur, on average, at least once per week for 3 months. With BN, weight is usually within or slightly above normal parameters.
- Individuals may not have a body image distortion or may actually see themselves not as heavy as they actually are.
- Psychosocial factors may include family conflict or ineffective coping during stressful times, such as when entering high school or college. Conversely, an individual feels "power or control" while participating with weight-control behaviors, especially if there are secondary rewards, such as compliments or acceptance by peers. The studies suggest that females in late childhood and adolescence who feel a need to diet or lose weight are at a risk for adopting harmful eating disorders.

Diagnostic and Statistical Manual of Mental Disorders, Fifth Edition: Diagnostic Criteria

- Repeated episodes of binge eating, in a discrete period of time, the volume of food consumed is definitely bigger than what most individuals would consume in a similar amount of time under similar circumstances. During the episode, the individual has a sense of lacking any control over eating during the episode.
- Repeated inappropriate compensatory behaviors to prevent gaining weight. Examples include self-induced vomiting; misuse of medications such as laxatives or diuretics; excessive exercise; or fasting.
- Both the compensatory behaviors and binge eating occur an average of at least once a week for 3 months.
- Self-evaluation is disproportionately influenced by body shape and weight.
- The BN episodes do not occur exclusively during AN episodes.
- The diagnosis should include specifications of (1) remission status, partial or full, and (2) severity status, which is initially based on the frequency of inappropriate compensatory behaviors per week, with 1 to 3 episodes a week constituting mild severity; 4 to 7, moderate; 8 to 13, severe; and 14 or more considered extreme severity.

Associated Features

- BN may occur as part of experimentation with induced vomiting, use of laxatives, fasting, or rigorous exercise to prevent weight gain.
- The patient's perceptions of body shape and body size have become distorted.
- Purging is the compensatory behavior most often used to avoid weight gain. Binge eating, however, is the defining element of the diagnosis.
- In adolescents, purging includes self-stimulation of the upper pharynx, pressure put on the abdomen, and the use of ipecac and laxatives.
- Adolescents may also use rigorous exercise and fasting to prevent weight gain.
- The individual with BN may exhibit attitudes of self-deprecation or have depressed mood after becoming aware of their anomalous eating patterns.

Etiology

- The pathogenesis believed to occur with an imbalance of serotonin is that at the hypothalamus, higher levels of 5-HT tend to decrease appetite and food intake, whereas lower levels are associated with decreased satiety. The CNS precursor to serotonin, 5-hydroxyindoleacetic acid (5-HIAA), is lower in patients with AN when they are ill but returns to a higher level during recovery from AN. A similar process occurs with BN.
- Two other factors associated with BN are sexual trauma and depression. Patients with BN have histories of depression. There is a higher incidence of sexual trauma among adolescents who have BN than in the general population. Depression is difficult to determine if it precedes BN or is associated with affective disorder.
- BN has been associated with dissatisfaction with one's body after sexual abuse, poor attachment to others, and insecurity.
- Athletes of any gender, especially gymnasts and runners who have low self-esteem, are predisposed to eating disorders.
- Male patients with eating disorders, who constitute a much lower incidence than females, have either BN. Male athletes will often engage in binge eating and vomiting.
- Increased incidence or prevalence of BN may account for the increase in eating disorders.
- Increased media attention, better screening of patients for eating disorders, and less stringent diagnostic criteria may also be responsible for the apparent increase in eating disorders.
- Binge eating and purging allow patients to be in control when engaged in weight-control behaviors, especially if secondary gains occur.
- During binges, individuals tend to eat food high in calories or fat that they would otherwise avoid.
- Suicide risk is elevated in BN. A complete suicide assessment, including suicide-related ideation, behaviors, other risk factors, and history of attempts, should be conducted.

Demographics

Of patients with BN, 90% are female; 95% are White; and 75% first developed the disorder as adolescents. Binge-eating disorder (BED) also occurs more in females, with a prevalence rate of 3.5% for women and 2.3% for adolescent females compared to 2.0% for men and 0.8% for adolescent males.

- BN is more common in high school and college students, with a peak incidence occurring around 18 years of age.

- Many children do not meet stringent diagnostic criteria for BN but may exhibit partial symptoms.
- BN is found across racial and socioeconomic groups, with boys representing one fifth of adolescents and about one tenth of adult males. Recent data suggest that bingeing and/or purging may occur when the individual perceives an increase in food intake and not on a regular basis. Lifetime prevalence rates for BN in the Latinx population is higher (2.0%) than the non-Latinx White population (0.51%).
- Twenty-five percent of adolescents regularly engage in self-induced purging as a means to control weight.
- There is an increase in prevalence for eating disorders primarily due to media attention and improved detection.
- BN is thought to be a learned behavior, acquired from modeling of peer groups.
- The mortality rate for BN is 17%, with almost a quarter as a result of suicide.

Risk Factors
Age
- Adolescents in high school and college; young adults.
- Athletes who have specific weight requirements.
- Patients with BN often have episodes of dieting to lose weight rapidly.
- Patients may use the excuse of bingeing as an attempt to bulk up for sports repeatedly and then use purging or vomiting as an attempt to avoid weight gain.

Gender
- Although both genders are at risk, female adolescents are more likely to participate in BN or BED.
- Postpubertal females constitute 5% to 10% of cases of mild variants of eating disorders.

Family History
- Genetic studies have indicated an underlying biological influence on eating disorders, especially in twins. There is an association with BN and being a twin in up to 35% to 50% of cases.
- Overweight parents, especially fathers.

Having Another Mental Health Disorder
Ninety-five percent of individuals with BN have one mental health comorbid disorder, and 64% have three or more comorbid diagnoses.

- Those with other mental health disorders, such as depression or substance abuse (alcoholism or drug abuse), have an increased risk for suicide or suicidal tendency. It is estimated that 30% of individuals seeking medical care are depressed or have depressive episodes such as sadness, depressed mood, lack of interest or enjoyment, or reduced energy or fatigability.
- Individuals with a history of sexual abuse in childhood are at risk for developing BN.

Diagnosis
Differential Diagnosis
- AN, binge-eating/purging type
- Major depressive disorder with atypical features

- Borderline personality disorder
- Kleine-Levin syndrome
- Bipolar disorder
- Insulin resistance
- Sleep apnea/daytime somnolence
- Pseudotumor cerebri
- Hyperthyroidism
- Inflammatory bowel disease
- Malignancy, CNS neoplasm
- Pregnancy
- AIDS/acute onset
- Systemic lupus erythematosus
- Substance abuse
- Obesity

ICD-10 Code
Bulimia nervosa (F50.2)

Diagnostic Workup
- Physical, mental, and psychosocial evaluation.
- Nutritional intake history and assessments for weight loss or weight cycling.
- Blood plasma protein levels and prealbumin (determine malnourishment).
- Erythrocyte sedimentation rate is usually normal and may be elevated with organic illness, such as inflammatory bowel disease.
- Thyroid function studies—may be depressed.
- Cholesterol levels may be elevated, with starvation due to depressed T3, cholesterol binding with globulin is low, and there is possible fatty infiltration and leakage of cholesterol into the hepatic system.
- CBC with differential, elevated hemoglobulin levels may be related to dehydration and hemoconcentration.
- *Transferrin and iron levels*: Levels may be normal.
- Electrolyte studies often indicate hypokalemia, hypochloremia, and/or metabolic alkalosis due to recurrent vomiting. The absence of abnormality in electrolytes does not exclude BN.
- Hypomagnesium may be present with excessive use of laxatives or water-diarrheal stools.
- CMP-14—biochemical profiles, especially for presence of electrolyte imbalance, such as hypoglycemia, hypomagnesemia, and hypokalemia.
- Liver function studies may be elevated with severe dehydration, as much as two times the normal.
- Electrocardiogram (EKG): presence of bradycardia and prolonged QT interval when BN occurs in low-weight individuals. U waves may be present secondary to hypokalemia and if cardiomyopathy has occurred due to alkaloid emetine contained in syrup of ipecac.
- Screening with appropriate instruments for depression.

Clinical Presentation
- Binge eating
  - Weight gain or weight fluctuation
  - Bloating

- Lethargy
  - Salivary gland enlargement (if vomiting)
  - Guilt
  - Depression
  - Anxiety
- Low self-esteem
- Purging
  - Weight loss
  - Fatigue
- Arrhythmia or palpitations
  - Decreased skin turgor, elevated urine specific gravity, dry mucous membranes
  - Guilt
  - Depression
  - Anxiety/guilt
- Low self-esteem
  - Knuckle calluses (vomiting)
  - Dental enamel erosion (vomiting)
  - Any form of self-mutilation, such as cutting
  - Frequent overeating used for coping
  - Self-induced vomiting, hematemesis
  - Excessive exercise
  - Salivary gland enlargement
  - Conjunctival hemorrhage
  - Epigastric pain, constipation, bloating, and oral sores
  - Xerosis

Diagnostic Guidelines

In BN, recurrent episodes of binge eating are characterized by the following:

- Eating amounts of food that are unquestionably larger than what most persons would consume in the same time period and under similar circumstances.
- Absence of self-control during the episodes.
- Presence of compensatory behaviors to prevent weight gain: induced vomiting, use of laxatives and diuretics, use of enemas, use of other medications, fasting, rigorous exercise.
- Binge eating and the accompanying compensatory behaviors, both occurring at least twice a week for 3 months.
- Self-evaluation is unduly influenced by body shape and weight.
- The episodes of BN do not occur exclusively during episodes of AN.

Treatment Overview

- Obtain a history and a physical that are comprehensive, with a review of the patient's height and weight history; restrictive and binge eating and exercise patterns and their changes; purging and other compensatory behaviors; core attitudes regarding weight, shape, and eating; and associated psychiatric conditions (Recommendation I).
- Obtain a family history of eating disorders or other psychiatric disorders, including alcohol and other substance-use disorders; a family history of obesity; the family's reactions or interactions in relation to the eating disorder; and family attitudes toward eating, exercise, and appearance (Recommendation I).

- It is important to determine stressors that may trigger the eating disorders in order to facilitate amelioration of the eating disorder.
- When assessing children and adolescents, it is essential to involve parents, significant others, and, when appropriate, school personnel and health professionals who routinely work with the patient (Recommendation I).
- With older adults, although spouses and significant others should be part of the treatment program, the clinician should consider whether others should be involved. Assess vital signs, especially for hypothermia and for presence of orthostatic hypotension.
- Assess for hypovolemia.
- Dental assessment for presence of dental enamel erosion.
- Assess for Russell sign—abrasion or callus of metacarpophalangeal joint of the index of middle finger of dominant hand.
- Assessment for alopecia.
- Assess for edema, especially peripheral, which is indicative of poor capillary integrity due to malnutrition.
- Assessment of weight and height is done by using standard growth charts for children or for those younger than 10 years old; calculate BMI. Children, especially boys, have an increase in BMI with age. It is best to use standard growth charts. BMI = (weight in kg)/(height in m^2).
- Assess for gastrointestinal irritability secondary to esophageal tears.
- Auscultate for cardiac arrhythmias.

Acute Treatment

- Treatment is multifaceted and interprofessional, including a mental health professional, a primary care provider or medical person, a dietitian, school personnel, and religious persons, if indicated.
- The medical personnel work to correct and manage medical issues, such as electrolyte imbalances and dental problems.
- The dietitian is essential in providing nutritional education and a rationale for selection of certain foods and a meal plan. In some organizations, a dietitian is supplemented by a sports physiologist or trainer to assist individuals with weight management.
- If exercise therapy is needed, proceed cautiously as excessive exercising could occur along with binge–purge eating in susceptible individuals.
- The nutritional intake for those requiring a weight gain should consist of 2 to 3 lbs/wk (0.9–1.4 kg) of controlled weight gain; for outpatients, it is 0.5 to 1 lbs/wk. The intake should start at 3,040 kcal/kg (1,000–1,500 kcal/d) and advance progressively.
- In severe situations, acute inpatient treatment for BN may be indicated for life-threatening conditions. Some of these conditions include cardiac arrhythmias, severe dehydration or electrolyte imbalance, arrested development, failure of outpatient treatment, acute food refusal, suicidal ideation, comorbid diagnosis such as depression, or severe family dysfunction.
- Intensive care has been instituted for life-threatening situations.
  - Total parenteral nutrition may be indicated along with intravenous replacement of electrolytes.
  - Albumin may be given to prevent sudden refeeding syndrome—a potentially fatal condition resulting from rapid changes in fluids and electrolytes in malnourished individuals given oral, enteral, or parenteral feeding. Monitor for hypophosphatemia occurring as a result of glycolysis.

- Hypophosphatemia can result in impairment of myocardial contractility.
- Heart failure can occur in the presence of fluid retention with an inadequate cardiac status.
- Hypokalemia may also result from insulin secretion in response to an increase in calories, which shifts the potassium into the cells.
- A daily multivitamin with thiamine should be used to prevent Wernicke's encephalopathy.
- Nasogastric feeding may be necessary to replenish caloric requirements once the acute phase for refeeding occurs.
- Caution should be provided that some patients may gain weight rapidly due to fluid retention, possibly due to low protein levels.
- Treat electrolyte or nutritional deficits first; inpatient treatment may be indicated.
  - CBT emphasizes that thoughts and feelings may lead to distorted eating patterns. CBT has higher efficacy and lower cost, dropout rates, and relapse rates than pharmacological treatments.
  - A combination of psychotherapy and antidepressant medications provide the best chance for remission.
  - Self-help programs have been found to be beneficial in the treatment of BN.
  - Appetite suppressants and psychological treatment have been effective in the treatment of individuals who are overweight or who have bulimia.

Chronic Treatment

- Multidisciplinary approach with a psychologist, primary care provider, and a dietitian is essential. Any therapy can last for over 1 year while the individual attempts to gain insight into triggers that can induce the eating-disorder behavior.
  - Use screening tools to determine the presence of depression, child abuse, or sexual abuse in older adolescents and use the SCOFF questionnaire:
    - S—Do you make yourself Sick because you feel uncomfortably full?
    - C—Do you worry you have lost Control over how much you eat?
    - O—Have you recently lost more than One stone (14 lbs or 7.7 kg) in a 3-month period?
    - F—Do you believe yourself to be Fat when others say you are too thin?
    - F—Would you say that Food dominates your life?
  - Use of cognitive-behavioral interventions such as CBT, dialectical behavior therapy, participation in appropriate student organizations, journaling, identifying feelings, linking food and emotions to circumvent unwanted behavior, and an internet support program have proven beneficial.

Pharmacotherapy Overview

- Antidepressants, with SSRIs as the first category of choice, may be useful with BN to counteract the depressive symptoms associated with eating disorders. Fluoxetine (Prozac) is the only FDA-approved SSRI for the treatment of BN. An initial dose of 20 mg/d is administered for adults with the goal of reaching a maintenance dose of 60 mg/d.
- The *DSM-5* identifies depressive disorders as the most common comorbid states associated with both BN.
- Appropriate pharmacological therapy and CBT, individually or in combination, are effective in more than 85% of cases.
  - BZDs, such as alprazolam (Xanax) and clonazepam (Klonopin) are also considered first-line treatment options for BN; however, short-term use is recommended to prevent abuse and side effects, including drowsiness, slurred speech, and ataxia.

Mood-stabilizing anticonvulsants are considered a second-line treatment option for BN, which include topiramate (Topamax), carbamazepine (Tegretol), and zonisamide (Zonegran); they have been useful in individuals with BN to improve binge–purge behaviors as well as improve depressive symptoms.

Although tricyclic antidepressants, such as clomipramine (Anafranil) and amitriptyline (Elavil), have been prescribed to individuals with BN and BED as a third-line treatment option, cardiac toxicity due to electrolyte abnormality, as seen in patients who purge, can occur. This category of drugs can also cause sedation, tachycardia, constipation, dry mouth, and confusion.

- *Gastric motor activity:* Osmotic agents such as Gl-Lytely or Glycolax can help with constipation and bloating.
- Zinc supplementation alone, or along with a multivitamin, has been associated with weight gain.

Recurrence Rate

- Poorer outcomes have been associated with later age of onset of eating disorders.
- Low self-esteem can impact the recurrence of binge–purge behaviors. Thirty percent of individuals may continue to engage in bingeing–purging up to 10 years after follow-up if substance abuse is coupled with the eating behavior.

Patient Education

Patient education should include disease etiology, pathophysiology, diagnostic evaluation, and treatment options, including psychopharmacology and psychotherapy.

Drug Selection Table for Bulimia Nervosa

CLASS	DRUG
SSRIs	First-line drug therapy *Fluoxetine (Prozac) Citalopram (Celexa) Sertraline (Zoloft)
BZDs	Alprazolam (Xanax IR and ER) Clonazepam (Klonopin) Diazepam (Valium)
Mood-stabilizing anticonvulsants	Second-line drug therapy Carbamazepine (Tegretol) Zonisamide (Zonegran)
Tricyclic antidepressants	Third-line drug therapy Amitriptyline (Elavil, Endep, Vanatrip) Clomipramine (Anafranil)

*Food and Drug Administration (FDA)-approved for BN.
BZDs, benzodiazepines; SSRIs, selective serotonin reuptake inhibitors.

Medical/Legal Pitfalls

- A common finding in those who commit suicide is the presence of more than one mental health disorder.
- Mood disorder (i.e., depression), personality disorder, and other psychiatric disorders may be overlooked. As of May 2, 2007, the National Clearing House labeled antidepressant drugs with a black box warning on the prescribing information to include warnings about the increased risk of suicidal thinking and behavior in young adults aged 18 to 24 years during the first 1 to 2 months of treatment.

■ As of May 12, 2006, the National Clearing House labeled paroxetine (Paxil) and Paxil CR with a Clinical Worsening and Suicide Risk advisory in the prescribing information related to adult patients, especially younger adults.

BINGE-EATING DISORDER

Background Information

Definition of Disorder
■ BED occurs when a large amount of food is eaten in a short time period.

Diagnostic and Statistical Manual of Mental Disorders, Fifth Edition: Diagnostic Criteria
■ Recurrent episodes of binge eating, in a discrete period of time, an amount of food that is definitely larger than what most individuals would eat in a similar period of time under similar circumstances, and a sense of lack of control over eating during the episode, including the ability to stop eating, or what and how much to eat.
  ■ BED is not associated with any compensatory behaviors as seen in those with AN or BN (i.e., laxative use, vomiting, purging, excessive exercise).
  ■ BED does not occur exclusively during episodes of AN or BN.
  ■ The binge-eating episodes are associated with three or more of the following: (1) eating much more rapidly than normal; (2) eating until feeling uncomfortably full; (3) eating large amounts of food when not feeling physically hungry; (4) eating alone because of feeling embarrassed by how much one is eating; (5) feeling disgusted with oneself, depressed, or very guilty afterward.
■ Marked distress regarding binge eating is present.
■ The binge eating occurs on average at least once a week for 3 months.
■ The severity of the condition is based on the frequency of inappropriate compensatory behaviors per week, with 1 to 3 episodes a week constituting mild severity; 4 to 7 constituting moderate severity; and 8 to 13 constituting a severe condition; 14 or more is considered extreme severity.

Associated Features
■ Fifty percent of individuals with BED are overweight or obese, with the remaining 50% being of ideal body weight.
■ Individuals with BED may use compensatory methods to avoid weight gain when other attempts to avoid weight gain have failed.
■ Individuals with BED often eat alone, as they are embarrassed about bingeing.
■ BED can be distinguished from BN in that, in BED, there is a recurring compensatory weight-control habit, such as dieting, when overeating occurs.
■ BED has been associated with male athletes' attempts to control weight during sports events.

Etiology
■ The pathogenesis believed to occur with an imbalance of serotonin is that at the hypothalamus, higher levels of 5-HT tend to decrease appetite and food intake, whereas lower levels are associated with decreased satiety. The CNS precursor to serotonin, 5-HIAA, is lower in patients with AN when they are ill but returns to a higher level during recovery from AN. A similar process occurs with BN.

- Two other factors associated with BED are sexual trauma and depression. Patients with BED have histories of depression. There is a higher incidence of sexual trauma among adolescents who have BED than in the general population.
- Athletes of any gender, especially gymnasts and runners who have low self-esteem, are predisposed to eating disorders.
- Male patients with eating disorders, who constitute a much lower incidence than females, have either BN or BED. Male athletes with BED avoid weight gain or maintain a certain weight for sports activities. Male athletes will often engage in binge eating and vomiting.
- Increased media attention, better screening of patients for eating disorders, and less stringent diagnostic criteria may also be responsible for the apparent increase in eating disorders.
- Binge eating and purging allow patients to be in control when engaged in weight-control behaviors, especially if secondary gains occurs.
- During binges, individuals tend to eat food high in calories or fat that they would otherwise avoid.
- Suicide risk is elevated in BN. A complete suicide assessment, including suicide-related ideation, behaviors, other risk factors, and history of attempts, should be conducted.

Demographics
- BED also occurs more in females, with a prevalence rate of 2.6% and a 3:1 ratio for females to males.
- BED is more common in high school and college students, with a median age of onset of 23 years of age.
- BED is found across racial and socioeconomic groups.
- There is an increase in prevalence for eating disorders primarily due to media attention and improved detection.

Risk Factors
Age
- Adolescents in high school and college, young adults.
- Athletes who have specific weight requirements.
- BED patients often have episodes of dieting to lose weight rapidly.
- Patients who have BED often can be overweight and may have parents who are overweight; maternal control over feeding (restricting or urging) is seen.
- Children older than 2 years with a BMI of 85% are considered at risk for becoming overweight; children at the 95th percentile are overweight.

Gender
- Although both genders are at risk, female adolescents are more likely to participate in binge eating.
- Postpubertal females constitute 5% to 10% of cases of mild variants of eating disorders.

Family History
- Genetic studies have indicated an underlying biological influence on eating disorders, especially in twins. There is an association with BN and being a twin in up to 35% to 50% of cases.
- Overweight parents, especially fathers.

Having Another Mental Health Disorder

- Those with other mental health disorders have a higher incidence of BED. Seventy-nine percent of individuals with BED have one other comorbid mental health condition, and 49% have 3 or more mental health comorbid conditions. The most frequently seen comorbid conditions in individuals who suffer from BED include phobias, major depression, posttraumatic stress disorder, and alcohol abuse.

Diagnosis

Differential Diagnosis

- AN, binge-eating/purging type

Bulimia Nervosa

- Major depressive disorder with atypical features
- Borderline personality disorder
- Kleine-Levin syndrome
- Bipolar disorder
- Insulin resistance
- Sleep apnea/daytime somnolence
- Pseudotumor cerebri
- Hyperthyroidism
- Inflammatory bowel disease
- Malignancy, CNS neoplasm
- Pregnancy
- AIDS/acute onset
- Systemic lupus erythematosus
- Substance abuse
- Obesity

ICD-10 Code

Binge eating disorder (F50.8)

Diagnostic Workup

- Physical, mental, and psychosocial evaluation.
- Nutritional intake history and assessments for weight loss or weight cycling.
- Blood plasma protein levels and prealbumin (determine malnourishment).
- Erythrocyte sedimentation rate is usually normal and may be elevated with organic illness, such as inflammatory bowel disease.
- Thyroid function studies—may be depressed.
- Cholesterol levels may be elevated, with starvation due to depressed T3, cholesterol binding with globulin is low, and there is possible fatty infiltration and leakage of cholesterol into hepatic system.
- CBC with differential, elevated hemoglobulin levels may be related to dehydration and hemoconcentration.
- *Transferrin and iron levels*: Levels may be normal.
- CMP-14—biochemical profiles, especially for presence of electrolyte imbalance, such as hyperglycemia
- Screening with appropriate instruments for depression

Clinical Presentation
- Binge eating
  - Weight gain or weight fluctuation
  - Bloating
  - Lethargy
  - Salivary gland enlargement (if vomiting)
  - Guilt
  - Depression
  - Anxiety

    Low self-esteem

  - Excessive exercise
    Chronic pain
    Elevated B/P
    Obesity
    Polyuria, polydipsia, and polyphagia
    Glucosuria

Diagnostic Guidelines
In BED, recurrent episodes of binge eating are characterized by the following:

- Eating amounts of food that are unquestionably larger than what most persons would consume in the same time period and under similar circumstances.
- Absence of self-control during the episodes.
- Binge eating occurring at least once a week for 3 months.
- Marked distress over binge-eating episodes.
- The episodes of BN do not occur exclusively during episodes of AN.

Treatment Overview

- Obtain a history and a physical that are comprehensive, with a review of the patient's height and weight history; restrictive and binge eating and exercise patterns and their changes; purging and other compensatory behaviors; core attitudes regarding weight, shape, and eating; and associated psychiatric conditions (Recommendation I).
- Obtain a family history of eating disorders or other psychiatric disorders, including alcohol and other substance-use disorders; a family history of obesity; the family's reactions or interactions in relation to the eating disorder; and family attitudes toward eating, exercise, and appearance (Recommendation I).
- It is important to determine stressors that may trigger the eating disorders in order to facilitate amelioration of the eating disorder.
- When assessing children and adolescents, it is essential to involve parents, significant others, and, when appropriate, school personnel and health professionals who routinely work with the patient (Recommendation I).
- With older adults, although spouses and significant others should be part of the treatment program, the clinician should consider whether others should be involved. Assess vital signs, especially for hypothermia and for presence of orthostatic hypotension.
- Assess for hyperglycemia.
- Assessment of weight and height is done by using standard growth charts for children or for those younger than 10 years old; calculate BMI. Children, especially boys, have an increase in BMI with age. It is best to use standard growth charts. BMI = (weight in kg)/(height in m^2).

Acute Treatment

- Treatment is multifaceted and interprofessional, including a mental health professional, a primary care provider or medical person, a dietitian, school personnel, and religious persons, if indicated.
- The dietitian is essential in providing nutritional education and a rationale for selection of certain foods and a meal plan. In some organizations, a dietitian is supplemented by a sports physiologist or trainer to assist individuals with weight management.
- If exercise therapy is needed, proceed cautiously as excessive exercising could occur along with binge–purge eating in susceptible individuals.
- The nutritional intake for those requiring a weight gain should consist of 2 to 3 lbs/wk (0.9–1.4 kg) of controlled weight gain; for outpatients, it is 0.5 to 1 lb/wk. The intake should start at 3,040 kcal/kg (1,000–1,500 kcal/d) and advance progressively.
  - CBT emphasizes that thoughts and feelings may lead to distorted eating patterns. CBT has higher efficacy and lower cost, dropout rates, and relapse rates than pharmacological treatments.
  - A combination of psychotherapy and antidepressant medications provides the best chance for remission.
  - Self-help programs have been found to be beneficial in the treatment of BED.
  - Appetite suppressants and psychological treatment have been effective in the treatment of individuals who are overweight or who have bulimia.
  - Individuals with BED may need to be treated for other physical problems, such as sleep apnea, snoring, diabetes, hyperlipidemia, or cardiovascular disease.

Chronic Treatment

- A multidisciplinary approach with a psychologist, primary care provider, and dietitian is essential. Any therapy can last for over 1 year while the individual attempts to gain insight into triggers that can induce the eating-disorder behavior.
  - Use screening tools to determine the presence of depression, child abuse, or sexual abuse in older adolescents and use the SCOFF questionnaire:
    - S—Do you make yourself Sick because you feel uncomfortably full?
    - C—Do you worry you have lost Control over how much you eat?
    - O—Have you recently lost more than One stone (14 lbs or 7.7 kg) in a 3-month period?
    - F—Do you believe yourself to be Fat when others say you are too thin?
    - F—Would you say that Food dominates your life?
  - Use of cognitive-behavioral interventions such as CBT, dialectical behavior therapy, participation in appropriate student organizations, journaling, identifying feelings, linking food and emotions to circumvent unwanted behavior, and an internet support program have proven beneficial.

Pharmacotherapy Overview

- Antidepressants, with SSRIs as the first category of choice, may be useful with BED to counteract the depressive symptoms associated with both disorders.
- The *DSM-5* identifies depressive disorders as the most common comorbid states associated with both BED.
- Appropriate pharmacological therapy and CBT, individually or in combination, are effective in more than 85% of cases.

▪ Benzodiazepines (BZDs), such as alprazolam (Xanax) and clonazepam (Klonopin), are also considered first-line treatment options for BED; however, short-term use is recommended to prevent abuse and side effects include drowsiness, slurred speech, and ataxia.
Mood-stabilizing anticonvulsants are considered a second-line treatment option for BED, which include topiramate (Topamax), carbamazepine (Tegretol) and zonisamide (Zonegran), and have been useful in individuals with BN to improve binge–purge behaviors as well as improve depressive symptoms.

▪ Although tricyclic antidepressants, such as clomipramine (Anafranil) and amitriptyline (Elavil), have been prescribed to individuals with BED as a third-line treatment option, cardiac toxicity due to electrolyte abnormality, as seen in patients who purge, can occur. This category of drugs can also cause sedation, tachycardia, constipation, dry mouth, and confusion.

Recurrence Rate

▪ Poorer outcomes have been associated with later age of onset of eating disorders.
▪ Low self-esteem can impact the recurrence of binge–purge behaviors. Thirty percent of individuals may continue to engage in bingeing–purging up to 10 years after follow-up if substance abuse is coupled with the eating behavior.

Patient Education

Patient education should include disease etiology, pathophysiology, diagnostic and evaluation and treatment options, including psychopharmacology and psychotherapy.

Drug Selection Table for Bulimia Nervosa

CLASS	DRUG
SSRIs	First-line drug therapy *Fluoxetine (Prozac) Citalopram (Celexa) Sertraline (Zoloft)
BZDs	Alprazolam (Xanax IR and ER) Clonazepam (Klonopin) Diazepam (Valium)
Mood-stabilizing anticonvulsants	Second-line drug therapy Carbamazepine (Tegretol) Zonisamide (Zonegran)
Tricyclic antidepressants	Third-line drug therapy Amitriptyline (Elavil, Endep, Vanatrip) Clomipramine (Anafranil)

*Food and Drug Administration (FDA)-approved for BN.
BZDs, benzodiazepines; SSRIs, selective serotonin reuptake inhibitors.

Medical/Legal Pitfalls

▪ A common finding in those who commit suicide is the presence of more than one mental health disorder.
▪ Mood disorder (i.e., depression), personality disorder, and other psychiatric disorders may be overlooked. As of May 2, 2007, the National Clearing House labeled antidepressant drugs with a black box warning on the prescribing information to include warnings about the increased risk of suicidal thinking and

behavior in young adults aged 18 to 24 years during the first 1 to 2 months of treatment.

■ As of May 12, 2006, the National Clearing House labeled paroxetine (Paxil) and Paxil CR with a Clinical Worsening and Suicide Risk advisory in the prescribing information related to adult patients, especially younger adults.

BIBLIOGRAPHY

American Psychiatric Association. (2006). *Practice guideline for the treatment of patients with eating disorders* (3rd ed.). Washington DC: American Psychiatric Press.

Arcelus, J., Mitchell, A. J., Wales, J., & Nielsen, S. (2011). Mortality rates in patients with anorexia nervosa and other eating disorders: A meta-analysis of 36 studies. *Archives of General Psychiatry, 68*(7), 724–731.

Berkman, N. D., Lohr, K. N., & Bulik, C. M. (2007). Outcomes of eating disorders: A systematic review of the literature. *International Journal of Eating Disorders, 40*(4), 293–309.

Burns, C. E., Dunn, A. M., Brady, M. A., Starr, N. B., & Blosser, C. G. (2009). *Pediatric primary care* (4th ed.). Saunders.

Crow, S. J., Peterson, C. B., Swanson, S. A., Raymond, N. C., Specker, S., & Eckert, E. D. (2009). Increased mortality in bulimiass nervosa and other eating disorders. *American Journal of Psychiatry, 166*(12), 1342–1346.

Hoek, H. W., & van Hoeken, D. (2003). Review of the prevalence and incidence of eating disorders. *International Journal of Eating Disorders, 34*(4), 383–396.

Hudson, J. I., Hiripi, E., Pope, H. G., & Kessler, R. C. (2007). The prevalence and correlates of eating disorders in the National Comorbidity Survey Replication. *Biological Psychiatry, 61*(3), 348–358.

Klein, D., & Attia, E. (2017). Anorexia nervosa in adults: Clinical features, course of illness, assessment, and diagnosis. In J. Yager (Ed.), UpToDate. https://www-uptodate-com. regiscollege.idm.oclc.org/contents/anorexia-nervosa-in-adults-clinical-features-course-of-illness-assessment-and-diagnosis (accessed on February 22, 2019).

Marques, L., Alegria, M., Becker, A. E., Chen, C., Fang, A., Chosak, A., & Diniz, J. B. (2011). Comparative prevalence, correlates of impairment, and service utilization for eating disorders across U.S. ethnic groups: Implications for reducing ethnic disparities in health care access for eating disorders. *International Journal of Eating Disorders, 44*(5), 412–420.

Mehler, P. (2019). Anorexia nervosa in adults and adolescents: Medical complications and their management. In J. Yager (Ed.), UpToDate. https://www-uptodate-com.regiscol-lege.idm.oclc.org/contents/anorexia-nervosa-in-adults-and-adolescents-medical-com-plications-and-their-management/ (accessed on February 24, 2019)

Sanci, L., Coffey, C., Olsson, C., Reid, S., Carlin, J. B., & Patton, G. (2008). Childhood sexual abuse and eating disorders in females: Findings from the Victorian Adolescent Health Cohort Study. *Archives of Pediatrics and Adolescent Medicine, 162*(3), 261–167. https://doi. org/10.1001/archpediatrics.2007.58

Smink, F. R. E., van Hoeken, D., & Hoek, H. W. (2012). Epidemiology of eating disorders: Incidence, prevalence and mortality rates. *Current Psychiatric Reports, 14*(4), 406–414.

Stice, E., & Shaw, H. (2004). Eating disorder prevention programs: Ameta-analytic review. *Psychology Bulletin, 130,* 206.

Swanson, S. A., Crow, S. J., Le Grange, D., Swendsen, J., & Merikanga, K. R. (2011). Prevalence and correlates of eating disorders in adolescents: Results from the National Comorbidity Survey Replication Adolescent Supplement. *Archives in General Psychiatry, 68*(7), 714–713.

Yager, J., Devlin, M. J., Halmi, K. A., Herzog, D. B., Mitchell, J. E., Powers, P., & Zerbe, K. J. (2012). *Guideline watch: Practice guideline for the treatment of patients with eating disorders* (3rd ed.). Washington DC: American Psychiatric Press.

WEB RESOURCES

- National Alliance of Mental Illness: http://www.nami.org/template.cfm?section=by illness&template=/contentmanagement/. This useful site provides information with discussions on diagnosis, treatment, and patient education for individuals with eating disorders.
- National Eating Disorders Association: https://www.nationaleatingdisorders.org. This site provides information on eating disorders, screening tools, helpline, treatment locator and community outreach.
- National Institute of Mental Health: http://www.nimh.nih.gov/. This site is a primary reference source for identification and classification of major mental health illnesses. Navigating through the site can lead to information on treatment and guidelines.

17

Sleep Disorders

CIRCADIAN RHYTHM SLEEP DISORDER

Background Information

Definition of Disorder

Circadian rhythm disorder (CRSD) is a sleep disorder characterized by a discrepancy between the internal setting of one's circadian clock and the sleep wake schedule required by one's occupational/educational or social obligations. The sleep disruption leads to fatigue and/or insomnia. This disruption produces clinically significant distress or impairs ones social and/or occupational/education functioning. Subtypes are listed in the following. It can be defined as episodic (symptoms occur for at least 1 month but less than 3 months), persistent (symptoms persist for 3 or more months), or recurrent (two or more episodes occur within 1 year).

- *Delayed sleep phase type*: delayed onset of sleep and poor maintenance of sleep, with an inability to fall asleep or wake at the desired time.
- *Advanced sleep phase type*: in which sleep onset and awakening times are advanced, and the patient is unable to stay awake or remain asleep until the desired time.
- *Irregular sleep–wake type*: The sleep/wake cycle is disorganized, with variable sleep–wake periods during a 24-hour period.
- *Non-24-hour sleep–wake type*: a sleep–wake cycle that is consistent with the 24-hour cycle, with a consistent dally drift of progressively later sleep onset and wake times.
- *Shift work type*: insomnia secondary to shift work and/or fatigue that can include falling asleep unintentionally.
- *Unspecified type*: The sleep disturbance is related to the 24-hour circadian rhythm cycle, but the symptoms do not match the more specific diagnoses.

Epidemiology

- Approximately 7% to 10% of patients who complain of insomnia are diagnosed with a circadian rhythm sleep disorder.
- In adolescence, the prevalence is approximately 7%.
- The prevalence of CRSD is probably higher because total sleep time is typically normal in patients and they adjust their lifestyle to accommodate their sleep schedule and do not seek medical treatment.

- The is little to no difference in prevalence based on sex of patients aged 20 to 40 years. In persons older than 40 years, women are 1.3 times more likely than men to report CRSD.

Risk Factors
- First-order relative with CRSD
- Poor sleep hygiene
- Flextime or swing-shift work schedule
- Napping during the day or sleeping past one's usual rising time
- Jet lag

Diagnosis
Differential Diagnosis
- Inadequate sleep routine
- Primary insomnia
- Depression
- Seasonal affective disorder
- Sleep-disordered breathing
- Narcolepsy
- Hypersomnolence
- Nocturnal eating

Diagnostic Workup
- Complete medical and medication history, physical examination, neurological examination, and psychological assessment
- Overnight polysomnograph
- Environmental cues and sleep hygiene

Initial Assessment
- Duration of symptoms
- Pattern of sleep–wake cycle
- Total sleep time
- Daytime fatigue
- Peak alertness
- Assess affect, body mass index, craniofacial morphology, chest (barrel chest), digital clubbing

ICD-10 Codes
Circadian rhythm sleep disorder, unspecified type (G47.20)

Circadian rhythm sleep disorder, delayed sleep phase type (G47.21)

Circadian rhythm sleep disorder, advanced sleep phase type (G47.22)

Circadian rhythm sleep disorder, irregular sleep phase type (G47.23)

Circadian rhythm sleep disorder, free running type (G47.24)

Circadian rhythm sleep disorder, shift work type (G47.26)

Treatment Overview
- Treatment for CRSD includes behavioral modifications, bright light or chronotherapy, and pharmacotherapy.

Behavioral Modification
- Sleep hygiene measures
- Avoidance of light exposure before bed (delayed sleep phase type)
- Bright light therapy
- Chronotherapy

Pharmacotherapy for Circadian Rhythm Disorder
- *Delayed sleep phase type*: See Insomnia Disorder.
- *Advanced sleep phase type*: See Hypersomnolence Disorder.
- *Non-24-hour sleep–wake type*: Tasimelteon (Hetlioz), a melatonin receptor agonist.
- *Shift work type*: armodafinil (Nuvigil) or modafinil (Provigil), anti-narcoleptic agents.

Follow-Up
- Consider psychiatric evaluation if mental, emotional, or behavioral disorder is suspected.

Patient Education
- Encourage patient to establish a routine before sleep.
- For patient education, visit WebMD's Circadian Rhythm Disorders Center: www.webmd.com/sleep-disorders/circadian-rhythm-disorders-cause

INSOMNIA DISORDER

Background Information
Definition of Disorder
- Insomnia disorder is associated with physical factors and physiological disorder, excluding anxiety or depression.
- Trouble falling asleep or maintaining sleep for 1 month.
- Patient complains of not feeling rested.

Epidemiology
- Women are 1.4 times more likely to have insomnia-related office visits than men.
- Forty percent (40%) of women between the ages of 40 and 55 years report insomnia.
- Occurs predominantly between the ages of 18 and 64 years.
- Twelve to 17 percent of adults present with insomnia disorder in primary care.

Risk Factors
- Acute stress
- Depression
- Anxiety
- Medications (nonprescription and prescription)
- Obesity
- Geriatric considerations
  - Medications should be used only for short-term management.
  - Benzodiazepines (BZDs) or sedative hypnotics increase risk of confusion, delirium, and/or falls.

- Pregnancy considerations
  - Physiological changes associated with pregnancy may disrupt sleep.
  - Avoid medications.
  - Consider other comfort measures, such as a change to a softer bed or a change in sleeping position.

Diagnosis

Differential Diagnosis
- Thyroid disorders
- Anxiety/stress
- Drug interactions
- Substance abuse
- Hypersomnia
- Parasomnia

Diagnostic Workup
- Subjective complaints of inability to fall asleep or maintain sleep
- Feeling of not being rested
- Impacts daytime functioning

Initial Assessment
- Sleep hygiene.
- Related medical conditions.
- Data on snoring, sleep movements, irregular breathing patterns, length of sleep, and changes in mood should be obtained from family.
- Length of time with sleep disturbance, difficulty falling asleep, thoughts racing, repeated awakenings, or early-morning awakening history should be obtained.
- New stressors.
- New medications, over-the-counter (OTC) medicines, or herbal supplements.

Laboratory Tests
- Thyroid function studies (triiodothyronine [T3], thyroxine [T4], thyroid-stimulating hormone [TSH])
- Complete metabolic panel, including glucose, calcium, and albumin; total protein analysis; and levels of sodium, potassium, CO_2 (carbon dioxide, bicarbonate), chloride, blood urea nitrogen (BUN), creatinine, alkaline phosphatase (ALP), alanine amino transferase (ALT, also called serum glutamic pyruvic transaminase [SGPT]), aspartate amino transferase (AST, also called serum glutamic oxaloacetic transaminase [SGOT]), and bilirubin
- *Complete blood count (CBC) with differentials*: hemoglobin, hematocrit, red blood cell (RBC) count, white blood cell (WBC) count, WBC differential count, and platelet count

ICD-10 Code
Insomnia, unspecified (G47.0)

Diagnostic and Statistical Manual of Mental Disorders, Fifth Edition:, Diagnostic Guidelines
- Difficulty initiating and maintaining sleep.
- Present for at least 3 months or early-morning awakening with inability to return to sleep.
- Daily functioning is impaired.

■ Occurs at least 3 nights per week despite the opportunity for sleep.
■ The insomnia is not caused by anxiety, depression, drug abuse, adverse effect of a medication, or other medical conditions related to sleep, such as obstructive sleep apnea.

Treatment Overview

Behavioral Modification

■ Eliminate stressors or assist patient in developing coping strategies
■ No caffeine after 3 p.m.
■ No alcohol intake within 3 hours of bedtime
■ Daily exercise (avoid 4 hours prior to sleep)
■ Establish sleep routine

Pharmacotherapy for Sleep Disorders

Short-term use of non-BZD medications:

■ Adult treatment only
   ■ Eszopiclone (Lunesta)
   ■ Zaleplon (Sonata)
   ■ Zolpidem (Ambien, Ambien CR, Edluar, Intermezzo, Zolpimist)
   ■ Ramelteon (Rozerem)

Short-term use of BZD medications:

■ Flurazepam (Dalmane)
■ Temazepam (Restoril)
■ Triazolam (Halcion)
■ Estazolam (ProSom)
■ Pentobarbital (Nembutal)

Short-term use of analgesic plus first-generation antihistamine combinations:

■ Excedrin PM
■ Tylenol PM

Drug Selection Table for Sleep Disorders

CLASS	DRUG
Non-benzodiazepine GABA receptor agonists	First-line drug therapy Eszopiclone (Lunesta) Zaleplon (Sonata) Ramelteon (Rozerem) Zolpidem (Ambien)
BZDs	Second-line drug therapy Flurazepam (Dalmane) Temazepam (Restoril) Triazolam (Halcion) Estazolam (ProSom) Pentobarbital (Nembutal)
Analgesic + first-generation antihistamine combination	Excedrin PM (OTC) Tylenol PM (OTC)

BZDs, benzodiazepines; GABA, gamma-aminobutyric acid.

Follow-Up

■ Consider psychiatric evaluation if mental, emotional, or behavioral disorder is suspected.
■ Consider sleep laboratory evaluation if symptoms persist.

Patient Education

- Use bed for sleep or intimacy only.
- Encourage patient to establish a routine before sleep.
- No caffeine 6 hours before sleep.
- No exercise 4 hours before sleep.
- Evaluate response to medication within 7 days.
- Avoid diet high in protein or alcohol 3 to 6 hours before sleep.
- Exercise regularly at least 5 to 6 hours before bedtime.
- Avoid use of OTC antihistamines or alcohol to induce sleepiness.
- Create a calm, cool, quiet atmosphere for sleep.
- If unable to sleep for 30 minutes, leave bedroom and engage in a quiet activity, such as light reading.
- Pharmacological agents are for short-term or intermittent use only.

HYPERSOMNOLENCE DISORDER

Background Information

Definition of Disorder

- Self-reported excessive daytime sleepiness or prolonged nighttime sleep that impacts activities of daily living without central origin despite 7 hours of main sleep with at least one of the following:
  - Recurrent sleep period lapses within same day
  - Main sleep of more than 9 hr/d non-refreshing
  - Difficulty being fully awake after abrupt wakening
    - Occurs a minimum of 3 times weekly for at least 3 months
    - Accompanied by significant distress or impairment with regard to social, cognitive, or occupational functioning
    - Not explained by other sleep disorders, substance abuse, adverse effects of medications, or other conditions

Etiology

- Idiopathic.
- No genetic, environmental, or other relating factors are identified.

Demographics

- Most common onset is during adolescence.
- Rarely presents after age of 30 years.
- Affects male and females equally.
- Exact prevalence is unknown in the United States.
- Five to 10 percent of all patients referred to a sleep laboratory for evaluation are diagnosed with primary insomnia.

Risk Factors

- Acute stress
- Depression
- Anxiety
- Medications (nonprescription and prescription)
- Physiological changes associated with pregnancy may disrupt sleep
- Poor sleep hygiene

Diagnosis

Differential Diagnosis

- Sleep apnea
- Kleine-Levin syndrome
- Depression
- Head trauma
- Insomnia

ICD-10 Code

Primary hypersomnia (F51.11)

Diagnostic Workup

- Excessive daytime sleepiness requiring frequent naps
- Wakes up not feeling refreshed
- Nighttime sleep longer than 12 hours
- Difficult to awaken once asleep
- Sleep hygiene
- Related medical conditions
- Data on snoring, sleep movements, irregular breathing patterns, length of sleep, and changes in mood should be obtained from family
- Length of time with sleep disturbance
- New medications, OTC medicines, or herbal supplements

Laboratory Tests

- Thyroid function studies (T3, T4, TSH)
- Complete metabolic panel, including glucose, calcium, albumin; total protein count; levels of sodium, potassium, CO_2 (carbon dioxide and bicarbonate), chloride, BUN, creatinine, ALP, ALT, AST, and bilirubin
- *CBC with differentials*: hemoglobin, hematocrit, RBC count, WBC count, WBC differential count, and platelet count
- Confirmed by multiple sleep latency test (MSLT)
- Mean initial sleep latency of less than 8 minutes without early onset of rapid eye movement (REM) sleep
- Polysomnography (PSG) is used to exclude other sleep disorders
- Epworth Sleepiness Scale is used

Clinical Presentation

- Prolonged sleep patterns
- Sleep drunkenness
- Less common
  - Headache
  - Orthostatic hypotension
  - Syncope
  - Raynaud's phenomenon

Diagnostic and Statistical Manual of Mental Disorders, Fifth Edition: Diagnostic Guidelines

Additional coding descriptors:

- Specify if (1) with mental disorder, (2) with medical condition, (3) with another sleep disorder
- *Acute*: duration of less than 1 month

- *Subacute*: duration of 1 to 3 months
- *Persistent*: more than 3 months
  - *Mild*: occurring 1 to 2 days weekly
  - *Moderate*: occurring 3 to 4 days weekly
  - *Severe*: occurring 5 to 7 days weekly

Treatment Overview

Behavioral

- Stimulants at the lowest dose produce optimal alertness and minimize side effects
- Avoidance of sleep deprivation
- Establish regular sleep and wake times
- Work in a stimulating environment
- Avoid shift work

Acute Treatment

- Trial stimulants at the lowest dose to produce optimal alertness and minimize side effects in combination with lifestyle modifications and regular work routine. Typically requires long-term treatment.

Chronic Treatment

- Stimulants (nonamphetamine or amphetamine) at the lowest dose to produce optimal alertness
- Reevaluate as indicated to ensure treatment compliance and relief of symptomatology
  - Methylphenidate (Ritalin)
  - Amphetamine/dextroamphetamine (Adderall)
  - Dextroamphetamine (Dexedrine)
  - Modafinil (Provigil)

Follow-Up

- Consider psychiatric evaluation if mental, emotional, or behavioral disorder is suspected.
- Consider sleep laboratory evaluation if symptoms persist.

Drug Selection Table for Hypersomnolence Disorder

CLASS	DRUG
Stimulants, nonamphetamine	First-line drug therapy Modafinil (Provigil) Armodafinil (Nuvigil)
Amphetamines	Second-line drug therapy Amphetamine/dextroamphetamine (Adderall) Dextroamphetamine (Dextrostat) Methylphenidate (Ritalin)

Prognosis

- Responds poorly to treatment
- Disabling

Patient Education

- Eat three meals every day.
- Exercise regularly.

- Avoid use of OTC antihistamines or alcohol before bedtime.
- Use bedroom for sleep or intimacy only.

NARCOLEPSY

Background Information
Definition of Disorder
- Chronic REM sleep disorder of central origin characterized by excessive daytime sleepiness.
- Classic presenting symptoms include excessive daytime sleepiness, sleep paralysis, cataplexy, and hypnagogic hallucinations.
- Nocturnal sleep disturbances are common.

Etiology
- Associated with specific human leukocyte antigen (HLA) haplotypes.
- Possible autoimmune etiology resulting in the discrete loss of brain cells that produce hypocretin. Other factors include infections, exposure to toxins, dietary factors, stress, hormonal changes, and alterations in a person's sleep schedule.

Demographics
- Male to female ratio is 1.64:1.
- First-degree relatives have a 10- to 40-fold higher risk than the general population.
- Age of peak presentation is 15 years.
- Narcolepsy is reported in children as young as 2 years.
- Affects 0.02% to 0.18% of the United States and Western population.
- Increases to 25 to 56 per 100,000 when cataplexy is not a required symptom for diagnosis.

Risk Factors
- Positive family history.
- Age.
- At risk for motor vehicle accidents and injuries.
- Pregnancy considerations.
- *Pediatric consideration*: Children rarely present with all four symptoms.

Diagnosis
Differential Diagnosis
- Absence seizures
- Benign childhood epilepsy
- Brainstem glioma
- Complex partial seizures
- Periodic limb movement disorder
- REM sleep behavior disorder
- Tonic-clonic seizures
- Transient global amnesia
- Syncope and related paroxysmal spells

ICD-Code
Narcolepsy (G47.419)

Diagnostic Workup
- Symptoms
  - Nocturnal sleep disturbances.
  - Short and frequent refreshing napping episodes.
  - Excessive daytime sleepiness for 3 months or longer.
  - Loss of muscle tone briefly.
  - Extraocular movements (EOMs) and respiratory function remain intact with cataplexy.
  - If cataplexy event is severe and generalized, patient may fall.
  - Cataplexy is often triggered by changes in emotions such as laughter or anger episodes.

Initial Assessment
- Sleep hygiene
- Related medical conditions
- Data on snoring, sleep movements, irregular breathing patterns, length of sleep, and changes in mood should be obtained from family
- Length of time with sleep disturbance
- New medications, OTC medicines, or herbal supplements

Laboratory Tests
- Thyroid function studies (T3, T4, TSH)
- Complete metabolic panel, including glucose, calcium, albumin; total protein count; levels of sodium, potassium, CO_2 (carbon dioxide and bicarbonate), chloride, BUN, creatinine, ALP, ALT, AST, and bilirubin
- *CBC with differentials*: hemoglobin, hematocrit, RBC count, WBC count, WBC differential count, and platelet count
- Confirmed by MSLT as demonstrated by sleep latency of less than 8 minutes accompanied by REM sleep occurring within 15 minutes of sleep onset during at least 2 out of 4 nap opportunities
- Epworth Sleepiness Scale
- PSG
- Actigraphy
- HLA typing
- Cerebrospinal fluid hypocretin-1 analysis

Diagnostic and Statistical Manual of Mental Disorders, Fifth Edition: Diagnostic Guidelines
- The individual falls asleep irresistibly, occurring 3 times per week for at least 3 months.
- The presence of one or both of the following:
  1. Cataplexy (abrupt loss of muscle tone)
     - *Patients with long-standing disease*: cataplexy without loss of consciousness, precipitated by laughter or joking
     - *Patients with onset of symptoms within 6 months*: spontaneous facial grimacing and tongue movement without an emotional trigger
  2. *Hypocretin deficiency*: confirmed with cerebrospinal fluid analysis without evidence of acute brain injury or meningitis
  3. Confirmed REM sleep latency 15 minutes or less
     Specify:
     Mild: cataplexy occurring 1 episode per week or less, napping twice daily, less disturbed nocturnal sleep (vivid dreams, movement during sleep and insomnia)

Moderate: cataplexy occurring daily or every few days, multiple napping episodes throughout the day, disturbed nocturnal sleep

Severe: drug-resistant cataplexy, frequent daily episodes, nearly continual drowsiness with disturbed nocturnal sleep

- Consistent incursions of elements of REM sleep into the transitions between sleep and wakefulness
- The disturbance is not the direct physiological effect of use of a substance or of other medical conditions.

Treatment Overview

Behavioral

- Sleep hygiene
- Scheduled naps
- Reassurance for patient and family
- Exercise programs
- Avoidance of foods high in sugar

Psychopharmacotherapy Overview for Narcolepsy

Armodafinil (Nuvigil), sodium oxybate (Xyrem) as well as the following:

- Adjunct agents for cataplexy—fluoxetine (Prozac); imipramine (Tofranil); nortriptyline (Aventyl, Pamelor); protriptyline (Vivactil); venlafaxine (Effexor)

Acute Treatment

- Trial stimulants at the lowest dose to produce optimal alertness and minimize side effects in combination with lifestyle modifications and regular work routine. Typically requires long-term treatment.

Chronic Treatment

- Stimulants (nonamphetamine or amphetamine) at the lowest dose to produce optimal alertness.
- Reevaluate as indicated to ensure treatment compliance and relief of symptomatology.

Follow-Up

- Pediatric patients should be followed by a pediatrician and pediatric neurologist.

Drug Selection Table for Narcolepsy

CLASS	DRUG
Stimulants, nonamphetamine	First-line drug therapy Modafinil (Provigil) Armodafinil (Nuvigil) Sodium oxybate (Xyrem)
Amphetamines	Second-line drug therapy Amphetamine/dextroamphetamine (Adderall) Dextroamphetamine (Dextrostat) Methylphenidate (Ritalin)

Prognosis

- With medications and treatment, the patient may lead a productive life.

Complications
- Adverse effects of medications
- Injury

Patient Monitoring
- Monthly follow-up is recommended to monitor response to medications.

Patient Education
- Advise adult patients regarding driving responsibilities.
- Educate patient regarding long-term effects of medications and need for safety precautions.

NIGHTMARE DISORDER

Background Information

Definition of Disorder
Is associated with REM sleep

- Occurs at any age.
- Patient describes bizarre dream plot.
- Patient is arousable from sleep.
- Remembers event.
- Nightmare disorder is exacerbated by stress.

Etiology
- Occurs equally in males and females.
- Twenty to 39% of children between ages 5 and 12 years are affected.
- Five to 8% of adults are affected.

Risk Factors
- Stress
- Sleep deprivation
- Psychiatric and neurological disorders in adults
- Medications affecting neurotransmitter levels, such as antidepressants, narcotics, or barbiturates

Diagnosis

Differential Diagnosis
- Sleep terrors
- Sleep-disordered breathing
- Restless leg syndrome (RLS)

ICD-10 Code
Nightmare disorder (F51.5)

Initial Assessment
- Sleep hygiene.
- Related medical conditions.
- Data on snoring, sleep movements, irregular breathing patterns, length of sleep, and changes in mood should be obtained from family.

- Length of time with sleep disturbance, difficulty falling asleep, repeated awakenings, or early-morning awakening history should be obtained.
- New stressors.
- New medications, OTC medicines, or herbal supplements.

Clinical Presentation
- Abrupt awakening
- Frightened and able to describe fears

Diagnostic and Statistical Manual of Mental Disorders, Fifth Edition: Diagnostic Guidelines
- Frequent awakenings from major sleep or naps, with detailed recall of extended and ominous dreams (usually involving threats to survival, personal security, or self-esteem).
- The awakenings generally occur during the latter part of the sleep period.
- On waking, the person rapidly becomes oriented and alert.
- The disturbance that is experienced on waking causes notable distress for the individual or impairment of social functioning.
- The nightmares do not occur concurrently with and exclusively during the course of another mental health disorder (e.g., delirium, posttraumatic stress disorder) and are not the direct physiological effect of substance use or another medical condition.
- Coexisting mental and medical disorders do not explain dysphoric dreams.
- Specify if
  - during sleep onset,
  - with associated nonsleep disorder,
  - associated with other medical conditions, and
  - associated with other sleep disorders.
- Specify if
  - acute—frequency of nightmares is 1 month,
  - subacute—frequency of nightmares greater than 1 month and less than 6 months, and
  - persistent—frequency of nightmares greater than 6 months.
- Specify if
  - *mild*: less than 1 episode weekly,
  - *moderate*: 1 or more episodes per week, not occurring nightly, and
  - *severe*: occurring nightly.

Treatment Overview
Behavioral
- Comfort and reassurance are given.
- Behavioral strategies or counseling if episodes are frequent and severe.

Pharmacotherapy
- None indicated

Follow-Up
- Referral to psychiatrist may be indicated if a psychiatric disturbance is suspected.
- Referral to sleep laboratory if history does not correlate with clinical findings to rule out sleep-disordered breathing, parasomnia, or restless legs syndrome.
- Nightmares should resolve with time.
- Insomnia from fear of sleeping may occur.

- Daytime sleepiness may occur.
- Cognitive dysfunction with protracted sleep disruption.

Patient Education
- Reassure parents that the disorder should resolve with maturity.
- Reinforce the need for security to parents.
- Adult patients should decrease stressors.

RESTLESS LEG SYNDROME

Background Information
Definition of Disorder
In the *Diagnostic and Statistical Manual of Mental Disorders*, Fifth Edition (*DSM-5*; American Psychiatric Association, 2013), RLS is noted as having the following criteria:

- An urge to move the legs that is usually accompanied by or occurs in response to uncomfortable and unpleasant sensations in the legs, characterized by all of the following: (1) the urge to move the legs begins or worsens during periods of rest or inactivity; (2) the urge is partially or totally relieved by movement; and (3) the urge to move legs is worse in the evening or at night than during the day or occurs only in the evening or at night.
- Symptoms occur at least 3 times per week and have persisted for at least 3 months.
- Symptoms cause significant distress or impairment in social, occupational, educational, academic, behavioral, or other areas of functioning.
- The symptoms cannot be attributed to another mental disorder or medical condition (e.g., leg edema, arthritis, leg cramps) or behavioral condition (e.g., positional discomfort, habitual foot tapping).
- The disturbance cannot be explained by the effects of a drug of abuse or medication.

Epidemiology
- RLS affects about 5% to 15% of the general population of the United States.
- RLS becomes more prevalent with age; however, it has a variable age of onset and can occur in children.
- In patients with severe RLS, 33% to 40% had their first symptom before the age of 20 years.
- RLS usually progresses slowly to daily symptoms and severe disruption of sleep after age 50 years.
- Individuals with familial RLS tend to have onset of symptoms before age 45 years.
- Women are affected more commonly than men, in a ratio of almost 2:1.
- RLS is estimated to affect 25% to 40% of pregnant women and 25% to 50% of patients with end-stage renal disease.

Risk Factors
- Idiopathic central nervous system (CNS) disorder
- Iron deficiency
- Peripheral neuropathy

- Folate or magnesium deficiency
- Amyloidosis
- Diabetes mellitus
- Lumbosacral radiculopathy
- Lyme disease
- Monoclonal gammopathy of undetermined significance
- Rheumatoid arthritis
- Sjögren syndrome
- Uremia
- Vitamin B12 deficiency
- Frequent blood donation
- Pregnancy
- Vitamin B12 deficiency
- Frequent blood donation

Diagnosis
Differential Diagnosis
- Akathisia
- Neuropathy
- Nocturnal leg cramps
- Vascular disease
- Radiculopathy

Diagnostic Workup
- Periodic movement during sleep
- Dysesthetic sensations variously described as "pins and needles," an "internal itch," or a "creeping or crawling" sensation
- Difficulty falling asleep at night
- Involuntary, repetitive, periodic, jerking limb movements (while asleep or awake)
- Daytime fatigue
- Impacts daytime functioning

Initial Assessment
- Sleep hygiene
- Related medical conditions
- Periodic leg movements of sleep (PLMS) index score
- New stressors
- New medications, OTC medicines, or herbal supplements

Laboratory Tests
- Iron panel (iron, ferritin, transferrin saturation, total iron-binding capacity)
- If a secondary cause of RLS is suspected on the basis of the history, abnormal findings on neurological examination, or a poor response to treatment, other laboratory tests should be done:
  - CBC
  - BUN
  - Fasting blood glucose
  - Magnesium
  - TSH

- Vitamin B12
- Folate
- Other studies
  - Needle electromyography (EMG)
  - PSG

ICD-10 Code
Restless legs syndrome (G25.81)

Treatment Overview
Behavioral Modification
- Sleep hygiene measures
- Avoidance of caffeine, alcohol, and nicotine
- Discontinuation of any offending medications (when possible)
- Daily exercise (avoid 4 hours prior to sleep)
- Sleep routine

Pharmacotherapy for Restless Leg Syndrome
In some patients, RLS symptoms occur sporadically, with spontaneous remissions lasting weeks or months. The use of pharmacotherapy on an irregular basis is warranted in such cases. Continuous pharmacological treatment should be considered if patients complain of having RLS symptoms at least 3 nights each week.

- Medications
  - Dopamine receptor agonists
  - Gamma aminobutyric acid analogs

Drug Selection Table for Restless Legs Disorder

CLASS	DRUG
Dopamine receptor agonists	First-line drug therapy Ropinirole (Requip) Pramipexole dihydrochloride (Mirapex) Rotigotine (Neupro)
Gamma aminobutyric acid analogs	Second-line drug therapy Gabapentin (Gralise, Neurontin) Gabapentin enacarbil (Horizant)

Recurrence Rate
- Cure is possible only for secondary RLS.

Patient Education
- Encourage patient to establish a routine before sleep.
- Pharmacological agents are for short-term or intermittent use only.
- For patient education, visit WebMD's Restless Leg Center: www.webmd.com/brain/restless-legs-syndrome/default.htm.

BIBLIOGRAPHY

American Psychiatric Association. (2013). *Diagnostic and statistical manual of mental disorders* (5th ed.). American Psychiatric Press.

Bozorg, A. M. (2017). *Restless legs syndrome*. https://emedicine.medscape.com/article/1188327-overview#a1

Cataletto, M. E. (2015). *Circadian rhythm disorder*. https://emedicine.medscape.com/article/1188944-overview

Chawla, J. (2020). *Insomnia*. https://emedicine.medscape.com/article/1187829-overview

Sadock, B., Sadock, V., & Ruiz, P. (2015). *Kaplan & Sadock's synopsis of psychiatry* (11th ed.). Wolters Kluwer.

Tusaie, K., & Fitzpatrick, J. (2017). *Advanced practice psychiatric nursing* (2nd ed.). Springer Publishing Company.

WEB RESOURCES

- American Academy of Sleep Medicine: https://aasm.org/
- American Sleep Association: https://www.sleepassociation.org/
- Centers for Disease Control and Prevention: https://www.cdc.gov/sleep/resources.html
- Sleep Foundation: https://www.sleepfoundation.org/

18

Personality Disorders

ANTISOCIAL PERSONALITY DISORDER

Background Information

Definition of Disorder

- Persistent pattern of disregard for and defiance of the rights of others that begins in childhood or early adolescence and remains consistent into adulthood.
- Deceit and manipulation are central features whereby the individual also lacks empathy as they have a tendency to disregard the feelings, rights, and suffering of others.
- History of pathological lying.
- Inflated sense of self that appears confident and assured but is often to the detriment of others as affected persons tend to be opinionated, coarse, and verbose, rambling about topics to impress others.
- Cannot be diagnosed until the age of 18 years.

Etiology

- Also known as sociopathy or psychopathy.
- Previous research has debated whether the disorder is due to nature or nurture.
- Biological studies have identified that there are no known genetic risk factors for personality disorders in the cluster A, B, and C classifications.
- Psychosocial studies have identified that the lack of socialization; the increasing incidence of childhood traumas; and childhood maltreatment and neglect such as abuse, lack of empathy poverty, family instability, and community violence may be related to the development of this disorder.

Demographics

- Thirty to seventy percent of childhood psychiatric admissions are for disruptive behavior disorders. A small percentage of antisocial children grow up to become adults with antisocial personality disorder (ASPD), whereas the remainder of those individuals persist with severe problems with authority, maintaining gainful employment, and/or satisfying relationships.
- ASPD affects approximately 0.7% to 4.1% of the US population.
- ASPD is 3 times more prevalent in men than in women.
- Higher incidence in correctional and substance abuse facilities and forensic settings.

Risk Factors
- Usually begins in childhood or adolescence
- Has been linked with head injuries in childhood
- Predominately affects males
- Low socioeconomic status and living in urban settings
- More common among first-degree biological relatives
- Familial linkage to female relatives is higher than to male relatives
- Increased risk for children adopted into homes with parents who have ASPD

Diagnosis

Differential Diagnosis
- Pathological gambling
- Anxiety disorders
- Substance-related disorders
- Malingering
- Somatoform and factitious disorders
- Developmental and pervasive disorders
- Attention deficit hyperactivity disorder (ADHD)
- Schizophrenia and psychotic disorders
- Bipolar, mania

ICD-10 Code
Antisocial personality disorder (F60.2)

Diagnostic Workup
- Complete history and physical examination with consideration of previous neurological trauma.
- No laboratory tests are indicated for this diagnosis.
- Psychiatric evaluation should specifically include a thorough focus on personal and social history as this area will highlight the individual's lack of empathy and their disregard of the feelings, rights, and suffering of others (i.e., multiple marriages, relationships, criminal history, lack of long-term plans or goals).
- Individuals will have underlying beliefs about the self, and this will be manifested in their behaviors. The consideration of these beliefs or cognitive schemas can also be a useful way to validate the diagnosis. Therefore, here are a few examples of beliefs, thoughts, or sentiments that the individual may share with the provider as part of the diagnostic interview:
  - Force and cunning are the best ways to get things done.
  - People will get at me if I don't get them first.
  - It is not important for me to keep promises or honor debts.
  - What others think of me really does not matter.
  - I can get away with things, so I do not need to worry about bad consequences.
  - If it was not me, it would be someone else (on raping a woman).

Clinical Presentation
- Failure to conform to rules in society so that often behaviors are in direct violation with the law
- Deceitful; tells lies and distortions to the pleasure and advantage of the self
- Lack of empathy and disregard for others

- May be initially pleasant and cooperative but then becomes nasty and difficult
- Impulsive, irritable, and aggressive physically as well as verbally
- Lacks the ability to plan ahead; lacks goals
- Consistently irresponsible and has lack of remorse for deviant activities and behaviors
- Pathological lying

Diagnostic and Statistical Manual of Mental Disorders, Fifth Edition: Diagnostic Guidelines
- Since the age of 15 years, there has been a disregard for and violation of the rights of others as well as a disregard for those rights considered normal by the local culture.
- At least three of the following must be present:
  - Failure to conform to the rules of society and disrespect for the law, leading to repeated acts that are the grounds for arrest
  - Deceitfulness (pathological lying, use of aliases, manipulation of others for personal profit or pleasure)
  - Inability to plan ahead or to set goals; engages in impulsive behaviors
  - History of assaults, aggressiveness, and irritability related to violent acts
  - Disregard for the safety of self and others; reckless
  - Irresponsible; unable to meet obligations; does not honor debts or meet financial obligations
  - Lack of regret or shame; indifferent regarding any hurt, damage, or theft
- At least 18 years of age
  - Evidence exists of conduct disorder with onset before the age of 15 years.
  - The incidence of the antisocial behaviors is not exclusively during the course of schizophrenia or a manic episode.

Treatment Overview

Acute Treatment
- There is no acute treatment for this disorder as personality disorders such as ASPDs in part are persistent and pervasive patterns of maladaptive behaviors that require chronic treatment in the form of psychotherapy.
- The individual with this personality disorder often ends up in the prison system or substance abuse treatment facility, where the treatment focuses on detainment (due to their criminal activity) or withdrawal from substances (that they have become addicted to, not for the treatment of their antisocial behaviors).

Chronic Treatment
- Previous studies have suggested that long-term intervention is the only form of treatment for this individual, whether incarceration or long-term psychotherapy. There is no psychopharmacological treatment indicated specifically for ASPD.
- Cognitive-behavioral therapy (CBT) is one example of a modality of psychotherapy that has been suggested for individuals who present with antisocial behaviors and ASPD.
- Rather than attempt to change the *moral structure* of the individual as evidence in psychodynamic psychotherapy, CBT instead can be implemented to focus on improving moral and social *behaviors* through enhancement of cognitive functioning.
- Individuals with ASPD would need to (1) identify and address the possible negative outcomes for their behaviors and (2) have an increased awareness of their

dysfunctional beliefs about themselves, the world, and the future before making cognitive changes. CBT would focus on assisting the individual with ASPD to make a transition from their concrete beliefs to a broader spectrum of possibilities and outcomes.

■ A small percentage of children who have conduct disorder (about 3% of males and 1% of females) grow up to become adults with ASPD while the remainder of those individuals persist with severe problems with authority, maintaining gainful employment, and/or satisfying relationships.

■ Individuals do not have episodes of a personality disorder; rather, they have these traits as lifelong behavioral patterns.

Patient Education

■ Individuals would have to make personal life changes to correct their deviant behaviors through psychosocial education, CBT, ongoing long-term psychotherapy, and/or incarceration.

■ In general, most individuals with this disorder have no interest in changing or understanding their behaviors. Education would most likely occur for family and friends who have been injured, deceived, or in some way manipulated by these individuals.

■ Family therapy for those who have been affected by an individual with ASPD would include (1) understanding the diagnosis; (2) identifying the behaviors that are manipulative and deceitful; (3) being able to set limits with the individual with ASPD so as to not be hurt, abused, or deceived in the future.

Medical/Legal Pitfalls

■ These individuals are dangerous and often can fool even the most experienced clinician. It is best to consider a forensic evaluation or consultation with a forensic specialist (psychiatrist or psychologist) for further direction.

■ Forensic psychiatry is a branch of medicine that focuses on the interface of law and mental health.

■ Forensic psychiatrists have additional education, training, and/or experience related to the various interfaces of mental health (or mental illness) with the law and are able to distinguish between a personality disorder or a clinical syndrome (i.e., when violent and hostile/aggressive behaviors are criminal or immoral).

■ Forensic psychiatrists often determine whether an individual is "clinically competent" to stand trial for their actions or provide expert evidence about their actions and behaviors.

■ Clinicians can be at risk for violence directed at them by individuals through threats, physical or emotional abuse, or harm.

■ Forensic research has identified three key principles when confronted with an individual with ASPD who is violent or has a history of violence: (1) In general, ASPDs are rarely ego dystonic; (2) most patients and violent situations associated with clinical issues involve comorbid conditions; and (3) violence and violence risk are often associated with intoxication. In other words, most individuals with ASPD will not seek treatment for their symptoms of this personality disorder; rather, they will present to healthcare providers for other symptoms, illnesses, and/or treatment (i.e., related to their violent behaviors). In addition, treating or managing the coexisting conditions (which may include illness, substance abuse, or environmental factors such as being arrested and imprisoned) may alleviate some violence potential if they are incarcerated as

they are out of the general public community. Finally, their outcome or prognosis for treatment of their substance abuse or dependence is poor.

■ Risk assessment includes being aware of a history of violence with the following antisocial behaviors: (1) *Purposeful, instrumental violence* refer to acts in which
violence is a means to a conscious, gainful end such as a robbery as well as violence
designed to manipulate or mislead another into some wanted behavior; (2) *purposeful, noninstrumental violence* is exemplified in seeking the pleasure of a stimulating
or antisocial activity but the actual injuring of others is not integral to the activity's
purpose; and (3) *purposeful, targeted, defensive violence* is identified in an individual
who fears abandonment or humiliation and strikes out in illogical ways, such as
murder or injury. Examples are "paranoid stalkers," who follow their "victims"
and are threatened by anything getting between their victims and themselves (i.e.,
police, children, spouse of victim).

■ Clinicians need to understand the importance of identifying these signs and
symptoms in clinical practice and how their relationship is defined in terms of the
individual with ASPD.

■ The key is to recognize and assess risk in order to remain safe.

BORDERLINE PERSONALITY DISORDER

Background Information

Definition of Disorder

■ Persistent pattern of mood instability, intense interpersonal relationships, impulsivity, identity disturbance, recurrent suicidal acts and/or self-mutilating behaviors, intense anger, and rage as well as the potential for dissociation and psychosis.

■ This disorder begins in adolescence and the behaviors vary throughout adulthood.

■ Fear of abandonment.

■ Idealizes and devalues people.

■ Sees the world in black and white ("no gray areas").

■ Three specific components help to conceptualize the disorder: (1) an unstable sense
of self, (2) impulsive thoughts, and (3) sudden shifts of mood.

■ Often confused with bipolar disorder due to impulsivity and mood instability.

Etiology

■ During the past 20 years, the literature has expanded with multiple reasons for the
development of this personality disorder.

■ Includes a history of childhood abuse, unstable or otherwise detrimental family
environment, and family history of psychopathology.

■ Childhood sexual abuse (CSA) is the most significant correlation with severity;
chronicity and age of onset of sexual abuse and co-occurrence (and severity) of
other forms of abuse and neglect take a second place in the determination.

■ Psychoanalytic theories focus on poor parental/caretaker attachment and the individual's resulting difficulty with separation.

Demographics

■ Borderline personality disorder (BPD) affects about 0.7% to 2.7% of the general
population.

■ BPD is 3 times more common in women than in men.

■ No difference is found in ethnic origin or socioeconomic status.

Risk Factors

- Childhood physical, sexual, and emotional abuse.
- Children who experience childhood sexual abuse are 4 times more likely to have BPD than those who have not.
- Severity, chronicity, and age of onset of sexual abuse (the younger the abuse, the poorer the prognosis) as well as the co-occurrence of other forms of abuse and neglect place the individual at greater risk.
- Family factors such as difficult relationships, poor attachment, and poor parental care.
- Social factors such as low socioeconomic status of family, being raised in a single-parent family, welfare support of family, parental death, and social isolation.
- Temperament has been studied, and findings suggest that children and adolescents who cope by "internalizing" symptoms such as anxiety and depression and "externalizing" symptoms such as impulsivity, defiance, and oppositional behavior are at greater risk for a poorer prognosis.
- Genetic factors play a role in the potential for individual differences in BPD features in Western society. This finding surmised that the symptoms and presentation of this disorder were consistent across three countries studying twins.
- Poor parenting and lack of attachment are frequently associated with the development of the symptoms of BPD in childhood, adolescence, and into adulthood.

Diagnosis

Differential Diagnosis

- Frequently comorbid with Axis I disorders, especially substance-use disorders in males, eating disorders in females, anxiety disorders, and mood disorders; therefore, it is often missed or misdiagnosed.
- Due to the mood instability, impulsivity, and psychotic symptoms, bipolar disorder is often mistaken for personality disorder (although individuals can have both).

ICD-10 Code

Borderline personality disorder (F60.3)

Diagnostic Workup

- Complete history and physical examination with consideration of previous neurological trauma and careful assessment of the potential for seizure disorder (i.e., temporal lobe epilepsy)
- Psychiatric evaluation with a focus on personal and social history, including history of abuse
- Physical and mental evaluation
- Thyroid function studies (thyroid-stimulating hormone [TSH], triiodothyronine [T3], thyroxine [T4])
- Complete metabolic panel glucose, calcium, albumin; total protein; sodium; potassium; CO_2 (carbon dioxide, bicarbonate); chloride; blood urea nitrogen (BUN); creatinine
- Alkaline phosphatase (ALP), alanine aminotransferase (ALT, also called serum glutamic pyruvic transaminase [SGPT]), aspartate amino transferase (AST, also called serum glutamic oxaloacetic transaminase [SGOT]), bilirubin
- *CBC with differential*: hemoglobin, hematocrit, red blood cell (RBC) count, white blood cell (WBC) count; WBC differential count, platelet count

■ Careful assessment for cuts, bruises, and scars where patient could have caused self-harm through cutting, burning, or self-injury

Clinical Presentation
■ Three specific components help to conceptualize the disorder: (1) an unstable view of self; (2) impulsive thoughts; and (3) sudden shifts of mood.
■ Reports mood instability, intense interpersonal relationships, impulsivity, identity disturbance, recurrent suicidal acts, and/or self-mutilating behaviors, intense anger, and rage as well as the potential for dissociation and psychosis.
■ Relates interpersonal issues in terms of extremes (black or white, good or bad, idealized or failed parenting or relationships).

Diagnostic and Statistical Manual of Mental Disorders, Fifth Edition: Diagnostic Guidelines
A pervasive pattern of instability in interpersonal relationships, self-image, and affects; marked impulsivity beginning by early adulthood and present in a variety of contexts, as indicated by five (or more) of the following:
1. Frantic efforts to avoid real or imagined abandonment
2. A pattern of unstable and intense interpersonal relationships characterized by alternating between extremes of idealization and devaluation
3. *Identity disturbance*: markedly and persistently unstable self-image or sense of self
4. Impulsivity in at least two areas that are potentially self-damaging (e.g., spending, sex, substance abuse, reckless driving, binge eating)
5. Recurrent suicidal behavior, gestures, or threats or self-mutilating behavior
6. Affective instability due to a marked reactivity of mood (e.g., intense episodic dysphoria, irritability, or anxiety usually lasting a few hours and only rarely more than a few days)
7. Chronic feelings of emptiness
8. Inappropriate, intense anger or difficulty controlling anger (e.g., frequent displays of temper, constant anger, recurrent physical fights)
9. Transient, stress-related paranoid ideation or severe dissociative symptoms

Treatment Overview

Acute Treatment
■ Establish a trusting interpersonal professional relationship.
■ Stabilize symptoms that are the most distressing to the individual (mood instability, psychosis, suicidal thoughts and actions).
■ May consider atypical antipsychotics to assist with the transient psychosis and mood instability as well as selective serotonin reuptake inhibitors (SSRIs) for depression. Stay away from tricyclic and monoamine oxidase inhibitor (MAOI) antidepressants as they have a higher risk for overdose and lethality.
■ Crisis intervention is frequently the most common acute treatment along with brief hospitalizations for threats to self (i.e., suicidal ideation, plan, and intent) and others (homicidal ideation, plan, and intent); self-mutilating behaviors; and brief psychosis.
■ If the individual is not in therapy, it is best to consider initiating this or referring to an experienced outpatient therapist as these individuals will present in crisis and need to know that there is a contact person.
■ Prescribe medications for short periods of time to avoid the potential for overdose of medications when individual is in crisis or impulsive.
■ If not the therapist or prescriber, maintain an ongoing collaborative relationship with the therapist or prescriber as individuals with this disorder often split and play one against the other.

Chronic Treatment

■ Studies have shown that long-term psychodynamic psychotherapy is the most useful if not the most successful long-term form of treatment.

■ Dialectical behavior therapy (DBT) is also very successful but often individuals need to repeat the group and individual sessions on a long-term basis to acquire the necessary skills to learn how to cope with their thoughts and feelings.

■ Medications for symptom relief are useful, such as SSRIs and/or mood stabilizers for management of mood instability. Cautious use of benzodiazepines or other addictive substances is needed.

■ This is a long-term pervasive personality disorder that does not "go away" and come back. It is frequently "crisis driven" and individuals with this disorder need to learn to live with the symptoms as well as learn to cope appropriately with their internalized emotions as well as the externalized behaviors.

■ Some individuals do mature and can move toward a healthier way of living and coping with stresses. This seems to be an outcome of long-term psychotherapy if the patient has insight and a willingness to change.

Patient Education

■ Books that may help include the following:
  1. *I Hate You, Don't Leave Me: Understanding the Borderline Personality* (1991; classic text; ISBN-10: 0380713055; ISBN-13: 978–0380713059)
  2. *Stop Walking on Eggshells: Taking Your Life Back When Someone You Care About Has BPD* (1998; whole series of books for individuals, families, and groups; ISBN-10: 157224108X; ISBN-13: 978–1572241084)
  3. *Surviving a Borderline Parent: How to Heal Your Childhood Wounds & Build Trust, Boundaries, and Self-Esteem* (2003; ISBN-10: 1572243287; ISBN-13: 978–1572243286)
  4. *Understanding the Borderline Mother: Helping Her Children Transcend the Intense, Unpredictable, and Volatile Relationship* (2002; ISBN-10: 0765703319; ISBN-13: 978–0765703316)
  5. *Skills Training Manual for Treating BPD* (a whole series of books by Marsha Linehan, related to assessment and treatment using various psychotherapies, including DBT, starting in 1993; ISBN-10: 0898620341 ISBN-13: 978–0898620344)

Medical/Legal Pitfalls

■ It is extremely important to understand that patients who suffer from this disorder have difficulty with boundaries (personal, social, and professional) and will "test" the limits in their relationships.

■ Hugging and/or touching the patient without some discussion of its meaning can be very dangerous for the clinician. It is best *not* to have physical contact with the patient and set this boundary early on in treatment.

■ Individuals with BPD are, for the most part, likely to provoke various kinds of boundary violations, including sexual acting out and testing your "affection" for them (e.g., they may invite you to an event that they are attending or offer you tickets to a theater production).

■ These individuals (sadly) also represent the majority of those patients who falsely accuse therapists of sexual involvement, touching, and inappropriate contact. Many clinicians choose not to work with these patients and also demoralize them because of their own lack of skill. Therefore, be aware of your own scope of practice and if you are not skilled, refer them to someone who is trained and/or skilled.

- In general, therapists can take advantage of developing an awareness of any repeating patterns of behaviors that occur with these individuals and in how they respond (both the patient and the clinician). With this knowledge, clinicians can then steer clear of the highly destructive litigation that can ensue.

NARCISSISTIC PERSONALITY DISORDER

Background Information

Definition of Disorder

- A persistent pattern of grandiosity (in fantasy or behavior), need for admiration, and lack of empathy, beginning by early adulthood and presenting in a variety of contexts
- Grandiose sense of self-importance (e.g., exaggerates achievements and talents, expects to be recognized as superior without commensurate achievements)
- Preoccupation with fantasies of unlimited success, power, brilliance, beauty, or ideal love
- Believes that they are "special" and unique and can only be understood by, or should associate with, other special or high-status people (or institutions)
- Requires excessive admiration
- Sense of entitlement, that is, unreasonable expectations of especially favorable treatment or automatic compliance with their expectations
- Interpersonally exploitative, that is, takes advantage of others to achieve their own ends
- *Lacks empathy*: is unwilling to recognize or identify with the feelings and needs of others
- Often envious of others or believes that others are envious of them
- Shows arrogant, haughty behaviors or attitudes

Etiology

- As with all personality disorders, early childhood development plays a role in the progression of the pathology that is inherent in each of the maladaptive behaviors listed in the definition of narcissistic personality disorder (NPD).
- Some theories (i.e., psychoanalytic) focus on the lack of paternal availability and the strength (or lack) of the relationship between the mother and father as a determinant in the development of a narcissistic child, adolescent, and adult as well as an outcome of the insufficient gratification of the normal narcissistic needs of infancy and childhood.
- Neo-analytical thinking takes an antithetical view that narcissism is the outcome of narcissistic over-gratification during childhood. This view focuses on parents who overindulge their child, protect the child from disappointment and failure, and minimize the criticisms of others about their child. This disorder also presents in the child who displays difficulties in self-esteem regulation with a tendency toward massive externalization of emotions.

Demographics

- Less than 1% of the general population suffer from NPD.
- Between 50% and 75% of patients with NPD are males.

Risk Factors
- There are no known genetic factors contributing to risk.
- An oversensitive temperament as a young child.
- Children who are adopted and therefore struggle to cope with the loss and rejection of their biological parents, especially if there is dysfunction within the current family of origin.
- Various developmental pathways may present a special risk for the formation of NPD: (1) having narcissistic parents, (2) being adopted, (3) being abused, (4) being overindulged, (5) having divorced parents, and/or (6) losing a parent through death.
- Some theorists believe that this is learned behavior and narcissistic children come from narcissistic parents or caretakers.

Diagnosis

Differential Diagnosis
- Histrionic personality disorder (HPD)
- ASPD
- Obsessive-compulsive personality disorder (OCPD)

ICD-10 Code
Narcissistic personality disorder (F60.81)

Diagnostic Workup
- Complete history and physical examination with consideration of previous neurological trauma.
- No laboratory tests are indicated for this diagnosis.
- Psychiatric evaluation, including a focus on personal and social history.

Clinical Presentation
- The essential features are grandiosity, lack of empathy, and need for admiration.
- A sense of superiority, a sense of uniqueness, exaggeration of talents, boastful and pretentious behavior, grandiose fantasies, self-centered and self-referential behavior, need for attention and admiration, arrogant and haughty behavior, and sense of high achievement.
- Individuals with NPD can be at high risk for suicide during periods when they are not suffering from clinical depression periods.
- The individual learns to use defenses, including projection and splitting into all good and all bad, along with idealization.

Diagnostic and Statistical Manual of Mental Disorders, Fifth Edition: Diagnostic Guidelines
NPD is defined as a pervasive pattern of grandiosity (in fantasy or behavior), need for admiration, and lack of empathy, beginning by early adulthood and presenting in a variety of contexts, as indicated by five (or more) of the following:

- Has a grandiose sense of self-importance (e.g., exaggerates achievements and talents, expects to be recognized as superior without commensurate achievements)
- Is preoccupied with fantasies of unlimited success, power, brilliance, beauty, or ideal love
- Believes that they are "special" and unique and can only be understood by, or should associate with, other special or high-status people (or institutions)

- Requires excessive admiration
- Has a sense of entitlement, that is, unreasonable expectations of especially favorable treatment or automatic compliance with their expectations
- Is interpersonally exploitative, that is, takes advantage of others to achieve their own ends
- *Lacks empathy*: is unwilling to recognize or identify with the feelings and needs of others
- Is often envious of others or believes that others are envious of them
- Shows arrogant, haughty behaviors or attitudes

Treatment

Acute Treatment

- Currently, there are no medications that have been developed specifically for the treatment of NPD.
- Patients with NPD who are also depressed or anxious may be given medications for relief of those symptoms.
- There are subjective reports in the literature that the SSRIs may reinforce narcissistic grandiosity and lack of empathy with others and thus worsen the disorder.

Chronic Treatment

- Intensive psychoanalytic psychotherapy; requires referral to therapist with extensive training to implement this type of treatment.
- The goals of treatment are to work on (1) the grandiose self, (2) the pathological defense mechanisms that interfered with the patient's normal development, and (3) the patient's manipulative interactions with family and friends.
- CBT can be implemented in some cases to assist the individuals to identify their negative behaviors and replace them with more functional ways of interacting with others.
- Most individuals who suffer from NPD cannot form a sufficiently deep bond with a therapist to allow healing of early childhood injuries, so treatment is usually long term if the individual can tolerate it.
- This is a long-term pervasive personality disorder that originates in childhood and/or adolescence and is retained throughout adulthood.

Patient Education

Books

- Brown, N. (2001). *Children of the self absorbed: A grown-up's guide to getting over narcissistic parents.* New Harbinger Publications.
- Golomb, E. (1995). *Trapped in the mirror.* William Morrow & Company.
- Miller, A. (1996). *The drama of the gifted child: The search for the true self.* Basic Books.

Medical/Legal Pitfalls

- Significant relationships were found between NPD and incarceration for violent crimes; therefore, a thorough social and legal history should be obtained.

BIBLIOGRAPHY

American Psychiatric Association. (2013). *Diagnostic and statistical manual of mental disorder* (5th ed.) Washington, DC: American Psychiatric Publishing.

Beck, A., & Freeman, A. (2003). *Cognitive therapy of personality disorders* (2nd ed.). Guilford Press.

Bienenfeld, D. (2016). *Personality disorders*. https://emedicine.medscape.com/article/294307-overview#a2

Bradley, R., Jenei, J., & Westen, D. (2005). Etiology of borderline personality disorder disentangling the contributions of intercorrelated antecedents. *Journal of Nervous & Mental Disorders, 193*, 24–31.

Cohen, P. (2008). Child development and personality disorder. *Psychiatric Clinics of North America, 31*(3), 477–93, vii.

Distel, M. A., Trull, T. J., Derom, C. A., Thiery, C. W., Grimmer, M. A., Martin, N. G., Willemsen, G., & Boomsma, D. I. (2008). Heritability of borderline personality disorder features is similar across three countries. *Psychological Medicine, 38*(9), 1219–1229.

Fonagy, P., & Bateman, A. (2008). The development of borderline personality disorder: A mentalizing model. *Journal of Personality Disorders, 22*(1), 4–21.

Gutheil, T. A. (1989). Borderline personality disorder, boundary violations, and patient-therapist sex: Medicolegal pitfalls. *American Journal of Psychiatry, 146*, 597–602.

Kendler, K. S., Aggen, S. H., Czajkowski, N., Røysamb, E., Tambs, K., Torgersen, S., Neale, M. C., & Reichborn-Kjennerud, T. (2008). The structure of genetic and environmental risk factors for DSM-IV personality disorders: A multivariate twin study. *Archives General Psychiatry, 65*(12), 1438–1446.

Paris, J. (2009). The treatment of borderline personality disorder: Implications of research on diagnosis, etiology, and outcome. *Annual Review of Clinical Psychology, 5*, 277–290.

Reid, W. H., & Thorne, S. A. (2007). Personality disorders and violence potential. *Journal of Psychiatric Practice, 13*(4), 261–268.

Sadock, B., Sadock, V., & Ruiz, P. (2015). *Kaplan & Sadock's synopsis of psychiatry* (11th ed.). Wolters Kluwer.

Smith, C. A., Ireland, T. O., Thornberry, T. P., & Elwyn, L. O. (2008). Childhood maltreatment and antisocial behavior: Comparison of self-reported and substantiated maltreatment. *American Journal of Orthopsychiatry, 78*(2), 173–186.

Torgersen, S., Kringlen, E., & Cramer, V. (2001). The prevalence of personality disorders in a community sample. *Archives of General Psychiatry, 58*, 590–596.

Tusaie, K., & Fitzpatrick, J. (2017). *Advanced practice psychiatric nursing* (2nd ed.). Springer Publishing Company.

Wheeler, K. (2014). *Psychotherapy for the advanced practice psychiatric nurse* (2nd ed.). Springer Publishing Company.

19

Neurodevelopmental Disorders

ATTENTION DEFICIT HYPERACTIVITY DISORDER

Background Information

Definition of Disorder

A biochemically based disorder of behavior and attention that results in a persistent pattern of difficulty affecting a child's functioning at home and school and socially. Symptoms must be outside of the range of normal behavior for the developmental level.

- An inability to pay attention or to sustain attention.
- Always on the move, as if driven by a motor.
- Impulsivity—verbally and physically.
- Symptoms interfere with multiple life domains:
  - School, social, home, or work.
  - Symptoms must be present before the age of 7 years.

Etiology

- Attention deficit hyperactivity disorder (ADHD) is not fully understood.
- It is hypothesized that inefficient neurochemical processing in the following areas account for the complex symptoms of ADHD:
  - Dorsal anterior cingulate cortex—selective attention
  - Dorsal lateral prefrontal cortex—sustained attention and problem solving
  - Prefrontal motor cortex—hyperactivity
  - Orbital frontal cortex—impulsivity

Demographics

- About 6.1% of school-age children have ADHD.
- ADHD is 3 to 5 times more common in boys than in girls. Some studies report an incidence ratio as high as 5:1.
  - This may be secondary to boys having higher rates of disruptive behavior due to hyperactivity and impulsivity.
  - Girls are less likely to be hyperactive and if they have good social skills, they often do not come to the attention of parents, teachers, or healthcare providers.
- The prevalence rate in adults has been estimated at 2% to 7%.

Risk Factors

Gender
- Male

Family History
- Family members with ADHD.
- Heritability is estimated at greater than or equal to 75%.

Precipitating Factors
- Infections
- Head injury
- Hypoxia
- Exposure to drugs or alcohol in utero
- Low birth weight

Comorbidity Factors
- Higher incidence of chronic health conditions than in nonaffected children.
- High incidence of substance use and abuse.
- Persons with ADHD are six times more likely to have psychiatric comorbidities:
  - ODD and conduct disorder
  - Developmental disorders
  - Learning disorders
  - Anxiety disorders
  - Mood disorders
  - Sleep problems
  - Difficulty winding down and falling asleep

Socioeconomic Factors
- Children from single-mother families are more likely to have an ADHD diagnosis.
- Children with Medicaid are more likely to have an ADHD diagnosis than privately insured children.
- Adolescents with ADHD are more likely to drop out of school.
- Higher rates of pregnancy among high school girls.
- Higher incidence of legal involvement.
- Higher incidence of auto accidents.

Diagnosis

ICD-10 Codes

Attention deficit hyperactivity disorder, predominantly inattentive type (F90.0)

Attention deficit hyperactivity disorder, predominantly hyperactive type (F90.1)

Attention deficit hyperactivity disorder, combined type (F90.2)

Attention deficit hyperactivity disorder, other type (F90.8)

Attention deficit hyperactivity disorder, unspecified type (F90.9)

Diagnostic Workup
- Vision and hearing screen may be indicated.
- Complete blood count (CBC), complete metabolic panel, thyroid-stimulating hormone (TSH), free thyroxine (T4), liver function test (LFT) are all recommended.

- Complete physical may be indicated.
- Consider an EKG if contemplating using a stimulant (this is not standardized practice).
- A complete psychiatric assessment is recommended.
  - Overall behavior, mood, sleep, drug, and alcohol use/abuse.
- Rating scales for ADHD
  - Parents and teachers to complete the rating scale:
    - ADHD rating scale (ages 6–12 years)
    - Conners Parent and Teacher Rating Scale (reliable with criterion validity)
    - Strengths and Weaknesses of ADHD Symptoms and Normal Behavior (SWAN) Rating Scale (helps differentiate type of ADHD)
    - Vanderbilt (ages 6–12 years with parent and teacher scales)
- School records

Initial Assessment
- Prenatal and postnatal care
- Growth and development
- Medical history
- Onset of symptoms
- Establish baseline symptoms
- Severity of symptoms
  - At home, school, work, and socially

Clinical Presentation
Symptom clusters: inattention, impulsive, and hyperactive.

- Combined type has features of inattention, impulsivity, and hyperactivity.
- Children often do not grasp how their behavior impacts others.
  - Kids can feel demoralized by how their symptoms affect their ability to function at home, school, and play.

Diagnostic and Statistical Manual of Mental Disorders, Fifth Edition: Diagnostic Guidelines
Inattention Symptoms
- Six or more of the following symptoms of inattention are present for at least 6 months, to a degree that is maladaptive:
  - The individual fails to give attention to details, in schoolwork or other activities.
  - Has difficulty in sustaining attention in performance of tasks.
  - Does not seem to be listening when spoken to directly.
  - Fails to follow through on instructions and fails to complete schoolwork or other duties (with failures not attributable to confrontational behavior or failure to understand instructions).
  - Has difficulty in organizing tasks and other activities.
  - Seeks ways to circumvent tasks that require mental effort.
  - Often loses things.
  - Individual is easily distracted by stimuli of many kinds.
  - Individual is more often than not forgetful in daily activities.

The *Diagnostic and Statistical Manual of Mental Disorders*, Fifth Edition (*DSM-5*) lists these symptoms as being diagnostic of ADHD:

- Has difficulty finishing any activity that requires concentration
- Does not seem to listen to anything said to them

- Is excessively active—running or climbing at inappropriate times, squirming in or jumping out of their seats
- Is very easily distracted
- Talks incessantly, often blurting out responses before questions are finished
- Has serious difficulty waiting their turn in games or groups
- May have specific learning disabilities

Hyperactivity–Impulsivity Symptoms

- Six or more of the following symptoms have persisted for at least 6 months, to a degree that is maladaptive:
  - Fidgets or squirms when seated
  - Leaves seat in classroom or in other situations in which remaining seated is required
  - Runs about in environments in which it is inappropriate to do so
  - Has difficulty in engaging in leisure activities quietly
  - Is always on the go
  - Talks excessively
  - Gives answers to questions before questions have been fully verbalized
  - Has difficulty in waiting for their turn
  - Interrupts the speech of others or intrudes in the activities of others
  - *In adolescents and adults*: the presence of feelings of extreme restlessness
- Symptoms are present before the age of 7 years.
- Social deficits are present in two or more settings.
- Clear evidence of impairment exists in social functioning.
- The symptoms do not occur concurrently with and exclusively during the course of a pervasive development disorder (PDD), schizophrenia, or other psychotic disorder and are not more readily ascribed to another psychiatric condition.

Treatment Overview

Acute Care

- Healthcare providers should be familiar with the multiple medications available to treat ADHD. Stimulant medications are first-line agents. Atomoxetine (*Strattera*) is a second-line agent and has been shown to be effective in placebo-controlled trials. Other medications with less extensive evidence to support their use include alpha-2-agonists (*Intuniv*).

Chronic Care

- Behavior modification, also called behavior therapy, is recommended as part of a total treatment.
- Plan for ADHD
- It is based on rewarding an individual for desired behaviors and having consequences for undesired behaviors. Rewards and point systems are effective when used consistently at school and home.
- It can help build self-esteem and guide the patient toward good behavior patterns.
- Create schedules and follow routines daily.
- Keep tasks simple.
- Help the child become organized.
- Use brief and clear instructions.
- Limit distractions (e.g., TV, radio, games) when the child is doing homework.

- Set SMART goals to track the child's progress:
  S, Specific: Develop specific goals that are clearly stated.
  M, Measurable: A goal is measurable if progress is made toward reaching it.
  A, Agreed upon: Talk about the goal with the child and agree on actions.
  R, Realistic: The goals should be within reach.
  T, Timely: A timely goal is one that can be achieved within a time frame that is meaningful.
- Stimulants
  - Immediate release.
  - Extended release.
    - Medications to treat ADHD can create sleep disturbance.
    - They can rebound appetite.
  - Twenty percent of patients do not respond to stimulants.
  - For patients with substance abuse issues, choose stimulants with nonabuse formulations.
    - Lisdexamfetamine (*Vyvanse*)
    - Dexmethylphenidate (*Focalin*)

Drug Selection Table for Attention Deficit Hyperactivity Disorder

CLASS	DRUG
Amphetamines	Short-acting stimulants Dextroamphetamine/amphetamine (*Adderall*) Dextroamphetamine (*Dexedrine* and *Dextrostat*) Long-acting stimulants Dextroamphetamine (*Spansule*) Dextroamphetamine/amphetamine (*Adderall XR*) Lisdexamfetamine (*Vyvanse*)
Methylphenidates (amphetamine derivatives)	Short-acting stimulants Dexmethylphenidate (*Focalin*) Methylphenidate (*Methylin*) Methylphenidate (*Ritalin SR* and *LA*) Intermediate-acting stimulants Methylphenidate (*Metadate ER* and *CD*) Methylphenidate (*Methylin ER*) Methylphenidate (*Ritalin SR* and *LA*) Long-acting stimulants Methylphenidate (*Concerta*) Methylphenidate transdermal (*Daytrana Patch*) Dexmethylphenidate (*Focaclin XR*)
SNRIs	Nonstimulant Atomoxetine (*Strattera*)
SARIs	Nonstimulant Guanfacine (*Intuniv*)
Aminoketones	Nonstimulant Bupropion HBr (*Aplenzin*) Bupropion HCl (*Forfivo XL, Wellbutrin, Wellbutrin SR* and *XL*)
Other Agents	Nonstimulant Clonidine (Catapres) SARIs, selective alpha-2a-adrenergic receptor agonist; SNRIs, serotonin-norepinephrine reuptake inhibitors.

- Nonstimulants
  - Atomoxetine (*Strattera*)
    - Black box warning
    - Analysis of 12 studies revealed that 4 out of 1,000 children experienced suicidal thoughts. There were no actual suicides in the studies.
  - Bupropion (*Wellbutrin*)
    - Contraindicated in patients with anorexia nervosa and bulimia nervosa
    - Can exacerbate tics
    - *Caution*—lowers seizure threshold
  - Guanfacine (Intuniv)
    - Longer duration of action than with clonidine (*Catapres*)
    - Immediate and extended release formulation
    - Clonidine (Catapres)

Recurrence Rate

- ADHD is a lifelong condition.
  - Hyperactive symptoms often dissipate with age as the brain matures and patients develop coping skills.
    - Symptoms of inattention persist into adulthood.
  - For an algorithm for treating ADHD by American Academy of Pediatrics, go to http://aappolicy.aappublications.org/cgi/reprint/pediatrics;108/4/1033.pdf

Patient Education

- Nonpharmacological intervention
  - Psychoeducation
    - Understanding of ADHD
    - Coping skills
      - Preplanning
      - Organize study time
      - Break up big tasks into smaller parts
    - Parenting strategies
      - Give one direction at a time.
      - A light touch can help refocus attention.
      - Provide a predictable and consistent schedule.
      - Get kids ready for school the night before.
      - Keep in close contact with teachers to proactively solve problems.
  - Psychosocial support for child and parent
    - Higher rates of divorce are found among parents of children with ADHD.
- Urge structure, structure, structure.

Medical/Legal Pitfalls

- *Comorbid illness*: medical and psychiatric.
- Treating ADHD with stimulants can exacerbate other conditions, such as bipolar mood disorder, thought disorders, and chemical dependency issues.
- Off-label prescribing:
  - Medication education includes indications, dose, route, schedule, potential side effects, class effects, off-label use, black box warnings, and alternatives.
- Diversion of stimulants for abuse:
  - A new fad among adolescent babysitters is to go through medicine cabinets and steal prescription medications.

- Persons diagnosed with ADHD are protected under the Americans With Disabilities Act of 1990 and have recourse, should they experience discrimination at school or work.

AUTISM SPECTRUM DISORDER

Background Information

Definition of Disorder

Spectrum disorders now include autistic disorders, Asperger's syndrome, childhood disintegrative disorder, and PDD. Autism is a PDD, is usually evident in the initial years of life (by age 3 years), and is often observed with other medical abnormalities, such as chromosomal abnormalities, congenital infections, and central nervous system (CNS) abnormalities. According to the *Diagnostic and Statistical Manual of Mental Disorders*, Fifth Edition (*DSM-5*), symptoms of autism include the following:

- Markedly abnormal or impaired development of social interaction, including at least two of the following:
  - Impaired nonverbal behaviors (e.g., eye contact, facial expression, body postures, and gestures)
  - Failure to develop age-appropriate peer relationships
  - Lack of spontaneous activity to share enjoyment, interests, or achievements with others (e.g., play)
- Marked impairment in communication as indicated by at least one of the following:
  - Delay or lack of development of spoken language
  - In individuals with adequate speech, the lack of ability to initiate or sustain conversations
  - Stereotyped or repetitive use of language or idiosyncratic language
  - Lack of spontaneous play
- Restricted repetitive or stereotyped patterns of behavior, as indicated by at least one of the following:
  - Narrowed range of interests
  - Inflexible adherence to specific, nonfunctional routines or rituals
  - Stereotyped and repetitive motor mannerisms
  - Persistent preoccupation with parts of objects

Etiology

There is no one known single cause of autism, but it is generally accepted that it is caused by abnormalities in the brain structure or functioning.

- A number of theories are being investigated, including the links among heredity, genetics, and medical problems. In many families, there appears to be a pattern of autism or related disabilities, further supporting a genetic basis for the disorder, but no one gene has been identified as causing autism.
- It also appears that some children are born with a susceptibility to autism, but researchers have not yet identified a single "trigger" that causes autism to develop. It is possible that under certain conditions a cluster of unstable genes may interfere with brain development.
- Other research focuses on pregnancy or delivery problems as well as environmental problems, including viral infections, metabolic imbalances, and exposure to environmental chemicals.

Demographics
- It is estimated that approximately 1 in 54 children in the United States are diagnosed with autism spectrum disorder (ASD).
- Boys are four times more likely to be diagnosed with autism than girls.
- Most children are diagnosed after age 4, though it can be reliably diagnosed as early as age 2.
- Autism affects all ethnic and socioeconomic groups; however, minority groups tend to be diagnosed later and less often.
- Early intervention affords the best opportunity to support healthy development and deliver benefits across the life span.

Risk Factors
- *Gender*: Rates are four to five times higher in males. Females with the disorder are more likely to exhibit more severe intellectual disability.
- *Familial pattern*: increased risk of autism among siblings (approximately 5%) and some risk for various developmental difficulties in affected siblings.
- Stressors
  - Having another mental disorder.
  - In most cases, there is an associated diagnosis of mental retardation (MR), ranging from mild to profound.
  - Having a child with autism can be a significant stressor for families.
  - Change in routine can be a major stressor for the autistic child.

Diagnosis
Differential Diagnosis
- Rett disorder
- Childhood disintegrative disorder
- ASD
- Selective mutism (SM)
- Language disorders
- MR
- Stereotypic movement disorder
- ADHD
- Schizophrenia

ICD-10 Code
Childhood autism (F84.0)

Diagnostic Workup
- Autism tends to occur more frequently than expected among children with certain medical conditions, including Fragile X syndrome, tuberous sclerosis, congenital rubella syndrome, and untreated phenylketonuria (PKU).
- Some harmful substances ingested during pregnancy also have been associated with increased risk of autism.
- Seizures may develop, especially in adolescence, in up to 25% of cases.
- Microcephaly and macrocephaly may be observed.

Initial Assessment
- Medical history, including assessing for the following:
  - Maternal infections, bleeding, or other problems during gestation

- Experiences in pre-, peri-, and neonatal periods
- Potentially brain-damaging events in the postnatal period
- Medical illnesses of infancy
- Growth patterns normal
- Physical examination, including head circumference, weight, and height measurements for growth patterns, and neurological examination

Considerations include posture, gait, and what the child is grasping in their hand. Is child rocking or whirling? Or catatonic? Observe for movements, such as self-biting, hands over ears, hand flapping, clasping, wringing, and clapping. Fingers or other objects in the mouth? Is there facial grimacing? Is child performing visual self-stimulation on a pattern in your office? Note and record any myoclonic jerks. If possible, observe spontaneous handedness. Record spoken language by child, if any. Observe information processing, overstimulation, or distraction by visual/auditory information, tactile defensiveness, or delay in response.

- Hearing tests can determine whether hearing problems may be causing developmental delays, especially those related to social skills and language use.
- Behavioral questionnaires are commonly used, and use varies according to age and informant, and presenting symptoms. Commonly used tests are as follows:
  - *Modified Checklist for Autism in Toddlers*: evaluates infants who are at least 24 months old and is used to identify milder autistic symptoms.
  - *Pervasive Development Disorders Screening Test*: This questionnaire is completed by parents to evaluate early signs of autism.
  - *Autism Screening Questionnaire*: used for children 4 years and older.
  - *Autism Behavior Checklist*: a screening tool that is completed by the teacher.
  - *Childhood Autism Rating Scale*: rates how much a child's behavior differs from that of other children of the same age (older than 24 months).
  - *Autism diagnostic interview*: Parents provide information about their child's behaviors during this wide-ranging, structured interview.
  - *Autism observation schedule*: observation of the child performing activities, including communication, interaction, play, and other behaviors.
- If a metabolic disorder is suspected, the DAN (Defeat Autism Now!) protocol may be used to pinpoint it; see www.healing-arts.org/children/assessment.htm#Metabolic for more information/

Clinical Presentation

- Symptoms of autism vary but contain core deficiencies in social and communication skills and behaviors, as previously described. CNS abnormalities will typically be present.
- Assess for known medical conditions, and refer for specialty assessment.
- When other medical conditions are present, note on Axis III.
- Assess for sleep problems, as fatigue and attention deficits are often the result of sleep problems or exacerbated behavioral problems.
- There is an increased frequency of gastroesophageal reflux disease (GERD), food allergies, and vitamin deficiencies in children with ASD.
- Assess for pain related to a wide range of physical and physiological risk factors, as pain can be a contributor to an increase in emotional and behavioral problems.

Laboratory Tests

When autism is associated with a general medical condition, laboratory findings consistent with the general medical condition will be tested.

- There are no medical tests for autism, but it should be diagnosed with a team of professionals.
- There are some differences with measures of serotonergic activity, but no specific pattern is clearly identified.
- Imaging studies may be abnormal.
- EEG abnormalities are common, even in the absence of a seizure disorder.
- A laboratory and clinical assessment of malabsorption problems and nutritional deficiencies is prudent, especially if nutrition supplements are being considered.
- Test for lead poisoning, especially if a condition called pica (a craving for substances that are not food, such as dirt or flecks of paint) is present. Children with developmental delays usually continue putting items in their mouths after this stage has passed. This practice can result in lead poisoning, which should be identified and treated as soon as possible.

Treatment Overview

Autism follows a continuous course. Language skills and intelligence are the strongest factors related to progress. In the school-age years, gains in some areas are common; however, some adolescents deteriorate and some improve. In general, autistic children respond best to highly structured and specialized treatment. A program that addresses helping parents and caregivers in improving communication, social, behavioral, adaptive, and learning aspects of a child's life will be most successful. Treatments can be broken down into the following five categories.

Behavioral and Communication Approaches
- Use positive reinforcement, self-help, and social skills training to improve behavior and communication.
- Many types of treatments have been developed, including applied behavioral analysis (ABA), treatment and education of autistic and related communication-handicapped children (TEACCH), and sensory integration.

Biomedical and Dietary Approaches
- Medicines are most commonly used to treat related conditions and problem behaviors, including depression, anxiety, hyperactivity, and obsessive-compulsive behaviors.
- Some studies (most of them unreplicated) have found the following supplements to improve functioning: cod liver oil (with vitamins A and D), vitamins C and B, biotin, selenium, zinc, and magnesium.
- Other studies suggest avoiding copper and taking extra zinc to boost the immune system and a need for more calcium.

Community Support and Parent Training
- Educating family members about autism and on how to effectively manage the symptoms has been shown to reduce family stress and improve the functioning of the child with autism.
- Some families will need more outside assistance than others, depending on their internal functioning, established support systems, and financial situation.

Specialized Therapies
- Speech, occupational, and physical therapies are important for managing autism and should all be included in various aspects of the child's treatment program.

- Speech therapy improves language and social skills.
- Occupational and physical therapy can help improve coordination and motor skills and help in learning to process information from the senses (sight, sound, hearing, touch, and smell) in more manageable ways.

Complementary Approaches

- Music, play, art, and animal therapy may be used.
- All can help to increase communication, develop social interaction, and provide a sense of accomplishment; these therapies can provide a nonthreatening way to develop a positive relationship with a therapist in a safe environment. Art and music are useful in sensory integration, providing tactile, visual, and auditory stimulation. Music therapy enhances speech development and language comprehension. Songs can teach language and increase the ability to put words together.
- Art therapy can provide a nonverbal, symbolic way for expression.
- Animal therapy, including horseback riding, provides improved coordination and motor development while creating a sense of well-being and self-confidence.

Note: With most complementary approaches, there may be little scientific research that has been conducted to support the particular therapy.

Chronic Treatment

- There is no known cure, and chronic treatment is necessary and depends on associated symptoms. There are no approved medications for autism. Targeted therapies for specific symptoms have included selective serotonin reuptake inhibitors (SSRIs) for rituals and compulsive behaviors, stimulants for attentive problems, neuroleptics for agitation and aggression, and benzodiazepines for anxiety.
- Be aware of interactions among multiple medications and assess for interactions.
- Treatment needs often change over time, as growth and development occur, and include the previously mentioned treatment approaches as well as vocational training and independent living skills, when appropriate, for older youth.

Recurrence Rate

- Follow-up studies indicate that only a small percentage of individuals with autism live and work independently as adults.
- In about one-third of cases, partial independence is possible, and in the highest functioning adults some degree of social and communication problems exists, along with markedly restricted interests and activities.

Drug Selection Table for Autism Spectrum Disorder

CLASS	DRUG
Amphetamines	Short-acting stimulants Dextroamphetamine/amphetamine (*Adderall*) Dextroamphetamine (*Dexedrine* and *Dextrostat*) Long-acting stimulants Dextroamphetamine (*Spansule*) Dextroamphetamine/amphetamine (*Adderall XR*) Lisdexamfetamine (*Vyvanse*)

Drug Selection Table for Autism Spectrum Disorder (*continued*)

CLASS	DRUG
Methylphenidates (amphetamine derivatives)	Short-acting stimulants Dexmethylphenidate (*Focalin*) Methylphenidate (*Methylin*) Methylphenidate (*Ritalin SR* and *LA*) Intermediate-acting stimulants Methylphenidate (*Metadate ER* and *CD*) Methylphenidate (*Methylin ER*) Methylphenidate (*Ritalin SR* and *LA*) Long-acting stimulants Methylphenidate (*Concerta*) Methylphenidate transdermal (*Daytrana Patch*) Dexmethylphenidate (*Foaclin XR*)
SNRIs	Nonstimulant Atomoxetine (*Strattera*)
SARIs	Nonstimulant Guanfacine (*Intuniv*)

SARIs, selective alpha-2a-adrenergic receptor agonist; SNRIs, serotonin-norepinephrine reuptake inhibitors.

Patient Education

It is important for families to actively seek assistance from whatever sources are available. The following measures are helpful for all families who have a member with autism:

- Schedule breaks for caregivers. Daily demands of caring for an autistic child can be overwhelming. Trained personnel can relieve family members from these duties as needed. Breaks can help families communicate in a less stressful context and allow parents to focus on their relationships with other children and significant others. Regular breaks may also help a family continue to care for a child at home, rather than considering out-of-home care. Government programs exist to help families with limited resources.
- Seek assistance for a child with autism who is entering adolescence. Community services and public programs can help families during what can be an especially difficult time for their child. An adolescent child may benefit from group home situations, special employment, and other programs designed to help the transition into adulthood.
- Make contact with other families who have a child with autism. Local and national groups can help connect families and provide much-needed sources of information. The internet and targeted websites (e.g., www.autism-society.org) can be an important tool that helps individuals with limited community resources (e.g., in rural areas) to connect with others.

Medical/Legal Pitfalls

- Given the complexity of medications, drug interactions, and the unpredictability of how each patient may react to a particular drug, parents should seek out and work with a provider with expertise in the area of medication management and experience with individuals with ASD.
- The Food and Drug Administration (FDA) has advised that antidepressants may increase the risk of suicidal thinking in some patients, especially children and adolescents, and all young people being treated with them should be monitored closely for unusual changes in behavior.

■ Individuals with ASD may be eligible for specialized education services under the Individuals With Disabilities Education Act (IDEA), which mandates the creation of an individualized education program (IEP). The IEP sets goals and objectives and describes what services a child will receive as part of their special education program. There is a process to determine eligibility; refer patient to locate school district.

CHILDHOOD-ONSET FLUENCY DISORDER

Background Information

Definition of Disorder
■ Speech disorder characterized by disruptions in speech
■ Syllable repetition
■ Syllable prolongation
■ Halted or interrupted flow of speech

Etiology
■ The disorder is not fully understood.
■ Research suggests heritability: chromosome 12q.
■ Pathology is the lack of integration between language development and the motor ability needed for a forward flow in speech production.
■ Auditory processing has also been implicated as a potential factor in stuttering.
■ Dysfluency can be normal in children just learning to talk and stuttering can abate on its own.
■ Stuttering is not caused by an emotional disturbance.

Demographics
■ Occurs in 1% of the general population.
■ About 2.5% of preschoolers are afflicted.
■ Male-to-female ratio is 3:1.
■ Some research supports higher prevalence in African American children.

Risk Factors
■ Age of onset is prior to ages 3 to 3.5 years.
■ Male gender.
■ Brain damage.
■ Twice as likely in families with a history of stuttering.

Diagnosis

Differential Diagnosis
■ *Normal stuttering*: Dysfluency beginning before 3 years of age is likely to abate on its own.

ICD-10 Code
Childhood onset fluency disorder (F80.81)

Diagnostic Workup
■ Functional hearing evaluation
■ Oral examination

Initial Assessment
- Prenatal care.
- Labor and delivery.
- Growth and development.
- Age of onset of dysfluency.
- Has stuttering lasted longer than 6 to 12 months?
- Symptoms of anxiety relating to speaking situations.
- Does the child stutter while singing, whispering, or talking to a pet?
- Previous treatment for stuttering.

Degrees of Dysfluency
Following is a guideline; the actual degree of impairment is to be determined by a speech pathologist.
- Normal stuttering (onset prior to the age of 3 years):
  - Occasional repetition of sounds, syllables, or short words
  - Periodic hesitation or insertion of fillers ("uh, um")
  - Increases when the child is tired
  - No distress to the child
- Mild stuttering:
  - Frequent repetition of sound, long syllables, or short words
  - *Physical manifestations*: closing eyes, muscle strain in lips
  - Occurs more of the time than not
  - No distress to mild frustration noted in the child
- Severe stuttering:
  - *Recurring long, repeated sounds*: prolongations and blockages
  - Pitch of utterances may increase
  - Difficulty in most speaking circumstances
  - Anxious, fearful, or embarrassed when speaking

Clinical Presentation
- Onset between the ages of 2 and 7 years with a peak occurrence at 5 years
- Difficulty starting a word
- Repeating the sound of a letter or word (usually vowels)
- Repeating sounds more than once every 8 to 10 sentences
- Use of filler words or utterances ("um, uh")
- Change in pitch
- Rapid blinking
- Facial grimacing
- Lip pressing
- Hands about the face
- Use of physical gestures to get words out
- Looking to the side when speaking
- Emotional distress or embarrassment when speaking

Diagnostic and Statistical Manual of Mental Disorders, Fifth Edition: Diagnostic Guidelines
- Abnormalities in the fluency, rhythms, and intonations of speech, characterized by frequent occurrences of one or more of the following:
  - Sound and/or syllable repetitions
  - Sound prolongations
  - Interjections, outbursts

- Pauses within a word
- Blocking (filled or unfilled pauses in speech)
- Circumlocutions (word substitutions as a way of avoiding problematic words)
- Exhibits a notable stress in the utterances of words
- The deficits in language fluency impede academic and occupational achievement.
- If a motor deficit related to speech or sensory deficit is present, the difficulties with language fluency are in excess of those usually associated with these deficits.

Note: If a motor deficit related to speech, sensory deficit, or neurological condition is present, the condition should be diagnosed as such.

Treatment Overview

- Refer to a speech/language pathologist (SLP)—first-line treatment.
- SLPs evaluate speech and language issues and establish a hierarchy of speaking challenges.
- SLPs may recommend mechanical devices such as delayed or altered auditory feedback: Patients with dysfluency can often speak fluently when talking in unison with someone else. These devices resemble a hearing aid with a pocket converter. The converter feeds back the patient's voice on a slight delay or an altered pitch and replicates the experience of speaking in unison.
- There is no gold standard pharmacological intervention for stuttering.
- Assess for comorbid psychiatric disorders and implement appropriate pharmacological treatments (i.e., anxiety).
- Medication studies for stuttering are for adults.
- No medication has been shown to consistently improve, decrease, or mediate the social, emotion, or cognitive symptoms of stuttering.
- All medications prescribed for stuttering are "off label" and not FDA approved for the treatment of dysfluency—especially in children.
- Dopamine antagonist
  - Risperidone (*Risperdal*): 0.25 to 1.0 mg daily.
  - Monitor for sedation, hypotension, dystonia, akathisia, oculogyric crisis, elevated prolactin, galactorrhea, amenorrhea, insulin resistance, and weight gain.
  - Monthly, administer an abnormal involuntary movement scale (AIMS) or the Dyskinesia Identification System: Condensed User Scale (DISCUS) rating scale to monitor for side effects.
  - Educate parents about the risk–benefit profile of an atypical antipsychotic.
  - Educate parents on how to recognize extrapyramidal side effects.

Patient Education

- Help the child to feel less anxious or self-conscious.
- Wait while the child finishes a sentence.
- Speak slowly to the child.
- Limit questions to the child.
- Practice talking and listening sessions with the child.
- Foster acceptance.
- Collaborate with schoolteachers and counselors—kids who stutter are often teased.

■ Support the child in practicing fluency skills.
■ Clarify that the word *therapy* in speech therapy does not relate to counseling.
■ The child's course of dysfluency often follows a family pattern in terms of whether stuttering abates on its own or requires treatment.

Medical/Legal Pitfalls
■ The child is protected under the Individuals With Disabilities Act and antidiscrimination laws. Go to www.stutterlaw.com/index.htm/

CONDUCT DISORDER

Background Information
Definition of Disorder
■ Conduct disorder is a group of behavioral and emotional problems that usually begin during the childhood or teenage years.
■ A long-term and continued pattern of behavior that violates the rights of others or goes against society's norms.

Etiology
■ Impairment in the prefrontal lobe and amygdala has been linked to conduct disorder, causing an inability to plan future actions, a lack of impulse control, and an inability to learn from past negative experiences.
■ More common in caregivers who have a history of bipolar, depressive, or alcohol use disorder.

Demographics
■ Males are typically more likely to express aggressive behavior, but females are more likely to be deceitful and violate rules.
■ There are three types differentiated by the age at which symptoms first begin: childhood onset before the age of 10 years; adolescent onset during the teenage years; and unspecified onset when the age of onset is unknown.
■ Most people with this disorder remit by adulthood.

Risk Factors
■ Alcohol abuse is a risk factor for further development of adult antisocial behavior. This excessive intake of alcohol or illicit drugs results in structural and functional changes in the brain, especially in the prefrontal area, which modulates emotional and behavioral self-regulation.
■ Temperamental risk factors include difficult under-controlled infant temperament.
■ Lower-than-average intelligence, especially regarding verbal IQ.
■ Family risk factors include parental rejection and neglect, inconsistent child-rearing practices, harsh discipline, physical or sexual abuse, lack of supervision, early institutional living, frequent changes of caregivers, large family size, incarcerated parent, exposure to violence in neighborhood, peer rejection, substance-related disorders, peer group of delinquents, and familial psychopathology.

Diagnosis

Differential Diagnosis
- Oppositional defiant disorder (ODD)
- ADHD
- Impulsive explosive disorder
- Adjustment disorder

ICD-10 Codes

Conduct disorder, childhood-onset type (F91.1)

Conduct disorder, adolescent-onset type (F91.2)

Conduct disorder, unspecified (F91.9)—to qualify for this, an individual must have displayed at least two of the following characteristics persistently over at least 12 months in multiple relationships and settings: lack of remorse or guilt, callousness or lack of empathy, lack of concern about performance, shallow or deficient affect.

Diagnostic Workup
- Cognitive function assessment
- Assessment of financial problems in family or divorce of parents
- Complete psychiatric examination
- Developmental assessment
- The Broadband Rating Scale testing to provide data regarding severity of the child's behaviors relative to same-aged peers
- Routine labs including thyroid panel

Initial Assessment
- Interview questions should include the following:
  - Have you had any run-ins with the police; if so, what were the circumstances?
  - Have you been in physical fights; if so, what were the circumstances?
  - Have you ever been suspended or expelled from school?
  - Have you ever runaway from home? Overnight? How many times?
  - Do you smoke, drink alcohol, or use street drugs? If so, what is the drug(s), duration, frequency?
  - Are you sexually active?
  - What kind of relationship do you have with your parents/teachers?
  - What is discipline like in your home?

Clinical Presentation
- Initially, there may be poor parent–child connections, difficulty in school, or close relationships with poor role models
- Aggressive conduct that causes or threatens harm to others or to animals
- Bullies or intimidates others, initiates fights, or may have used a weapon that can cause physical clinic referral to people and/or animals
- Deliberately engaged in fire setting or destroyed another's property
- Broken into someone's home or car or stolen items from others
- Serious violation of rules—stolen while confronting a victim, forced someone into sexual activity, or truant from school before the age of 13

Diagnostic and Statistical Manual of Mental Disorders, Fifth Edition: Diagnostic Guidelines
- Conduct disorder is a repetitive and persistent pattern of behavior in which the rights of others, as well as societal rules, are violated. This diagnosis is confirmed based on at least 3 of the following in the past 12 months:
  Aggression to people and animals—bullies, threatens, intimidates others; engages in physical fights and has used a weapon to cause serious harm to others; has been physically cruel to people/animals; has stolen while confronting a victim, as in a purse snatching, mugging, extortion, and/or armed robbery
  Destruction of property—engaged in fire setting or deliberately destroyed someone's property
  Deceitfulness or theft—broken into someone else's house, building, or car; lies to obtain favors or goods to avoid obligations, as in conning someone; has stolen items of nontrivial value without confronting the victim, as in shoplifting or forgery
  Serious violations of rules—stays out at night despite parental prohibitions before age 13 years
- Is truant from school beginning at 13 years—has run away from home overnight at least twice while living in the parent/custodian's home, or once without returning for a lengthy period

Treatment
- Pharmacotherapy—The risks of cognitive deficits with lithium or antipsychotics should be weighed against potential benefits:
  - Lithium with haloperidol showed significant improvement.
  - Other possible drugs to use include the following: methylphenidate, risperidone, quetiapine, thioridazine, divalproex sodium, and carbamazepine. These medications have some efficacy for the disorder.
- Psychotherapy
  - Behavioral therapy
  - Family-based therapy
  - Parental skills training
  - Cognitive-behavioral therapy (CBT)
- Complementary therapy
  - Yoga
  - Mindfulness
  - Meditation
  - Teaching grounding techniques
  - Aroma therapy and reprocessing
  - Eye movement desensitization
  - Relaxation exercises
  - Massage therapy
- Community activities/skill training/animal therapy
  - Big Brothers Big Sisters
  - Sports teams
  - Art projects
  - Volunteer work for Habitat for Humanity
  - Learning new skills like woodworking/cooking
  - Animal-assisted therapy

Chronic Treatment
- Educate patient and family on the diagnosis.
- Treat any comorbid conditions.
- Structure the daily routine to include pleasing activities.
- Emphasize parental monitoring and whom they are with.
- Demonstrate clear and specific parental communication therapies.
- Teach positive coping skills.
- Reward good behavior.
- Establish consequences for noncompliance.
- Consider pharmacotherapy for children who are highly aggressive or impulsive or both.
- Teach relaxation and stress management.

Prognosis/Recurrence Rate
- The earlier the onset, the worse the prognosis.
- If the behavior intensifies and continues beyond the age of 18, a diagnosis of antisocial personality disorder is made.
- Patients are at risk for later mood disorders, anxiety disorders, posttraumatic stress disorder, and impulse-control in adults.

Medical/Legal Pitfalls
- Serious injury or death due to unlawful activity
- Incarceration due to violation of society's rules

DYSLEXIA

Background Information
Definition of Disorder
- Dyslexia is a language-based reading disorder.
- Difficulty with written language: writing, spelling, and reading.
- Combination of phonological and letter-processing errors.
- Persons with reading disorders have normal intellect.

Etiology
- Neurobiological disorders
- Inherited genetic connections

Demographics
- Evenly distributed among sexes, cultures, and social groups.
- All languages are affected.
- Twenty percent of any given population is likely to have some degree of reading difficulty.

Risk Factors
- Boys are affected twice as much as girls.
- Family history of reading and learning disabilities.
- Families with histories of autoimmune disease (asthma and diabetes).

Diagnosis

ICD-10 Code

Specific reading disorder (F81.0)

Diagnostic Workup
- Functional hearing examination.
- Functional eye examination.
  Testing is standardized: Refer to a psychologist, education specialist, or specialist dyslexia teacher.

Initial Assessment
- Was there any birth trauma?
- *Growth and development*: Were milestones met on time for speaking?
- Is there a family history of learning disabilities?
- History of chronic ear infections.
- Has the child attended school regularly?
- Specialist referral.

Clinical Presentation
- Delay in language acquisition—late to speak.
- Does not hear sound patterns.
- Difficulty with learning the names and sounds of letters.
- Can read a word on one page but cannot recognize it on another.
- Reading comprehension is well below expected grade level: inaccurate, slow, and effortful reading.
- Classic warning signs of dyslexia before the age of 5 years are as follows:
  - Speech delay
  - Slow to get words out
- Warning signs in school-age children:
  - Stuttering and articulation issues
  - Mixes up letters
  - Produces sounds out of sequence (animal = aMinal)
  - Difficulty with the letters R, L, M, and N
  - Adds or eliminates words while reading
  - Difficulty with learning how to write
  - Difficulty with memorizing sequences
  - Poor written expression that lacks clarity
  - Difficulties remembering number facts
  - Inaccurate mathematical reasoning

Diagnostic and Statistical Manual of Mental Disorders, Fifth Edition: Diagnostic Guidelines
- An individual's ability to read is impaired.
- Reading achievement, as measured by standardized tests of reading accuracy and comprehension, is substantially below age-appropriate reading achievement levels.
- The deficit in reading achievement interferes with academic achievement and activities of daily living that require reading skills.
- If a sensory deficit is also present, the impaired reading ability is in excess of impairments associated with the sensory deficit.
- *Note*: If a general medical condition (e.g., a neurological condition) or sensory deficit is present, the disorder should be classified as such.

- *DSM-5* states that an individual's specific learning disorder (SLD) is diagnosed by the following:
  - Clinical review of the individual's developmental, medical, educational, and family history.
  - Reports of test scores and teacher observations.
  - Response to academic interventions.
  - The diagnosis requires persistent difficulties in reading, writing, and arithmetic or mathematical reasoning skills during formal years of schooling.

Treatment Overview

- Individual education should plan for accommodations at school.
- Small-group education.
- Focus on repetition.
- Therapies that integrate auditory, visual, and motor inputs.

Patient Education

- Dyslexia is a lifelong condition.
- Severity of disability is variable.
- Treatment is important as children who have difficulty learning often believe they are incapable of learning, give up, and risk failure.
- Foster the child's strengths and creativity.

Medical/Legal Pitfalls

- Higher incidence of autoimmune disease in families with a history of language disorders
- Protected under the IDEA; visit http://idea.ed.gov/

INTELLECTUAL DISABILITY

Background Information

Definition of Disorder

- Disorder of intellectual functioning.
- Limitations in adaptive skills, such as communication, self-care, and social skills.
- Mild MR is IQ of 50 to 55 through 70.
- Moderate MR is IQ of 35 to 40 through 50 to 55.
- Severe MR is IQ of 20 to 25 through 35 to 40.
- Profound MR is IQ below 20 to 25.

Etiology

- Thirty-five percent of cases have a genetic cause.
- Ten percent are caused by malformation syndrome.
- Thirty-three percent are external or trauma related (prenatal, perinatal, or postnatal factors).
- Causes of 20% of cases are unknown.

Demographics

- One percent of total population are affected.
- Eighty-five percent have mild MR.
- Two times more likely to have medical conditions than other populations with mental issues.

Risk Factors
- Parental age at birth
- Congenital heart disease
- Parental education/occupation/income
- Trauma
- PKU
- Hydrocephalus
- Infection
- Increased lead levels
- Pre- or postcerebral hemorrhage

Diagnosis

Comorbidities
- Increased level of MR severity—increased medical comorbidity.
- Hypothyroidism, congenital cataracts, or cardiac defects.
- Fifteen to 30 percent have seizures.
- Twenty to 30 percent have a motor handicap such as cerebral palsy.
- Ten to 20 percent have a sensory impairment such as a vision handicap.
- Five times more likely to have a diagnosable psychiatric illness.
- Anxiety disorder, conduct disorder, depression, eating disorder (pica and ruminations).
- Seventy-five percent of autistic children have comorbid MR.
- Seventy-five percent of people with Down syndrome may have Alzheimer's by the age of 60 years.
- ADHD rates are similar to those of the general population.

ICD-10 Codes
Mild MR (F70)

Moderate MR (F71)

Severe MR (F72)

Profound MR (F73)

Diagnostic Workup
- IQ testing
- Physical examination
- Chromosomal analysis
- Brain imaging (MRI or CT)
- EEG
- Urinary amino acids, blood organic acids, lead levels
- Biochemical tests for inborn errors of metabolism

Initial Assessment
- Parent/child early development
- Prenatal or perinatal development, postnatal development
- Physical assessment
- Milestones
- Motor/coordination
- Medical history
- Onset of symptoms
- Severity of symptoms (communication, social, behavioral)

Assessment Tools
- The Aberrant Behavior Checklist—moderate to severe MR
- The Reiss Scales—eight psychopathology scales and six maladaptive behaviors

Clinical Presentation
- Decreased cognitive functioning
- Concrete thinking
- May have stereotypical movements
- Difficulty with change/transitions

Diagnostic and Statistical Manual of Mental Disorders, Fifth Edition: Diagnostic Guidelines
- *Notably substandard intellectual functioning*: IQ of approximately 70 or below (for infants, a judgment of substandard intellectual functioning must be based on a clinical evaluation).
- The individual cannot fulfill standards of adaptive functioning for their age group. Presence of deficits in adaptive functioning in at least two of the following areas: communication, care of self, home living, social and interpersonal skills, self-direction, use of community resources, academic skills, work, leisure, health, and safety.
- The onset is prior to 18 years.

ICD-10 Codes: Based on Degree of Severity Reflecting Level of Intellectual Impairment
- *Mild MR*: IQ level, 50 to 55 through approximately 70 (F70)
- *Moderate MR*: IQ level, 35 to 40 through 50 to 55 (F71)
- *Severe MR*: IQ level, 20 to 25 through 35 to 40 (F72)
- *Profound MR*: IQ level below 20 to 25 (F73)
- MR, severity inspecified: when there is strong presumption of MR but the person's intelligence cannot be tested using standard IQ tests (F79)

Treatment Overview
- Parent education programs.
- Habilitation focusing on attempts to care for individuals in the community.
- Behavior therapy.
- Social skills training.
- Special education.
- Ancillary therapies—occupational therapy and physical therapy.
- There are no specific medicines used for MR; medicines treat coexisting medical and psychological conditions. There are no FDA-approved medications for use in children with MR.
- Neuroleptic/antipsychotics such as risperidone (*Risperdal*) have been used as first-line treatment for behavior problems associated with MR but due to the patients' limited verbal skills, monitoring side effects is difficult. Strongly weigh the risk–benefit of these medicines.
- People with Down syndrome are particularly sensitive to anticholinergics.
- People with MR may be disinhibited by sedative-hypnotics and benzodiazepines, which is a paradoxical reaction.
- Benzodiazepines are not used as first-line treatment.

Patient Education
- Educate about diagnosis, including prognosis
- Treatment options

- Available community resources
- Importance of support systems for the family

Medical/Legal Pitfalls

- Most people with MR will require guardianship as they enter adulthood.
- IDEA guarantees children with disabilities diagnostic, educational, and support service until the age of 21 years.
- Public Law 94 to 142 mandates provision of free appropriate education up to the age of 21 years.
- Informed consent is required for medications; most are not FDA approved for use in children; this should be part of consent.

MIXED RECEPTIVE–EXPRESSIVE LANGUAGE DISORDER

Background Information

Definition of Disorder

- A mixed receptive–expressive language disorder is a language disability that causes impairment in both the understanding and the expression of language.

Etiology

- Communication disorders may be developmental or acquired.
- The cause is believed to be based on biological problems, such as abnormalities of brain development, or possibly by exposure to toxins during pregnancy, such as abused substances or environmental toxins such as lead.
- A genetic factor is sometimes considered a contributing cause in some cases.
- Some causes of speech and language disorders include hearing loss; neurological disorders; brain injury; intellectual disability; drug abuse; physical impairments, such as a cleft lip or palate; and vocal abuse or misuse.
- Frequently, however, the cause is unknown.
- For unknown reasons, boys are diagnosed with communication disorders more often than girls.
- Children with communication disorders frequently have other developmental disorders as well.
- Most children with communication disorders are able to speak by the time they enter school; however, they continue to have problems with communication. School-age children often have problems understanding and formulating words.
- Teens may have more difficulty with understanding or expressing abstract ideas.
- The diagnosis for receptive–expressive language disorder is as follows:
  - Most children with communication disorders are first referred for speech and language evaluations when their delays in communicating are noted.
  - A child psychiatrist is usually consulted, especially when emotional or behavioral problems are also present.
  - A comprehensive evaluation also involves psychometric testing (testing designed to assess logical reasoning abilities, reactions to different situations, and thinking performance, not tests of general knowledge) and psychological testing of cognitive abilities.
  - There are varied language disorders—for example, receptive language may be mildly delayed and expressive language may be severely delayed.

- Knowing the type of mixed receptive–expressive language delay is important because the split may impact academics.
- The child may exhibit severely delayed receptive language skills and only mildly delayed expressive language.
- The receptive language difficulties will most likely have a significant impact on being able to follow directions and understand classroom instruction.
- Children with this condition will need extra help (written directions, one-on-one time) in order to be successful.
- Many speech problems are developmental rather than physiological, and as such they respond to remedial instruction.
- Language experiences are vital to a young child's development. In the past, children with communication disorders were routinely removed from the regular class for individual speech and language therapy.
- This is still the case in severe instances, but the trend is toward keeping the child in the mainstream as much as possible.
- In order to accomplish this goal, teamwork among the teacher, the speech and language therapist, the audiologist, and parents is essential.
- Speech improvement and correction are blended into the regular classroom curriculum and the child's natural environment.
- It is a communication disorder in which both the receptive and expressive areas of communication may be affected in any degree, from mild to severe.
- If someone is being assessed on the Wechsler Adult Intelligence Scale, for instance, this may show up in relatively low scores for information, vocabulary, and comprehension (perhaps below the 25th percentile). If the person has difficulty with spatial concepts, such as "over," "under," "here," and "there," they may have arithmetic difficulties, difficulty in understanding word problems and instructions, or have difficulties using words.
- They may also have a more general problem with words or sentences, both understanding and speaking them.
- If someone is suspected to have a mixed receptive–expressive language disorder, then that person can go to a speech therapist or pathologist and receive treatment. Most treatments are short term and rely on accommodations made in the person's environment, so as to interfere minimally with work and school functioning.
- Three to 5 percent of all children have a receptive or an expressive language disorder or both.
- These children have difficulty understanding speech (language receptivity) and using language (language expression).
- The cause is unknown, but there may be genetic factors, and malnutrition may play a role.
- Problems with receptive language skills usually begin before the age of 4 years.
- Some mixed-language disorders are caused by brain injury, and these are sometimes misdiagnosed as developmental disorders.

Diagnosis

Differential Diagnosis
- Dyslexia
- Autism
- SLD
- Intellectual disability

ICD-10 Code
Mixed receptive–expressive language disorder (F80.2)

Clinical Presentation
The following are the most common symptoms of communication disorders. However, each child may experience symptoms differently.

- May not speak at all or may have a limited vocabulary for their age.
- Has difficulty in understanding simple directions or is unable to name objects.
- Shows problems with socialization.
- Inability to follow directions but shows comprehension with routine, repetitive directions.
- Echolalia (repeating back words or phrases either immediately or at a later time).
- Difficulty in responding appropriately to "yes/no" questions, "either/or" questions, "who/what/where" questions, or "when/why/how" questions.
- Repeats back a question first and then responds to it.
- High activity level and not attending to spoken language.
- Jargon (e.g., unintelligible speech) is used.
- Uses "memorized" phrases and sentences.
- The child may have a problem with words or sentences, in both understanding and speaking them.
- Learning problems and academic difficulties occur.
- Although many speech and language patterns can be called baby talk and are part of a young child's normal development, they can become problems if they are not outgrown as expected.
- In this way, an initial delay in speech and language or an initial speech pattern can become a disorder, which can cause difficulties in learning. Because of the way the brain develops, it is easier to learn language and communication skills before the age of 5 years.
- The symptoms of communication disorders may resemble other problems or medical conditions.
- Always consult your child's physician for diagnosis of the following:
  - Problems with language comprehension
  - Problems with language expression
  - Speech containing many articulation errors
  - Difficulty recalling early sight or sound memories

Diagnostic and Statistical Manual of Mental Disorders, Fifth Edition: Diagnostic Guidelines
- Impairment in both receptive and expressive language development, as demonstrated by lowered scoring on standardized tests (e.g., IQ tests)
- Characterized by reductions in receptive language skills whereby a child has difficulty in extracting usable information from spoken language
- Characterized by reductions in expressive language skills whereby a child has a diminished vocabulary, has difficulty in producing words and sentences, and uses verb tenses incorrectly
- *Note*: Measures/tests of language development must be appropriate to and relevant to language use in the specific cultural group.
- Onset is generally before the age of 4 years. However, this disorder can also occur if there is physical trauma later in childhood, for example, head injury.
- With positive input, some affected children may develop normal language.
- Associated features and disorders are as follows:

- Conversational skills (e.g., waiting one's turn to speak, staying with a topic of conversation) are lacking.
- A deficit in some aspect of sensory information processing is common (especially in auditory information processing).
- Difficulties with the language's sound system are often present.
- SLD is often present.
- Memory impairments.
- May occur concurrently with ADHD, developmental coordination disorder, or enuresis.
- The ability to process verbal output is reduced. The individual may find it difficult to absorb and recall a simple list of instructions.
- There may be high levels of competence in non-language-based problem solving.
- *Note*: A school psychologist, clinical psychologist, psychiatrist, or other qualified specialist should make this diagnosis. If there is a head injury or another medical problem (e.g., encephalitis), a physician should be on the diagnostic team.
- This is applicable to developmental dysphasia or aphasia, receptive type, and developmental Wernicke aphasia.
- Type 1 excludes central auditory processing disorder, dysphasia or aphasia NOS, expressive language disorder, expressive type dysphasia or aphasia, and word deafness.
- Type 2 excludes acquired aphasia with epilepsy, pervasive developmental disorders, SM, and intellectual disabilities.

Laboratory Tests

- Standardized receptive and expressive language tests can be given to any child suspected of having this disorder.
- An audiogram should also be given to rule out the possibility of deafness as it is one of the most common causes of language problems.
- All children diagnosed with this condition should be seen by a neurologist or a developmental pediatric specialist to determine whether the cause can be reversed.
- If someone is being assessed on the Wechsler Adult Intelligence Scale, for instance, this may show up in relatively low scores for information, vocabulary, and comprehension (perhaps below the 25th percentile). If the person has difficulty with spatial concepts, such as "over," "under," "here," and "there," they may have arithmetic difficulties, have difficulty understanding word problems and instructions, or have difficulties using words.

Treatment Overview

- Speech and language therapy are the best approaches to this type of language disorder.
- A coordinated effort among parents, teachers, and speech/language and mental health professionals provides the basis for individualized treatment strategies that may include individual or group remediation, special classes, or special resources.
- Special-education techniques are used to increase communication skills in the areas of the deficit.
- A second approach helps the child build on their strengths to overcome their communication deficit.
- Specific treatment for communication disorders will be determined by the child's physician, special-education teachers, and speech/language and mental health professionals on the basis of the following:

- The child's age, overall health, and medical history.
- Extent of the disorder.
- Psychotherapy is also recommended because of the possibility of associated emotional or behavioral problems.
  - Type of disorder
  - The child's tolerance for specific medications or therapies
  - Expectations for the course of the disorder
- SLPs assist children who have communication disorders in various ways.
  - They provide individual therapy for the child, consult with the child's teacher about the most effective ways to facilitate the child's communication in the class setting, and work closely with the family to develop goals and techniques for effective therapy in class and at home.
  - Early detection and intervention can address the developmental needs and academic difficulties to improve the quality of life experienced by children with communication disorders.
  - The SLP may assist vocational teachers and counselors in establishing communication goals related to the work experiences of students and suggest strategies that are effective for the important transition from school to employment and adult life.

Patient Education

- The outcome varies based on the underlying cause.
- Brain injury or other structural pathology is generally associated with a poor outcome with chronic deficiencies in language, whereas other, more reversible causes can be treated effectively.
- The outcome varies based on the underlying cause.
- Difficulty in understanding and using language can cause problems with social interaction and ability to function independently as an adult.

OPPOSITIONAL DEFIANT DISORDER

Background Information

Definition of Disorder
- ODD is complex and is explained through multiple perspectives—psychoanalytical, neurobiological, behavioral, and developmental.
- There is a failure of motor inhibition, acceptance of immediate small rewards versus delayed large ones, and risky behavior in terms of impulsive decision-making.

Etiology
- ODD is linked to complex and multifactorial etiologies.
- Biological, psychological, social, and developmental factors each contribute in different degrees to the development and clinical course.
- Enhanced expression of the L/L variant of the serotonin transporter gene was found in ODD.
- Elevated testosterone and androstenedione were related to higher levels of acting out.

- Evidence of monoamine neurotransmitter dysfunction has been identified in some adults and children.
- Low levels of 5-hydroxyindoleacetic acid (5-HIAA) have been found to be associated with violent, aggressive behavior and loss of impulse control.

Demographics
- Prevalence of ODD is 1% to 11% with an average prevalence of 3.3%.
- Male-to-female ratio is 1.4:1 prior to adolescence.

Risk Factors
- Temperament of high levels of emotional reactivity and poor frustration tolerance have been predictive of this disorder.
- Harsh, inconsistent, or neglectful child-rearing practices have been linked to the development of ODD.
- Neurobiological markers such as lower heart rate and skin conductance reactivity; reduced basal cortisol reactivity; and abnormalities in the prefrontal cortex and amygdala have been found in these children.
- No differences have been found across cultures.

Diagnosis
Differential Diagnosis
- Conduct Disorder
- ADHD
- Depressive and bipolar disorders
- Disruptive mood dysregulation disorder
- Intermittent explosive disorder
- Intellectual disability
- Language disorder
- Social anxiety disorder

ICD-10 Code
Oppositional defiant disorder (F91.3)

Diagnostic Workup
- Careful and detailed mental status exam
- Physical examination
- Labs as needed to evaluate physical complaints:
  - Thyroid function studies (T3, T4, TSH)
  - *CBC with differentials*: hemoglobin, hematocrit, red blood cell (RBC) count, white blood cell (WBC) count, WBC differential count and platelet count
  - Complete metabolic panel, including glucose, calcium, albumin; total protein count; levels of sodium, potassium, CO_2 (carbon dioxide and bicarbonate), chloride, blood urea nitrogen (BUN), creatinine, alkaline phosphatase (ALP), alanine amino transferase (ALT), aspartate amino transferase (AST), and bilirubin
- Psychological examination to include possible screening:
  - The Child Behavior Checklist
  - Iowa Conners Aggression Factor
  - Modified Overt Aggression Scale

Initial Assessment
- Mental status examination to rule out other disorders.
- Diagnostic interviews.
- Review of pertinent records from the school and clinics.
- Information about cognitive style, family structure and functioning, and physical signs and symptoms.
- These patients can arouse countertransference in clinicians.

Clinical Presentation
- Symptoms of ODD may begin during the preschool years but may develop later.
- Common behaviors include being angry, irritable, argumentative, defiant, and vindictive.
- The disorder can be mild (occur in only one setting), moderate (occur in at least two settings) or severe (occur in three or more settings).
- Children usually present with parental concern about the child's behavior due to disruption within the family unit.
- School-age children present because of problems with their teachers.
They may have poor grades, be unable to make friends at school, or have trouble following school rules.

Diagnostic and Statistical Manual of Mental Disorders, Fifth Edition: Diagnostic Guidelines
- Pattern of angry/irritable mood.
- Often loses temper, often touchy or easily annoyed.
- Argumentative/defiant behavior.
- Argues with authority figures, actively defies or refuses to comply with requests from authority figures or with rules.
- Deliberatively annoys others.
- Blames others for their mistakes or misbehavior.
- Has been spiteful or vindictive at least twice within the past 6 months.
- Causes distress in immediate social contacts or impacts negatively in important areas of functioning.
- Behaviors do not occur exclusively during a psychotic, substance, depressive, or bipolar disorder.

Treatment
- Parent training to incorporate parenting skills that are more positive and less frustrating for the family.
- Parent–child interaction therapy (PCIT) involves coaching parents while they observe interactions with the child via a one-way mirror using an audio device with an ear bud to guide the parent.
- CBT is used to help the child identify and change thought patterns that are destructive. Problem-solving approaches are used where parent and child work together to come up with solutions that are acceptable to both.
- Social skills training helps the child to interact more positively and effectively with peers.
- Unconditional love involves helping the parent to show acceptance of the child.
- Reinforce with praise to identify small successes to make the child feel good about the treatment.

Pharmacotherapy
- No medications have been approved for ODD.
- Stimulants have been used in this disorder because of the high comorbidity rate with ADHD, such as methylphenidate and D-amphetamine.
- Antipsychotics such as risperidone are used as a second- or third-line option because of their adverse effects.
- Alpha-2 agonists such as clonidine and guanfacine have shown some efficacy.
- Atomoxetine has been shown to have limited efficacy.

Ongoing Treatment
- Praise good behavior and model the behavior you want in the child.
- Pick your battles and avoid power struggles.
- Set limits and have consistent reasonable consequences.
- Develop a routine where you spend time with your child.
- Ensure consistent appropriate discipline.
- Be prepared for challenges as child's behavior may worsen during the initial treatment phases.

Prognosis/Recurrence Rate
- This condition will resolve in most children. Two-thirds of the children will no longer have significant behavioral problems after 3 years, and about 70% will have no behavioral problems by the age of 18.
- About 10% of all children with ODD will go on to develop conduct disorder.
- ODD has been shown to predict depression and anxiety and borderline personality disorder.

Medical/Legal Pitfalls
- Of children/adolescents diagnosed with ODD, the following occurred:
  - A total of 18.95% had been arrested or detained by the police in the past year.
  - A total of 16% reported illegal drug use.
  - A total of 32.4% had serious injuries in the form of severe burns or severe cuts, head injuries, or internal injuries.
  - injuries/broken bones
  - A total of 7.8% had a gunshot or stabbing injury within the last 5 years.
  - A total of 11.3% had two or more health problems.
  - A total of 28.7% had their license suspended.

REACTIVE ATTACHMENT DISORDER

Background Information

Definition of Disorder

Reactive attachment disorder (RAD) is a developmental disorder that is a direct response to abuse, neglect, and disruptions in early caretaking. Attachment and social interaction are rooted in infancy and early childhood. Failures of attachment occur when a child's basic needs for emotional and physical safety, security, and predictability are not met. This failure to attach results in children being incapable of developing normal loving relationships, and they exhibit maladaptive and disruptive behaviors. This disorder can be diagnosed as early as 1 month of age.

Etiology
- Maternal deprivation.
- Birth to 36 months is a hallmark period for attachment.

Demographics
Estimate of prevalence is 1% of the general population. This is hard to estimate as abuse and neglect are seriously underreported in the United States.

Risk Factors
- Birth to the age of 5 years.
- Emotional, physical, sexual abuse, and inconsistent care providers.
- Genetic vulnerability is unclear.
- Being removed from neglectful or abusive homes.
- Children do attach to abusive caregivers.
- Postpartum depression in a mother.
- Unwanted pregnancy.
- Living in an orphanage or institution.
- Parents with abuse histories, mental illness, MR, substance abuse, and behavioral disturbance.
- Long medical hospitalizations with separation from parent.
- Failure to thrive.
- Poverty.

Diagnosis

Differential Diagnosis
- ADHD
- Autistic disorder
- Conduct disorder
- MR
- ODD
- PDD

ICD-10 Code
Reactive attachment disorder of infancy or early childhood (F94.1)

Diagnostic Workup
- Full psychological evaluation with a multidisciplinary approach
  - Psychosocial history
  - Intellectual functioning
  - Psychometric assessment

Initial Assessment
- Destruction of property.
- Hoarding food.
- Highly controlling of others and situations.
- Lying about things or issues that the child does not need to lie about or when it would be easier to tell the truth.
- Refusal to make eye contact.
- Does not seek comfort from caregiver.
- Failure to initiate or respond to social interactions.

- Being demonstrative with strangers and refusing to be separated from new acquaintances.
- Dangerous behavior with a lack of remorse.
  - Assaulting others
  - Fire setting
  - Injury to self
    - Head banging
    - Hitting and biting oneself
  - Stealing
  - Sexual acting out
  - Learning problems
  - Stereotyped behaviors
    - Nose picking
    - Nail biting
    - Rocking
- The child's negative behaviors are much easier to assess than their attachment.
- Ask parents whether they are afraid of their child.
- The Randolph Attachment Disorder Questionnaire (RADQ) is standard.

Clinical Presentation
- *Inhibited*: inability to initiate or respond to social interactions
  - Emotionally withdrawn
  - Guarded
  - Disinterested in others
  - Does not seek comfort
  - Minimal eye contact
  - Avoidance of physical touch
- *Disinherited*: inability to identify an appropriate attachment figure
  - Indiscreet and superficial attachments to others
  - Exaggerates need for help
  - Anxious—seeks reassurance
  - Excessive childlike behaviors

Diagnostic and Statistical Manual of Mental Disorders, Fifth Edition: Diagnostic Guidelines
- There are two types:
  - *Inhibited type*: if inhibitions predominate in the clinical presentation
  - *Disinhibited type*: if indiscriminate sociability predominates in the clinical presentation
- Disturbed and developmentally inappropriate ways of relating to others, beginning before the age of 5 years, as evidenced by either of the following:
  - Failure to initiate social interaction or failure to respond in a developmentally appropriate fashion to many social stimuli, as manifested by excessively inhibited or ambivalent/contradictory responses
  - Indiscriminate sociability, with the individual showing a marked inability to form appropriate selective attachments (e.g., excessive familiarity with strangers).
- The social deficits cannot be ascribed to developmental delay (as in MR) and do not meet criteria for a PDD.
- Care of the child or infant is very likely to have included at least one of the following:
  - Persistent disregard of the child's basic emotional needs; disregard of the child's need for affection

- Persistent disregard of the child's physical needs
- Repeated changes of primary caregiver (e.g., frequent changes in foster care setting)
- There is a presumption that the unmet needs are responsible for the failures of social interaction.

Treatment Overview

Behavioral
- There is no gold standard treatment for RAD.
- Focus treatment effort on parents or primary caregiver.
- Play therapy for patient.
- Residential treatment.
- Behavior management therapy:
  - Provides psychoeducation and parenting strategies
- Holding therapy:
  - This is not well researched and is highly controversial.
- It is not mandatory that children be removed from their previously neglectful parents if those parents have changed their behavior and are now capable of providing a loving, stable relationship and environment.

Psychopharmacotherapy Overview
- Mood stabilizer/antiseizure medications—off label
  - Aggression
  - Mood instability
- Atypical antipsychotics—off label
  - Mood stabilization
  - Disorganized behavior
  - Behavior disturbance
  - Comorbid diagnosis
  - See specific diagnosis

Recurrence Rates
- Lifelong condition

Patient Education
- Children with RAD need consistent, predictable relationships and a stable environment.
- Parents must be flexible.
- Coach parents on how the child's behavior is not personal and rather a response to failures of empathy and protection.
- Older children with RAD often have behavioral disturbances resulting in legal difficulties.
- Parents are encouraged to spend time and money resources on themselves as children will get the benefit of parents who feel capable and supported.
- Work closely with school and incorporate interventions into the child's individual education plan.

Medical/Legal Pitfalls
- It is not unusual that adopted children with RAD will be "un-adopted" by their families.
- Follow mandatory reporting guidelines for abuse and neglect.

SELECTIVE MUTISM

Background Information

Definition of Disorder

SM is a condition in which children are unable to speak in situations where talking is an expected behavior. These children are able to talk freely at home and in situations where they are comfortable. They may have articulation problems or a medical condition that affects speech, but overall SM is an anxiety-based disorder.

Etiology
- The exact etiology is unknown.
- Children with SM are likely to have issues related to shyness, avoidance, and anxiety.

Demographics
- About 0.2% to 2% of population

Risk Factors
- *Age*: onset between the ages of 3 and 6 years
- *Gender*: boys and girls
- Family history
  - Parent with history of SM
  - Parents with anxiety disorders
- Precipitating factors
  - Traumatic events during the time of language development
  - Multiple moves in homes or school
  - Being threatened or bullied at school

Diagnosis

Comorbidities
- Developmental disorders
- Elimination disorders
- Learning disabilities
- ODD
- Separation anxiety disorder
- Social phobia

ICD-10 Code

Selective mutism (F94.0)

Diagnostic Workup
- Dental examination.
- Hearing evaluation.
- Rule out language disorders:
  - Consultation with a speech language pathologist
- Rule out medical causes:
  - Asthma—being short of breath makes it difficult to speak.
- Rating scales:
  - Anxiety Disorder Interview Schedule for Children
  - Social Anxiety Scale for Children–R

Initial Assessment

- Baseline level of functioning.
- Onset of symptoms.
  - Difficulties may not come into focus until the child enters school.
- Environments and situations where the child is mute.
- How does the child communicate at home, at school, and in social situations?
  - Gestures, writing, whispering
  - Will the child talk on the phone?
  - Will the child talk to people in one situation but not in another?
    - Talks to a friend in the child's home but not at school.

Clinical Presentation

- Refuses to speak in situations where talking is appropriate and expected.

Diagnostic and Statistical Manual of Mental Disorders, Fifth Edition: Diagnostic Criteria

- Consistent inability to speak in specific social situations in persons who are capable of speech in other situations.
- The disturbance interferes with educational/occupational/social functioning.
- A duration of at least 1 month (excluding the first month of school attendance).
- The failure cannot be ascribed to a lack of familiarity or comfort with the spoken language.
- The disturbance is not more easily ascribed to a communication disorder (e.g., stuttering) and does not occur concurrently with and exclusively during the course of a PDD, schizophrenia, or other psychotic disorder.

Treatment Overview

- Individual and family therapy
- Behavioral therapy
- Cognitive therapy
- Exposure therapy
- Skills training
  - Communication skills
  - Anxiety management
- Speech language pathologist
- SSRIs may be appropriate to treat anxiety symptoms
  - Case studies report benefit
    - Fluoxetine is most studied
- Coordinate services with school

Patient Education

- SM can remit on its own without treatment.
- Treatment may take several months before benefit is noted.
- Positive accomplishment should be reinforced.
- Educational pitfalls.
- Hinders social development.
- Interferes with reading language developmental tasks.
- Hinders a child's ability to engage in regular and extracurricular activities.

SEPARATION ANXIETY DISORDER

Background Information

Definition of Disorder

- Anxiety disorder of childhood and early adolescence
- Characterized by unrealistic fear of separation from attachment figures
- Interferes significantly with daily life and development
- Begins before the age of 18 years

Etiology

- Genetic link but only in girls
- Temperamental traits
- Parental rearing styles
- Caregiver stress/support
- Life events

Demographics

- Most common anxiety disorder in childhood.
- Prevalence is 2.4%.
- Peak onset is 7 to 9 years of age.

Risk Factors

- Female
- Family history of anxiety disorder or depression
- African American
- Lower-socioeconomic-status homes
- Child temperament
- Parenting styles
- Life events such as death or threat of separation

Diagnosis

Comorbidities

- Another anxiety disorder such as OCD
- Depression

ICD-10 Code

Separation anxiety disorder (F93.0)

Diagnostic Workup

- Clinical interview using *DSM-5* criteria
- Anxiety disorder interview schedule for *DSM-5*—child/parent (ADIS-C/P)
- Screen for child anxiety-related emotional disorders (SCARED)—parent and child

Initial Assessment

- Growth and development
- Current or recent life stressors for child and caregivers

- Significant losses
- Onset of symptoms
- Severity of symptoms
- Medical history
- School reports

Clinical Presentation
- Physical complaints involving stomach aches or headaches, particularly on school days
- Distress upon separation
- Fears that something bad will happen to parent(s) or attachment figure
- School refusal
- Severe anxiety/worry
- Difficulty with sleep

Diagnostic and Statistical Manual of Mental Disorders, Fifth Edition: Diagnostic Guidelines
- Disproportionate or extreme anxiety related to separation from home or from persons to whom the individual is attached, as manifested by three or more of the following:
  - Distress for the individual, when separation from home or "attachment figures" occurs or is anticipated
  - Frequent worry about losing attachment figures; worry about harm coming to attachment figures
  - Frequent worry that an untoward event will lead to separation from attachment figures (e.g., getting lost)
  - Reluctance or refusal to go to school or elsewhere because of fear of separation
  - Reluctance or refusal to be alone or without attachment figures, at home or in other settings
  - Reluctance or refusal to go to sleep in the absence of proximity to an attachment figure or to sleep away from home
  - Repeated nightmares that include the element of separation
  - Physical symptoms (such as headache, nausea, vomiting) when separation from attachment figures occurs or is anticipated
- A duration of 4 weeks or more.
- Onset before age of 18 years.
- The disturbance causes significant distress for the individual or impairment in social functioning.
- The disturbance does not occur exclusively during the course of a PDD, schizophrenia, or other psychotic disorder.
- In adults and adolescents, the disturbance is not more easily ascribed to panic disorder with agoraphobia.

Treatment Overview
- Consensus exists that CBT is the treatment of choice.
- Exposure-based CBT is preferable—refer out.
- Psychopharmacology is the recommended treatment for resistant separation anxiety disorder.
- SSRI antidepressants are effective.
- Sertraline (*Zoloft*) and fluoxetine (*Prozac*) have been shown to be effective in randomized controlled trials (RCTs).
- Fluoxetine (*Prozac*; if older than 7 years), initiate 10 mg/d; adolescents, initiate 20 mg/d; FDA approved for use in depression and OCD.

- Sertraline (*Zoloft*; if older than 6 years), initiate 25 mg/d; FDA approved for use in OCD.
- Monitor antidepressants for side effects such as nausea, agitation, sleep disturbance, suicidal thoughts, changes in appetite, and drowsiness.
- SSRIs carry black box warning for increased suicidal ideation.
- Results on tricyclic antidepressants (TCAs) are mixed—increased risks for cardiac problems.
- Benzodiazepines are effective but, due to risk–benefit considerations, are not often used in the pediatric population.

Drug Selection Table Separation Anxiety Disorder

CLASS	DRUG
SSRIs	First-line drug therapy Sertraline (*Zoloft*) Fluoxetine (*Prozac*) Paroxetine (*Paxil*) Paroxetine mesylate (*Pexeva*) Fluvoxamine (*Luvox*) Citalopram (*Celexa*) Escitalopram (*Lexapro*)
TCAs	Drugs for treatment-resistant cases Imipramine (*Tofranil*) Desipramine (*Norpramin*) Clomipramine (*Anafranil*)
BZDs	Drugs used for short-term treatments Alprazolam (*Xanax/Xanax XR/Niravam*) Lorazepam (*Ativan*) Diazepam (*Valium*) Chlordiazepoxide (*Librium*)

BZDs, benzodiazepines; SSRIs, selective serotonin reuptake inhibitors; TCAs tricyclic antidepressants.

Patient Education

- About diagnosis.
- Treatment options.
- Strategies for management of symptoms such as school refusal; accommodation of symptoms makes the problem worse.
- Community/national resources and supports.

Medical/Legal Pitfalls

- School refusal may lead to problems with truancy.

SPECIFIC LEARNING DISORDER

Background Information

Definition of Disorder

- SLD is diagnosed when achievements on standardized tests are substantially below (at least 2 standard deviations) what is expected for the age, schooling, and level of intelligence, and learning problems significantly interfere with academic achievement and activities of daily living.
- These can be categorized as reading disorder, mathematics disorder, and disorder of written expression.

- Children with SLD have specific impairments in acquiring, retaining, and process-ing information. Standardized tests place them well below their IQ range in their area of difficulty.
- If a sensory deficit is present, the difficulties are in excess of those usually associ-ated with it.
- Problematic areas may include the following:
  - Language development and language skills (listening, speaking, reading, writ-ing, and spelling)
  - Social studies
  - Mathematics
  - Social skills
  - Motor skills (fine motor skills as well as coordination)
  - Cognitive development and memory
  - Attention and organization
  - Test taking

Etiology

- There may be abnormalities in cognitive processing, including deficits in visual perception, linguistic processes, attention, or memory that precede or are associated with SLD.
- CNS damage (prenatal or postnatal).
- SLD may also be caused by such medical conditions as a traumatic brain injury or brain infections, such as encephalitis or meningitis.
- SLD is frequently found in association with a variety of general medical conditions (e.g., lead poisoning, fetal alcohol syndrome, or fragile X syndrome).
- Prenatal factors that may play a role in SLD include eclampsia, placental insuffi-ciency, cord compression, malnutrition, and bleeding during pregnancy.
- School dropout rates for children with SLD are 40% (or 1.5 times the average).
- Prevalence of specific disorders is difficult to determine because many studies focus on the prevalence of SLD in general.
- Reading disorders are the most common form of SLD.
- *Gender*: From 60% to 80% of children with reading disorders are males; but when stringent criteria are used, the disorder has been found to occur at more equal rates in males and females. Males more often display disruptive behaviors in association with SLD.
- *Family history*: SLD aggregates among family members and 40% of first-degree biological relatives of children with SLD have SLD themselves.
- Demoralization, low self-esteem, and social skill deficits are associated with SLD.
- Inadequate teaching.
- Learning problems are often stressful for family members and can strain relationships.
- Children with SLD are more likely to have disruptive behavior disorders.

Diagnosis

Differential Diagnosis

- Differentiate from normal variations in academic achievement, lack of opportunity, poor teaching, and cultural factors.
- Impaired vision or hearing may affect learning, and the learning disability cannot be due to sensory impairment.
- Intellectual disability.

- ASD.
- Math and written-expression disorders most commonly occur in combination with reading disorders.
- ADHD.
- Rule out substance use as the most common feature of substance abuse is an impairment in psychosocial and academic functioning.

ICD-10 Codes

Specific reading disorder (F81.0)

Mathematics disorder (F81.2)

Disorder of written expression (F81.81)

Developmental disorder of scholastic skills, unspecified (F81.9)

Diagnostic Workup

- Individualized testing reflecting attention to ethnic or cultural background.
- Rule out inadequate teaching and cultural barriers to learning.
- Because standardized group testing is not accurate enough, it is important that special, psychoeducational tests be individually administered to the child to determine whether they have an SLD. In administering the test, give special attention to the child's ethnic and cultural background.
- Commonly used tests include the Wechsler Intelligence Scale for Children (WISC-III), the Woodcock-Johnson Psychoeducational Battery, the Peabody Individual Achievement Test-Revised (PIAT-R), and the California Verbal Learning Test (CVLT).
- Substance use as indicated by assessment.
- Rule out acute infection when problems occur abruptly.

Initial Assessments

- Medical history and physical examination, including hearing and vision tests.
- Psychological assessment to include screening for self-esteem and self-confidence.
- Youth with SLD may also have conduct disorder, ADHD, or depression.
- A complete medical examination is needed to rule out an organic cause of the problem. This may include an eye examination by an ophthalmologist, a psychological examination by a psychologist, and an otolaryngology examination.

Treatment Overview

Behavioral

- Because youth with SLD have higher rates of depression and anxiety and behavior disorders, concurrent treatment for these symptoms must be considered.
- Skill development specific to the child's limitations (e.g., social skills, problem solving, study skills, anger control, and leisure skills).
- SLD is treated with special educational methods and students with SLD frequently benefit from individualized tutoring focusing on their specific learning problem.
- Initial strategies focus on improving a child's recognition of the sounds of letters and language through phonics training. Later strategies focus on comprehension, retention, and study skills. Students with disorders of written expression are often encouraged to keep journals and to write with a computer keyboard instead of a pencil. Instruction for students with mathematical disorders emphasizes real-world uses of arithmetic, such as balancing a checkbook or comparing prices.

- In the academic setting, short, brief assignments with time for feedback, preferential seating, reduced written tasks, support in organization and study skills, untimed tests and assignments, and colored cued materials and techniques.
- Symptoms may occur as early as kindergarten.
- Up to 40% of youth with SLD drop out of school, so chronic counseling, special education services, and other support are often needed.

Recurrence Rate

- SLD can continue into adulthood, but with treatment and special accommodations, symptoms can be decreased.
- Children with undiagnosed SLD or who are improperly treated/educated may never achieve functional literacy. They often develop serious behavior problems as a result of their frustration with school.

Patient Education

- Parents of children with SLD should stay in close contact with educators and school administrators to ensure that their child's IEP undergoes a regular review and continues to provide the maximum educational benefit.
- School evaluations that include observations of the child in class can offer crucial information about coexisting issues.
- Mental health services may be required in addition to special academic services. Issues addressed in counseling children with SLD can include frustration, anxiety related to school performance, poor peer relationships, and depression.

Medical/Legal Issues

- Federal legislation mandates that testing be done free of charge within the public school system. The IDEA guides the actions of school committees on special education in determining the eligibility for special services of students through the age of 21 years.
- Parents may need legal assistance to ensure that their child's needs are met by the school system.

BIBLIOGRAPHY

American Academy of Child and Adolescent Psychiatry. (2007). Practice parameters for the assessment and treatment of children and adolescents with anxiety disorders. *Journal of American Academy of Child and Adolescent Psychiatry, 46*(2), 267–283.

American Psychiatric Association. (2013). *Diagnostic and statistical manual of mental disorder* (5th ed.). Washington, DC: American Psychiatric Publishing.

Barkley, R., & Benton, C. (1998). *Your defiant child.* Guilford Press.

Berninger, V. W., Abbott, R. D., Abbott, S. P., Graham, S., & Richards, T. (2002). Writing and reading: Connections between language by hand and language by eye. *Journal of Learning Disabilities, 35*(1), 39–56.

Biederman, J. (2005). Attention-deficit/hyperactivity disorder: A selective overview. *Biological Psychiatry, 57,* 1215–1220.

Bothe, A. K., Davidow, J. H., Bramlett, R. E., Franic, D. M., & Ingham, R. J. (2006). Stuttering treatment research 1970–2005: II. Systemic review incorporating trial quality assessment of pharmacological approaches. *American Journal of Speech-Language Pathology, 15*(4), 342–352.

Buckner, J. D., Lopez, C., Dunkle, S., & Joiner, T. E. Jr. (2008). Behavior management training for the treatment of reactive attachment disorder. *Child Maltreatment, 13*(3), 289–297.

Carr, E. G., & Herbert, M. R. (2008). Integrating behavioral and biomedical approaches: A marriage made in heaven. *Autism Advocate, 50*(1), 46–52.

Farone, S. V., Perlis, R. H., Doyle, A. E., Smoller, J. W., Goralnick, J. J., Holmgren, M. A., & Sklar, P. (2005). Molecular genetics of attention-deficit/hyperactivity disorder. *Biological Psychiatry, 57,* 1313–1323.

Ferguson-Noyes, N., & Wilkinson, A. M. (2008). *Caring for individuals with ADHD throughout the lifespan: An introduction to ADHD.* Delaware Media Group.

Filipek, P. (2005) Medical aspects of autism. In F. Volkmar, R. Paul, A. Klin, & C. Donald (Eds.), *Handbook of autism and pervasive developmental disorders* (pp. 534–578). Wiley.

Fombonne, E. (2002). Prevalence of childhood disintegrative disorder. *Autism, 6*(2), 149–157.

Hall, S. E. K., & Geher, G. (2003). Behavioral and personality characteristics of children with reactive attachment disorder. *Journal of Psychology, 137*(2), 145–163.

Kearny, C. A., & Vecchio, J. L. (2007). When a child won't speak. *Journal of Family Practice, 56*(11), 917–921.

Kessler, R. C., Adler, L., Barkley, R., Biederman, J., Connors, C. K., Demler, O., Faraone, S. V., Greenhill, L. L., Howes, M. J., Secnik, K., Spencer, T., Ustun, T. B., Walters, E. E., & Zaslavsky, A. M. (2006). The prevalence and correlates of adult ADHD in the United States: Results from the National Comorbidity Survey Replication. *American Journal of Psychiatry, 163*(4), 716–723.

Kristensen, H. (2000). Selective mutism and comorbidity with developmental disorder/delay, anxiety disorder, and elimination disorder. *Journal of the American Academy of Child and Adolescent Psychiatry, 39*(2), 249–256.

MacDonald, H. Z., Beeghly, M., Grant-Knight, W., Augustyn, M., Woods, R. W., Cabral, H., Rose-Jacobs, R., Saxe, G. N., & Frank, D. A. (2008). Longitudinal association between infant disorganized attachment and childhood posttraumatic stress symptoms. *Developmental Psychopathology, 20*(2), 493–508.

Muter, V., & Snowling, M. J. (2009). Children at familial risk of dyslexia: Practical implications for an at-risk study. *Children and Adolescent Mental Health, 14*(1), 37–41.

Sadock, B., Sadock, V., & Ruiz, P. (2015). *Kaplan & Sadock's synopsis of psychiatry* (11th ed.). Wolters Kluwer.

Sakolsky, D., & Birmaher, B. (2008). Pediatric anxiety disorders: Management in primary care. *Current Opinion in Pediatrics, 20*(5), 538–543.

Silverman, W. K., & Dick-Niederhauser, A. (2004). Separation anxiety disorder. In T. L. Morris & J. S. March (Eds.), *Anxiety disorders in children and adolescents* (2nd ed., pp. 212–240). Guilford Press.

Silverman, W. K., & Ollendick, T. H. (2005). Evidence-based assessment of anxiety and its disorders in childhood. *Journal of Clinical Child and Adolescent Psychology, 34*(3), 380–411.

Seida, J. K., Ospina, M. B., Karkhaneh, M., Hartling, L., Smith, V., & Clark, B. (2009). Systematic reviews of psychosocial interventions for autism: an umbrella review. *Developmental Medicine and Child Neurology, 51*(2), 95–104.

Swiezy, N., & Korzekwa, P. (2008). Bridging for success in autism: Training and collaboration across medical, educational, and community systems. *Child and Adolescent Psychiatric Clinics of North America, 17*(4), 907–922, xi, Review.

Tusaie, K., & Fitzpatrick, J. (2017). *Advanced practice psychiatric nursing* (2nd ed.). Springer Publishing Company.

Wheeler, K. (2014). *Psychotherapy for the advanced practice psychiatric nurse* (2nd ed.). Springer Publishing Company.

Wiener, J., & Dulcan, M. (2004). *Textbook of child and adolescent psychiatry* (3rd ed.). American Psychiatric Publishing.

Ziegler, J. C., Castel, D., Georget-Pech, C., George, F., Alario, F. X., & Perry C. (2008). Developmental dyslexia and the dual role model of reading: Simulating individual differences and subtypes. *Cognition, 107*, 151–178.

WEB RESOURCES

- American Academy of Child and Adolescent Psychiatry: http://www.aacap.org/
- American Association on Intellectual and Developmental Disabilities (AAIDD) for professionals: http://www.aaidd.org/
- American Psychiatric Association: http://www.psych.org/
- American Speech-Language-Hearing Association: http://www.asha.org/
- Anxiety Disorders Association of America (ADAA): http://www.adaa.org/
- ARC of the United States: http://www.thearc.org/
- Association for the Treatment and Training in the Attachment of children: http://www.ATTACh.org/
- Autism Society of America: www.autism-society.org/
- CHADD (Children and Adults with Attention Deficit Hyperactivity Disorder): http://www.chadd.org/
- International Dyslexia Association: http://www.interdys.org/
- National Alliance on Mental Illness: http://www.nami.org/
- National Autism Association: http://www.nationalautismassociation.org/
- Selective Mutism Foundation Inc.: http://www.selectivemutismfoundation.org/

PART TWO

Psychopharmacological Drug Monographs

This part includes drug monographs for common drug therapies. Note that not every drug within a classification is included. For some drugs, off-label use is reported. It is the responsibility of the clinician to evaluate the efficacy of such use. It is also the responsibility of the clinician to carefully review the package inserts accompanying each drug and check whether the dosage schedules therein or the contraindications stated by the manufacturer differ from the statements made in this book. Such examination is particularly important with drugs that either are rarely used or have been newly released on the market.

20

Drug Monographs

ACAMPROSATE (Campral)

Classification
Gamma-aminobutyric acid (GABA) Taurine Analog

Indications
Used to treat alcohol dependence, dependence, and withdrawal syndrome. Campral does not eliminate or diminish alcohol withdrawal symptoms.

Available Forms
Tablet (extended-release [XR]), 333 mg

Dosage
- *Adults*: 666 mg TID; begin therapy during abstinence; continue during relapse; CrCl 30 to 50 mL/min: maximum 333 mg TID; CrCl < 30 mL/min; contraindicated.
- *Children younger than 18 years*: not recommended.

Administration
- Do not crush, chew, or break a delayed-release tablet. Swallow the tablet whole.
- Take with or without food.
- Take medication for the full prescribed length of time, even in relapse.
- Store at room temperature away from moisture and heat.

Side Effects
- *Central nervous system*: amnesia, dizziness, headache, paresthesia, somnolence, syncope, taste perversion, tremor.
- *Cardiovascular*: chest pain, hypertension (HTN), palpitations, peripheral edema, vasodilation.
- *Dermatological*: pruritus, maculopapular rash, rash, sweating.
- *Eyes, ears, nose, throat* (EENT): abnormal vision.
- *Gastrointestinal*: diarrhea, abdominal pain, constipation, dry mouth, dyspepsia, flatulence, nausea, vomiting.

- *Genitourinary*: frigidity, impotence.
- *Hematological*: anemia, eosinophilia, lymphocytosis, thrombocytopenia.
- *Hepatic*: uncommon—alanine aminotransferase (ALT) increased, aspartate aminotransferase (AST) increased, bilirubinemia, hepatitis, liver cirrhosis, liver function tests abnormal.
- *Hypersensitivity*: allergic reaction.
- *Immunological*: flu syndrome, infection.
- *Metabolic*: anorexia, increased appetite, weight gain.
- *Musculoskeletal*: arthralgia, back pain, myalgia.
- *Psychiatric*: abnormal thinking, anxiety, depression, insomnia, libido decreased, suicide attempt.
- *Renal*: creatinine increased, kidney calculus.
- *Respiratory*: bronchitis, cough increased, dyspnea, pharyngitis, rhinitis.

Drug Interactions
- Acamprosate does not affect the pharmacokinetics of alcohol. The pharmacokinetics of acamprosate are not affected by alcohol, diazepam, or disulfiram, and clinically important interactions between naltrexone and acamprosate were not observed.
- See manufacturing label for full list of interactions.

Pharmacokinetics
- *Metabolism*: nil
- *Half-life*: 20 to 33 hours
- Renal excretion

Precautions
- Contraindicated in patients who previously have exhibited hypersensitivity to acamprosate calcium or any of its components.
- Contraindicated in patients with severe renal impairment (creatinine clearance [CrCl] of ≤30 mL/min).
- In controlled clinical trials of Campral, adverse events of a suicidal nature (suicidal ideation, suicide attempts, completed suicides) were infrequent overall but were more common in Campral-treated patients than in patients treated with placebo (1.4% vs. 0.5% in studies of 6 months or less; 2.4% vs. 0.8% in year-long studies). Completed suicides occurred in 3 of 2,272 (0.13%) patients in the pooled acamprosate group from all controlled studies and 2 of 1,962 patients (0.10%) in the placebo group. Adverse events coded as "depression" were reported at similar rates in Campral-treated and placebo-treated patients. Although many of these events occurred in the context of alcohol relapse, and the interrelationship between alcohol dependence, depression, and suicidality is well recognized and complex, no consistent pattern of relationship between the clinical course of recovery from alcoholism and the emergence of suicidality was identified. Alcohol-dependent patients, including those patients being treated with Campral, should be monitored for the development of symptoms of depression or suicidal thinking. Families and caregivers of patients being treated with Campral should be alerted to the need to monitor patients for the emergence of symptoms of depression or suicidality and to report such symptoms to the patient's healthcare provider.

Patient and Family Education
- Remind patients that Campral will not treat or prevent alcohol withdrawal symptoms.
- Advise patients to alert clinician to any thoughts of suicide.

Special Populations

- *Pregnancy*: category C. There are no adequate and well-controlled studies in pregnant women. Campral should be used during pregnancy only if the potential benefit justifies the potential risk to the fetus.
- *Pediatric*: not for use in children.
- *Older adults*: This drug is known to be substantially excreted by the kidney, and the risk of toxic reactions to this drug may be greater in patients with impaired renal function. Because older adult patients are more likely to have decreased renal function, care should be taken in dose selection, and it may be useful to monitor renal function.

ALPRAZOLAM (Xanax/Xanax Xr/Niravam; Also Apo-Alpraz, Apo-Alpraz Ts, Novo-Alprazol, Nu-Alpraz)

Classification
Benzodiazepine (BZD), anxiolytic

Indications
Short-acting BZD is used to treat generalized anxiety disorder (GAD) and panic disorder. It may be used as a short-term adjunct to a selective serotonin reuptake inhibitor (SSRI) while waiting for the therapeutic effects of the SSRI to develop.

Available Forms
Tablet, 0.25, 0.5, 1, and 2 mg; orally disintegrating tablets (ODTs), 0.25, 0.5, 1, 2, and 3 mg; XR capsule, 0.5, 1, and 2 mg; melt, 0.25, 0.5, 1, 2, and 3 mg.

Dosage
- *Xanax*: starting dose, 0.25 to 0.5 mg up to 2 to 3 times daily; maximum, 4 mg daily. It can be increased every 3 to 4 days. Treatment should be limited to as short a period as possible (<4 months) and/or reevaluated for continued use.
- *Xanax XR*: starting dose, 0.5 to 1 mg PO, daily. Increase at intervals of at least 3 to 4 days by up to 1 mg/d. Taper no faster than 0.5 mg every 3 days; maximum 10 mg/d. When switching from immediate-release alprazolam, give total daily dose of immediate-release once daily.
- *Niravam* (*melt*): starting dose, 0.25 to 0.5 mg up to 2 to 3 times daily; maximum, 4 mg daily; may titrate every 3 to 4 days; maximum 4 mg/d.

Administration
- PO with a glass of water.
- Do not crush, cut, or chew XR tablets.
- Orally disintegrating form (*Niravam*) has special instructions.

Side Effects
- Drowsiness, light-headedness, dry mouth, headache, changes in bowel habits, diarrhea, amnesia, changes in appetite, changes in sexual desire, constipation, increased saliva production, tiredness, trouble concentrating, unsteadiness, and weight changes.
- Some other side effects are syncope, tachycardia, seizures, respiratory depression, dependency, withdrawal syndrome, suicidal ideation, and hypomania/mania.

Drug Interactions
- Contraindicated in patients with known sensitivity to this drug or other benzylpiperazines (BZPs).
- Avoid grapefruit juice when using this drug.
- It may be used in patients with open-angle glaucoma who are receiving appropriate therapy but is contraindicated in patients with acute narrow-angle glaucoma.
- This is contraindicated with ketoconazole and itraconazole, as these medications significantly impair the oxidative metabolism mediated by cytochrome P450 3A (CYP3A).

Pharmacokinetics

The drug metabolizes in the liver (CYP450) and is excreted in the urine. It binds to BZP receptors and enhances GABA effects.

BZDs enhance the activity of GABA, a major CNS neurotransmitter, known to open central nervous system (CNS) Cl-channels, leading to an inhibition of subsequent CNS neuronal signaling. BZDs with similar action can differ in their potency and rate of absorption.

- *Metabolism*: by the liver in the CYP450 3A4.
- *Excretion*: urine.
- *Peak*: 1 to 2 hours.
- *Half-life*: Xanax half-life-immediate release: 11.2 hours; XR: 10.7 to 15.8 hours; 13 hours for oral disintegrating tablets.

Precautions

- Do not abruptly stop taking the medication.
- It is not prescribed for children.
- Use lowest effective dose for shortest duration.
- It can be habit forming; do not increase dosage without checking patient compliance and review of chief complaints.
- Keep out of light in a tightly closed container.
- Store securely at room temperature.
- See patients as often as necessary to ensure that the drug is working on the panic attacks, determine compliance, and review side effects.
- Instruct patients and their families to watch for worsening depression or thoughts of suicide. Also, watch out for sudden or severe changes in feelings, such as feeling anxious, agitated, panicky, irritated, hostile, aggressive, impulsive, severely restless, overly excited, hyperactive, or not being able to sleep. If this happens, especially at the beginning of antidepressant treatment or after a change in dose, patient should call the healthcare provider.
- *Drowsiness or dizziness*: Patients should not drive or use machinery or do anything that needs mental alertness until the effects of this medicine are known.
- Caution patients not to stand or sit up quickly, especially if older. This reduces the risk of dizziness or fainting spells. Alcohol may interfere with the effect of this medicine. Avoid alcoholic drinks.
- Do not abruptly withdraw this drug as it may cause seizures.
- Caution should be exercised in the following:
  - Major depressive disorder (MDD), psychosis, or bipolar affective disorder
  - Respiratory disease
  - Sleep apnea
  - Heart disease
  - Liver disease
  - Seizures (convulsions)
  - Suicidal thoughts, plans, or attempts by patients or a family member
  - An unusual or allergic reaction to alprazolam, other medicines, foods, dyes, or preservatives

Patient and Family Education

- Tell the healthcare provider of glaucoma, hepatic or renal impairment, drug-abuse history, salivary flow decrease (interferes with ODT absorption), or pregnancy.
- Missed doses should be taken as soon as possible; however, if it is too close to the next dose, then it should be skipped.

- Take the medicine as prescribed and do not stop it abruptly, without first discussing with healthcare provider.
- Store alprazolam at room temperature away from moisture, heat, and light. Remove any cotton from the bottle of disintegrating tablets, and keep the bottle tightly closed. Discard liquid 90 days after first opening.
- Before taking this medicine, tell the healthcare provider of medical history of liver disease, kidney disease, lung/breathing problems, drug or alcohol abuse, or any allergies.
- Do not drive, operate heavy machinery, or perform dangerous activities until it is known how this medicine will exert its effects.
- This drug may be habit forming and should be used only by the person for whom it was prescribed. Alprazolam should never be shared with another person, especially someone who has a history of drug abuse or addiction. Keep the medication in a secure place where others cannot get to it.

Special Populations

- *Older adults*: Older patients may be more sensitive to the effects of BZDs. Give 0.25 mg PO BID or TID. Use lowest, most effective dose. Dose adjustment is necessary for patients with liver impairment and/or renal disease due to excessive metabolites excreted by the kidney. Due to increased risk of sedation leading to falls and fractures, all BZDs are included on the Beers List of Potentially Inappropriate Medications for Geriatrics.
- *Renal impairment*: No adjustment needed.
- *Hepatic impairment*: With advanced hepatic disease, start at 0.25 mg PO BID or TID and titrate gradually.
- *Pregnancy*: category D; can cause teratogenic fetal effects. Infants born to mothers taking BZDs may be at risk for withdrawal symptoms contraindicated in the postnatal period.
- *Lactation*: excreted in human breast milk; infants can become lethargic and lose weight.
- *Children*: not indicated for use in children younger than 18 years of age.

ALPROSTADIL (Caverject, Caverject Impulse, EDEX)

Classification
Phosphodiesterase type 5 (PDE5) inhibitor, CGMP specific

Indications
Used to treat erectile dysfunction.

Available Forms
Cartridge, 10, 20, and 40 mcg (2 cartridge starter and refill packs); syringe, 5, 10, 20, and 40 mcg (4/pck); vial, 5, 10, 20, and 40 mcg/vial (powder for reconstitution w. diluent); vial: 5, 10, 20, and 40 mcg/vial (6/pck).

Dosage
- Inject over 5 to 10 seconds into the dorsal lateral aspect of the proximal third of the penis; avoid visible veins; rotate injection sites and sides; if no initial response, may give next higher dose within 1 hour; if partial response, give next higher dose after 24 hours; maximum 60 mcg and 3 self-injections/week; allow at least 24 hours between doses; reduce dose if erection lasts >1 hour.

Administration
- Clinician should instruct patient on how to use the urethral suppository.
- Wash hands before and after use.
- Store at room temperature away from moisture, heat, and light.
- Medication most effective if urine is passed before using.
- Keep pellets in their original foil pouch in the refrigerator. Store pouch at cool room temperature for up to 14 days. Protect from freezing or extreme heat. Do not store in a closed automobile or in luggage while traveling.
- Store injection vials at cool room temperature. The 40-mcg strength should be used within 3 months or before the expiration date on the label.
- After mixing a Caverject injection, keep it at room temperature and use within 24 hours.

Side Effects
- Side effects include bleeding and pain at the injection site, (short-term) painful erection, headache, flushing, nasal congestion, rhinitis, dyspepsia, and diarrhea.
- *Serious*: curving of penis with pain during erection, erection continuing for 4 to 6 hours, erection continuing longer than 6 hours with severe and continuing pain of the penis, swelling in or pain of the testes; heart attack symptoms—chest pain or pressure, pain spreading to jaw or shoulder, nausea, sweating, vision changes or sudden vision loss; ringing in ears or sudden hearing loss; pain, swelling, warmth, or redness in one or both legs; shortness of breath; swelling in hands or feet; light-headed feeling; erection that is painful or lasts 4 hours or longer.

Drug Interactions
- Contraindicated in patients with a known hypersensitivity to alprostadil or any component of the medication.
- Contraindicated in men with anatomical deformation or fibrotic conditions of the penis (e.g., angulation, cavernosal fibrosis, or Peyronie disease) or penile implants.

Pharmacokinetics

- *Metabolism*: IV: ~70% to 80% by oxidation during a single pass through the lungs; metabolite is active and has been identified in neonates.
- *Half-life*: 30 seconds to 10 minutes.
- *Excretion*: primarily urine (90% as metabolites) within 24 hours.

Precautions

- There is a potential for cardiac risk during sexual activity in patients with preexisting cardiovascular (CV) disease. Contraindicated in patients for whom sexual activity is inadvisable because of their underlying CV status. Due to system vasodilatory properties, it is not recommended for patients who have underlying CV status.
- Intracavernous injections can increase peripheral blood levels of alprostadil, resulting in hypotension. Syncope has also been reported. Avoid use in men with known cavernosal venous leakage. Patients must be cautioned to avoid tasks such as operating machinery or driving following administration where injury could result if hypotension or syncope were to occur.
- Discontinue use in men who develop penile angulation or cavernosal fibrosis.
- Contraindicated in men who have conditions that predispose them to priapism.
- *Muse*: Urethral abrasion resulting in minor bleeding or spotting may occur from improper administration.
- *Caverject and Caverject Impulse*: A superfine needle is used for administration. Needle breakage (a portion of the needle remaining in the penis) has been reported; hospitalization and surgical removal may be necessary.

Patient and Family Education

- Advise patients to not use more than two pellets per day. Do not use more than 3 injections per week. Wait at least 24 hours between each injection.
- Advise patients to prepare an injection only when ready to give it. Do not use if the medicine looks cloudy, has changed colors, or has particles in it.
- Remind patients to use a needle and syringe only once and place them in a puncture-proof "sharps" container. Follow state or local laws about how to dispose of this container. Keep it out of the reach of children and pets.
- Remind patients to call the clinician if a needle breaks during injection. If patient is able to grasp the broken end, they should remove the needle right away.
- Advise patients on proper storage and administration.

AMITRIPTYLINE (Elavil)

Classification
Tricyclic antidepressant (TCA)

Indications
The drug is used to treat adults with depression. It has been used off label for anxiety disorders, post-herpetic neuralgia, prevention of chronic headache, prevention of migraine, and fibromyalgia.

Available Forms
Tablet, 10, 25, 50, 75, 100, and 150 mg.

Dosage
- *Adults and adolescents*: between 25 and 75 mg PO at bedtime. Dosage can be increased by 25 to 50 mg/d every week up to 200 mg until desired effect occurs. Maximum daily dose for hospitalized patients is 300 mg.
- *Older adults*: starting dose, 10 to 25 mg PO at night in older adult patients; dosage can be increased by 10 to 25 mg/d every week. Maximum daily dose is 150 mg/d.
- *Children (9–12 years old)*: not recommended.

Administration
- PO with a glass of water.
- Do not abruptly stop taking the medication.
- Use lowest effective dose for shortest duration.

Side Effects
- *Most common*: drowsiness, dry mouth, dizziness, constipation, blurred vision, palpitations, tachycardia, lack of coordination, appetite increase, nausea/vomiting, sweating, weakness, disorientation, confusion, restlessness, insomnia, anxiety/agitation, urinary retention/urinary frequency, rash/urticaria, pruritus, weight gain, libido changes, impotence, gynecomastia, galactorrhea, tremor, hypo/hyperglycemia, paresthesias, and photosensitivity.
- *Less common*: HTN or orthostatic hypotension, ventricular arrhythmias, extrapyramidal symptoms (EPS), thrombocytopenia.

Drug Interactions
- Coadministration of TCAs with SSRIs requires extreme caution.
- There are many drugs that may interact with amitriptyline.
- Some of the most common drugs that react with amitriptyline are arbutamine, disulfiram, levodopa, thyroid supplements, and other drugs that can cause bleeding/bruising (including antiplatelet drugs such as clopidogrel, [NSAIDs]) such as ibuprofen, "blood thinners" such as warfarin), anticholinergic drugs (such as benztropine, belladonna alkaloids), some antihypertensive drugs such as clonidine, guanabenz, reserpine.
- Avoid taking monoamine oxidase inhibitors (MAOIs) (isocarboxazid, linezolid, methylene blue, moclobemide, phenelzine, procarbazine, rasagiline, selegiline,

tranylcypromine) within 2 weeks before, during, and after treatment with this medication.

- Avoid cimetidine, fluconazole, terbinafine, drugs to treat irregular heart rate (such as quinidine/propafenone/flecainide), and antidepressants (such as SSRIs, including paroxetine/fluoxetine/fluvoxamine). These drugs can affect the removal of amitriptyline from the body, thereby affecting how amitriptyline works.
- Many drugs besides amitriptyline may affect the heart rhythm (QT prolongation in the EKG), including amiodarone, cisapride, dofetilide, pimozide, procainamide, quinidine, sotalol, macrolide antibiotics (such as erythromycin), among others.
- Avoid drugs that may cause drowsiness, such as alcohol, antihistamines (such as cetirizine, diphenhydramine), drugs for sleep or anxiety (such as alprazolam, diazepam, zolpidem), muscle relaxants, and narcotic pain relievers (such as codeine).
- Seizure risk may increase when amitriptyline is combined with isoniazid (INH), phenothiazines (such as thioridazine), theophylline, or TCAs (such as nortriptyline), among others.

Pharmacokinetics

- TCAs are thought to work by inhibiting reuptake of norepinephrine and serotonin in the CNS, which potentiates the neurotransmitters. They also have significant anticholinergics, antihistaminic, and alpha-adrenergic activity on the cardiac system. These classes of antidepressants also possess class 1A antiarrhythmic activity, which can lead to depression of cardiac conduction, potentially resulting in heart block or ventricular arrhythmias.
- *Metabolism*: extensively by the liver within the CYP450: 1A2, 2D6 (primary), 3A4 substrate; active metabolites include nortriptyline.
- *Peak*: 2 to 12 hours.
- *Excretion*: Primarily in urine (18% unchanged), feces.
- *Half-life*: 10 to 50 hours (amitriptyline).

Precautions

- See patients as often as necessary to ensure that the drug is working on the panic attacks, determine compliance, and review side effects.
- Instruct patients and families to watch for worsening depression or thoughts of suicide. Also, watch out for sudden or severe changes in feelings, such as feeling anxious, agitated, panicky, irritated, hostile, aggressive, impulsive, severely restless, overly excited, hyperactive, or not being able to sleep. If this happens, especially at the beginning of antidepressant treatment or after a change in dose, the patient should call the healthcare provider.
- *Drowsiness or dizziness*: Patients should not drive, use machinery, or do anything that needs mental alertness until the effects of this medicine are known. Caution patients not to stand or sit up quickly, especially if older. This reduces the risk of dizziness or fainting spells. Alcohol may interfere with the effect of this medicine. Avoid alcoholic drinks.
- Do not abruptly withdraw this drug, as it may cause headache, nausea, and malaise.
- Advise to protect skin from ultraviolet light due to increased skin sensitivity.
- Grapefruit and grapefruit juice may interact with drug. Caution should be exercised in the following:
  - MDD, psychosis, or bipolar affective disorder
  - Contraindicated in patients with a recent myocardial infarction

- Blood dyscrasias
- Respiratory disease
- Heart disease
- Liver disease, diabetes mellitus, asthma, and increased intracranial pressure
- Seizures (convulsions)
- Suicidal thoughts, plans, or attempts by patients or a family member

Patient and Family Education

- Do not stop taking this medicine without notifying the healthcare provider.
- Notify doctor or pharmacist promptly if any of these effects persist or worsen.
- To relieve dry mouth, suck on (sugarless) hard candy or ice chips, chew (sugarless) gum, drink water, or use a saliva substitute.
- To prevent constipation, maintain a diet adequate in fiber, drink plenty of water, and exercise. In case of constipation, consult pharmacist for help in selecting a laxative (e.g., stimulant type with stool softener).
- Inform clinician immediately if any of these unlikely but serious side effects occur: mental/mood changes (e.g., confusion, depression, hallucinations, memory problems), enlarged/painful breasts, unwanted breast milk production, irregular/painful menstrual periods, muscle stiffness/twitching, feelings of restlessness, ringing in the ears, sexual problems (e.g., decreased sexual ability, changes in desire), shakiness (tremors), numbness/tingling of the hands/feet, trouble urinating, and severe vomiting.
- Inform clinician immediately if any of these rare but very serious side effects occur: easy bruising/bleeding, signs of infection (e.g., fever, persistent sore throat), unusual/uncontrolled movements (especially of the tongue/face/lips), severe stomach/abdominal pain, dark urine, and yellowing of eyes/skin.
- Seek immediate medical attention if any of these rare but very serious side effects occur: black stools, chest pain, fainting, high fever, slow/fast/irregular heartbeat, seizures, vomit that looks like coffee grounds.
- Store amitriptyline at room temperature away from moisture and heat.
- Stopping this medication suddenly could result in unpleasant side effects.
- Take the missed dose as soon as remembered. If it is almost time for the next dose, skip the missed dose and take the medicine at the next regularly scheduled time. *Do not* take extra medicine to make up the missed dose.

Special Populations

- *Older adults*: Older adult patients may need a reduced dose for they may be more sensitive to usual dosages. For older adult patients, 10 to 25 mg each day with increases of 10 to 25 mg at bedtime every 2 to 3 days may be sufficient. Amitriptyline is included in the Beers List of Potentially Inappropriate Medications for Geriatrics.
- *Renal impairment*: Use with caution when renal impairment is suspected. Confer with renal specialist.
- *Hepatic impairment*: Dosing in the presence of hepatic dysfunction is not given; caution is advised; strong anticholinergic properties; lower dosage initially and cautious titration recommended.
- *Pregnancy*: Safety has not been established. Use with category C caution.
- *Lactation*: Excreted in human breast milk.
- *Children*: Monitor closely for suicidal ideation with children, adolescents, and young adults with major depressive or other psychiatric conditions. Not recommended in children under 12 years.

ARIPIPRAZOLE (Abilify, Abilify Discmelt, Abilify Maintena)

Classification
Second-generation (atypical) antipsychotic, quinolone derivative

Indications
Schizophrenia (13 years and older), manic and mixed episodes associated with bipolar I disorder, adjunctive treatment to antidepressants for MDD, agitation associated with schizophrenia or bipolar disorder, manic or mixed.

Available Forms
Tablet, 2, 5, 10, 15, 20, and 30 mg; ODT, 15 mg; vial, 300, 400 mg XR powder for intramuscular (IM) injection after reconstitution; 300, 400 mg single-dose prefilled dual-chamber syringes.

Dosage
- Initially 15 mg once daily; may increase to maximum 30 mg/d.
- IM 9.75 mg as a single dose (range: 5.25–15 mg). Repeated doses may be given with or without food.
- Parenteral administration is intended for IM use only at >2-hour intervals to maximum of 30 mg/d.
- Maintain IM once monthly at 300 or 400 mg. This preparation needs a 14-day overlapping oral antipsychotic treatment for first dose.
- Not indicated for children under age 10 years.
- Ten to 17 years and older: initially 2 mg/d in a single dose for 2 days; then increase to 5 mg/d in a single dose for 2 days; then increase to target dose of 10 mg/d in a single dose; may increase by 5 mg/d at weekly intervals as needed to maximum 30 mg/d.

Administration
- IM or PO; do not administer IV or SC; inject slowly, deep into muscle mass.
- *IM injection has not been evaluated in children.*
- Oral solution may be substituted for tablets on a mg-per-mg basis up to a 25-mg dose. Patients receiving 30-mg tablets should receive 25 mg of solution.
- Dosing for the ODT is the same as the oral tablet.
- Do not open the ODTs until ready to administer. The ODT should be taken without liquid. Do not split the ODT.
- Use oral aripiprazole 10 to 30 mg/d instead of IM aripiprazole as soon as possible if ongoing therapy is indicated.

Side Effects
Nausea, vomiting, dizziness, insomnia, akathisia, activation, headache, asthenia, sedation, constipation, orthostatic hypotension (occasionally during initial phase), increased risk of death and cerebrovascular events in older adults with dementia-related psychosis, tardive dyskinesia (TD), neuroleptic malignant syndrome (NMS) (rare), seizures (rare), metabolic syndrome, corrected QT interval (QTc) prolongation, suicide risk increase, bradycardia.

Drug Interactions
Major substrate of CYP450 3A4, CYP2D6, and CYP3A4. Caution with other CYP2D6 inhibitors (e.g., nefazodone, fluvoxamine, fluoxetine) and CYP450 2D6 or CYP3A4

inhibitors. Avoid with metoclopramide (e.g., paroxetine, fluoxetine, duloxetine) and quinidine. It may increase plasma levels of aripiprazole.

- Carbamazepine and other CYP450 3A4 inducers may decrease plasma levels of aripiprazole.
- Aripiprazole may enhance effects of antihypertensive medications by causing orthostatic hypotension.
- Aripiprazole may antagonize levodopa and dopamine agonists.
- *Alert*: This list may not describe all possible interactions. Instruct clients to provide a list of all medicines, herbs, nonprescription drugs, or dietary supplements they use.

Pharmacokinetics

- *Excretion*: About 25% of a single oral dose is excreted in urine (<1% unchanged) and 55% is excreted in feces (18% as unchanged drug).
- *Metabolism*: It is primarily metabolized by CYP450 2D6 and CYP450 3A4. Hepatic 50% to 60% glucuronidation.
- *Absorption*: IM, 100%; PO, 87%.
- *Onset*: IM, 1 hour; PO, 1 to 3 weeks.
- *Peak*: IM, 1 to 3 hours; PO, 3 to 5 hours.
- *Duration*: 2 hours for injectable.
- *Half-life*: 75 hours (aripiprazole) and 94 hours (active aripiprazole metabolite).

Precautions

- CV disease; dementia.
- Dysphagia is associated with use of aripiprazole. Use with caution in patients who are at risk for aspiration pneumonia.
- Use with caution in patients with conditions that may develop hypotension (dehydration, overheating, etc.).
- Do not use in patients who are allergic to aripiprazole, seizures; Parkinson's disease; sedation.

Patient and Family Education

- Store aripiprazole at 59°F to 86°F (15° C to 30° C). It can be used for up to 6 months after opening. Protect injection from light by storing in carton until use.
- Same precautions are to be taken for neonates as with other antipsychotics.
- If client becomes pregnant, contact provider. Discuss with provider if you have any of these conditions. A dose adjustment or special tests to safely take aripiprazole may be needed:
  - Liver or kidney disease
  - Heart disease, high blood pressure (BP), heart rhythm problems
  - History of heart attack or stroke
  - History of low white blood cell (WBC) counts
  - History of breast cancer
  - Seizures or epilepsy
  - A personal or family history of diabetes
  - Trouble swallowing
- Client should be encouraged to talk to provider if they have signs of hyperglycemia, such as increased thirst or urination, excessive hunger, or weakness. If they have diabetes, check blood sugar levels on a regular basis while taking aripiprazole.
- *Avoid alcohol*: Maintain adequate hydration; caution when changing position from lying to sitting.

Special Populations

There is a black box warning (BBW) for use with older adults with dementia with psychosis.

- *Older adults*: Dosage adjustment is generally not required. Older adults with dementia-related psychosis treated with atypical antipsychotics are at higher risk for death and cerebrovascular events.
- *Renal impairment*: No dosage adjustment is needed.
- *Hepatic impairment*: No dosage adjustment is required.
- *Cardiac impairment*: Use with caution because of the risk of orthostatic hypotension.
- *Lactation*: Although there are no data on the excretion of aripiprazole into human milk, it is suggested that women receiving aripiprazole should not breastfeed.
- *Children and adolescents*: approved for schizophrenia (age 13 years and older) and manic/mixed episodes (age 10 years and older). It should be monitored more frequently than adults. Children may tolerate lower doses better.
- *Pregnancy*: category C.

ARMODAFINIL (Nuvigil)

Classification
Central nervous system (CNS) stimulant

Indications
It is *used* primarily to treat sleep disorders that result in excessive sleepiness, such as narcolepsy, obstructive sleep apnea, hypopnea syndrome, and shift work sleep disorder.

Available Forms
Tablet, 50, 150, and 250 mg

Dosage
- *Narcolepsy/obstructive sleep apnea (adults and children 17 years and older)*: PO, 150 or 250 mg as a single dose in the morning.
- *Shift work sleep disorder (adults and children 17 years and older)*: PO, 150 mg daily approximately 1 hour prior to the start of work shift.
- *Pediatric*: Younger than 17 years, not recommended; ≥17 years, same dosage as adult.
- *Older adults*: PO, consider using lower doses.
- *Hepatic function impairment*: PO, reduce dose in severe hepatic impairment.

Administration
- PO with a glass of water. Take in morning to get maximum effects during waking hours and to avoid sleep later in the evening.
- Take without food.

Side Effects
Palpitations, increased heart rate, headache, insomnia, dizziness, anxiety, depression, fatigue, agitation, attention disturbance, depressed mood, migraine, nervousness, paresthesia, tremor, rash, contact dermatitis, hyperhidrosis nausea, dry mouth, diarrhea, dyspepsia, upper abdominal pain, anorexia, constipation, decreased appetite, loose stools, vomiting, increased gamma-glutamyl transferase (GGT), increased alkaline phosphatase, dyspnea, influenza-like illness, pain, polyuria, pyrexia, seasonal allergy, and thirst.

Drug Interactions
- Avoid concomitant use with alcohol.
- When used with dextroamphetamine/methylphenidate, absorption may be delayed approximately 1 hour; the same effect may be applicable to armodafinil.
- Drugs metabolized by CYP2C19 (e.g., clomipramine, diazepam, midazolam, omeprazole, phenytoin, propranolol, triazolam) for plasma concentration may be elevated by armodafinil, increasing the risk of adverse reactions.
- Drugs metabolized by CYP3A4/5 (e.g., cyclosporine, ethinyl estradiol, midazolam, triazolam) for plasma concentrations may be reduced by armodafinil, decreasing efficacy.
- Food may delay the armodafinil T_{max} by approximately 2 to 4 hours. Because the delay in T_{max} is associated with elevated plasma concentrations later in time, food can potentially affect the onset and time course of the pharmacological action of armodafinil.

- The efficacy of hormonal contraceptives may be reduced during and for 1 month after armodafinil coadministration. Use of alternative or concomitant methods of contraception is recommended during and for 1 month after coadministration with armodafinil.
- Use caution when administering MAOIs and armodafinil.
- Potent inducers of CYP3A4/5 (e.g., carbamazepine, phenobarbital, rifampin) may reduce drug efficacy.
- Potent inhibitors of CYP3A4/5 (e.g., erythromycin, ketoconazole) may increase drug concentration, increasing the risk of adverse reactions.
- Possible decrease in armodafinil levels due to prazosin; larger doses of armodafinil may be needed.
- A pharmacodynamic interaction cannot be ruled out. Monitor prothrombin time (PT) and international normalized ratio (INR) more frequently when armodafinil is administered with warfarin.

Pharmacokinetics

- This medicine is a stimulant; the exact mechanism of action is unknown. It is believed to have similar wake-promoting actions as sympathomimetic agents.
- There is rapid absorption in absence of food.
- Peak plasma levels are reached in 2 hours in the fasted state: food delays peak plasma concentrations by 2 to 4 hours.
- Steady state reached within 7 days of dosing.
- *Excretion*: urine 80%.
- *Half-life*: Average is 15 hours once steady state is reached.

Precautions

- See client as often as necessary to ensure drug is promoting wakefulness, determine compliance, and review side effects.
- Advise patient to report any new rashes immediately.
- Discontinue drug immediately if any rash is reported.
- Advise patient of risk for transient psychosis-like symptoms (ideas of reference, paranoid delusions, and auditory hallucinations).
- May experience transient palpitations and EKG changes.
- Avoid using in clients with left ventricular hypertrophy or mitral valve prolapsed.

Patient and Family Education

- Do not operate heavy machinery or equipment until reasonably certain that drug will not affect ability to engage in such activities.
- Discontinue medication immediately if a rash is noted and follow up with provider.
- Patients may experience palpitations.
- Have patient monitor BP at home and notify provider of persistent BP elevations.
- Store securely at room temperature between 20°C and 25°C (68°F and 77°F).

Special Populations

- *Older adults*: Clearance has been reduced in older adults. Use lowest effective dose. Safety in those above the age of 65 years has not studied.
- *Hepatic impairment*: Modify dosage by one-half accordingly.
- *Pregnancy*: category C.
- *Lactation*: No human studies have been performed. The medicine is not recommended in breastfeeding mothers.
- *Children*: This medicine is not for use in pediatric patients.

ASENAPINE (Saphris)

Classification
Dopamine and serotonin antagonist; antipsychotic drug, atypical (second generation)

Indications
Schizophrenia, manic or mixed episodes associated with bipolar I disorder as monotherapy or as adjunctive therapy with either lithium or valproate.

Available Forms
Sublingual tablets, 5 and 10 mg.

Dosage
Initial dose, 5 mg BID; after 1 week may increase to 10 mg BID. Can decrease back to 5 mg BID based on tolerability.

Administration
- The drug comes in tablet form. Place the tablet under the tongue and allow to dissolve completely.
- The tablet dissolves within seconds.
- Do not eat or drink anything for 10 to 30 minutes after administration.
- Tablets should not be crushed, chewed, or swallowed.

Side Effects
Akathisia, oral hypoesthesia (numbness); somnolence; dizziness; other EPS excluding akathisia; weight gain; insomnia; headache; may induce orthostatic hypotension and syncope in some patients, especially early in treatment; rare NMS (rare); TD (rare); and metabolic changes.

Drug Interactions
- The drug may enhance the effects of certain antihypertensive drugs because of its alpha-1-adrenergic antagonism with potential for inducing hypotension.
- Inhibitor of P450 CYP2D6: subject also to induction/inhibition of 1A2. Manufacturer recommends caution with other QTc drugs; may contribute to increased levels of other drugs acting as substrates of 2D6.
- It appears to decrease prolactin from baseline.

Pharmacokinetics
- Rapidly absorbed within 0.5 to 1.5 hours.
- *Half-life*: approximately 24 hours.

Precautions
- Caution should be used when the drug is taken in combination with other centrally acting drugs or alcohol. EKG should be taken prior to starting this medication.
- Caution should be used with other drugs that are both substrates and inhibitors for CYP 2D6. For example, CYP2D6 may double the level of paroxetine.

- The drug may cause transient increases in serum transaminase; therefore, it needs to be monitored during the initial months.
- Older adult patients with dementia-related psychosis treated with antipsychotic drugs are at an increased risk of death. Asenapine is not approved for the treatment of patients with dementia-related psychosis. Note the BBW.
- Patients with a preexisting low WBC or a history of drug-induced leukopenia/ neutropenia should have their complete blood count (CBC) monitored frequently during the first few months of therapy, and asenapine should be discontinued at the first sign of decline in WBC in the absence of other causative factors.
- The use of asenapine should be avoided in combination with other drugs known to prolong the QTc interval, including class 1A antiarrhythmics (e.g., quinidine, procainamide) or class 3 antiarrhythmics (e.g., amiodarone, sotalol), antipsychotic medications (e.g., ziprasidone, chlorpromazine, thioridazine), and antibiotics (e.g., gatifloxacin, moxifloxacin).
- Like other drugs that antagonize dopamine D2 receptors, asenapine can elevate prolactin levels, and the elevation can persist during chronic administration. As with other antipsychotic drugs, asenapine should be used with caution in patients with a history of seizures or with conditions that potentially lower the seizure threshold, for example, Alzheimer's dementia. Conditions that lower the seizure threshold may be more prevalent in patients 65 years or older.

Patient and Family Education

- Take exactly as prescribed by the provider. Do not take in larger or smaller amounts or for longer than recommended.
- Asenapine tablets must be placed under the tongue and be allowed to dissolve. Do not crush, chew, or swallow.
- No eating or drinking for at least 10 to 30 minutes after the drug is absorbed.
- *Avoid drinking alcohol.*
- *Stop using this medication and call provider immediately* if you have very stiff (rigid) muscles, high fever, sweating, confusion, fast or uneven heartbeats, tremors; feel like you might pass out; have jerky muscle movements you cannot control, trouble swallowing, problems with speech; have blurred vision, eye pain, or see halos around lights; have increased thirst and urination, excessive hunger, fruity breath odor, weakness, nausea, and vomiting; have fever, chills, body aches, and flu symptoms; or have white patches or sores inside your mouth or on your lips.
- Do not stop taking this drug suddenly without first talking to your provider, even if you feel fine. You may have serious side effects if you stop taking the drug suddenly.
- Call provider if symptoms do not improve or get worse.
- Store at room temperature away from moisture and heat.

Special Populations

- *Older adults:* Older adults may tolerate lower doses better and are more sensitive to adverse effects. It is not approved for treatment of older adult patients with dementia-related psychosis, and such patients are at increased risk for CV events and death.
- *Renal impairment*: No adjustment is needed.
- *Hepatic impairment*: Lower dose for mild-to-moderate impairment is to be administered. It is not recommended with severe liver impairment.
- *Cardiac impairment*: Use with caution due to risk of orthostatic hypotension and QTc potential prolongation.

- *Pregnancy*: category C. There are no adequate and well-controlled studies of asenapine in pregnant women. It is not recommended for this population.
- *Lactation*: Asenapine is excreted in the milk of rats during lactation. It is not known whether asenapine or its metabolites are excreted in human milk. As many drugs are excreted in human milk, caution should be exercised when asenapine is administered to a nursing woman. It is recommended that women receiving asenapine should not breastfeed.
- *Children and adolescents*: This medicine is not indicated for use in children.

ATOMOXETINE HYDROCHLORIDE (Strattera)

Classification
Serotonin-norepinephrine reuptake inhibitor (SNRI), attention deficit hyperactivity disorder (ADHD) drug

Indications
This is the first nonstimulant drug approved for the treatment of ADHD of children aged 6 years and above and adults. Although nonstimulants are considered second-line therapy, they may be a safer alternative than stimulants for patients with a history of substance abuse.

Available Forms
Capsule, 10, 18, 25, 40, 60, 80, and 100 mg.

Dosage
- Dosage should be individualized according to the therapeutic needs and response of the patient.
- *Adults*: 80 mg QAM; start, 40 mg PO QAM × 3 days, then increase to 80 mg PO QAM; may increase to 100 mg/d after 2 to 4 weeks if needed. Maximum: 100 mg/d.
- *Children younger than 6 years*: not recommended.
- *Children older than 6 years*: Less than 70 kg: start, 0.5 mg/kg PO QAM × 3 days, then increase to 1.2 mg/kg PO QAM; maximum, 1.4 mg/kg/d or 100 mg/d (whichever is less), doses >0.5 mg/kg/d may be divided BID. More than 70 kg: start, 40 mg PO QAM × 3 days, then increase to 80 mg PO QAM; may increase to 100 mg/d after 2 to 4 weeks if needed; maximum, 100 mg/d.

Administration
Taking the drug with food may alleviate gastrointestinal (GI) side effects; requires slower titration if patient is a poor CYP2D6 metabolizer or on a strong CYP2D6 inhibitor. For poor CYP2D6 metabolizers, initiate at 40 mg/d but do not exceed 80 mg/d. Periodically reassess need for treatment during maintenance.

Side Effects
Nausea and/or vomiting, fatigue, decreased appetite, abdominal pain, somnolence, constipation, dry mouth, insomnia, priapism, urinary hesitancy or retention or dysuria, dysmenorrheal, hot flashes, severe liver injury, serious CV events (myocardial infarction, stroke, sudden death), rapid heart rate and increased BP, suicidal ideation, allergic reactions, and decreased growth.

Drug Interactions
The drug may interact with MAOIs, CYP2D6 inhibitors, SSRIs, quinidine BP agents, albuterol, and other beta-2 agonists. The action of albuterol on CV system can be potentiated.

Pharmacokinetics
- The precise mechanism by which atomoxetine produces its therapeutic effect is unknown.

- Its therapeutic effect may be related to selective inhibition of the presynaptic norepinephrine transporter.
- Minimally affected by food intake.
- Maximal plasma concentration is reached within 1 to 2 hours after dosing.
- Mainly excreted in the urine (80%); feces (17%).
- *Half-life*: approximately 21 hours.
- *Bioavailability*: 63% to 94%.

Precautions

- Healthcare providers should monitor patients taking this medication for clinical worsening, suicidality, and unusual changes in behavior, particularly within the first few months of initiation or during dose changes.
- Do not prescribe to patients with cardiomyopathy and pheochromocytoma.
- Hypersensitivity to atomoxetine or other constituents of the product.
- Use within 2 weeks of taking or discontinuing MAOIs.
- Narrow-angle glaucoma.

Patient and Family Education

- Do not crush, open, or chew capsules.
- *Avoid touching a broken capsule*: Powder is a known ocular irritant, and if it gets into eyes it needs to be flushed out immediately.
- It can be taken with or without food.
- Do not double the dose if a day is missed.
- Call poison control/seek medical attention for overdose.
- Seek medical attention for chest pain, shortness of breath, elevated BP, erections that last more than 4 hours, or any other concerning symptoms.
- Children, adolescents, or adults who are being considered for treatment with atomoxetine should have a careful history (including assessment for a family history of sudden death or ventricular arrhythmia) and physical exam to assess for the presence of cardiac disease and should receive further cardiac evaluation if findings suggest such disease (e.g., EKG and echocardiogram). Patients who develop symptoms such as exertional chest pain, unexplained syncope, or other symptoms suggestive of cardiac disease during atomoxetine treatment should undergo a prompt cardiac evaluation.
- Store at room temperature.
- Routinely assess weight and BP.

Special Populations

- *Older adults*: Safety has not been studied in geriatric patients.
- *Pregnancy*: category C
- *Lactation*: Safety is unknown in lactating mothers.
- *Children*: not recommended for use in children younger than 6 years.

AVANAFIL (Stendra)

Classification
Phosphodiesterase type 5 (PDE5) inhibitor, CGMP specific

Indications
Used to treat erectile dysfunction

Available Forms
Tablet, 50, 100, and 200 mg.

Dosage
- Initially 100 mg taken 30 minutes prior to sexual activity; may decrease to 50 mg or increase to 200 mg based on response; maximum 1 administration/day.

Administration
- Take with or without food.
- Do not take this medicine more than once a day. Allow 24 hours to pass between doses.
- Store at room temperature away from moisture, heat, and light.

Side Effects
- Side effects include headache, flushing, nasal congestion, rhinitis, dyspepsia, and diarrhea.
- *Serious*: vision changes, sudden vision loss; ringing in ears or sudden hearing loss; pain, swelling, warmth, or redness in one or both legs; shortness of breath; swelling in hands or feet; light-headed feeling; erection that is painful or lasts 4 hours or longer.

Drug Interactions
- Concomitant use of nitrates in any form is contraindicated.
- Concomitant use of strong CYP3A4 inhibitors (including ketoconazole, ritonavir, atazanavir, clarithromycin, indinavir, itraconazole, nefazodone, nelfinavir, saquinavir, and telithromycin) is contraindicated.
- Contraindicated in patients who are using a GC stimulator, such as riociguat. PDE5 inhibitors, may potentiate the hypotensive effects of GC stimulators.
- If avanafil is coadministered with an alpha-blocker, patients should be stable on alpha-blocker therapy prior to initiating treatment with Stendra, and Stendra should be initiated at the 50 mg dose.
- For patients taking concomitant moderate CYP3A4 inhibitors (including erythromycin, amprenavir, aprepitant, diltiazem, fluconazole, fosamprenavir, and verapamil), the maximum recommended dose of Stendra is 50 mg, not to exceed once q24h.

Pharmacokinetics
- *Metabolism*: nil
- *Half-life*: 20 to 33 hours
- Renal excretion

Precautions

- There is a potential for cardiac risk during sexual activity in patients with preexisting CV disease. Contraindicated in patients for whom sexual activity is inadvisable because of their underlying CV status. Patients with left ventricular outflow obstruction and those with severely impaired autonomic control of BP can be particularly sensitive to the actions of vasodilators. Not recommended for patients who have suffered a myocardial infarction, stroke, life-threatening arrhythmia, or coronary revascularization within the past 6 months; patients with resting hypotension or HTN; patients with unstable angina, angina with sexual intercourse, or New York Heart Association class 2 or greater congestive heart failure.
- Use with caution in patients with anatomical deformation of the penis (such as angulation, cavernosal fibrosis, or Peyronie disease) or in patients who have conditions that may predispose them to priapism (such as sickle cell anemia, multiple myeloma, or leukemia).

Patient and Family Education

- Advise patients to seek emergency medical help if they have signs of allergic reaction—hives; difficulty breathing; swelling of face, lips, tongue, or throat; or have sudden vision loss.
- Advise patients to seek emergency medical help if they have become dizzy or nauseated or have pain, numbness, or tingling in chest, arms, neck, or jaw during sexual activity.
- Remind patients that it should be taken only when needed, about 15 to 30 minutes before sexual activity.
- Remind patients that sexual response is needed for a response to treatment. An erection will not occur just by taking a pill.
- Advise patients that drinking alcohol can increase certain side effects of avanafil. Avoid drinking more than three alcoholic beverages while taking medication.
- Advise patients to avoid the use of grapefruit products.

Special Populations

- *Pregnancy*: not indicated for use in females
- *Renal and hepatic impairment*: not for use patients in patients with severe hepatic or renal disease or those on dialysis

B COMPLEX (Vitamin B1/Thiamine Hydrochloride)

Classification
Vitamin

Indications
Treat and prevent thiamine deficiency, including thiamine-specific deficiency, and Wernicke-Korsakoff syndrome (common in patients diagnosed with
alcoholism)

Available Forms
Tablets, 50, 100, 250, and 500 mg; injection, 100 mg/mL; enteric coated tablets, 20 mg.

Dosage
1 to 2 mg of thiamine per day is commonly used. The daily recommended daily allow-
ances (RDAs) are as follows:
- *Infants*: 0 to 6 months: 0.2 mg; 7 to 12 months: 0.3 mg
- *Children*: 1 to 3 years: 0.5 mg; 4 to 8 years: 0.6 mg
- *Males*: 9 to 13 years: 0.9 mg; 14 years and older: 1.2 mg
- *Females*: 9 to 13 years: 0.9 mg; 14 to 18 years: 1 mg; over 18 years: 1.1 mg; pregnant
  women: 1.4 mg; lactating breastfeeding women: 1.5 mg

Administration
- PO with a glass of water.
- It may be taken with or without food.

Side Effects
Feelings of warmth, restlessness, nausea, and pruritus.

Drug Interactions
None indicated.

Pharmacokinetics
The drug is widely distributed. It is eliminated in urine.

Precautions
- Watch for anaphylaxis reaction.

Patient and Family Education
- Take medication at same time every day.

Special Populations
- *Older adults*: no contraindications.
- *Renal impairment*: Use with caution.
- *Hepatic impairment*: Use with caution.
- *Pregnancy*: category A.

- *Lactation*: The American Academy of Pediatrics classifies thiamine as compatible with breastfeeding.
- *Children and adolescents*: multivitamin use in children determined by nutritional deficiency noted. Dose contingent is based on weight.

BISMUTH SUBSALICYLATE (Pepto-bismol)

Classification
Antidiarrheal

Indications
- Used for mild, nonspecific diarrhea

Available Forms
- Tablets (chewable), 262 mg.
- Liquid, 262 mg/15 mL (4, 8, 12, and 16 oz).
- Oral suspension, 525 mg/15 mL (4, 8, 12, and 16 oz).

Dosages
For patients with mild, nonspecific diarrhea:
- *Adults and children age 12 years and older*: 2 tablets or 30 mL every 30 to 60 minutes, up to maximum of 8 doses, no longer than 2 days
- *Children aged 9 to 11 years*: 15 mL or 1 chewable tablet every 30 to 60 minutes, up to maximum of 8 doses, no longer than 2 days
- *Children aged 6 to 8 years*: 10 mL or two-thirds chewable tablet PO every half hour to an hour up to maximum of 8 doses, no longer than 2 days
- *Children aged 3 to 5 years*: 5 mL or one-third chewable tablet PO every 30 to 60 minutes, up to 8 doses
- *Children younger than 3 years (14–18 lbs)*: 2.5 mL every 30 to 60 minutes, up to 6 doses

Administration
- Shake liquid well before administration. Have patient chew or dissolve tablets in the mouth.
- Liquid formulation works more effectively for relief of severe symptoms.
- Avoid use prior to radiological procedures because drug is radiopaque and may interfere with x-rays.
- Liquid form is preferred for children to give more accurate dosing.

Side Effects
- *Gastrointestinal*: temporary darkening of tongue and stools, salicylic with high doses
- *Effects on lab test results*: none reported

Drug Interactions
- *Aspirin/other salicylates*: may cause salicylate toxicity. Monitor patient.
- *Oral anticoagulants, oral antidiabetics*: may increase effects of these drugs after high doses of bismuth. Monitor patient closely.
- *Tetracycline*: may decrease tetracycline absorption. Separate doses by at least 2 hours.

Pharmacokinetics
- Drug may have antisecretory, antimicrobial, and antiinflammatory effects against bacterial and viral enteropathogens.
- *Onset of action*: 1 hour, peak unknown, duration and half-life unknown.

Precautions

- It is contraindicated in patients hypersensitive to salicylates.
- Use the drug cautiously in patients taking aspirin.
- Stop therapy if tinnitus occurs.
- Use cautiously in children and in patients with bleeding disorders or salicylate sensitivity.

Patient and Family Education

- Advise patient that drug contains salicylate.
- Instruct patient to shake liquid before measuring dose and to chew tablets well before swallowing.
- Tell patient to call prescriber if diarrhea lasts longer than 2 days, accompanied by high fever.
- Advise patient to drink plenty of clear fluids to avoid dehydration, which may accompany diarrhea.
- Avoid red-colored hydration fluids as this may be misinterpreted as bleeding from rectum.
- Inform the patient that tongue and stools may temporarily turn gray-black.
- Urge patient to consult with prescriber prior to giving the drug to children or teenagers during or after recovery from flu or chicken pox.
- Tell the patient to watch for hives, ringing in the ears, or rectal bleeding.

Special Populations

- *Older adults*
  - Caution is recommended for older adults because of the risk of fluid and electrolyte loss; also, older adults are more likely to have age-related renal function impairment, which may increase the risk of salicylate toxicity.
  - Bismuth is more likely to cause impaction in older adult patients.
- *Pediatric*
  - Avoid use in children or teenagers who have recovered or are recovering from influenza or varicella.
  - *Use cautiously in infants and debilitated patients due to increased risk of constipation with impaction.*
  - Use cautiously in children and in patients with bleeding disorders or salicylate sensitivity.
- *Pregnancy*
  - Drug has not been officially assigned to a pregnancy category.
  - The effects of the drug are unknown.

BROMOCRIPTINE MESYLATE (Parlodel, Cycloset)

Classification
Ergot derivative with potent dopamine receptor agonist activity; antiparkinsonian

Indications
Hyperprolactinemia-Associated Dysfunctions
- Indicated in disorders associated with hyperprolactinemia, including amenorrhea with or without galactorrhea, infertility or hypogonadism, with prolactin-secreting adenomas.

Acromegaly
- It is indicated in the treatment of acromegaly.
- The drug is used alone or as adjunctive therapy with pituitary irradiation or surgery.

Parkinson's Disease
- The drug is used for the treatment of the signs and symptoms of idiopathic or post-encephalitic Parkinson's disease.
- It is used as adjunctive treatment to levodopa (alone or with a peripheral decarboxylase inhibitor).
- It is also used for traumatic brain injury.

Available Forms
Tablet, 2.5 mg; capsule, 5 mg.

Dosage
Hyperprolactinemia
Initial: 1.25 to 2.5 mg PO daily
Titration: Add 2.5 mg PO, as tolerated, to the treatment dosage every 2 to 7 days
Maintenance: 2.5 to 15 mg PO daily

Acromegaly
Initial: 1.25 to 2.5 mg PO once daily, with food, at bedtime for 3 days
Titration: Add 1.25 to 2.5 mg PO, as tolerated, to the treatment dosage every 3 to 7 days
Maintenance: 20 to 30 mg PO daily
  The maximum dosage should not exceed 100 mg/d.

Parkinson's Disease
Initial: 1.25 mg BID with meals
Titration: Add 2.5 mg/d, with meals, to dosage regimen every 14 to 28 days
Maximum dosage: 100 mg/d

Hyperprolactinemia
For 11- to 15-years-olds:
Initial: 1.25 to 2.5 mg PO daily
Maintenance: 2.5 to 10 mg PO daily

Administration

PO: Take the drug with food to avoid GI distress; take in evening with food to minimize adverse reactions.

Drug Interactions

- Metoclopramide will antagonize the effects of this drug and should be avoided.
- Use with caution ergot alkaloids (e.g., ergonovine); "triptans" (e.g., sumatriptan, frovatriptan); medications for high BP (e.g., methyldopa, reserpine, beta-blockers such as metoprolol/propranolol); antipsychotic medication (e.g., haloperidol, pimozide); metoclopramide; nitrates (e.g., nitroglycerin); octreotide; cimetidine; delavirdine; efavirenz; telithromycin; azole antifungals, including ketoconazole; macrolide antibiotics, including erythromycin; HIV protease inhibitors, such as ritonavir; rifamycins, including rifabutin, can affect concentrations of the drug. Salicylates may increase adverse reactions.
- St. John's wort; certain antiseizure medicines, including carbamazepine; drugs that cause drowsiness, such as certain antihistamines (e.g., diphenhydramine), antiseizure drugs (e.g., phenytoin), medicine for sleep or anxiety (e.g., alprazolam, diazepam, zolpidem), and muscle relaxants; narcotic pain relievers (e.g., codeine); psychiatric medicines (e.g., chlorpromazine, risperidone, nortriptyline, trazodone) will also affect efficacy.
- Patients need to check the labels on all their medicines (e.g., cough-and-cold products) because they may contain drowsiness-causing ingredients.

Pharmacokinetics

- *Absorption:* 28% bioavailable
- *Onset:* 1 to 3 hours
- *Peak:* 8 hours
- *Metabolism:* Via CYP3A4 (major)
- *Excretion:* 85% feces; urine 2.5% to 5%
- *Half-life:* 15 hours

Precautions

- Bromocriptine is contraindicated for use in patients with uncontrolled HTN due to risk of acute myocardial infarction. It is also contraindicated for use in the prevention of physiological lactation.
- Bromocriptine should be used with caution in patients with a history of psychosis or CV disease.
- Patients should be evaluated frequently during dose titration to determine the lowest dosage possible to achieve the desired therapeutic effects.
- Patients treated with pituitary irradiation should be withdrawn from bromocriptine therapy on a yearly basis to assess both the clinical effects of radiation on the disease process and the effects of bromocriptine. Usually a 4- to 8-week withdrawal period is adequate for this purpose.
- With older adults, start at the lower end of the dose range, reflecting the greater frequency of decreased hepatic, renal, or cardiac function of concomitant disease, or other drug therapy in this population.
- Patients with cardiac valvular fibrosis and other CV diseases need to be carefully assessed to determine risk and benefit.
- This drug may cause impulse control disorders.
- It may increase the risk of melanoma

Patient and Family Education

- The patient needs to know that they should not discontinue this medicine without consulting the prescriber.
- Take with meals to avoid GI distress.
- Urine or perspiration may appear darker.

Special Populations

- *Older adults*: Clinical studies for Parlodel did not include sufficient numbers of subjects aged 65 years and older to determine whether older adults respond differently from younger subjects.
- *Pregnancy*: category B. Withdraw unless medically impossible—such as rapidly expanding macroadenoma that necessitates continued use.
- *Lactation*: Breastfeeding is not recommended.
- *Children:* The safety and effectiveness of bromocriptine for the treatment of prolactin-secreting pituitary adenomas have been established in patients aged 16 years to adult. There are available data on bromocriptine use in pediatric patients under the age of 8 years. This medicine is not indicated for children under the age of 11 years.

BUPRENORPHINE, BUPRENORPHINE HCL, BUPRENEX, BUTRANS, AND NALOXONE HCL DIHYDRATE (Subutex, Suboxone)

Classification
Opiate partial agonists, opioid analgesic

Indications
- The drug is used sublingually for treatment of opiate dependence.
- It is preferred for the initial (i.e., induction) phase of opiate-dependence treatment.
- It is also used for controlling pain (acute and chronic).

Available Forms
Sublingual tablets, Subutex: 2 and 8 mg; Suboxone: 2 mg/0.5 mg, 4 mg/1 mg, 8 mg/2 mg, and 12 mg/3 mg; injectable, Subutex: 0.3 mg/mL; transdermal patch, 5 mcg/hr, 10 mcg/hr, and 20 mcg/hr.

Dosage
Pediatric
Intravascular or IM

- *Children 2 to 12 years of age*: 2 to 6 mcg/kg q4h to q6h; monitor effects of the drug before establishing fixed doses.
- *Children 13 years of age or older*: 0.3 mg given at intervals of up to q6h prn (pro re nata). Can repeat initial dose (up to 0.3 mg) once in 30 to 60 minutes, if control is not achieved.
- Exercise particular caution with IV administration, especially with initial doses.

Adults
Intravascular or IM

- Administer 0.3 mg q6h prn. Repeat initial dose (up to 0.3 mg) once in 30 to 60 minutes, if needed.
- A regimen including an initial dose of 0.3 mg followed by another 0.3-mg dose repeated in 3 hours is as effective as a single 0.6-mg dose in relieving postoperative pain.
- Decrease dosage by approximately 50% in patients who are at increased risk for respiratory depression.

Opiate Dependence
Induction

Sublingual
- Begin with 8 mg on day 1 and 16 mg on day 2. From day 3 onward, administer buprenorphine in fixed combination with naloxone at the same buprenorphine dose as on day 2.
- To avoid precipitating withdrawal, give the first dose when the patient is objective and clear signs of opiate withdrawal are evident.
- Manufacturer recommends that an adequate maintenance dosage, titrated to clinical effectiveness, be achieved as rapidly as possible to prevent undue opiate withdrawal symptoms.

Maintenance

Sublingual

- Target dosage of buprenorphine in fixed combination with naloxone is 16 mg daily; however, dosages as low as 12 mg daily may be effective in some patients. Adjust dosage in increments/decrements of 2 or 4 mg daily to a dosage that suppresses opiate withdrawal symptoms and ensures that the patient continues treatment.
- *Usual dosage*: 4 to 24 mg daily depending on the individual patient.
- If switching between buprenorphine/naloxone sublingual tablets and sublingually dissolving strips, continue same dosage. However, not all doses and dose combinations are bioequivalent; monitor for efficacy and tolerability and adjust dosage if needed.

Administration

- Administer sublingually as a single agent or in fixed combination with naloxone for management of opiate dependence.
- Also administered by continuous IV infusion by IM or IV injection using a patient-controlled infusion device and by epidural injection for pain relief. Incompatibilities: diazepam, furosemide, lorazepam.

Sublingual Tablets

- Place tablets under the tongue and allow to dissolve; swallowing the tablets reduces bioavailability. Drinking warm fluids prior to administration may aid dissolution.
- For doses requiring more than two tablets, all the tablets may be placed under the tongue at once.
- Alternatively, patients may place two tablets under the tongue at a time if unable to place more than two tablets comfortably.
- To ensure consistent bioavailability, patients should adhere to the same dosing schedule with continued use.

IV Injection
Rate of Administration

Administer over greater than or equal to 2 minutes.

Transdermal

- Apply the transdermal system to a dry, intact, nonirritated, hairless, or nearly hairless surface on the upper chest, upper back, side of chest, or upper outer arm.
- Firmly press the system by hand for 15 seconds with the adhesive side touching the skin and ensuring that contact is complete, particularly around the edges.
- Clip do not shave hair at the application site prior to application, if indicated.
- Only water should be used if the site must be cleaned before transdermal application; do *not* use soaps, oils, lotions, alcohol, or abrasive devices that could alter absorption of the drug.
- System is intended to be worn continuously for 7 days.
- Apply subsequent systems to a different site each time administered.
- At least 21 days should elapse before reusing any single application site.

Restricted Distribution Program
The Drug Addiction Treatment Act (DATA) of 2000 allows qualifying physicians to prescribe and dispense opiates in Schedules III, IV, and V of the Federal Controlled Substances Act, which have been approved by the FDA for detoxification or maintenance treatment of opiate dependence.

Side Effects

- Somnolence, dizziness, alterations in judgment, or alteration in level of consciousness, including coma.
- Use with caution in comatose patients or in patients with CNS depression.
- It may impair mental alertness and/or physical coordination needed to perform potentially hazardous activities, such as driving or operating machinery.
- Concurrent use of other CNS depressants may potentiate CNS depression, increased intracranial pressure, and bradycardia.

Drug Interactions

- CNS depression.
- Respiratory depression.
- Diazepam may cause respiratory distress or cardiac arrest.
- Macrolide antibiotics may increase drug levels.

Pharmacokinetics

- *Metabolism*: liver by CYP 3A4
- *Peak*: IV, 2 minutes; IM, 1 hour; sublingual, unknown; transdermal, 3 to 6 days
- *Half-life*: 37 hours; transdermal, 26 hours

Precautions

- Watch for respiratory depression.
- Supervise ambulation due to sedative effects.

Patient and Family Education

- Do not drive or engage in other hazardous activities until response to drug is known.
- Avoid alcohol or other CNS depressants.
- It may cause constipation.

Special Populations

- *Older adults*: Use with caution due to sedative effects.
- *Renal impairment*: Use with caution.
- *Hepatic impairment*: Use with caution; patients may require lower dosage.
- *Pregnancy*: category C.
- *Lactation*: Safety has not been established.
- *Children and adolescents*: Safety has not been established.

BUPRENORPHINE/NALOXONE (Suboxone)

Classification
Opioid (narcotic) partial agonist–antagonist

Indications
It is indicated for maintenance treatment of opioid dependence.

Available Forms
Sublingual film, 2 mg/0.5 mg; 4 mg/1 mg; 8 mg/2 mg; 12 mg/3 mg.

Dosage
- Recommended dosage is 16 mg/4 mg a day as a single daily dose.
- Dosage adjusted in increments/decrements of 2 mg/0.5 mg or 4 mg/1 mg to a level that obtains optimum results and avoids withdrawal.
- Maintenance dose is 4 mg/1 mg to 24 mg/6 mg per day.

Administration
- It cannot be cut, chewed, or swallowed.
- It should be placed under the tongue until the film is completely dissolved.
- Rotate places where film is placed.
- Do not move film once it is placed under tongue.

Side Effects
- Most common side effects are headache, stomach pain, constipation, vomiting, difficulty falling asleep or staying asleep, and sweating.
- Some side effects can be serious. The following symptoms are uncommon but serious possible effects:
  - Hives, skin rash, itching, difficulty breathing or swallowing, slowed breathing, upset stomach, extreme tiredness, unusual bleeding or bruising, lack of energy, loss of appetite, pain in the upper right part of the stomach, yellowing of the skin or eyes, and flu-like symptoms.

Drug Interactions
- MAOIs
- Itraconazole, ketoconazole, erythromycin, clarithromycin, ritonavir, indinavir
- Saquinavir
- Local anesthetics
- Avoid use with BZDs
- Alcohol
- Medicine for sleep
- Antianxiety drugs
- Narcotic pain relievers
- Phenothiazines
- Tricyclics
- Antiseizure drugs
- Muscle relaxants
- Antihistamines

Pharmacokinetics

- Mean elimination half-life from plasma ranging from 24 to 42 hours.
- Naloxone has a mean elimination half-life from plasma ranging from 2 to 12 hours.

Precautions

- Check all known allergies.
- Use with extreme caution in patients with histories of lung disease, liver disease, serious head injury or CNS diseases, hypothyroidism, Addison's disease, psychosis, BPH, acute alcoholism, kyphoscoliosis, and biliary tract disease.
- Check for a history of vertigo and syncope.
- Avoid alcoholic beverages.
- Respiratory depression.
- Lethargy.
- New studies show difficulty in weaning patients off Suboxone.
- *For patients with hepatic impairment:* higher plasma levels in patients with moderate and severe hepatic impairment.
- Dosage should be adjusted and patients should be watched for signs and symptoms of opioid withdrawal.
- *Patients with renal impairment:* Effects are unknown.

Patient Education

- Instruct patient that if they miss a dose to take it as soon as possible unless it is almost time for next dose; if so, then patient needs to be instructed to wait until then to use the medicine and skip the missed dose. Do not use extra medicine to make up for a missed dose.
- Medication should be stored in a closed container at room temperature, away from heat, moisture, and direct light.
- *Over-the-counter (OTC) medications should not be used without conferring with provider. This includes vitamins and herbal products.*
- Do not drink alcohol while you are using this medicine.
- Be aware that there are numerous drug–drug interactions with this drug.
- Explore with patient history of any mental or emotional problems.
- This medication cannot be abruptly stopped. Provider will slowly decrease dose before stopping it completely.
- All dentists and providers need to be aware that patient is on this drug.
- Necessary to draw blood levels at specific intervals; therefore, all appointments need to be kept.

Special Populations

- *Older adults*
  - There is little clinical data on safety and efficacy in older adults.
  - If used in older adults, do so with caution. Start at the low end of the dosing range and monitor carefully.
  - There are higher plasma levels in patients with moderate and severe hepatic impairment.
  - Dosage should be adjusted and patients should be watched for signs and symptoms of opioid withdrawal. For those with renal impairment, providers need to use caution for its unknown effects.

- *Pregnancy: category C*
  - There is no adequate information regarding efficacy and safety in pregnant women.
  - This drug should be used during pregnancy only if the potential benefit justifies the potential risk to the fetus.
- *Nursing Mothers*
  - Drug passes into breast milk.
  - Breastfeeding is not recommended.
- *Pediatric*
  - It is not recommended for pediatric patients. Safety and effectiveness have not been established in pediatric patients.

BUPROPION (Wellbutrin) BUPROPION HYDROBROMIDE (Aplenzin) AND BUPROPION HYDROCHLORIDE (Wellbutrin, Wellbutrin SR, Wellbutrin XL, Zyban)

Classification

Norepinephrine/dopamine reuptake inhibitor (NDRI); antidepressant, aminoketone

Indications

Used for the treatment of major depression of adults; used for smoking cessation, seasonal affective disorder (SAD)

Available Forms

Tablet, 75 and 100 mg; sustained-release (SR) tablet, 100 and 150 mg; XR tablet, 100, 150, 200, and 300 mg; 450 mg XL newly available. Plain bupropion is still available.

Dosage

Adults: 100 mg PO TID; start, 100 mg PO BID, dose increase after 3 days; maximum, 150 to 450 mg/dose, 450 mg/d.

Administration

Depending on formulation prescribed, taken TID (rapid release), BID; second dose not to be given within 5 to 6 hours of bedtime to avoid insomnia (SR) and to prevent seizures. SR without food and XL formulations are most commonly used, and XL formulation is recommended if available. XR formulations to be taken once daily.

Side Effects

- Dry mouth, headache, agitation
- Seizure threshold significantly decreased particularly at >300 to 450 mg/d dosage. Use of SR or XL formulation is also helpful in reducing risk of seizure, suicidal behavior, and arrhythmias.
- Headache, anxiety, tremor, tachycardia, and insomnia; cognitive impairment and mental clouding; delayed hypersensitivity reactions; tachycardia; nausea; increased sweating; blurred vision; dry mouth; weight loss.

Drug Interactions

It can be fatal when combined with MAOIs. *Caution:* Use with Phenergan with codeine, Linezolid, and ethanol. Avoid other medications that lower seizure threshold, including BZD withdrawal.

- The drug can elevate TCA activity; use with caution.
- It potentially increases plasma levels of other 2D6 metabolites.
- Risk of seizure may be increased by concomitant use of inhibitors of CYP2D6 (e.g., desipramine, sertraline, paroxetine, fluoxetine), due to increased bupropion blood levels. Nausea; dizziness; constipation; tremor; sweating; abnormal dreams; insomnia; tinnitus; pharyngitis; anorexia; weight loss; infection; abdominal pain; diarrhea; anxiety; flatulence; rash; palpitations; myalgia/arthralgia; chest pain; blurred vision; urinary frequency; suicidality; depression, worsening; psychiatric disorder exacerbation; behavioral disturbances; agitation; psychosis; hallucinations; paranoia; mania; seizures; hepatotoxicity; arrhythmias; tachycardia; HTN, severe;

elevated intraocular pressure; migraine; Stevens-Johnson syndrome (SJS); erythema multiforme; anaphylactic/anaphylactoid reactions.

Pharmacokinetics

- It inhibits activity of CYP450 2D6, potentially increasing plasma levels of other 2D6 metabolites.
- It has been converted to an active metabolite.
- Mechanism for smoking cessation is unknown.
- The exact mechanism of action for depression is unknown.
- The drug inhibits neuronal uptake of norepinephrine and dopamine.
- *Metabolism*: liver, excreted mainly in the urine.
- *Half-life*: parent compound, 10 to 24 hours; active metabolite, 20 to 24 hours.
- 8 to 24 hours, peak: 3 to 5 hours.

Precautions

- Use with caution in patients with CV disease, hepatic impairment, or renal impairment.
- Do not use in patients with seizure disorders, alcoholism, or hypersensitivity to drug/class.
- Do not use with MAOI until off the drug for 14 days.
- Seizure disorder.
- Bulimia.
- Anorexia nervosa.
- Sexual dysfunction: less sexual dysfunction with bupropion.
- *Black box warning*: Drug may cause hostility, agitation, and depressed mood. It may increase risk of suicidal thinking and behavior in children, adolescents, and young adults with MDD or other psychiatric disorders. It is not for use in children. Bupropion hydrobromide (Aplenzin) is not approved for smoking cessation.
- *Patients at risk for seizure disorders:* The drug may lower seizure threshold.
- Avoid combinations with other CNS stimulants, injury/intracranial lesion, alcohol or drug abuse, psychiatric disorder, bipolar disorder, suicidality history, suicidal ideation.
- Use with caution in case of diabetes mellitus, cirrhosis, severe hepatic impairment, renal impairment, recent myocardial infarction, and HTN.

Patient and Family Education

- The medicine should be taken about the same time every day, preferably in the morning (for XL formulation) with or without food.
- If taking rapid-release or SR formulation, take last dose more than 5 to 6 hours from bedtime, as late dosing can precipitate insomnia.
- The drug may take up to 4 to 8 weeks to show its maximum effect, but some may see symptoms of dysthymia improving in as few as 2 weeks.
- If patient plans on becoming pregnant, discuss the benefits versus the risks of using this medicine while pregnant.
- This medicine is excreted in the breast milk, and hence, nursing mothers should not breastfeed while taking this medicine without prior consultation with a psychiatric nurse practitioner or psychiatrist. Newborns may develop symptoms, including feeding or breathing difficulties, seizures, muscle stiffness, jitteriness, or constant crying.
- Do not stop taking this medication unless your healthcare provider directs you to do so. Report side effects or worsening dysthymia symptoms to your healthcare provider promptly.

- Treatment should continue for 6 to 12 months following last reported dysthymic experience.
- Keep these medications out of the reach of children and pets.
- Store at room temperature.
- Monitor the patient for worsening psychiatric complaints.

Special Populations

- *Older adults*: Older individuals tend to be more sensitive to medication side effects, such as hypotension and anticholinergic effects. They often require adjustment of medication doses for hepatic or renal dysfunction. Begin at a lower dosage; XL formulation is recommended. Caution with use due to polypharmacy and comorbid conditions.
- *Pregnancy*: Psychotherapy is the initial choice for most pregnant patients with depression disorder (DD). Category C; not recommended during pregnancy, especially first trimester, as there are no adequate studies during pregnancy.
- *Lactation:* unsafe.
- *Children:* It is recommended that the dose begin in the lower range. Monitor the patient closely for suicidal ideation. Psychiatric consultation is recommended due to BBW of increased suicidal ideation using SSRI therapy in children. It may be useful in treating children with comorbid ADHD, ages 6 to 17 years.

CARBAMAZEPINE (Tegretol, Carbatrol, Tegretol XR, Equetro)

Classification
Mood-stabilizing anticonvulsant, iminostilbene derivative

Indications
Used alone or in combination with other medications for seizures and neuropathic pain. Additional uses include the treatment of trigeminal neuralgia. It can be used as XR capsules to treat episodes of mania or mixed episodes in patients with bipolar I disorder. It can be also used for tonic–clonic seizures, complex partial seizures, mixed seizure patterns (except Carbatrol and Equetro), borderline personality disorder (BPD), and alcohol withdrawal.

Available Forms
Tablet, 100 and 200 mg; chew tablets, 100 mg; XR capsule, 100, 200, and 300 mg; oral suspension, 100 mg/5 mL; XR tablets, 100, 200, and 400 mg.

Dosage
Trigeminal Neuralgia
- Carbatrol
  - *Adults*: initially 200 mg BID; may increase weekly as needed by 200 mg/d; usual maintenance, 800 mg to 1.2 gm/d.
  - *Children older than 15 years*: initially 200 mg BID; may increase weekly as needed by 200 mg/d; usual maintenance, 800 mg to 1.2 gm/d.
  - *Children 12 to 15 years*: maximum 1 gm/d in 2 divided doses; >15 years; usual maintenance, 1.2 gm/d in 2 divided doses.
  - *Children younger than 12 years*: maximum <35 mg/kg/d; use XR form 400 mg/d.
- Tegretol
  - *Adults*: initially 100 mg BID or 1/2 teaspoon suspension QID; may increase dose by 100 mg q12h or by 1/2 teaspoon suspension q6h; usual maintenance 400 to 800 mg/d; maximum 1,200 mg/d.
  - *Children older than 6 years*: initially 100 mg BID; increase weekly as needed by 100 mg/d in 3 to 4 divided doses; maximum 1 gm/d in 3 to 4 divided doses.
  - *Children younger than 6 years*: initially 10 to 20 mg/kg/d in 2 divided doses; increase weekly as needed in 3 to 4 divided doses; maximum 35 mg/kg/d in 3 to 4 divided doses.
- *Maintenance*: at least once every 3 months throughout the treatment period; attempts should be made to reduce the dose to the minimum effective level or even to discontinue the drug.

Epilepsy
Adults and Children Above 12 Years of Age
- *Initial*: either 200 mg BID for tablets and XR tablets or 1 teaspoon QID for suspension (400 mg/d).
- Increase at weekly intervals by adding up to 200 mg/d using a BID regimen of Tegretol-XR or a TID or QID until the optimal response is obtained.
- It should not exceed 1,000 mg daily in children 12 to 15 years of age and 1,200 mg daily in patients above 15 years of age.
- *Maintenance*: Usually 800 to 1,200 mg daily.

Children 6 to 12 Years of Age

- *Initial:* either 100 mg BID for tablets or XR tablets or 1/2 teaspoon QID for suspension (200 mg/d).
- Increase at weekly intervals by adding up to 100 mg/d BID of Tegretol-XR or TID or QID of other formulations until the optimal response is obtained.
- Dosage generally should not exceed 1,000 mg daily.
- *Maintenance:* usually 400 to 800 mg daily. Maximum dose can be 1,000 mg/d.

Children Below 6 Years of Age

- *Initial:* 10 to 20 mg/kg/d BID or TID as tablets, or QID as suspension.
- Increase weekly to achieve optimal clinical response administered TID or QID.
- *Maintenance:* Optimal clinical response is achieved at daily doses below 35 mg/kg. If satisfactory clinical response has not been achieved, plasma levels should be measured to determine whether or not they are in the therapeutic range.

Bipolar Disorder

- *Adults:* initially 400 mg/d in 2 divided doses; adjust in increments of 200 mg/d; maximum 1.6 gm/d. XR oral forms should be swallowed whole; may open caps and sprinkle on applesauce (do not crush or chew beads).
- *Children older than 12 years:* initially 400 mg/d in 2 divided doses; adjust in increments of 200 mg/d; maximum 1.6 gm/d. XR oral forms should be swallowed whole; may open caps and sprinkle on applesauce (do not crush or chew beads).
- *Children younger than 12 years:* not recommended.
- *Older adults:* Reduce initial dose and titrate slowly; oral doses are preferred.

Administration

- Store at room temperature.
- Give with meals to reduce the risk of GI distress.
- Shake oral suspension well.
- Do not administer with grapefruit juice.
- Do not crush capsules or tablets. If switching from tablets to capsules, maintain the same dose.
- Contents of XR capsules may be sprinkled over applesauce if the patient faces difficulty in swallowing.

Side Effects

- *Central nervous system:* Fatigue, lethargy, coma, epileptiform seizures, tremors, drowsiness, headache, confusion, restlessness, dizziness, psychomotor retardation, blackouts, electroencephalogram changes, worsened mental syndrome, impaired speech, ataxia, and incoordination.
- *Cardiovascular:* Arrhythmias, bradycardia, reversible EKG changes, and hypotension.
- *EENT:* Tinnitus and blurred vision.
- *Gastrointestinal:* Vomiting, anorexia, diarrhea, thirst, nausea, metallic taste, dry mouth, abdominal pain, flatulence, and indigestion.
- *Genitourinary:* Polyuria, renal toxicity with long-term use, glycosuria, decreased CrCl, and albuminuria.
- *Hematological:* anemia, agranulocytosis, and leukocytosis with leukocyte count of 14,000 to 18,000/mm.

- *Metabolic*: transient hyperglycemia, goiter, hypothyroidism, and hyponatremia.
- *Musculoskeletal*: muscle weakness.
- Serious and sometimes fatal dermatologic reactions, including toxic epidermal necrolysis (TEN) and SJS, have been reported with Tegretol treatment.
- *Psychiatric*: Increases the risk of suicidal thoughts or behavior; possibility of activation of a latent psychosis and, in older adults, of confusion or agitation should be borne in mind.
- *Other*: mild anticholinergic activity; use with caution in patients with increased intraocular pressure.
- The use of Tegretol should be avoided in patients with a history of hepatic porphyria (e.g., acute intermittent porphyria, variegate porphyria, and porphyria cutanea tarda).

Drug Interactions

- CYP 3A4 inhibitors inhibit Tegretol metabolism, which can increase plasma carbamazepine levels.
- Drugs that increase plasma carbamazepine levels include cimetidine, danazol, diltiazem, macrolides, erythromycin, troleandomycin, clarithromycin, fluoxetine, fluvoxamine, nefazodone, trazodone, loxapine, olanzapine, quetiapine, loratadine, terfenadine, omeprazole, oxybutynin, dantrolene, INH, niacinamide, nicotinamide, ibuprofen, propoxyphene, azoles (e.g., ketoconazole, itraconazole, fluconazole, voriconazole), acetazolamide, verapamil, ticlopidine, grapefruit juice, protease inhibitors, valproate.
- CYP 3A4 inducers can increase the rate of Tegretol metabolism.
- Drugs that decrease plasma carbamazepine levels include cisplatin, doxorubicin HCl, felbamate, fosphenytoin, rifampin, phenobarbital, phenytoin, primidone, methsuximide, theophylline, and aminophylline.
- Tegretol is a potent inducer of hepatic CYP 3A4 and may therefore reduce plasma concentrations of other drugs mainly metabolized by 3A4 through induction of their metabolism, resulting in decreased levels of the following: acetaminophen, alprazolam, bupropion, dihydropyridine calcium channel blockers (e.g., felodipine), citalopram, cyclosporine, corticosteroids (e.g., prednisolone, dexamethasone), clonazepam, clozapine, dicumarol, doxycycline, ethosuximide, everolimus, haloperidol, imatinib, itraconazole, lamotrigine, levothyroxine, methadone, methsuximide, midazolam, olanzapine, oral and other hormonal contraceptives, oxcarbazepine, phensuximide, phenytoin, praziquantel, protease inhibitors, risperidone, theophylline, tiagabine, topiramate, tramadol, trazodone, TCAs (e.g., imipramine, amitriptyline, nortriptyline), valproate, warfarin, ziprasidone, zonisamide.
- Coadministration of carbamazepine with nefazodone results in insufficient plasma concentrations of nefazodone and its active metabolite to achieve a therapeutic effect. Coadministration of carbamazepine with nefazodone is contraindicated.
- Concomitant administration of carbamazepine and lithium may increase the risk of neurotoxic side effects.
- Concomitant use of carbamazepine and INH has been reported to increase INH-induced hepatotoxicity.
- Concomitant medication with Tegretol and some diuretics (hydrochlorothiazide, furosemide) may lead to symptomatic hyponatremia.
- Carbamazepine may antagonize the effects of non-depolarizing muscle relaxants.
- Alterations of thyroid function have been reported in combination therapy with other anticonvulsant medications.

■ Concomitant use of Tegretol with hormonal contraceptive products (e.g., oral and levonorgestrel subdermal implant contraceptives) may render the contraceptives less effective because the plasma concentrations of the hormones may be decreased.

■ Breakthrough bleeding and unintended pregnancies have been reported. Alternative or back-up methods of contraception should be considered.

■ Lamotrigine (may lower lamotrigine level and increase carbamazepine level).

■ *Peak action*: 30 minutes to 1 hour; PO, 1.5 to 12 hours; PO XR, 4 to 8 hours.

■ *Half-life*: 18 hours (adolescents); 36 hours (older adults); 25 to 65 hours with single dose, 8 to 29 hours with long-term use.

■ *Excretion*: urine.

Precautions

■ Before initiating therapy, perform a detailed history and physical examination.

■ Use with caution in patients with a mixed seizure disorder that includes atypical absence seizures due to increased frequency of seizures.

■ Use with caution in patients with a history of cardiac conduction disturbance, including second- and third-degree AV heart block; cardiac, hepatic, or renal damage; adverse hematological or hypersensitivity reaction to other drugs, including reactions to other anticonvulsants.

■ There are possible elevations of liver enzymes.

■ Before initiating the drug, obtain a history of hypersensitivity reactions to other drugs for there is a high probability of sensitivity to this drug.

■ Patients of Asian background should be screened for serious skin reactions before starting carbamazepine.

■ *Black box warning*: Aplastic anemia and agranulocytosis have been reported. Obtain complete pretreatment hematological testing as baseline. If patient in course of treatment exhibits low or decreased WBC or platelet counts, monitor closely. The drug may have to be discontinued if there is significant bone marrow depression.

Patient and Family Education

■ Patients should be made aware of the early toxic signs and symptoms of a potential hematological problem, as well as dermatological, hypersensitivity, or hepatic reactions.

■ The patient should be advised that they must report any occurrence of side effects immediately to the provider.

■ In addition, the patient should be advised that any side effects should be reported, even if mild or when occurring after extended use.

■ Patients, their caregivers, and families should be counseled on increased risk of suicidal thoughts and behavior or worsening of symptoms of depression; any unusual changes in mood or behavior; or the emergence of suicidal thoughts, behavior, or thoughts about self-harm.

■ Patients should be advised that serious skin reactions have been reported in association with Tegretol. In the event a skin reaction should occur while taking Tegretol, patients should consult with their physician immediately.

■ Tegretol may interact with some drugs. Therefore, patients should be advised to report to their doctors the use of any other prescription or nonprescription medications or herbal products.

■ Caution should be exercised if alcohol is taken in combination with Tegretol therapy, due to a possible additive sedative effect.

■ Grapefruit and grapefruit juice may increase the effects of this medicine by increasing the amount in the body. You should not eat grapefruit or drink grapefruit juice while you are taking this medicine.

Special Populations

■ *Older adults*: Use with caution in men with benign prostatic hyperplasia (BPH) due to increased urinary retention; monitor for dizziness and falls secondary to sedation.

■ *Pregnancy/lactation*: Do not use if breastfeeding.

■ *Children*: approved for use in epilepsy; therefore, safety profile exists. Used off label for aggression.

CHLORDIAZEPOXIDE HYDROCHLORIDE (Librium)

Classification
Benzodiazepine (BZD), anxiolytic

Indications
Used to achieve sedation during hypnosis, relieve anxiety, and prevent withdrawal from alcohol; used on a temporary (tapering) basis.

Available Forms
Capsule, 5, 10, and 25 mg; injection 100 mg.

Dosage
Adults: 5 to 10 mg PO TID to QID for moderate symptoms.

Children aged 6 years or older: 5 mg BID or QID; increase to 10 mg BID or TID.

Children younger than 6 years: not recommended.

For withdrawal symptoms of acute alcoholism: 50 to 100 mg PO, up to 300 mg/d.

Administration
- Administered PO.
- Use exactly as prescribed.
- Do not increase the dose, take it more frequently, or use it for a longer period of time.
- Take with full glass of water.
- The drug should not be stopped abruptly but tapered off slowly.
- When used for an extended period of time, this medicine may not work as well and may require different dosing.
- Write prescription for the shortest duration possible to prevent potential dependence.
- *Missed dose*: Take as soon as remembered. Skip the missed dose if it is almost time for the next scheduled dose. Do not take extra medicine.

Side Effects
Drowsiness, ataxia, confusion, skin eruptions, edema, menstrual irregularities, nausea, constipation, extrapyramidal effects, libido changes, paradoxical stimulation, depression, fatigue, sedation, dizziness, slurred speech, weakness, confusion, nervousness, hyperexcitability, hypersalivation, dry mouth, hallucinations (rare), and agranulocytosis.

Drug Interactions
- Avoid sodium oxybate as it can stimulate CNS and respiratory rate.
- There are increased CNS depressive effects when taken with other CNS depressants.
- Fluconazole and similar drugs can increase and prolong chlordiazepoxide levels. Avoid its use altogether.
  - *Cimetidine*: This medicine may decrease chlordiazepoxide clearance and increase risk of adverse reactions.
  - *Digoxin*: It may increase digoxin level and risk of toxicity.
  - *Disulfiram*: It may decrease clearance and increase half-life of chlordiazepoxide.
  - *Herbs*: Kava may increase sedation.

Pharmacokinetics

- *Half-life*: 5 to 30 hours. Metabolites can range from 14 to 100 hours. It can last for weeks in the blood after the initial dosing interval.
- *Peak*: 0.5 to 4 hours.
- Metabolized in the liver (CYP450) and excreted in the urine.
- Binds to BZD receptors and enhances GABA effects.

Precautions

In general, concomitant administration of chlordiazepoxide and other psychotropic drugs is not recommended. Caution should be exercised in administering chlordiazepoxide to patients with a history of psychosis, depression, suicidal ideation, porphyria, or alcohol/drug substance abuse.

- Use with caution in patients with pulmonary impairment/disease.
- History of substance abuse increases risk of dependency.
- Some patients present with disinhibiting behaviors after administration.
- Since dependence may develop, use with caution in patients with history of depression. The action of BZDs may be potentiated by barbiturates, narcotics, phenothiazines, MAOIs, or other antidepressants and can be used if depression, porphyria, suicidal ideation, alcohol/drug-abuse, or psychosis is present.

Patient and Family Education

- Inform the healthcare provider of glaucoma, hepatic or renal impairment, drug-abuse history, salivary flow decrease, or pregnancy.
- Take medicine as prescribed and do not abruptly stop without first consulting with provider.
- Before taking this medicine, tell provider of medical history of liver disease, kidney disease, lung/breathing problems, drug or alcohol abuse, or any allergies.
- Do not drive, operate heavy machinery, or perform dangerous activities until it is known how this medicine will exert its effects.
- This drug may be habit forming and should be used only by the person for whom it was prescribed.
- It can be taken with or without food.
- Do not drink alcohol while on medication.
- Smoking may decrease the drug's effectiveness.

Special Populations

- *Older adults*: Start with 5 mg every day BID and then gradually increase to 5 mg PO BID or QID. Due to the sedative effects and increased risk of falls, all BZDs are included on the Beers List of Potentially Inappropriate Medications for Geriatrics.
- Use with caution; it may require smaller dosage due to comorbid modalities.
- *Renal impairment*: CrCl ≥10, no dose adjustment needed; for <10, decrease by 50%.
- *Hepatic impairment*: Use with caution with hepatic impairment.
- *Pregnancy*: category D; positive evidence of human fetal risk.
- *Lactation*: It is contraindicated for breastfeeding mothers.
- *Children and adolescents*: This drug is not recommended for children below 6 years of age.

CITALOPRAM HYDROCHLORIDE (Celexa)

Classification
Selective serotonin reuptake inhibitor (SSRI), antidepressant

Indications
This medicine is used for MDD, premenstrual disorders, and obsessive-compulsive disorder (OCD).

Available Forms
Oral tablet, 10, 20, and 40 mg; oral solution, 10 mg/5 mL (120 mL)

Dosage
- *Adults*: initially, 20 mg once daily; may increase after 1 week to 40 mg; maximum 40 mg
- *Children older than 12 years*: initially, 20 mg once daily; may increase after 1 week to 40 mg; maximum 40 mg
- *Children younger than 12 years*: not recommended
- *Older adults*: maximum 20 mg/d

Administration
- Give PO with a glass of water.
- Take the medicine with or without food.
- Scored tablets may be crushed.
- Take at regular intervals.
- Caution patients not to stop taking drug except on provider's advice.
- This drug is not prescribed for children younger than 12 years of age.
- Instruct patients to take missed dose as soon as possible. If it is almost time for the next dose, advise to take only that dose.

Side Effects
Most common: The most common side effects are somnolence, headache, asthenia, dizziness, sweating, dry mouth, drowsiness, tremor, diarrhea, abnormal ejaculation, decreased libido, nausea, agitation, and suicide attempt.

Drug Interactions
Linezolid or MAOIs may cause anorexia, nervousness, anxiety, abnormal vision change in appetite, change in sex drive or performance, diarrhea, constipation, indigestion, and nausea.

- *Less common*: The less common side effects are suicidality, worsening depression, serotonin syndrome, seizures, hyponatremia, EPS, priapism, and acute-angle glaucoma.
- Most of the interactions occur with OTC cough-and-cold preparations. This medicine may also interact with the following medications:
  - Absolute contraindications include concurrent use with MAOIs such as phenelzine (Nardil), tranylcypromine (Parnate), isocarboxazid (Marplan), and selegiline (Eldepryl).
  - Avoid using with other SSRIs due to serotonin effect; SNRI drugs such as desvenlafaxine (Pristiq) and venlafaxine (Effexor); drugs with sympathomimetic

properties, such as phenylpropanolamine, pseudoephedrine, St. John's wort, diazepam (Valium), any other antidepressants; and clopidogrel (Plavix), amoxicillin, erythromycins, and lansoprazole (Prevacid).

- Exercise caution with cold medications, NSAIDs, and drugs used for analgesia with opioid properties, diabetes (DM), and serotonin syndrome.
- Use with caution due to increased risk of bleeding with NSAIDs, aspirin (acetylsalicylic acid [ASA]).
- *Alert:* This list may not describe all possible interactions. Instruct patients to provide a list of all medicines, herbs, nonprescription drugs, or dietary supplements used and whether they smoke, drink alcohol, or use illegal drugs.

Pharmacokinetics

- *Onset:* 1 to 2 weeks
- *Peak:* 4 hours
- *Metabolism:* Citalopram is extensively metabolized in the liver into DCT, DDCT, and citalopram-N-oxide. The CYP enzymes that are responsible for the metabolism of citalopram are CYP2C19 and CYP3A4.
- *Excretion:* primarily excreted in the urine (10% unchanged), feces liver in CYP450 2C19, 3A4 substrate; 2D6 (weak) inhibitor.
- *Half-life:* 35 hours.

Precautions

Contraindications
Sensitivity to citalopram; MAOI use within 14 days.

Cautions
While prescribing this drug, be cautious of hepatic/renal impairment, history of seizures, mania, and hypomania.

- Use should be avoided in patients with certain conditions because of the risk of QT prolongation; EKG monitoring and/or electrolyte monitoring should be performed if citalopram must be used in such patients.
- Patients with congenital long QT syndrome are at particular risk of torsade de pointes, ventricular tachycardia, and sudden death when given drugs that prolong the QT interval.
- Citalopram should be discontinued in patients who are found to have persistent QTc measurements >500 ms.
- See patients as often as necessary to ensure that the drug is working on the panic attacks, determine compliance, and review side effects.
- Make sure patients realize that they need to take prescribed doses even if they do not feel better right away. It can take several weeks before they feel the full effect of the drug.
- Instruct patients and their families to watch for worsening depression or thoughts of suicide. Also, watch out for sudden or severe changes in feelings, such as feeling anxious, agitated, panicky, irritated, hostile, aggressive, impulsive, severely restless, overly excited, or hyperactive or not being able to sleep. If this happens, especially at the beginning of antidepressant treatment or after a change in dose, patient should call the healthcare provider.
- *Drowsiness or dizziness:* Patients should not drive or use machinery or do anything that needs mental alertness until the effects of this medicine are known.

■ Caution patients not to stand or sit up quickly, especially if older. This reduces the risk of dizzy or fainting spells. Alcohol may interfere with the effect of this medicine. Avoid alcoholic drinks.

■ Caution patients not to treat themselves for coughs, colds, or allergies without asking a healthcare professional for advice. Some ingredients, such as dextromethorphan, can increase possible side effects.

■ Dry mouth: chewing sugarless gum, sucking hard candy, and drinking plenty of water may help. Contact healthcare provider if the problem persists or is severe.

■ Caution should be exercised in the following:
  ▪ Bipolar disorder or a family history of bipolar disorder
  ▪ Diabetes
  ▪ Heart disease
  ▪ Liver disease
  ▪ Electroconvulsive therapy
  ▪ Seizures (convulsions)
  ▪ Suicidal thoughts, plans, or attempts by patients or a family member
  ▪ An unusual or allergic reaction to citalopram, other medicines, foods, dyes, or preservatives
  ▪ Pregnancy or trying to get pregnant
  ▪ Breastfeeding

Patient and Family Education

■ Do not stop taking medication abruptly or increase dosage without notifying healthcare provider.

■ Store at room temperature. Avoid alcohol use.

■ Avoid tasks that require alertness and motor skills until response to drug is established.

■ Try to take the medicine at the same time each day. Follow the directions on the prescription label. To get the correct dose of liquid citalopram, measure the liquid with a marked measuring spoon or medicine cup, not with a regular tablespoon. If there is no dose-measuring device available, ask the pharmacist for one.

Special Populations

■ *Older adults*: Older adults are more sensitive to anticholinergic effects. They are more likely to experience dizziness, sedation, confusion, hypotension, and hyperexcitability. The maximum recommended dose of citalopram is 20 mg per day for patients older than 60 years of age.

■ *Children*: Citalopram may cause increased anticholinergic effects and hyperexcitability. It is not indicated for children under 12 years of age.

■ *Renal and hepatic impairment*: The initial dose should be reduced in patients with severe renal and/or hepatic impairment. Half-life is doubled in patients with hepatic impairment. Titration upward should be slow and at intervals.

■ *Pregnancy*: category C; potential for persistent pulmonary HTN if the patient is at more than 20 weeks' gestation.

■ *Lactation*: Drug is excreted in human breast milk; some reports of infant somnolence. Lactation is not recommended.

CLOMIPRAMINE (Anafranil)

Classification
Tricyclic antidepressant (TCA)

Indications
- This drug is not used much anymore; it is off many formularies due to high risk of suicidality and completion.
- It is indicated for OCD.

Available Forms
Capsule, 25, 50, and 75 mg

Dosage
- *Adults*: initially 25 mg daily in divided doses; gradually increase to 100 mg during first 2 weeks; maximum 250 mg/d; total maintenance dose may be given at HS.
- *Children older than 10 years*: initially 25 mg daily in divided doses; gradually increase; maximum 3 mg/kg or 100 mg (whichever is smaller).
- *Children younger than 10 years*: not recommended.

Administration
Take this medicine PO with or without food. Do not abruptly discontinue medication.

Side Effects
Dry mouth, nausea, vomiting, diarrhea, constipation, nervousness, decreased sexual ability, decreased memory or concentration, headache, stuffy nose, and change in appetite or weight. *The following side effects should be immediately reported to the clinician:* extrapyramidal syndrome/dystonia seizures; fast, irregular, or pounding heartbeat; difficulty urinating or loss of bladder control; believing things that are not true, hallucinations (seeing things or hearing voices that do not exist), eye pain; shakiness; difficulty breathing or fast breathing; severe muscle stiffness, unusual tiredness or weakness; and sore throat, fever, and other signs of infection.

Drug Interactions
- The following drugs are contraindicated: antiarrhythmics class IA such as procainamide, quinidine gluconate, quinidine sulfate, disopyramide (Norpace) as these may increase risk of side effects or increase the risk of a QT prolongation.
- Specific medications that may interact with the agent include cimetidine (Tagamet); guanethidine monosulfate (Ismelin; methylphenidate [Concerta, Ritalin, Daytrana]); phenytoin (Dilantin); warfarin (Coumadin); heart or BP medication, such as clonidine (Catapres) or digoxin (Lanoxin); heart rhythm medications, such as flecainide (Tambocor), quinidine (Cardioquin, Quinidex, Quinaglute); or antipsychotic medications, such as chlorpromazine (Thorazine), haloperidol (Haldol), thioridazine (Mellaril), clozapine (Clozaril), olanzapine (Zyprexa, Zydis), quetiapine (Seroquel), risperidone (Risperdal), or ziprasidone (Geodon). Cisapride (Propulsid) may increase risk of QT prolongation, cardiac arrhythmias; dronedarone (Multaq) may increase TCA levels and risk of adverse effects, increase risk of QT prolongation, cardiac arrhythmias; it may increase risk of cardiac arrhythmias, seizures.

- MAOIs such as selegiline (Eldepryl/Zelapar), procarbazine (Matulane), phenelzine (Nardil), tranylcypromine (Parnate), isocarboxazid (Marplan), selegiline transdermal (Eldepryl/Zelapar), and rasagiline (Azilect) may result in CNS overstimulation, hyperpyrexia, seizures, or death.
- Pimozide (Orap) may increase risk of CNS depression and psychomotor impairment, QT prolongation, arrhythmias, anticholinergic effects, and hyperpyrexia; potassium salts such as potassium acid phosphate, potassium citrate, potassium chloride, potassium iodide, potassium phosphate/sodium phosphate, potassium acid, phosphate/sodium acid phosphate, and potassium phosphate are contraindicated for solid potassium dose forms.
- Weigh risk–benefit of thyroid protection with solid iodide salt forms; may delay solid potassium passage through GI tract and increase risk of ulcerative/stenotic lesions.
- Use with caution in patients with altered GI motility.
- Monitor the patient for anticholinergic symptoms.

Pharmacokinetics

This drug is presumed to influence obsessive and compulsive behaviors through its effects on serotonergic neuronal transmission.

- It is metabolized in the liver extensively (CYP450, 1A2, 2C19, 2D6) and is excreted in the urine (66%) and in the feces (32%).
- *Half-life*: 32 hours.
- *Peak*: 2 to 6 hours.
- The exact neurochemical mechanism of action is unknown, but its capacity to inhibit the reuptake of serotonin (5-HT) is thought to be important.

Precautions

- It is contraindicated with recent myocardial infarction.
- Do not use the drug if MAOI is used within past 14 days.
- Do not use the drug if patient is allergic to similar drugs (TCAs).
- Monitor the patient for suicidal thoughts.
- Report new or worsening symptoms of mood or behavior changes, anxiety, panic attacks, insomnia, or feelings of impulsivity, irritability, agitation, hostility aggressiveness, restlessness, hyperactivity, increased depression, or suicidal thoughts. It inhibits norepinephrine and serotonin reuptake.

Patient and Family Education

- Anxiety symptoms may temporarily worsen when you first start taking clomipramine.
- Do not stop taking this medicine without notifying the healthcare provider.
- Anxiety symptoms may temporarily worsen when first starting.
- Notify doctor or pharmacist promptly if any of these effects persist or worsen.
- To relieve dry mouth, suck on (sugarless) hard candy or ice chips, chew (sugarless) gum, drink water, or use a saliva substitute.
- To prevent constipation, maintain a diet adequate in fiber, drink plenty of water, and exercise. In case of constipation, consult your pharmacist for help in selecting a laxative (e.g., stimulant-type with stool softener).
- Notify your clinician immediately if any of these unlikely but serious side effects occur: mental/mood changes (e.g., confusion, depression, hallucinations, memory problems), enlarged/painful breasts, unwanted breast milk production,

irregular/painful menstrual periods, muscle stiffness/twitching, feelings of restlessness, ringing in the ears, sexual problems (e.g., decreased sexual ability, changes in desire), shakiness (tremors), numbness/tingling of the hands/feet, trouble urinating, and severe vomiting.

■ Notify your clinician immediately if any of these rare but very serious side effects occur: easy bruising/bleeding, signs of infection (e.g., fever, persistent sore throat), unusual/uncontrolled movements (especially of the tongue/face/lips), severe stomach/abdominal pain, dark urine, and yellowing of eyes/skin.

■ Seek immediate medical attention if any of these rare but very serious side effects occur: black stools, chest pain, fainting, high fever, slow/fast/irregular heartbeat, seizures, vomit that looks like coffee grounds.

Special Populations

■ *Older adults*: Lower doses are recommended.
■ *Renal impairment*: Significant caution is warranted with renal impairment.
■ *Hepatic impairment*: Caution is advised in children with hepatic impairment.
■ *Pregnancy/lactation*: This is a category C drug; animal studies have shown adverse fetal effects.
■ *Children and adolescents 12 to 17 years*: There is an increased risk of suicidality in children, adolescents, and young adults. Gradual increase in dose is recommended.

CLONAZEPAM (Klonopin)

Classification
Benzodiazepine (BZD)

Indications
- This is an antianxiety medication.
- It is also used to prevent seizures.

Available Forms
Tablets, 0.5, 1, and 2 mg; disintegrating wafers, 0.125, 0.25, 0.5, 1, and 2 mg

Dosage
- Seizures: initially 1.5 mg daily in 3 divided doses; increase by 0.5 to 1 mg daily every 3 days until seizures are controlled or side effects preclude further increases in dose; maximum 20 mg/d
- *Panic disorder*: initially 0.25 mg BID; increase to 1 mg/d after 3 days; maximum 1 mg/d

Administration
- The dose is tailored to the patient's needs.
- It can be taken with or without food.

Side Effects
- Sedation, dizziness weakness, and unsteadiness
- Depression, loss of orientation, headache, and sleep disturbance

Drug Interactions
- Other BZDs can accentuate the effects of other drugs that slow the brain's processes, such as alcohol, barbiturates, and narcotics, and lead to increased sedation.

Pharmacokinetics
- Act by enhancing the effects of GABA in the brain. GABA inhibits brain activity.
- Excessive activity in the brain can cause anxiety or mood disorders.

Precautions
- Sudden cessation of the drug can cause seizures, tremors, muscle cramping, vomiting, and/or sweating, severe depression, agitation, and insomnia.
- The dose should be reduced slowly.
- It can cause increased risk of suicidal thinking and behavior.
- Observe patient for clinical worsening, suicidal thoughts, or unusual changes in behavior.

Patient Education
- This drug can cause physical dependence.
- Never stop taking the drug, as sudden cessation of the drug can cause serious side effects.
- Report all side effects to provider.

Special Populations

- *Older adults*: Older adults are more sensitive to this drug's CNS effects.
- *Pregnancy*: category D.
  - There is documented evidence of fetal damage, including congenital malformations, when taken by pregnant women in their first trimester.
  - It is not recommended throughout pregnancy.
- *Lactation*
  - BZDs are secreted in breast milk.
  - It is not recommended for mothers who are breastfeeding.
- *Children*: The drug is not indicated for treatment of panic disorder.

CLONIDINE HYDROCHLORIDE (Catapres, Catapres-TTS, Kapvay, Nexiclon XR)

Classification

Alpha-agonist, antihypertensive

Indications

- Essential and renal HTN, severe cancer pain, ADHD as monotherapy or adjunct to stimulant medications.
- It is used for ADHD and control of pain and has been used off label for control of withdrawal symptoms for opiates and ETOH.

Available Forms

- Tablet, 0.1, 0.2, and 0.3 mg; 0.025, 0.1, 0.2, and 0.3 mg; XR tablets, 0.1, 0.17, 0.2, and 0.26 mg; oral suspension, 0.09 mg/mL; patch (7-day administration), 0.1, 0.2 mg/d (12/carton); 0.3 mg/d (4/carton).

Dosage

- Catapres
  - *Adults*: 4 to 5 mcg/kg/d
  - *Children older than 12 years*: 4 to 5 mcg/kg/d
  - *Children younger than years*: not recommended
- Catapres-TTS
  - *Adults*: initially 0.1 mg patch weekly; increase after 1 to 2 weeks if needed; maximum 0.6 mg/d
  - *Children older than 12 years*: initially 0.1 mg patch weekly; increase after 1 to 2 weeks if needed; maximum 0.6 mg/d
  - *Children younger than 12 years*: not recommended
- Kapvay
  - *Adults*: not indicated
  - *Children 6 to 12 years*: initially 0.1 mg at bedtime × 1 week; then 0.1 mg BID × 1 week; then 0.1 mg AM and 0.2 mg PM × 1 week; then 0.2 mg BID; withdraw gradually by 0.1 mg/d at 3 to 7 day intervals.
  - *Children younger than 6 years*: not recommended
- Nexiclon XR
  - *Adults*: initially 0.18 mg (2 mL) suspension or 0.17 mg tab once daily; usual maximum 0.52 mg (6 mL suspension) once daily
  - *Children older than 12 years*: initially 0.18 mg (2 mL) suspension or 0.17 mg tablet once daily; usual maximum 0.52 mg (6 mL suspension) once daily
  - *Children younger than 12 years*: not recommended

Administration

Oral: Take the medicine with a full glass of water; it may be taken with or without food.

Topical: Apply patch on skin without hair. Leave it in place for 7 days. It may require special covering. Take last dose immediately before bedtime.

Side Effects

Dry mouth, sedation, dizziness, constipation, weakness, fatigue, insomnia, headache, impotence, loss of libido, major depression, hypotension, nervousness, agitation, nausea, vomiting, rashes with patches, bradycardia, and severe rebound HTN are the side effects of the drug.

Drug Interactions

- Do not administer the medicine with a beta-blocker due to CV symptoms. It may cause the paradoxical hypertensive effect.
- It causes increased sedative and depressive symptoms when given with another CNS depressant.
- Administration with drugs that affect sinus node or AV function may result in bradycardia or AV block. Herbs such as capsicum and ma huang may reduce antihypertensive effectiveness; digoxin, verapamil, and diuretics may increase hypotensive effect; levodopa may reduce effectiveness of levodopa; MAOIs may decrease antihypertensive effect.

Pharmacokinetics

- Inhibit central vasomotor centers, lowering peripheral vascular resistance, BP, and heart rate
- *Metabolism*: liver, excreted by kidney (urine 72%)
- *Peak*: PO, 2 to 4 hours; transdermal, 2 to 3 days
- *Half-life*: 6 to 20 hours

Precautions

- There have been rare cases of hypertensive crisis and stroke after abrupt discontinuation.
- If used with a beta-blocker, the beta-blocker should be stopped several days before tapering drug.

Patient and Family Education

- Make position changes slowly and in stages. Dangle feet over bed prior to standing.
- Lie down immediately if feeling faint or dizzy.
- Avoid potentially hazardous activities until effect of medication has been determined.
- *Missed dose*: Take the dose as soon as remembered. If it is almost time for next dose, wait until next regularly scheduled dose. Do not take extra medicine to make up the missed dose.

Special Populations

- *Older adults*: Use with caution due to sedative effects.
- *Renal impairment*: Use with caution. It may require smaller dosage.
- *Hepatic impairment*: Use with caution.
- *Pregnancy*: category C.
- *Lactation*: Some drug is found in mother's breast milk; discontinue drug or bottle-feed.
- *Children and adolescents*: Safety and efficacy not established for children under 12 years; children are more likely to experience CNS depression with overdose.

CLORAZEPATE (Tranxene)

Classification
Benzodiazepine (BZD)

Indications
Clorazepate is used to achieve sedation during hypnosis and to relieve anxiety, panic disorder, and alcohol withdrawal syndrome.

Available Forms
Tablet, 3.75, 7.5, and 15 mg

Dosage
Adults: 30 mg/d in divided doses; maximum 60 mg/d

Children older than 9 years: 30 mg/d in divided doses; maximum 60 mg/d

Children younger than 9 years: not recommended

Administration
The drug is taken as per PO. It should not be abruptly stopped. To discontinue this drug, client must consult with healthcare provider.

Side Effects
Drowsiness, dizziness, various GI complaints, nervousness, blurred vision, dry mouth, headache, and confusion.

Drug Interactions
- Avoid antacids.
- Avoid sodium oxybate as it can increase CNS and respiratory depression.
- Avoid chloramphenicol, cimetidine (Tagamet), clarithromycin (Biaxin), conivaptan (Vaprisol), cyclosporine (Gengraf/Neoral), delavirdine (Rescriptor), imatinib (Gleevec), INH, itraconazole (Sporanox), ketoconazole, nefazodone (Serzone), posaconazole (Noxafil), protease inhibitors, telithromycin (Ketek), voriconazole (Vfend), and use of antacids for they may increase BZD levels, risk of CNS depression, and psychomotor impairment.
- The action of BZDs may be potentiated by barbiturates, narcotics, phenothiazines, MAOIs, or other antidepressants. The concomitant use of other CNS-depressant drugs is contraindicated.

Pharmacokinetics
- Drug is metabolized in the liver (CYP 450) and excreted primarily through the urine and feces.
- This drug has depressant effects on the CNS by binding to BZD receptors and enhancing GABA effects.
- *Half-life*: 40 to 50 hours.
- *Onset*: 1 to 2 hours.
- *Duration*: Variable 8 to 24 hours.

Precautions

Serious reactions to the drug include hepatotoxicity, respiratory depression, seizure exacerbation, suicidality, dependency, and abuse.

Patient and Family Education

- Do not abruptly stop taking the drug without consulting the prescriber; the dose must be carefully tapered.
- It may increase the risk of suicidal thoughts and behavior; be alert for the emergence of or worsening of signs and symptoms of depression, unusual changes in mood or behavior, or emergence of suicidal thoughts.
- Avoid taking this drug if there is a known hypersensitivity to the drug or if there is acute narrow-angle glaucoma.
- Do not drive, operate heavy machinery, or do other dangerous activities until it is known how clorazepate exerts its effects.
- Do not drink alcohol or take other drugs that may cause sleepiness or dizziness while taking clorazepate without first talking to the provider.
- Avoid becoming pregnant while on this drug; if pregnancy occurs, alert healthcare provider immediately.

Special Populations

- *Older adults*: Older adults or debilitated patients need to start at 7.5 to 15 mg/d. Due to its sedative effect and increased risk of falls, all BZDs are included on the Beers List of Potentially Inappropriate Medications for Geriatrics.
- *Renal impairment*: No adjustment needed.
- *Hepatic impairment*: Not defined at this time.
- *Pregnancy*: category D; trimester specific. There is an increased risk of congenital malformations associated with the use of this drug during the first trimester of pregnancy.
- *Lactation*: It is probably safe during lactation but caution is advised.
- *Children*: It is not recommended for children under 9 years of age.

CLOZAPINE (Clozaril, Fazaclo)

Classification

Antipsychotic drug, atypical (second generation); dibenzapine derivative

Indications

It is used for treatment-resistant schizophrenia, reduction in risk of recurrent suicidal behavior in patients with schizophrenia, or schizoaffective disorder.

Available Forms

Tablet, 150 and 200 mg; ODT, 12.5, 25, 100, 150, and 200 mg

Dosage

Taper to goal dose.

Adults: initially 12.5 mg/d, taken as a single dose or two times per day; maximum 900 mg/d.

Children: This is a drug not for pediatric use.

Administration

The drug is subject to restricted distribution in the United States; permission for its use should be granted through the FDA. It requires registration. WBC levels should be drawn weekly and reported to the dispensing pharmacy prior to drug being dispensed. After 6 months of normal WBC counts, blood draws reduced to every 2 weeks; monitor CBC, glucose, and cholesterol throughout treatment course—WBC/absolute neutrophil count (ANC) at baseline, then every week × 6 months, then every 2 weeks × 6 months, then every 4 weeks for treatment duration and every week × 4 weeks after discontinuing drug; fasting glucose at baseline if diabetes is a risk factor, then periodically; see package insert for additional recommendations based on results of WBC/ANC monitoring.

Side Effects

Hypotension, severe; syncope; EPS, severe; TD; NMS; hyperglycemia, severe; diabetes mellitus; seizures; priapism; stroke; transient ischemic attacks (TIA); QT prolongation; hypersensitivity reaction; anaphylactic reaction; angioedema; erythema multiforme; leukopenia; neutropenia; agranulocytosis; suicidality; somnolence; increased appetite; fatigue; rhinitis; upper respiratory infections; nausea/vomiting; cough; urinary incontinence; salivation; constipation; fever; dystonia; abdominal pain; anxiety; dizziness; dry mouth; tremor; rash; akathisia; dyspepsia; tachycardia; hyperprolactinemia/gynecomastia; weight gain; dysphagia.

Drug Interactions

- The drug interacts with Haldol, sodium oxybate, and ziprasidone. Caution is required with diabetes and HTN.
- Tablets may be given with or without food. Take the regular oral tablet with a full glass of water.
- The ODT FazaClo can be taken without water. Advise patients to keep the tablet in its blister pack until ready to take. The patient should gently peel back the foil from the blister pack and drop the tablet onto dry hand; place the tablet in mouth;

it will begin to dissolve right away; allow it to dissolve in the mouth without chewing; swallow several times as the tablet dissolves. If desired, advise patients to drink liquid to help swallow the dissolved tablet.

- If one half of an ODT is prescribed, advise patients to break the tablet in half and throw the other half away. *Do not* save the other half for later use.
- If patients stop taking clozapine for more than 2 days in a row, caution patients to call providers before starting to take it again.
- Store clozapine at room temperature away from moisture and heat.
- Risk or severity of bone marrow suppression may be increased if the drug is given in conjunction with medications that suppress bone marrow.
- Use with caution if given in conjunction with alcohol, CNS depressants, or general anesthesia.
- It may enhance effects of antihypertensive drugs.
- Clozapine dose may need to be reduced if given in conjunction with CYP450 1A2 inhibitors (e.g., fluvoxamine) or with smoking cessation.
- There may be a need to increase clozapine dose if given in conjunction with CYP450 1A2 inducers (e.g., cigarette smoke).
- CYP450 2D6 inhibitors (e.g., paroxetine, fluoxetine, and duloxetine) and CYP450 3A4 inhibitors (e.g., nefazodone, fluvoxamine, and fluoxetine) can raise clozapine levels, but usually dosage adjustment is not required.
- *Alert:* This list may not describe all possible interactions. Instruct clients to provide a list of all the medicines, herbs, nonprescription drugs, or dietary supplements they use.

Pharmacokinetics

- Exact mechanism of action is unknown.
- It antagonizes dopamine D2 receptors and serotonin 5-HT2 receptors.
- *Metabolism*: metabolized by multiple CYP450 enzymes, including 1A2, 2D6, and 3A4.
- *Half-life*: 5 to 16 hours.
- *Excretion*: Urine (50%), feces (30%).

Precautions

- Hypersensitivity to drug/class.
- Caution in case of renal impairment, hepatic impairment, dementia, Parkinson's disease, and NMS history.
- There is an increased risk of fatal myocarditis, especially during, but not limited to, the first month of therapy. Promptly discontinue clozapine if myocarditis is suspected.
- Life-threatening agranulocytosis can occur. Baseline WBC and ANC should be done before initiation of treatment, during treatment, and for at least 4 weeks after discontinuing treatment, every week × 6 months, then every 2 weeks for 6 more months, and monthly thereafter if blood work is acceptable.
- Use with caution in patients with glaucoma or enlarged prostate.
- *Do not use in patients with the following conditions:*
  - Myeloproliferative disorder.
  - Uncontrolled seizure history, cardiac disease, cerebrovascular disease, hypotension, hypovolemia, dehydration, aspiration pneumonia risk; it may impair body temperature regulation, phenylketonuria (PKU; phenylalanine-containing forms), diabetes mellitus or diabetes mellitus risk; caution is required with older adults, pediatric or adolescent patients, and patients with drug-induced leukopenia or neutropenia history and suicide risk.

- Granulocytopenia.
- Paralytic ileus.
- CNS depression.
- Allergic symptoms to clozapine.

Patient and Family Education

- Drug effects can linger for 7 to 8 weeks after last dose.
- Clozapine will only be provided in 1- to 4-week supplies depending on frequency of WBC monitoring. Follow-up visits and weekly blood cell counts are required to monitor therapy and to keep appointments.
- Take prescribed dose with or without food. Take with food if stomach upset occurs.
- Keep tablet in unopened blister until just before use. Remove tablet by peeling the foil from the back of the blister and then immediately place the tablet (or half tablet, if ordered) in mouth, allow the tablet to disintegrate, and then swallow with saliva.
- Do not stop taking clozapine when feeling better.
- If medication needs to be discontinued, it will be slowly withdrawn over a period of 1 to 2 weeks unless safety concerns (e.g., low WBC) require a more rapid withdrawal.
- *Immediately report to provider* if any of these conditions occur: altered mental status, change in personality or mood, chest pain, fever, flu-like symptoms, frequent urination, general body discomfort, involuntary body or facial movements, lethargy, mucous membrane sores or other signs of possible infection, muscle rigidity, pounding in the chest, rapid or difficult breathing, rapid or irregular heartbeat, seizures, sore throat, sweating, swelling of feet or ankles, unexplained fatigue, unexplained shortness of breath, unquenchable thirst, weakness, or weight gain.
- *If you have diabetes*, monitor blood glucose more frequently when drug is started or dose is changed and inform provider of significant changes in readings.
- *If you are taking antihypertensive drugs*, monitor BP at regular intervals.
- *If you have history of seizures or factors predisposing to seizures*, clozapine may cause seizures. Do not engage in any activity in which sudden loss of consciousness could cause serious risk to you or others (e.g., driving, swimming, climbing).
- *Avoid* strenuous activity during periods of high temperature or humidity.
- *Avoid* alcoholic beverages and sedatives (e.g., diazepam) while taking clozapine.
- Get up slowly from a lying or sitting position and avoid sudden position changes to prevent postural hypotension. Hot tubs and hot showers or baths may make dizziness worse.
- Take sips of water, suck on ice chips or sugarless hard candy, or chew sugarless gum if dry mouth occurs. Excess salivation can be treated; report to physician.
- Clozapine may impair your judgment, thinking, or motor skills, or it may cause drowsiness. Thus, use with caution while driving or performing other tasks requiring mental alertness until tolerance is determined.

Special Populations

- *Older adults*: Caution is required due to polypharmacy and comorbid conditions. Older adults may tolerate lower doses better. Older adults with dementia-related psychosis treated with atypical antipsychotics are at higher risk for death and cerebrovascular events.
- *Renal impairment*: Use with caution.
- *Hepatic impairment*: Use with caution.
- *Cardiac impairment*: Use with caution, especially if patient is taking concomitant medication.

- *Pregnancy*: category B; animal studies do not show significant evidence of safety.
- *Lactation*: It is not known whether clozapine is secreted in human breast milk. Discontinuing the drug or bottle-feeding is recommended. Infants of women who choose to breastfeed while on this drug should be monitored for possible adverse effects.
- *Children*: It is not for use in children who show adverse effects.

CYCLOBENZAPRINE (Amrix, Fexmid, Flexeril)

Classification
Muscle relaxant

Indications
It is used to treat short-term relief of muscle spasms associated with acute painful muscle and skeletal conditions, fibromyalgia, and temporomandibular joint (TMJ) disorder.

Available Forms
Tablet, 5, 7.5, and 10 mg; XR capsules, 15 and 30 mg

Dosage
- *Adult:* 10 mg TID; usual range 20 to 40 mg/d in divided doses; maximum 60 mg/d × 2 to 3 weeks or 15 mg XR once daily; maximum 30 mg XR/d × 2 to 3 weeks
- *Children older than 15 years:* 10 mg TID; usual range 20 to 40 mg/d in divided doses; maximum 60 mg/d × 2 to 3 weeks or 15 mg XR once daily; maximum 30 mg XR/d × 2 to 3 weeks
- *Children younger than 15 years:* not recommended

Administration
- The drug is to be taken by mouth with or without food.
- It should usually be administered once daily.
- Swallow the capsules whole.
- Capsules cannot be crushed or chewed. Doing so can release all of the drug at once, increasing the risk of side effects.
- The dosage is based on medical condition and response to treatment.
- It should only be used short term (for 3 weeks or less).

Side Effects
- Drowsiness, dry mouth, fatigue, headaches, and dizziness.
- Nausea, vomiting, GI upset with constipation, acid reflux, and abdominal pain.
- Blurred vision, agitation/nervousness, confusion.
- The patient needs to understand not to stop taking this drug especially if they have taken it for over 3 weeks, for it could cause withdrawal symptoms.

Drug Interactions
The following products may cause serious drug-to-drug interactions:
- TCAs.
- Avoid MAOIs both 2 weeks before treatment and during treatment with this medication.
- Avoid taking this drug with other products that cause drowsiness, such as alcohol, antihistamines, drugs for sleep or antianxiety agents, other muscle relaxants, and narcotic pain relievers.

Pharmacokinetics
- The drug is metabolized and excreted via the kidney.
- The drug is eliminated quite slowly, with an effective half-life of 18 hours (range 8–37 hours; $n = 18$).
- Plasma clearance is 0.7 L/min.

Precautions

- This drug should be used with caution with patients with liver disease, hyperthyroidism, irregular heartbeat, heart block, heart failure, recent history of myocardial infarction, BPH, and glaucoma.
- It may cause dizziness or drowsiness.
- Patients are advised not to drive, use machinery, or do any activity that requires alertness until effects of the drug are known.
- The patients should not indulge in alcoholic beverages while taking this medication.

Patient and Family Education

- If patient has used an MAOI such as isocarboxazid (Marplan), tranylcypromine (Parnate), phenelzine (Nardil), or selegiline (Eldepryl, Emsam) within the past 14 days, they should not use this drug.
- Do not use this drug if patient has a significant cardiac history with a heart rhythm disorder, congestive heart failure, heart block, or an overactive thyroid.
- This drug may impair thinking or reactions.
- Avoid driving or doing anything that requires alertness.
- Avoid drinking alcohol, which can increase side effects of cyclobenzaprine.

Special Populations

- *Pregnancy*: There are no adequate studies of use in pregnant women.
- *Nursing mothers*: It is not known whether the drug is secreted in milk. However, since it is related to the TCAs, some of which are excreted in breast milk, caution is advised in using this medication in women who are breastfeeding.
- *Older adults:*
  - The plasma concentration of cyclobenzaprine is increased in older adults.
  - Older adults may also be more at risk for CNS adverse events.
  - Cardiac events.
  - Falls.
  - *Note*: For these reasons, in older adults, cyclobenzaprine should be used only if clearly needed. In older adults, initiate dose at 5 mg and titrate upward slowly.
- *Pediatric*: Safety and effectiveness have not been established in pediatric patients younger than 15 years of age.

CYPROHEPTADINE (Periactin)

Classification
Antihistamine

Indications
This drug is used to treat hay fever; nightmares, including nightmares related to posttraumatic stress disorder (PTSD); serotonin syndrome; and cases of hyperserotoninemia. It can also be used as a preventive measure against migraine in children and adolescents. It can relieve SSRI-induced sexual dysfunction and drug-induced hyperhidrosis (excessive sweating). It can also be used in the treatment of cyclical vomiting syndrome and to stimulate the appetite and in the treatment of anorexia/cachexia.

Available Forms
Tablet, 4 mg; syrup, 2 mg/5 mL

Dosage
- *Adult:* initially 4 mg TID prn; then adjust as needed; usual range, 12 to 16 mg/d; maximum 32 mg/d
- *Children older than 14 years:* initially 4 mg TID prn; then adjust as needed; usual range, 12 to 16 mg/d; maximum 32 mg/d
- *Children 7 to 14 years:* 4 mg BID to TID prn; maximum 16 mg/d
- *Children 2 to 6 years:* 2 mg BID to TID prn
- *Children younger than 2 years:* not recommended

Administration
PO; take with food to avoid GI distress.

Drug Interactions
There are no interactions to avoid concomitant use.

Pharmacokinetics
- *Absorption:* Complete; peak 6 to 9 hours
- *Metabolism:* Hepatic
- *Half-life:* 1 to 4 hours

Precautions
- This drug is contraindicated in narrow-angle glaucoma.
- Concurrent use of MAOIs.
- Precaution must be taken in cases of bladder neck obstruction and GI obstruction.
- It may cause CNS depression.

Patient and Family Education
Avoid using this drug with other depressants and sleep-inducing medications unless approved by prescriber. It can cause possible dizziness and drowsiness (caution when driving or engaging in tasks requiring alertness).

Special Populations

- *Older adults:* It may be inappropriate for older adults due to anticholinergic effects although for short-term use weigh risk versus benefit.
- *Pregnancy:* pregnancy category B.
- *Lactation:* It is not indicated.
- *Pediatric:* not recommended in children younger than 2 years of age.
- *Outcome:* Symptoms improve in 24 hours although mental confusion can last for several days.

DESIPRAMINE (Norpramin)

Classification
Tricyclic antidepressant (TCA)

Indications
Desipramine is used to treat adults with depression.

Available Forms
Tablet, 10, 25, 50, 75, 100, and 150 mg

Dosage
- *Adult:* 100 to 200 mg/d in single or divided doses; maximum 300 mg/d
- *Children older than 12 years:* 100 to 200 mg/d in single or divided doses; maximum 300 mg/d
- *Children younger than 12 years:* not recommended

Administration
- PO with a glass of water.
- Do not abruptly stop taking the medication.
- Food can lessen GI upset.
- Not prescribed for children.
- Use lowest effective dose for shortest duration—shortest but adequate duration for an optimal trial. Duration is based on number of episodes of depression.

Side Effects
- *More common:* Drowsiness, dizziness, constipation, nausea/vomiting, urinary retention or frequency, libido changes, weight gain, general nervousness, galactorrhea, rash, and urticaria are the most common side effects of desipramine.
- *Less common:* Cardiac arrhythmias, EPS, clotting disturbances, worsening depression, suicidality, hyperthermia, and HTN are the less common side effects of desipramine.

Drug Interactions
- Absolute contraindications include class IA antiarrhythmics and MAOIs such as phenelzine (Nardil), tranylcypromine (Parnate), isocarboxazid (Marplan), and selegiline (Eldepryl).
- Avoid using with cimetidine, amiodarone, clarithromycin, erythromycin, haloperidol, and St. John's wort.
- *Alert:* This list may not describe all possible interactions. Instruct patients to provide a list of all medicines, herbs, nonprescription drugs, or dietary supplements used, and if they smoke, drink alcohol, or use illegal drugs.

Pharmacokinetics
- TCAs are thought to work by inhibiting reuptake of norepinephrine and serotonin in the CNS, which potentiates the neurotransmitters. They also have significant anticholinergics, antihistaminic, and alpha-adrenergic activity on the cardiac system. These classes of antidepressants also possess class 1A antiarrhythmic activity, which can lead to depression of cardiac conduction, potentially resulting in heart block or ventricular arrhythmias.

- *Metabolism*: Primarily in the liver.
- *Excretion*: Urine.
- *Half-life*: Seven to 60 hours with high variability due to first-pass effects of those taking the drug.

Precautions

- See patients as often as necessary to ensure that the drug is working on the panic attacks, determine compliance, and review side effects.
- Instruct patients and families to watch for worsening depression or thoughts of suicide. Also watch out for sudden or severe changes in feelings such as feeling anxious, agitated, panicky, irritated, hostile, aggressive, impulsive, severely restless, overly excited, or hyperactive or not being able to sleep. If this happens, especially at the beginning of antidepressant treatment or after a change in dose, patient should call the healthcare provider.
- *Drowsiness or dizziness*: Patients should not drive or use machinery or do anything that needs mental alertness until the effects of this medicine are known. Other medications that cause drowsiness can add to the drowsiness of desipramine.
- Caution patients not to stand or sit up quickly, especially if older. This reduces the risk of dizzy or fainting spells. Alcohol may interfere with the effect of this medicine. Avoid alcoholic drinks.
- Do not abruptly withdraw this drug as it may cause headache, nausea, and malaise.
- Advise to protect skin from ultraviolet light due to increased skin sensitivity.
- Caution should be exercised in the following:
  - MDD, psychosis, or bipolar affective disorder
  - Contraindicated in patients with a recent myocardial infarction
  - Blood dyscrasias
  - Respiratory disease
  - Heart disease
  - Liver disease
  - Seizures (convulsions)
  - Psychoses or schizophrenia
  - Suicidal thoughts, plans, or attempts by patients or a family member
  - Monitor for hypersensitivities

Patient and Family Education

- Store desipramine at room temperature away from moisture and heat.
- Stopping this medication suddenly could result in unpleasant side effects.
- Take the missed dose as soon as remembered. If it is almost time for the next dose, skip the missed dose and take the medicine at the next regularly scheduled time. *Do not* take extra medicine to make up the missed dose.

Special Populations

- *Older adults*: Older patients may be more sensitive to the effects of TCAs. The smallest effective dose should be used (beginning at 10–25 mg/d). Dose adjustment is necessary for patients with liver impairment.
- *Pregnancy*: category C; unknown effects as there is limited study.
- *Lactation*: The drug is excreted in human breast milk and hence should be used with caution.
- *Children*: It is not indicated for children younger than 12 years of age.

DESVENLAFAXINE (Pristiq)

Classification
Serotonin-norepinephrine reuptake inhibitor (SNRI)

Indications
Desvenlafaxine is used to treat MDD, panic disorder, anxiety disorder, and PTSD.

Available Forms
XR tablets, 50 and 100 mg

Dosage
- *Adult:* initially 50 mg once daily; maximum 120 mg/d (swallow whole)
- *Children older than 12 years:* initially 50 mg once daily; maximum 120 mg/d (swallow whole)
- *Children younger than 12 years:* not recommended
- Doses >50 mg/d are rarely more effective; maintenance may increase adverse drug reaction risk; consider a dose of 50 mg every other day if poorly tolerated in older adults.

Administration
PO, can be taken with or without food. Do not crush, cut, or chew capsule or tablet.
- Take at regular intervals.
- Caution patients not to stop taking drug except on provider's advice.
- The drug is not prescribed for children.
- Instruct patients to take missed dose as soon as possible. If it is almost time for the next dose, advise to take only that dose.

Side Effects
- *Most common*: The most common side effects are nausea, vomiting, headache, insomnia, dizziness, somnolence, decreased libido and GI distress, sexual dysfunction, palpitations, nervousness, HTN, hyperhidrosis, constipation, and fatigue.
- *Less common*: The less common side effects are worsening depression, suicidality, hypersensitivity reactions, urinary retention, and increased BP.

Drug Interactions
- Absolute contraindications to this drug include MAOIs such as phenelzine (Nardil), tranylcypromine (Parnate), isocarboxazid (Marplan), and selegiline (Eldepryl).
- Avoid using with other SSRIs due to serotonin effect; SNRI drugs such as venlafaxine (Effexor) and all triptan agents. Exercise caution with cold medications, NSAIDs, and drugs used for analgesia with opioid properties.
- *Alert:* This list may not describe all possible interactions. Instruct patients to provide a list of all medicines, herbs, nonprescription drugs, or dietary supplements used and if they smoke, drink alcohol, or use illegal drugs.

Pharmacokinetics
- SNRI agents are potent inhibitors of neuronal serotonin and norepinephrine reuptake and weak inhibitors of dopamine reuptake.
- Relative to SSRIs, SNRI agents seem to be more effective in treating chronic pain issues that coexist with depression and may produce more stimulative effects.

■ Highly bound to plasma proteins and has a large volume of distribution.

■ *Metabolism*: liver inactivation via CYP 3A4.

■ *Excretion*: urine 64% to 69% (45% unchanged); 11 hours (*o*-desmethylvenlafaxine).

■ *Half-life*: 11 hours, 13 to 14 hours (moderate-to-severe hepatic impairment), 13 to 18 hours (mild-to-severe renal impairment), 23 hours (end-stage renal disease).

■ *Peak*: 7.5 hours.

■ The drug is not metabolized by P450s, so has more predictable plasma levels than many other antidepressants, including venlafaxine.

Precautions

■ See patients as often as necessary to ensure that the drug is working on the panic attacks, determine compliance, and review side effects.

■ Make sure patients realize that they need to take prescribed doses even if they do not feel better right away. It can take several weeks before depression resolves.

■ Instruct patients and families to watch for worsening depression or thoughts of suicide. Also watch for sudden or severe changes in feelings, such as feeling anxious, agitated, panicky, irritated, hostile, aggressive, impulsive, severely restless, overly excited, or hyperactive or not being able to sleep. If this happens, especially at the beginning of antidepressant treatment or after a change in dose, patient should call the healthcare provider.

■ *Drowsiness or dizziness*: Patients should not drive or use machinery or do anything that needs mental alertness until the effects of this medicine are known.

■ Caution patients not to stand or sit up quickly, especially if older. This reduces the risk of dizzy or fainting spells. Alcohol may interfere with the effect of this medicine. Avoid alcoholic drinks.

■ Caution patients not to treat themselves for coughs, colds, or allergies without asking the healthcare professional for advice. Some ingredients can increase possible side effects.

■ *Dry mouth*: Chewing sugarless gum, sucking hard candy, and drinking plenty of water may help. Contact a healthcare provider if the problem persists or is severe.

■ Caution should be exercised in the following:
   ■ Bipolar disorder or a family history of bipolar disorder
   ■ Diabetes
   ■ Heart disease
   ■ Liver disease
   ■ Seizures (convulsions)
   ■ Suicidal thoughts, plans, or attempts by patients or a family member
   ■ An unusual or allergic reaction to venlafaxine, other medicines, foods, dyes, or preservatives
   ■ Pregnancy or trying to get pregnant
   ■ Breastfeeding

Patient and Family Education

■ Store at room temperature. Take any unused medication after the expiration date to the local pharmacy on drug give-back day. Avoid discarding the medication into the environment.

■ Try to take the medicine at the same time each day. Follow the directions on the prescription label.

■ The medicine should be taken about the same time every day, morning or evening, and can be taken with or without food.

■ It may take up to 4 weeks to be fully effective, but patient may see symptoms of depression improving in as few as 1 to 2 weeks.

■ If patient plans on becoming pregnant, discuss the benefits versus the risks of using this medicine while pregnant. This medicine is excreted in breast milk; nursing mothers should not breastfeed while taking this medicine.

■ This medication should be used only when clearly needed during pregnancy. The patient should discuss the risks and benefits with the doctor.

■ If this medication is used during the last 3 months of pregnancy, the newborn may have feeding or breathing difficulties, seizures, muscle stiffness, jitteriness, or constant crying.

■ This medication should not be stopped unless the healthcare provider directs it. Report any adverse symptoms to the healthcare provider promptly.

■ Caution should be exercised when using this drug in older adults because they may be more sensitive to the effects of the drug.

■ Similar to other SNRIs.

■ Do not administer with MAOIs and use caution when combining with other drugs that have activating properties.

■ Use with caution in patients with a history of seizures or heart disease.

Special Populations

■ *Older adults:* Older individuals tend to be more sensitive to medication side effects, such as hypotension and anticholinergic effects, often requiring adjustment of medication doses for hepatic or renal dysfunction. Older adults may tolerate lower doses better, and there is a reduced risk of suicide. This medicine may assist in the treatment of chronic or depression-related physical pain.

■ *Pregnancy:* Psychotherapy is the initial choice for most pregnant patients with mild to moderate MDD. It is a category C drug, as there are no adequate studies during pregnancy. Particular caution is needed with exposure (avoid if possible) during first trimester. An individual risk–benefit analysis must be done to determine appropriate treatment in pregnant women with MDD.

■ *Children:* Monitor closely, as risk of suicidal ideation is greatest in adolescents. Monitor for excessive activation effects or undiagnosed bipolar disorder. Obtain consultation with a pediatric psychiatric specialist. Not recommended for children younger than 12 years of age.

DEXMETHYLPHENIDATE (Focalin, Focalin ER, Focalin XR)

Classification
Methylphenidate (amphetamine derivative)

Indications
Dexmethyphendidate is a stimulant indicated for the treatment of ADHD in children.

Available Forms
Capsule, 2.5, 5, and 10 mg; XR capsules, 5, 10, 15, 20, 25, 30, 35, and 40 mg

Dosage
Dosage should be individualized according to the therapeutic needs and responses of the patient. All stimulant preparations should be administered at the lowest effective dosage.

- *Children older than 6 years*: initially 2.5 mg BID; allow at least 4 hours between doses; may increase at 1 week intervals; maximum 20 mg/d
- *Children younger than 6 years*: not established
- *Adults*: not indicated

Administration
Do not crush or chew the drug; it may be given with or without food.

Side Effects
Decreased appetite, dizziness, dry mouth, irritability, insomnia, upper abdominal pain, nausea and/or vomiting, weight loss, headaches, anxiety, psychiatric events, increase in manic states for bipolar patients, aggression, tics, tremors, long-term growth suppression—patients should be monitored throughout treatment; if there appears to be growth suppression, the treatment should be discontinued—rash, pyrexia, palpitations, tachycardia, elevated BP, sudden death, myocardial infarction, cardiomyopathy, SJS and TEN, impotence, and libido changes.

Drug Interactions
There are over 242 drugs that can interact with dexmethylphenidate. Make sure to review patients' drug regimen before prescribing this drug.

Pharmacokinetics
- Drug is absorbed by the GI tract.
- Amphetamines are non-catecholamine-sympathomimetic amines with CNS-stimulant activity.
- The mode of therapeutic action in ADHD is not known. Amphetamines are thought to block the reuptake of norepinephrine and dopamine into the presynaptic neuron and increase the release of these monoamines into the extraneural space.
- *Metabolism*: liver; excreted in the urine.
- *Half-life*: 2 to 4.5 hours.

Precautions

- Advanced arteriosclerosis, symptomatic CV disease, moderate-to-severe HTN contraindicated in glaucoma, patients with motor tics, or diagnosis of Tourettes.
- Hyperthyroidism.
- Known hypersensitivity or idiosyncratic reaction to sympathomimetic amines.
- Contraindicated in patients with glaucoma-agitated states.
- *Patients with a history of drug abuse*: Amphetamines have a high potential for abuse. Administration of amphetamines for an extended period of time may lead to drug dependence. Particular attention should be paid to the possibility of patients obtaining this class of medication for nontherapeutic use or distribution to others, and the drugs should be prescribed or dispensed sparingly.
- During or within 14 days following the administration of MAOIs, hypertensive crisis may result.
- Use with caution in patients with preexisting psychosis.
- *Seizure history*: Some studies have shown that the drug has the potential for lowering the seizure threshold.

Patient and Family Education

- Store the drug at room temperature, protected from light.
- Keep out of reach of children.
- Seek medical care for any signs of heart problems (chest pain, shortness of breath), fainting, psychotic symptoms, overdose, or any other concerns.
- Routinely assess weight and BP.
- Treatment should be initiated at low dosages and then titrated over 2 to 4 weeks until an adequate response is achieved, or unacceptable adverse effects occur.
- If one stimulant is not effective, another should be attempted before second-line medications are considered. Although some children benefit from daily stimulant therapy, weekend and summer "drug holidays" are suggested for children whose ADHD symptoms predominantly affect schoolwork or to limit adverse effects (e.g., appetite suppression, abdominal pain, headache, insomnia, irritability, tics).

Special Populations

- *Older adults*: Use with caution for older adults with polypharmacy and comorbid conditions; the drug has not been studied for use in this population.
- *Pregnancy*: category C; based on animal data, drug may cause fetal harm.
- *Lactation*: It is possibly unsafe for breastfeeding.
- *Children*: It has not been studied in children younger than 6 years; it should not be used in children younger than 6 years.

DEXTROAMPHETAMINE AND AMPHETAMINE (Adderall, Adderall XR, Dexedrine, Dexedrine Spansule, DextroStat)

Classification

Amphetamine

Indications

The medicine is a stimulant indicated for the treatment of ADHD and narcolepsy in children and adults.

Available Forms

Tablet, 5, 7.5, 10, 12.5, 15, 20, and 30 mg; capsule (XR), 5, 10, 15, 20, 25, and 30 mg

Dosage

- Adderall
  - *Adult*: initially 10 mg daily; may increase weekly by 10 mg/d; usual maximum 60 mg/d in 2 to 3 divided doses; first dose on awakening; then q4h to q6h prn
  - *Children older than 12 years*: initially 10 mg daily; may increase weekly by 10 mg/d; usual maximum 60 mg/d in 2 to 3 divided doses; first dose on awakening; then q4h to q6h prn
  - *Children 6 to 12 years*: initially 5 mg daily; may increase by 5 mg/d at weekly intervals
  - *Children younger than 6 years*: not recommended
- Adderall XR
  - *Adult*: 20 mg PO once daily in AM; may increase by 10 mg/d at weekly intervals; maximum 60 mg/d
  - *Children 13 to 17 years*: 10 to 20 mg PO daily in the AM; may increase by 10 mg/d at weekly intervals; maximum 40 mg/d; do not chew; may sprinkle on apple sauce
  - *Children 6 to 12 years*: initially 10 mg daily in the AM; may increase by 10 mg/d at weekly intervals; maximum 30 mg/d
  - *Children younger than 6 years*: not recommended
- Dexedrine, Dexedrine Spansule, DextroStat
  - *Adult*: initially start with 10 mg daily; increase by 10 mg at weekly intervals if needed; may switch to daily dose with sust-rel spansules when titrated
  - *Children older than 12 years*: initially 10 mg daily; may increase by 10 mg/d at weekly intervals; maximum 40 mg/d
  - *Children 6 to 12 years*: initially 5 mg daily or BID; may increase by 5 mg/d at weekly intervals; usual maximum 40 mg/d
  - *Children 3 to 5 years*: 2.5 mg daily; may increase by 2.5 mg daily at weekly intervals if needed
  - *Children younger than 3 years*: not recommended
- Where possible, drug administration should be interrupted occasionally to determine whether there is a recurrence of behavioral symptoms sufficient to require continued therapy.

Administration

Swallow capsules whole with water or other liquids. If patient cannot swallow the capsule, open it and sprinkle the medicine over a spoonful of applesauce. Swallow all of the applesauce and medicine mixture without chewing immediately. Follow with a drink of water or other liquid. Never chew or crush the capsule or the medicine inside the capsule. It can be taken with or without food.

Side Effects

Decreased appetite, dizziness, dry mouth, irritability, insomnia, upper abdominal pain, nausea and/or vomiting, weight loss, headaches, anxiety, psychiatric events (increase in manic states for bipolar patients, aggression, tics, tremors), long-term growth suppression (patients should be monitored throughout treatment; if there appears to be growth suppression, the treatment should be discontinued), rash, pyrexia, palpitations, tachycardia, elevated BP, sudden death, myocardial infarction, cardiomyopathy, SJS and TEN, impotence, and libido changes.

Drug Interactions

This drug has too many drug interactions to mention. Provider must review patients' drug regimen to determine safety.

Pharmacokinetics

- The drug is absorbed by the GI tract.
- Amphetamines are non-catecholamine sympathomimetic amines with CNS-stimulant activity.
- The mode of therapeutic action in ADHD is not known. Amphetamines are thought to block the reuptake of norepinephrine and dopamine into the presynaptic neuron and increase the release of these monoamines into the extraneural space.
- *Excretion*: urine.
- *Half-life*: 9 *to* 14 hours.
- *Duration*: 4 to 6 hours; onset: 30 to 60 minutes.

Precautions

- Advanced arteriosclerosis, symptomatic CV disease, moderate-to-severe HTN.
- Hyperthyroidism.
- Known hypersensitivity or idiosyncratic reaction to sympathomimetic amines.
- Contraindicated in glaucoma.
- Agitated states.
- *Patients with a history of drug abuse*: Amphetamines have a high potential for abuse. Administration of amphetamines for an extended period of time may lead to drug dependence. Particular attention should be paid to the possibility of subjects obtaining this class of medication for nontherapeutic use or distribution to others, and the drugs should be prescribed or dispensed sparingly.
- During or within 14 days following the administration of MAOIs, hypertensive crisis may result.
- Use with caution in patients with preexisting psychosis.
- *Seizure history*: Some studies have shown that the drug has the potential for lowering the seizure threshold.

Patient and Family Education

- Store the drug at room temperature, protected from light.
- Keep out of reach of children.
- Seek medical care for any signs of heart problems (chest pain, shortness of breath), fainting, psychotic symptoms, overdose, or any other concerns.

- Routinely assess weight and BP.
- Treatment should be initiated at low dosages and then titrated over 2 to 4 weeks until an adequate response is achieved or unacceptable adverse effects occur.
- If one stimulant is not effective, another should be attempted before second-line medications are considered. Although some children benefit from daily stimulant therapy, weekend and summer "drug holidays" are suggested for children whose ADHD symptoms predominantly affect schoolwork or to limit adverse effects (e.g., appetite suppression, abdominal pain, headache, insomnia, irritability, tics).

Special Populations

- *Odults*: Use with caution for older adults with polypharmacy and comorbid conditions; it has not been studied for use in this population.
- *Pregnancy*: category C; based on animal data, they may cause fetal harm.
- *Lactation*: It is possibly unsafe for breastfeeding.
- *Children*: It is not recommended in children younger than 3 years of age.

DIAZEPAM (Valium, Valium injectable, Valium intensol oral solution, Valium oral solution, Diastat, Diastat acudial)

Classification
Benzodiazepine (BZD)

Indications
Diazepam is used to treat anxiety, acute alcohol withdrawal, and seizures.

Available Forms
Tablets, 2, 5, and 10 mg; oral solution, 5 mg/mL; vial, 5 mg/mL; ampule, 5 mg/mL; prefilled syringe, 5 mg/mL; rectal gel, 2.5, 10, and 20 mg

Dosage
- *Adult*: 2 to 10 mg BID to QID
- *Children older than 12 years*: 2 to 10 mg BID to QID
- *Children younger than 12 years*: not recommended

Administration
- Diazepam may be taken with or without food.

Side Effects
- Drowsiness, fatigue, and ataxia (loss of balance).
- Possible paradoxical reaction with excitability, muscle spasm, lack of sleep, and rage.
- Confusion, depression, speech problems, and double vision also are rare side effects.

Drug Interactions
- Alcohol or medications that cause sedation may add to the sedative effects of diazepam.
- Avoid use with other BZDs.
- Cimetidine (Tagamet), ketoconazole (Nizoral), itraconazole (Sporanox), omeprazole (Prilosec, Rapinex), erythromycin, clarithromycin (Biaxin), darunavir (Prezista), fluvoxamine (Luvox), and fluoxetine (Prozac) may prolong the effects of diazepam by inhibiting liver enzymes that eliminate diazepam.
- Dosages may need to be decreased when these drugs are used with diazepam.
- Carbamazepine (Tegretol), rifampin (Rifadin), and St. John's wort decrease levels of diazepam by increasing the elimination of diazepam by liver enzymes.

Pharmacokinetics
- Diazepam is metabolized by the liver and is excreted mainly by the kidney.
- Dosages of diazepam may need to be lowered in patients with abnormal kidney function.

Precautions
- The dosages need to be lowered in patients with abnormal kidney function.
- It can lead to addiction (dependency), especially when higher dosages are used over prolonged periods of time.

- Abrupt discontinuation may cause symptoms of withdrawal, light-headedness, sweating, anxiety, and fatigue.
- Seizures can occur in more severe cases of withdrawal. Therefore, after extended use, diazepam should be slowly tapered under a provider's supervision rather than abruptly stopped.
- This drug may make the patient dizzy and drowsy or cause blurred vision; use caution engaging in activities requiring alertness such as driving or using machinery.
- Limit alcoholic beverages.
- Caution is advised when using this drug in older adults because they may be more sensitive to the effects of the drug, especially the drowsiness effect.

Patient and Family Education

Inform the patient of the following:

- Provider should be made aware of all prescription and nonprescription/herbal products used, especially of antacids, certain antidepressant drugs that cause drowsiness, medicine for sleep (e.g., sedatives), muscle relaxants, and narcotic pain relievers.
- This product can affect the results of certain lab tests.
- Smoking can decrease the effectiveness of this drug.
- Not to start or abruptly stop any medicine without provider approval.

Special Populations

- *Older adults*: Adjust dose according to age.
- *Pregnancy*: It can cause fetal abnormalities and should not be used during pregnancy.
- *Nursing mothers*: It is excreted in breast milk and can affect nursing infants; it should not be used in mothers who plan to breastfeed.
- *Pediatric*: The use of this drug is not recommended in children younger than 12 years.

DICYCLOMINE (Bentyl)

Classification
Anticholinergic drug

Indications
Dicyclomine is used to treat abdominal cramping associated with opiate withdrawal.

Available Forms
Capsule, 10 mg; tablet, 20 mg; syrup, 10 mg/5 mL; vial, 10 mg/mL (10 mL); ampule, 10 mg/mL (2 mL)

Dosage
- *Adult*: initially 20 mg BID to QID; may increase to 40 mg QID PO; usual IM dose 80 mg/d divided QID; do not use IM route for more than 1 to 2 days.
- *Children older than 12 years*: initially 20 mg BID to QID; may increase to 40 mg QID PO; usual IM dose 80 mg/d divided QID; do not use IM route for more than 1 to 2 days.
- *Children younger than 12 years*: not recommended.

Administration
- PO with glass of water.
- Measure liquid medicine with a special dose-measuring spoon or cup, not a regular tablespoon.

Side Effects
Confusion, disrupted thoughts, palpitations and/or arrhythmias, decreased urination, drowsiness, dizziness, blurred vision, nausea and/or vomiting, anorexia, pruritus or rash, stuffy nose, and dry mouth are the various side effects for dicyclomine.

Drug Interactions
- The following medications may exacerbate side effects: amantadine, antiarrhythmic agents of class 1, antihistamines, antipsychotic agents, BZDs, MAOIs, narcotic analgesics, nitrites and nitrates sympathomimetic agents, and TCAs.
- The drug may antagonize the effects of antiglaucoma agents.
- It should be avoided when intraocular pressure is present and when taking corticosteroids.
- It may affect GI absorption of digoxin.
- The drug may antagonize the effects of metoclopramide.
- Avoid the use of dicyclomine simultaneously with the use of antacids.

Pharmacokinetics
- *Half-life*: 1.8 hour

Precautions
- The drug may increase risk of heat stroke by decreasing sweating.

Patient and Family Education
- Use with caution when driving or operating machinery.

- Avoid drinking alcohol.
- Avoid become overheated or dehydrated during exercise and hot weather.
- Tell healthcare provider about all prescription and OTC medications due to interaction.

Special Populations

- *Older adults*: Use with caution among older adults; dosage should start at the low end.
- *Renal impairment*: Use with caution.
- *Hepatic impairment*: Use with caution.
- *Pregnancy*: category B.
- *Lactation*: Contraindicated.
- *Children and adolescents*: not recommended in children younger than 12 years.
- *Other*: Use with caution in patients with the following: autonomic neuropathy, hepatic/renal disease, ulcerative colitis, hyperthyroidism, HTN, coronary heart disease, heart failure, cardiac tachyarrhythmia, hiatal hernia, and prostatic hypertrophy.

DIPHENHYDRAMINE HYDROCHLORIDE (Benadryl)

Classification
Antihistamine

Indications
This drug is used to treat rhinitis, allergy symptoms, motion sickness, Parkinson's disease

Available Forms
Chew tablets, 12.5 mg; capsules, 25 mg; liquid, 12.5 mg/5 mL; tablet, 25 mg; dye-free soft gel, 25 mg; dye-free liquid, 12.5 mg/5 ML

Dosage
- *Adults and children older than 12 years*: 25 to 50 mg PO q6h to q8h; maximum 100 mg daily
- *Children 6 to 12 years*: 12.5 to 25 mg PO q4h to q6h; maximum dose 150 mg daily
- *Children 2 to 6 years*: 6.25 mg PO q4h to q6h; maximum dose 37.5 mg daily
- *Children younger than 2 years*: not recommended
- Nighttime sleep aid
  - *Adults*: 50 mg PO at bedtime

Administration
- PO; give with food or milk to reduce GI distress.
- *IV*: Do not exceed 25 mg mg/min.
- *IV incompatibilities*: allopurinol, amobarbital, amphotericin B, cefepime, dexamethasone, foscarnet, haloperidol lactate, phenobarbital, phenytoin, thiopental.
- *IM*: Give deep injection into large muscle.
- Alternate injection sites to prevent irritation.

Side Effects
- *Central nervous system*: seizures, drowsiness, sedation, sleepiness, dizziness, incoordination, confusion, insomnia, headache, vertigo, fatigue, restlessness, tremor, and nervousness
- *Cardiovascular*: palpitations, hypotension, and tachycardia
- *EENT*: diplopia, blurred vision, nasal congestion, and tinnitus
- *Gastrointestinal*: dry mouth, nausea, epigastric distress, vomiting, diarrhea, constipation, and anorexia
- *Genitourinary*: dysuria, urine retention, and urinary frequency
- *Hematologic*: thrombocytopenia, agranulocytosis, and hemolytic anemia
- *Respiratory*: thickening of bronchial secretions
- *Other*: anaphylactic shock

Drug Interactions
- CNS depressants may increase sedation. Use together cautiously.
- MAOIs may increase anticholinergic effects. Avoid using together.
- Other products containing diphenhydramine may increase risk of adverse reactions. Drug lifestyle: Alcohol use may increase CNS depression. Discourage use together.
- Sun exposure may cause photosensitivity reaction. Avoid prolonged sunlight exposure.

■ *Effects of lab test results*: may decrease hemoglobin level and hematocrit, may decrease granulocyte and platelet counts, may prevent reduce or mask positive result in diagnostic skin test.

Pharmacokinetics

■ *PO onset*: 15 minutes, peak 1 to 4 hours, duration 5 to 8 hours.
■ IV onset immediate, peak 1 to 4 hours, duration 6 to 8 hours.
■ IM onset unknown, peak 1 to 4 hours, duration 6 to 8 hours.
■ It competes with histamine for H1 receptor sites.
■ Prevents but does not reverse histamine-mediated responses, particularly those of bronchial tubes, GI tract, uterus, and blood vessels.
■ It is structurally related to local anesthetics.
■ Drug provides local anesthesia and suppresses cough reflex.

Precautions

■ The drug is contraindicated in patients hypersensitive to the drug, newborns, and premature neonates.
■ Avoid with breastfeeding women; patients with angle-closure glaucoma, stenosing peptic ulcer, symptomatic prostatic hyperplasia, bladder neck obstruction, or pyloroduodenal obstruction; and those having an acute asthmatic attack.
■ Avoid the use of the drug in patients taking MAOIs.
■ Use with caution with patients with prostatic hyperplasia, asthma, chronic obstructive pulmonary disease, increased intraocular pressure, hyperthyroidism, CV disease, and HTN.
■ Overdose signs and symptoms are dry mouth, fixed or dilated pupils, flushing, and GI symptoms.
■ Stop drug 4 days before diagnostic skin testing. Injection form is for IV or IM administration only.
■ Dizziness, excessive sedation, syncope, toxicity, paradoxical stimulation, and hypotension are more likely to occur in older adults.

Patient and Family Education

■ Warn patients not to take this drug with other products containing diphenhydramine because of risk of adverse reactions.
■ Take drug half hour before travel to prevent motion sickness.
■ Take it with food or milk to reduce GI distress.
■ Avoid alcohol and hazardous activities that require alertness until CNS effects of drug are known.
■ Sugarless gum, hard candy, or ice chips may prevent dry mouth.
■ Notify prescriber if tolerance develops because a different antihistamine may need to be prescribed.
■ This drug can be found in many OTC sleep and cold products.
■ Consult prescriber before using these products.
■ Warn against possible photosensitive reactions.
■ Advise use of sun block when going outdoors.

Special Populations

■ *Older adults*: Be mindful of disease or age-related symptoms that may contraindicate usage.
■ *Pregnancy*: category B.
■ *Pediatric*: Children below age 12 years should use only as directed by prescriber.

DISULFIRAM (Antabuse)

Classification
Aversion therapy

Indications
Used to treat alcohol dependence, dependence, and withdrawal syndrome

Note
Disulfiram use requires informed consent.

Available Forms
Tablets, 250 and 500 mg; chew tablets, 200 and 500 mg

Dosage
- *Adults:* 500 mg once daily × 1 to 2 weeks; then 250 mg once daily
- *Children younger than 18 years:* not recommended

Administration
- Store at room temperature away from moisture, heat, and light.
- Take the missed dose as soon as you remember. Take the rest of the day's doses at evenly spaced intervals unless otherwise directed by your provider.

Side Effects
- *Central nervous system:* drowsiness, peripheral neuritis, encephalopathy, polyneuritis, peripheral neuropathy, headache, seizures, lethargy
- *Dermatologic:* skin eruptions, acneiform eruptions, allergic dermatitis, maculopapular rash
- *EENT:* Optic neuritis, eye pain or tenderness, changes in vision
- *Gastrointestinal:* nausea, vomiting, constipation, halitosis, metallic or garlic-like aftertaste, light gray-colored stools, severe stomach pain
- *Genitourinary:* decreased libido, darkening of urine
- *Hepatic:* altered liver function tests, hepatic cell damage, hepatitis (cholestatic and fulminant), hepatic failure resulting in transplant or death, jaundice, cirrhosis
- *Psychiatric:* psychotic reactions, depression, paranoia, schizophrenia, mania, confusion, personality changes, disorientation, memory impairment

Drug Interactions
- *Alcohol (ethyl):* Disulfiram may enhance the adverse/toxic effect of alcohol (ethyl). A disulfiram-like reaction may occur. Avoid combination.
- *Atazanavir:* may diminish the therapeutic effect of disulfiram. Monitor therapy.
- *Bacampicillin:* may enhance the adverse/toxic effect of disulfiram. Avoid combination.
- *Benznidazole:* may enhance the adverse/toxic effect of disulfiram. In particular, the risk for CNS toxicities such as psychosis may be increased. Avoid combination.
- *Chlordiazepoxide:* Disulfiram may increase the serum concentration of chlordiazepoxide. Monitor therapy.
- *Chlorzoxazone:* CYP2E1 inhibitors (strong) may increase the serum concentration of chlorzoxazone. Monitor therapy.

■ *Clozapine*: CYP1A2 inhibitors (weak) may increase the serum concentration of clozapine.

■ *Chlordiazepoxide*: Disulfiram may increase the serum concentration of chlordiazepoxide. Monitor therapy.

■ *Diazepam*: Disulfiram may increase the serum concentration of diazepam. Monitor therapy.

■ *Dronabinol*: Disulfiram may enhance the adverse/toxic effect of dronabinol. Specifically, disulfiram may produce severe intolerance to the alcohol contained in the dronabinol oral solution. Avoid combination.

■ *Fexinidazole*: may enhance the adverse/toxic effect of disulfiram. Avoid combination.

■ *Flunitrazepam*: Disulfiram may increase the serum concentration of flunitrazepam. Monitor therapy.

■ *INH*: CYP2E1 inhibitors (strong) may increase the serum concentration of INH. Monitor therapy.

■ *Metronidazole (systemic)*: Disulfiram may enhance the adverse/toxic effect of metronidazole (systemic). In particular, the risk for CNS toxicities such as psychosis may be increased. Avoid combination.

■ *Metronidazole (topical)*: may enhance the adverse/toxic effect of disulfiram. In particular, the risk for CNS toxicities such as psychosis may be increased. Management: Warn patients and monitor for the development of serious CNS toxicity if topical metronidazole is used in a patient taking disulfiram. Some manufacturers of vaginal metronidazole products list disulfiram use within 2 weeks as a contraindication. Consider therapy modification.

■ *Phenytoin*: Disulfiram may increase the serum concentration of phenytoin. Management: Avoid concomitant use of disulfiram and phenytoin when possible. Phenytoin dose adjustment will likely be necessary when starting and/or stopping concurrent disulfiram. Monitor phenytoin response and concentrations closely. Consider therapy modification.

■ *Theophylline*: Disulfiram may increase the serum concentration of theophylline. Monitor therapy.

■ *Theophylline derivatives*: CYP1A2 inhibitors (weak) may increase the serum concentration of theophylline derivatives. Exception: dyphylline. Monitor therapy.

■ *Tinidazole*: may enhance the adverse/toxic effect of disulfiram. Avoid combination.

■ *Tipranavir*: disulfiram may enhance the adverse/toxic effect of tipranavir. Avoid combination.

■ *Tizanidine*: CYP1A2 inhibitors (weak) may increase the serum concentration of tizanidine. Management: Avoid these combinations when possible. If combined use is necessary, initiate tizanidine at an adult dose of 2 mg and increase in 2- to 4-mg increments based on patient response. Monitor for increased effects of tizanidine, including adverse reactions. Consider therapy modification.

■ *Vitamin K antagonists (e.g., warfarin)*: Disulfiram may increase the serum concentration of vitamin K antagonists. Monitor therapy.

Pharmacokinetics

■ Reduction of disulfide linkage to diethyldithiocarbamic acid, followed by further metabolization via glucuronidation, nonenzymatic degradation, methylation, and oxidation.

■ *Half-life*: 60 to 120 hours.

■ Approximately 20% remains in the system for 1 week after discontinuation.

Precautions

- *Black box warning*: Disulfiram should never be administered to a patient in a state of alcohol intoxication or without their full knowledge. The clinician should instruct relatives accordingly. Do not administer disulfiram if alcohol has been consumed within the prior 12 hours.
- Contraindicated in patients with hypersensitivity to disulfiram or any component of the formulation or to other thiuram derivatives used in pesticides and rubber vulcanization; in patients receiving or using alcohol, metronidazole, paraldehyde, or alcohol-containing preparations (e.g., cough syrup, tonics); or in patients with psychosis or severe myocardial disease or coronary occlusion.
- Ingesting alcohol, even in small amounts, during treatment with disulfiram may result in flushing, throbbing in head and neck, nausea, copious vomiting, respiratory difficulty, diaphoresis, thirst, chest pain, palpitation, dyspnea, hyperventilation, tachycardia, hypotension, syncope, marked uneasiness, weakness, vertigo, blurred vision, and confusion. Severe reactions may involve respiratory depression, CV collapse, arrhythmias, myocardial infarction, acute congestive heart failure, unconsciousness, seizure, and death. The intensity of the reaction is generally proportional to the amounts of disulfiram and alcohol ingested. The reaction can last from 30 minutes to several hours in more severe cases, or as long as it takes the alcohol to be metabolized. Patients should avoid alcohol consumption for >12 hours prior to administration; disulfiram reactions can occur up to 14 days after taking disulfiram if alcohol is consumed.
- Severe (sometimes fatal) hepatitis and/or hepatic failure resulting in transplantation have been associated with use; may occur in patients with or without prior history of abnormal hepatic function. Monitor for hepatotoxicity and educate patients about signs and symptoms.
- Use with extreme caution in patients with cerebral damage.
- Evaluate patients with a history of rubber contact dermatitis for hypersensitivity to thiuram derivatives before administering disulfiram.
- Use with extreme caution in patients with diabetes mellitus.
- Use with extreme caution in patients with hepatic cirrhosis or impairment.
- Use with extreme caution in patients with hypothyroidism.
- Use with extreme caution in patients with acute or chronic nephritis.
- Use with extreme caution in patients with a history of seizure disorder.
- Monitor liver function tests.

Patient and Family Education

- Warn patients about the disulfiram reaction to alcohol and "disguised" forms of alcohol (e.g., tonics, mouthwashes, cough mixtures, sauces, vinegars, aftershave lotions, back rubs) and the duration of drug activity.
- Advise patients to avoid all alcohol while taking this medication.

Special Populations

- *Pregnancy*: category C
- *Pediatric*: Not for use in children

DIVALPROEX SODIUM (Depacon, Depakene, Depakote, Depakote ER, Depakote Sprinkle)

Classification

Mood-stabilizing anticonvulsant

Indications

Divalproex sodium is used for the treatment of the manic episodes of bipolar disorder and MDD and is taken long term for prevention of both manic and depressive phases of bipolar disorder, especially the rapid-cycling variant, and for the treatment of epilepsy, certain side effects of autism, chronic pain associated with neuropathy, and migraine headaches.

Available Forms

Capsule (delayed release), 125 mg, 250 mg, 250 mg/mL (16 oz); tablet (delayed-release), 125, 250, and 500 mg; table (XR), 250 and 500 mg

Dosage

Mania

- *Adults*: Take once daily; swallow XR form whole; initially 25 mg/kg/d in divided doses; maximum 60 mg/kg/d.
- *Older adults*: Take once daily; swallow XR form whole; initially 25 mg/kg/d in divided doses; maximum 60 mg/kg/d. Reduce initial dose and titrate slowly.
- *Children older than 12 years*: Take once daily; swallow XR form whole; initially 25 mg/kg/d in divided doses; maximum 60 mg/kg/d.
- *Children younger than 12 years*: not recommended.

To Prevent Migraine Headache

- *Adults*: delayed-release: initially 250 mg BID; titrate weekly to usual maximum 500 mg BID; XR: initially 500 mg once daily; may increase after 1 week to 1,000 mg once daily
- *Older adults*: Start at lower dosage. Increase dosage more slowly and with regular monitoring of fluid and nutritional intake and watch for dehydration, somnolence, and other adverse reactions.
- *Children older than 10 years*: delayed-release: initially 250 mg BID; titrate weekly to usual maximum 500 mg BID; XR: initially 500 mg once daily; may increase after 1 week to 1,000 mg once daily
- *Children younger than 10 years*: not recommended

Administration

- PO: Give the drug with food or milk to reduce adverse GI effects.
- Do not mix syrup with carbonated beverages, as the mixture may be irritating to oral mucosa.
- Capsules may be swallowed whole or opened and contents sprinkled on a teaspoonful of soft food. Patient should swallow the capsule immediately without chewing.
- Monitor drug level and adjust dosage as needed.

Side Effects

- *Central nervous system*: asthenia, dizziness, headache, insomnia, nervousness, somnolence, tremor, abnormal thinking, amnesia, ataxia, depression, emotional upset, fever, sedation

- *Cardiovascular*: chest pain, edema, HTN, hypotension, tachycardia
- *EENT*: blurred vision, diplopia, nystagmus, pharyngitis, rhinitis, tinnitus
- *Gastrointestinal*: abdominal pain, anorexia, diarrhea, dyspepsia, nausea, vomiting, pancreatitis, constipation, increased appetite
- *Hematologic*: bone marrow suppression, hemorrhage, thrombocytopenia, bruising, petechiae
- *Hepatic*: hepatotoxicity
- *Metabolic*: hyperammonemia, weight gain
- *Musculoskeletal*: back and neck pain
- *Respiratory*: bronchitis, dyspnea
- *Skin*: alopecia, flu syndrome, infection, erythema multiforme, hypersensitivity reactions, SJS, rash, photosensitivity reactions, pruritus

Drug Interactions

This drug interacts with aspirin, chlorpromazine, clonazepam, topiramate, cimetidine, felbamate, carbamazepine, lamotrigine, phenobarbital, phenytoin, rifampin, warfarin, and zidovudine. Alcohol use is discouraged.

Pharmacokinetics

- *Peak action*: oral, between 15 minutes and 4 hour. Facilitates the effects of the inhibitory neurotransmitter GABA
- *Half-life*: 6 to 16 hours

Precautions

- It may increase ammonia, ALT, AST, and bilirubin lab levels.
- It may increase eosinophil count and bleeding time. It may also decrease platelet, red blood cell, and WBC counts.
- The drug may cause false-positive results for urine ketone levels.
- It is contraindicated in patients hypersensitive to the drug, in those with hepatic disease or significant hepatic dysfunction, and in patients with a urea cycle disorder (UCD).
- Safety and efficacy of Depakote ER in children younger than age 10 years have not been established.
- Obtain liver function test results, platelet count, PT, and INR before starting therapy and monitor these values periodically.
- Adverse reactions may not be caused by valproic acid alone because it is usually used with other anticonvulsants.
- Never withdraw a drug suddenly, because sudden withdrawal may worsen seizures. Call the prescriber at once if adverse reactions develop.
- Patients at high risk for hepatotoxicity include those with congenital metabolic disorders, mental retardation, or organic brain disease; those taking multiple anticonvulsants; and children younger than 2 years of age.
- Notify the prescriber if tremors occur; a dosage reduction may be needed.
- Weight gain is common. Monitor body mass index and assess for prediabetes and dyslipidemia.
- Sedation is common.
- Therapeutic level is 50 to 100 mcg/mL.
- When converting patients from a brand-name drug to a generic drug, use caution because breakthrough seizures may occur.
- The drug may cause thrombocytopenia or tremors.

■ *Alert:* Sometimes fatal, hyperammonemic encephalopathy may occur when starting valproate therapy in patients with UCD and pancreatitis. Evaluate patients with UCD risk factors before starting valproate therapy. Patients who develop symptoms of unexplained hyperammonemic encephalopathy during valproate therapy should stop taking the drug, undergo prompt appropriate treatment, and be evaluated for underlying UCD.

■ *Alert:* Fatal hepatotoxicity may follow nonspecific symptoms, such as malaise, fever, and lethargy. If these symptoms occur during therapy, notify the prescriber at once, because patients who might be developing hepatic dysfunction must stop taking the drug.

■ *Alert:* Life-threatening pancreatitis has been reported following initiation of therapy as well as after prolonged use. Monitor the patient for developing symptoms and discontinue treatment if pancreatitis is suspected.

Patient and Family Education

■ Take the drug with food or milk to reduce adverse GI effects.
■ Do not chew capsules; irritation of mouth and throat may result.
■ It may take several weeks or longer to optimize mood-stabilizing effects.
■ Capsules may be swallowed whole or carefully opened and contents sprinkled on a teaspoonful of soft food. Swallow the capsule immediately without chewing.
■ Keep drugs out of children's reach.
■ Warn about the consequences of stopping drug therapy abruptly.
■ Women should call their prescriber if they become pregnant or plan to become pregnant during therapy.
■ Syrup should not be mixed with carbonated beverages; mixture may be irritating to mouth and throat.
■ Keep drug out of children's reach.
■ Do not stop drug therapy abruptly.
■ Call the prescriber if malaise, weakness, lethargy, facial swelling, loss of appetite, or vomiting occurs.

Special Populations

■ *Older adults:* Caution is advised when using this drug in older adults due to more sensitivity to the drug. Initiate treatment at a lower dose and then escalate the dose more slowly.
■ *Pregnancy:* category D; this medication should only be used when clearly needed or required utmost during pregnancy.
■ *Lactation:* The drug is secreted into breast milk. Increased risk of neural tube defects (1 in 20) and other major birth defects have been reported, especially when the fetus is exposed during first 12 weeks of pregnancy.
■ *Children:* Caution must be exercised when using this drug in a child or an adolescent.
■ *Alert:* Antidepressants increased the risk of suicidal thinking and behavior (suicidality) in short-term studies in children and adolescents with depression and other psychiatric disorders. Caution is advised when using this drug in children because they may be more sensitive to the side effects of the drug, especially loss of appetite and weight loss. It is important to monitor weight and growth in children who are taking this drug.

DONEPEZIL HYDROCHLORIDE (Aricept, Aricept ODT)

Classification

Cholinesterase inhibitor

Indications

Aricept is indicated for the treatment of dementia of the Alzheimer's type. Efficacy has been demonstrated in patients with mild, moderate, and severe Alzheimer's disease.

Available Forms

Tablet, 5, 10, and 23 mg; ODT, 5 and 10 mg

Dosage

- Initially 5 mg PO at bedtime; increase to 10 mg after 4 to 6 weeks as needed; maximum 23 mg/d.
- Effective dose range is 5 to 10 mg/d.

Administration

- Orally, once daily, just prior to retiring. Swallow tablets whole; do not crush, split, or chew. It may be given with or without food.
- *Rapidly dissolving tablet*: Place on tongue, allow to dissolve, and then swallow.
- *Oral solution*: Measure dose with a calibrated oral syringe.

Side Effects

- The side effects of this drug are nausea, vomiting, diarrhea, loss of appetite, weight loss, frequent urination, muscle cramps, joint pain, swelling, stiffness, pain, excessive tiredness, drowsiness, headache, dizziness, nervousness, depression, confusion, changes in behavior, abnormal dreams, difficulty falling asleep or staying asleep, discoloration or bruising of the skin, red, scaling, and itchy skin.
- *Serious side effects that require immediate medical attention*: Fainting, slow heartbeat, chest pain, black or tarry stools, red blood in stools, bloody vomit, vomit that looks like coffee grounds, inability to control urination, difficulty urinating or pain when urinating, lower back pain, fever, and seizures.

Drug Interactions

This medicine may interact with the following medications: other cholinesterase inhibitors, neuromuscular blockers, parasympathomimetics, amantadine, amiodarone, amoxapine, antiretroviral protease inhibitors, antimuscarinics, barbiturates, bosentan, carbamazepine, clozapine, cyclobenzaprine, digoxin, disopyramide, fluoxetine, fluvoxamine, fosphenytoin, general anesthetics, imatinib, ST I-571, ketoconazole, local anesthetics, maprotiline, nefazodone, nilotinib, NSAIDs, olanzapine, orphenadrine, oxcarbazepine, paroxetine, phenothiazines, phenytoin, ranolazine, rifampin, rifapentine, sedating H1 blockers, sertraline, St. John's wort, TCAs, troglitazone, cimetidine, clarithromycin, dalfopristin, delavirdine, dexamethasone, diltiazem, efavirenz, erythromycin, gefitinib, itraconazole, modafinil, nevirapine, propafenone, quinidine, verapamil, and voriconazole.

Pharmacokinetics

- Cholinesterase inhibitor selectively inhibits acetylcholinesterase.

- Peak plasma levels are reached in 3 to 4 hours.
- Bioavailability of 100%.
- *Half-life*: Average 70 hours.

Precautions

Parasympathetic effects may occur in patients with the following conditions: asthma, coronary disease, peptic ulcer, arrhythmias, epilepsy, parkinsonism, bradycardia, and intestinal; or urinary tract obstruction could be exacerbated by the stimulation of cholinergic receptors.

Patient and Family Education

Store the drug at controlled room temperature between 15°C and 30°C (59°F and 86°F).

Special Populations

- *Hepatic impairment*: No specific dosage adjustments are needed. Adjust dose to patient response and tolerance.
- *Pregnancy*: category C; the uterus could be stimulated along with induction of labor.

DOXEPIN (Sinequan)

Classification

Tricyclic antidepressant (TCA)

Indications

Doxepin is used for the treatment of anxiety/depression.

Available Forms

Capsule, 10, 25, 50, 75, 100, and 150 mg; oral concentrate, 10 mg/mL (4 oz. w/dropper)

Dosage

- *Adults*: usual optimum dose 75 to 150 mg/d; maximum single dose 150 mg; maximum 300 mg/d in divided doses
- *Older adults*: usual optimum dose 75 to 150 mg/d; lower initial dose and therapeutic dose; maximum single dose 150 mg; maximum 300 mg/d in divided doses
- *Children older than 12 years*: usual optimum dose 75 to 150 mg/d; maximum single dose 150 mg; maximum 300 mg/d in divided doses
- *Children younger than 12 years*: not recommended

Administration

Take this medication regularly and at the same time every day to get the most benefit. Do not stop taking this medication without consulting the healthcare provider. If this medicine should be taken only once a day, take at bedtime to reduce daytime sleepiness.

Side Effects

Common reactions include drowsiness, dry mouth, dizziness, constipation, blurred vision, palpitations, tachycardia, uncoordination, appetite increase, nausea/vomiting, sweating, weakness, disorientation, confusion, restlessness, insomnia, anxiety/agitation, urinary retention/frequency, rash/urticaria, pruritus, weight gain, libido changes, impotence, gynecomastia, galactorrhea, tremor, hypo/hyperglycemia, paresthesias, and photosensitivity.

Drug Interactions

- The following drugs are to be used cautiously with doxepin: antiarrhythmics class 1A, such as procainamide, quinidine gluconate, quinidine sulfate, especially if coadministration is medically necessary and with risk versus benefit fully assessed by the provider, and disopyramide (Norpace), which may increase risk of QT prolongation.
- Cisapride (Propulsid) may increase risk of QT prolongation and cardiac arrhythmias; dronedarone (Multaq) may increase TCA levels and risk of adverse effects and increase risk of QT prolongation and cardiac arrhythmias; flumazenil (Romazicon) may increase risk of cardiac arrhythmias and seizures.
- MAOIs, such as selegiline (Eldepryl/Zelapar), procarbazine (Matulane), phenelzine (Nardil), tranylcypromine (Parnate), isocarboxazid (Marplan), selegiline transdermal (Eldepryl/Zelapar), and rasagiline (Azilect), may result in CNS overstimulation, hyperpyrexia, seizures, and death. Separate by at least 14 days.

■ Wait at least 5 weeks after stopping fluoxetine (Prozac) before taking doxepin.
■ Pimozide (Orap) may increase risk of CNS depression, psychomotor impairment, QT prolongation, arrhythmias, and hyperpyrexia; potassium salts, such as potassium acid phosphate, potassium citrate, potassium chloride, potassium iodide, potassium phosphate/sodium phosphate, potassium acid, phosphate/sodium acid phosphate, and potassium phosphate, are contraindicated for solid potassium dose forms. Weigh risk–benefit of thyroid protection with solid iodide salt forms; may delay solid potassium passage through GI tract and increase risk of ulcerative/stenotic lesions.

Pharmacokinetics

■ The drug is metabolized extensively in the liver (CYP450, 2 C9/19, 2 D6) and is excreted in the urine.
■ The exact mechanism of action is unknown; it inhibits norepinephrine and serotonin reuptake.

Precautions

■ Glaucoma, urinary retention, bipolar disorder, lung disorders, long-term constipation and heartburn, and diabetes are contraindications to doxepin.
■ Avoid abrupt cessation.

Patient and Family Education

■ Take the drug with food or milk to reduce adverse GI effects.
■ Do not chew capsules; irritation of mouth and throat may result.
■ It may take several weeks or longer to optimize mood-stabilizing effects.
■ Capsules may either be swallowed whole or be carefully opened and contents sprinkled on a teaspoonful of soft food.
■ Keep drugs out of children's reach.
■ Warn about the consequences of stopping drug therapy abruptly.

Special Populations

■ *Pregnancy*: category C; use the drug with extreme caution.
■ *Lactation*: Doxepin is excreted in human milk. Due to the potential for serious adverse reactions in nursing infants from doxepin, a decision should be made whether to discontinue nursing or to discontinue the drug, taking into account the importance of the drug to the mother.
■ *Pediatric use*: not recommended for children under 12 years.
■ *Older adults*: Caution is advised when using this drug in older adults because they may be more sensitive to its side effects, especially dizziness, drowsiness, confusion, and difficulty urinating.

DULOXETINE (Cymbalta)

Classification
- Antidepressant, antianxiety
- Selective serotonin-norepinephrine reuptake inhibitor (SNRI)

Indications
This drug is used to treat the following:
- Depression, anxiety disorder
- Pain associated with diabetic peripheral neuropathy, or fibromyalgia

Available Forms
Delayed-release capsules, 20, 30, 40, and 60 mg

Dosage
- *Adults*: Swallow whole; initially 30 mg once daily × 1 week; increase to 60 mg once daily; maximum 120 mg/d
- *Children older than 12 years*: Swallow whole; initially 30 mg once daily × 1 week; increase to 60 mg once daily; maximum 120 mg/d
- *Children younger than 12 years*: not recommended

Administration
- The drug should be swallowed whole.
- It should not be chewed or crushed, nor should the capsule be opened and its contents sprinkled on food or mixed with liquids.
- It can be given without regard to meals.

Side Effects
- Nausea, dry mouth, constipation, diarrhea, fatigue, difficulty sleeping, and dizziness.
- Increased BP can occur and should be monitored.
- Seizures.
- Sexual dysfunction (decreased sex drive and delayed orgasm and ejaculation).
- The dose of duloxetine should be gradually reduced when therapy is discontinued.
- Antidepressants increased the risk of suicidal thinking and behavior (suicidality) in short-term studies in children and adolescents with depression and other psychiatric disorders.

Note: Closely observe for clinical worsening, suicidality, or unusual changes in behavior.

Drug Interactions
- This drug is not to be used with a MAOI or within 14 days of discontinuing the MAOI.
- Caution when using combinations of SNRIs and MAOIs for this can lead to serious, sometimes fatal, reactions, including very high body temperature, muscle rigidity, rapid fluctuations of heart rate and BP, extreme agitation progressing to delirium, and coma.
- Same side effects are also seen when this drug is used in combination with antipsychotics, TCAs, or other drugs that affect serotonin in the brain.

- It may increase the risk of bleeding, because duloxetine itself is associated with bleeding.
- Drugs that raise the pH in the GI system (e.g., omeprazole) may cause duloxetine to be released early, whereas conditions that slow gastric emptying (e.g., diabetes) may cause premature breakdown of duloxetine.
- Duloxetine may reduce the breakdown of desipramine, leading to increased blood concentrations of desipramine and potential side effects.

Pharmacokinetics

- This drug works by preventing the reuptake of serotonin and epinephrine.
- This reduced uptake increases the effect of serotonin and norepinephrine in the brain.

Precautions

- Hepatotoxicity
- Discontinuation of treatment
- Activation of mania or hypomania
  Note: Screen for risk of bipolar disorder (e.g., family history of suicide, bipolar disorder, and depression) prior to initiating treatment with Cymbalta.
- Seizures
- Effects on BP
- Hyponatremia
- Concomitant illnesses
- Urinary hesitancy and retention

Patient Education

- Antidepressant medications are used to treat a variety of conditions, including depression and other mental/mood disorders. These medications can help prevent suicidal thoughts/attempts and provide other important benefits. However, a small number of people (especially people younger than 25) who take antidepressants for any condition may experience worsening depression, other mental/mood symptoms, or suicidal thoughts/attempts. Therefore, it is very important to talk with the clinician about the risks and benefits of antidepressant medication (especially for people younger than 25), even if treatment is not for a mental/mood condition. The patient should tell the clinician right away if they notice worsening depression/ other psychiatric conditions, unusual behavior changes (including possible suicidal thoughts/attempts), or other mental/mood changes (including new/worsening anxiety, panic attacks, trouble sleeping, irritability, hostile/angry feelings, impulsive actions, severe restlessness, very rapid speech). Be especially watchful for these symptoms when a new antidepressant is started or when the dose is changed.
- Check for allergies in the patient.
- Check whether the patient feels dizzy or drowsy after using the drug.
- Avoid alcoholic beverages.
- It may affect blood sugar levels.
- Before having surgery, patient must let doctor or dentist know about all the products they use (including prescription drugs, nonprescription drugs, and herbal products).

Special Populations

- *Older adults*
  - Older adults may be more sensitive to the effects of this medicine; monitor for hyponatremia.

- Older adults may be at greater risk for bleeding while taking this drug.
- *Pregnancy: category C*
  - In animal studies, duloxetine has been shown to have adverse effects on fetal development.
  - There are no adequate studies in pregnant women.
- *Breastfeeding*
  - There are no adequate studies in women for determining infant risk when using this medication during breastfeeding.
  - Weigh the potential benefits against the potential risks before administering this medication to breastfeeding patients.
  - Duloxetine is excreted in the milk of lactating women.
  - As the safety of duloxetine in infants is not known, nursing while on duloxetine is not recommended.
- *Pediatric*: not recommended for children under 12 years.

ESCITALOPRAM (Lexapro)

Classification
Antidepressant; selective serotonin reuptake inhibitor (SSRI)

Indications
For treating MDD, GAD, and PTSD

Available Forms
Tablet, 5, 10, and 20 mg; oral solution, 1 mg/mL

Dosage
- *Adults*: initially 10 mg daily; may increase to 20 mg daily after 1 week; older adults or those with hepatic impairment, 10 mg once daily
- *Older adults*: 10 mg once daily
- *Children 12 to 17 years*: initially 10 mg daily; may increase to 20 mg daily after 3 weeks
- *Children younger than 12 years*: not recommended

Administration
- PO with a glass of water.
- Take with or without food.
- Take at regular intervals, preferably in the morning.
- Caution clients not to stop taking drug except on provider's advice.
- Safety not established for children younger than 18 years in GAD.
- Instruct client to take missed dose as soon as possible. If it is almost time for the next dose, advise to take only that dose.

Side Effects
- *Most common:* somnolence, headache, asthenia, dizziness, sweating, dry mouth, tremor, insomnia, anorexia, nervousness, anxiety, abnormal vision, change in appetite, change in sex drive or performance, diarrhea, constipation, indigestion, and nausea.
- *Less common:* Suicidality, worsening depression, serotonin syndrome, seizures, hyponatremia, EPS, priapism, and acute-angle glaucoma are less common side effects of escitalopram. The other side effects are nervousness, dry mouth, constipation, asthenia, diaphoresis, anxiety, headache, drowsiness, anorexia, dyspepsia, suicide risk, fatigue, fever, palpitations, hot flashes, nasal congestion, pharyngitis, sinusitis, nausea, diarrhea, abdominal pain, vomiting, flatulence, increased appetite, sexual dysfunction, weight loss, muscle pain, upper respiratory tract, infection, cough, respiratory distress, rash, pruritus, diaphoresis, and flu-like syndrome.

Drug Interactions
Most of the interactions occur with OTC cough-and-cold preparations.
- This medicine may also interact with the following medications:
  - Absolute contraindications include MAOIs such as phenelzine (Nardil), tranylcypromine (Parnate), isocarboxazid (Marplan), cyproheptadine, flecainide, carbamazepine, vinblastine, insulin, lithium, TCAs, phenytoin, tryptophan,

warfarin, and selegiline (Eldepryl). Avoid using with other SSRIs due to serotonin effect; SNRI highly protein-bound drugs due to increased risk of serotonin syndrome, such as desvenlafaxine (Pristiq) and venlafaxine (Effexor); St. John's wort; haloperidol diazepam (Valium); any other antidepressants; and clopidogrel (Plavix). Exercise caution with cold medications, NSAIDs, and drugs used for analgesia with opioid properties.

■ Concomitant use with SSRIs, SNRIs, or tryptophan is not recommended.
■ Use caution when concomitantly consuming drugs that affect hemostasis (NSAIDs, aspirin, cimetidine, warfarin).
■ *Alert*: This list may not describe all possible interactions. Instruct clients to provide a list of all medicines, herbs, nonprescription drugs, or dietary supplements used and state whether they smoke, drink alcohol, or use illegal drugs.

Pharmacokinetics

■ *Metabolism*: liver; CYP450, 2C19, 2D6, CYP 3A4 substrate; 2D6 (weak) inhibitor.
■ *Excretion*: only 10% excreted in urine.
■ SSRIs are metabolized in the liver by cytochrome P-450 MFO microsomal enzymes.
■ Highly bound to plasma proteins and have a large volume of distribution; peak plasma levels are reached in 5 hours.
■ Steady-state plasma levels are achieved in 1 week with escitalopram.
■ *Half-life*: 27 to 32 hours, but is increased by 50% in older adults.

Precautions

■ *Clinical worsening/suicide risk*: Monitor for clinical worsening, suicidality, and unusual change in patient behavior, especially during the initial few months of therapy or at times of dose changes.
■ *Serotonin syndrome*: Manage with immediate discontinuation and continue monitoring.
■ *Discontinuation of treatment with Lexapro*: A gradual reduction in dose rather than abrupt cessation is recommended whenever possible.
■ *Seizures*: Prescribe with care in clients with history of seizure.
■ *Activation of mania/hypomania*: Use cautiously in clients with a history of mania.
■ *Hyponatremia*: can occur in association with syndrome of inappropriate antidiuretic hormone (SIADH) secretion.
■ *Abnormal bleeding*: Use caution in concomitant use with NSAIDs, aspirin, warfarin, or other drugs that affect coagulation.
■ Interferes with cognitive and motor performance; patient should use caution when operating machinery.
■ Use in clients with concomitant illness: Use caution in clients with diseases or conditions that produce altered metabolism or hemodynamic response.
■ See client as often as necessary to ensure that the drug is working on the panic attacks, determine compliance, and review side effects.
■ Make sure clients realize that they need to take prescribed doses even if they do not feel better right away. It can take several weeks before they feel the full effect of the drug.
■ Watch out for sudden or severe changes in feelings, such as feeling anxious, agitated, panicky, irritable, hostile, aggressive, impulsive, severely restless, overly excited, and hyperactive or not being able to sleep. If this happens, especially at the beginning of antidepressant treatment or after a change in dose, clients should call the healthcare provider.

■ Caution clients not to stand or sit up quickly, especially if an older client. This reduces the risk of dizziness or fainting spells. Alcohol may interfere with the effect of this medicine. Avoid alcoholic drinks.

■ Caution clients not to treat themselves for coughs, colds, or allergies without asking the healthcare professional for advice. Some ingredients can increase possible side effects.

■ *Dry mouth*: Chewing sugarless gum or sucking hard candy and drinking plenty of water may help.

■ Caution should be exercised in the following:
  ■ In clients with bipolar disorder or a family history of bipolar disorder
  ■ Diabetes
  ■ Heart disease
  ■ Liver disease
  ■ Electroconvulsive therapy
  ■ Seizures (convulsions)
  ■ Suicidal thoughts, plans, or attempts by client or a family member
  ■ An unusual or allergic reaction to citalopram, sertraline, other medicines, foods, dyes, or preservatives
  ■ Women who are pregnant or trying to get pregnant
  ■ Breastfeeding

Patient and Family Education

■ Antidepressant medications are used to treat a variety of conditions, including depression and other mental/mood disorders. These medications can help prevent suicidal thoughts/attempts and provide other important benefits. However, a small number of people (especially people younger than 25) who take antidepressants for any condition may experience worsening depression, other mental/mood symptoms, or suicidal thoughts/attempts. Therefore, it is very important to talk with the clinician about the risks and benefits of antidepressant medication (especially for people younger than 25), even if treatment is not for a mental/mood condition. Tell the clinician right away if you notice worsening depression/other psychiatric conditions, unusual behavior changes (including possible suicidal thoughts/attempts), or other mental/mood changes (including new/worsening anxiety, panic attacks, trouble sleeping, irritability, hostile/angry feelings, impulsive actions, severe restlessness, very rapid speech). Be especially watchful for these symptoms when a new antidepressant is started or when the dose is changed.

■ Store at room temperature.

■ The patient should try to take the medicine at the same time each day. Follow the directions on the prescription label. To get the correct dose of liquid escitalopram, measure the liquid with a marked measuring spoon or medicine cup, not with a regular tablespoon. If there is no dose-measuring device available, ask the pharmacist for one.

■ Drug may cause dizziness or drowsiness. Warn client to avoid driving and other hazardous activities that require alertness and good psychomotor coordination until effects of drug are known.

■ Tell client to consult prescriber before taking other prescription or OTC drugs.

■ Advise client that full therapeutic effect may not be seen for 4 weeks or longer.

Special Populations

■ *Older adults*: A dose of 10 mg daily is recommended for geriatric clients. The initial dose should be reduced in clients with severe renal and/or hepatic impairment. Titration upward should be slow and at intervals.

- *Pregnancy*: category C; potential for persistent pulmonary HTN if >20-weeks' gestation; use in third semester may cause complications at birth.
- *Lactation*: The drug is excreted in human breast milk, and there are some reports of infant somnolence.
- *Children*: It may be given to children older than 12 years of age. Monitoring of suicidal ideation is important.

ESZOPICLONE (Lunesta)

Classification
Hypnotic, pyrrolopyrazine derivative; non-benzodiazepine gamma-aminobutyric acid (GABA) receptor agonist

Indications
Treatment of insomnia in the nondepressed patient and fibromyalgia

Available Forms
Tablet, 1, 2, and 3 mg

Dosage
- *Adults*: 1 to 3 mg; maximum 3 mg/d × 1 month; do not take if unable to sleep for at least 8 hours before requiring to be active again; delayed effect if taken with a meal
- *Children younger than 18 years*: not recommended

Administration
- PO with a glass of water immediately before bedtime.
- Drowsiness and/or dizziness will be exacerbated with concomitant alcohol consumption; alcohol should be avoided while taking this medication.
- Only to be used for 10 days to 2 weeks; not meant for long-term use.

Side Effects
- Hallucinations; behavior changes; SSRI-treated patients who take eszopiclone may experience impaired concentration, aggravated depression, and manic reaction.
- *Side effects that usually do not require medical attention*: unpleasant taste, nausea, daytime drowsiness, headache, vomiting, dizziness, infection, pain, and pharyngitis.

Drug Interactions
This medicine may interact with the following medications: antifungals, rifampin, ritonavir, SSRIs, and CNS depressants (including alcohol) and CYP3A4 inhibitors (clarithromycin, itraconazole, ketoconazole, nefazodone, nelfinavir, troleandomycin); olanzapine may impair cognitive function.

Pharmacokinetics
This is a non-benzodiazepine hypnotic. Mechanism of action is thought to occur at the level of the GABA receptor complex.
- Weakly bound to plasma proteins.
- Peak plasma levels are reached in 1 hour.
- Bioavailability is 80%.
- *Half-life*: Average is 6 hours.

Precautions
- See patient as often as necessary if long-term use is indicated.
- Ensure that patient is aware they are not to exceed maximum dosage and are not taking other CNS-depressant medications.
- Instruct patient to monitor for behavior changes.

- If patient is drowsy or dizzy, patient should not drive, use machinery, or attempt to accomplish any task that requires mental alertness.
- Avoid alcohol, as concomitant use may exacerbate symptoms.

Patient and Family Education

Store at room temperature between 15°C and 30°C (59°Fand 86°F). Throw away any unused medication after the expiration date. Avoid giving with high-fat meals.

Special Populations

- *Older adults*: recommended starting dose for older adults who have difficulty falling asleep is 1 mg. For older adults who have difficulty staying asleep, the recommended dose is 1 to 2 mg.
- *Hepatic impairment*: The starting dose should be 1 mg in patients with severe hepatic impairment. Monitor closely.
- *Pregnancy*: category C.
- *Lactation*: No human studies have been performed. Not recommended in breast-feeding mothers.
- *Children*: Safety and efficacy have not been established.

FLUOXETINE HYDROCHLORIDE (Prozac, Prozac weekly/Sarafem)

Classification
Antidepressant

Indications
This drug is used to treat MDDs, OCD, bulimia nervosa, premenstrual dysphoric disorder (PMDD), PTSD, BPD, panic disorder (short term), Raynaud phenomenon, and personality disorders.

Available Forms
Tablets, 10, 15, and 20 mg; capsules, 10, 20, and 40 mg; capsule (delayed-release), 90 mg; oral solution, 20 mg/5 mL

Dosage
Prozac
- *Adults:* initially 20 mg daily; may increase after 1 week; doses >20 mg/d should be divided into AM and noon doses; maximum 80 mg/d
- *Children older than 17 years*: initially 20 mg daily; may increase after 1 week; doses >20 mg/d should be divided into AM and noon doses; maximum 80 mg/d
- *Children 8 to 17 years*: initially 10 mg/d; may increase after 1 week to 20 mg/d; range 20 to 60 mg/d; range for lower-weight children, 20 to 30 mg/d
- *Children younger than 8 years*: not recommended

Prozac Weekly
- *Adults:* following daily fluoxetine therapy at 20 mg/d for 13 weeks, may initiate Prozac Weekly 7 days after the last 20-mg fluoxetine dose
- *Children older than 12 years*: following daily fluoxetine therapy at 20 mg/d for 13 weeks, may initiate Prozac Weekly 7 days after the last 20-mg fluoxetine dose
- *Children younger than 12 years*: not recommended

Sarafem
- *Adults:* Administer daily or 14 days before expected menses and through first full day of menses; initially 20 mg/d; maximum 80 mg/d
- *Children 8 to 17 years*: initially 10 or 20 mg/d; start lower-weight children at 10 mg/d; if starting at 10 mg/d, may increase after 1 week to 20 mg/d
- *Children younger than 8 years*: not recommended

Administration
- PO with a glass of water.
- Take the medicine with or without food.
- Take it at regular intervals.
- Caution patients not to stop taking drug except on provider's advice.
- Prozac Weekly may be prescribed for children as young as 7 years for selected conditions; precautions do apply.
- Do not prescribe Prozac Weekly for acute treatment.
- Instruct patients to take missed dose as soon as possible. If it is almost time for the next dose, advise to take only that dose.

- Do not take fluoxetine with grapefruit juice, as it may increase blood levels of the drug.
- Avoid use of herbs that have a sedative effect.
- Fluoxetine may increase the levels of phenytoin and TCAs or serotonin potential such as St. John's wort. Alcohol should be avoided while using fluoxetine.
- Use of buspirone, dextromethorphan, lithium, meperidine, nefazodone, paroxetine, pentazocine, sertraline, sumatriptan, tramadol, trazodone, tryptophan, and venlafaxine can cause a serotonin syndrome.
- Fluoxetine can be taken with or without food. It should be taken in the morning to reduce nervousness and insomnia.
- Be cautious while driving, riding a bicycle, or operating machinery, as this drug causes drowsiness.

Side Effects

- *Most common*: Suicidal ideation, dizziness, headache, insomnia, nervousness, anxiety, somnolence, and change in sex drive or performance are the most common side effects.
- *Less common*: The less common side effects are allergic reactions (skin rash, itching, or hives); swelling of the face, lips, or tongue; psoriasis; arthralgias; asthenia, diarrhea, anorexia; feeling faint or lightheaded, falls, nausea; dizziness, dry mouth; constipation; tremor, dyspepsia; suicidal thoughts or other mood changes; unusual bleeding or bruising; fatigue; tremor; change in appetite; increased sweating; indigestion, nausea; flu syndrome; ejaculatory dysfunction, libido decrease; rash; and abnormal vision and vivid dreams.

Drug Interactions

Most of the interactions occur with OTC cough-and-cold preparations. This medicine may also interact with the following medications:

- Absolute contraindications include MAOIs such as phenelzine (Nardil), tranylcypromine (Parnate), isocarboxazid (Marplan), and selegiline (Eldepryl).
- Avoid using with other SSRIs due to serotonin effect; SNRI drugs, such as desvenlafaxine (Pristiq) and venlafaxine (Effexor); drugs with sympathomimetic properties, such as phenylpropanolamine, pseudoephedrine. Avoid using the drug with St. John's wort, haloperidol, diazepam (Valium), any other antidepressants, and clopidogrel (Plavix). Exercise caution with cold medications; arrhythmia medications, such as flecainide, aspirin, and other NSAIDs; and drugs used for analgesia with opioid properties.
- *Alert:* This list may not describe all possible interactions. Instruct patients to provide a list of all medicines, herbs, nonprescription drugs, or dietary supplements used and state if they smoke, drink alcohol, or use illegal drugs. The following drugs are known to interact with fluoxetine:
  - Linezolid (Zyvox) may increase the risk of serotonin syndrome and neuroleptic syndrome and in combination with fluvoxamine (Luvox) may increase rasagiline (Azilect) levels.
  - MAOIs are contraindicated within 5 weeks of fluoxetine use because they may increase the risk of serotonin syndrome, neuroleptic syndrome, and in combination with fluvoxamine (Luvox) may increase rasagiline (Azilect) levels and risk of adverse effects.
  - Pimozide (Orap) may increase the risk of bradycardia, pimozide levels, risk of QT prolongation, and cardiac arrhythmias.

- Thioridazine (Mellaril) may increase thioridazine levels, risk of QT prolongation, and cardiac arrhythmias and may increase risk of SIADH, hyponatremia, serotonin syndrome, and neuroleptic and malignant syndrome.
- Tramadol may increase risk of serotonin syndrome.

Pharmacokinetics

- *Metabolism:* liver; CYP450 2C19, 2D6 (primary) substrate; 2C19, 3A4 (weak) inhibitor; active metabolite excreted in the urine (80%) and feces (15%).
- Selectively inhibits serotonin reuptake.
- *Half-life:* fluoxetine: 2 to 3 days, norfluoxetine: 7 to 9 days.

Precautions

- See patients as often as necessary to ensure that the drug is working on the panic attacks, determine compliance, and review side effects.
- Make sure patients realize that they need to take prescribed doses even if they do not feel better right away. It can take several weeks before they feel the full effect of the drug.
- Instruct patients and families to watch for worsening depression or thoughts of suicide. Also, watch out for sudden or severe changes in feelings such as feeling anxious, agitated, panicky, irritated, hostile, aggressive, impulsive, severely restless, overly excited, or hyperactive or not being able to sleep. If this happens, especially at the beginning of antidepressant treatment or after a change in dose, patient should call the healthcare provider.
- *Drowsiness or dizziness:* Patients should not drive or use machinery or do anything that needs mental alertness until the effects of this medicine are known.
- Caution patients not to stand or sit up quickly, especially if older. This reduces the risk of dizzy or fainting spells. Alcohol may interfere with the effect of this medicine. Avoid alcoholic drinks.
- Caution patients not to treat themselves for coughs, colds, or allergies without asking a healthcare professional for advice. Some ingredients can increase possible side effects.
- *Dry mouth:* Chewing sugarless gum, sucking hard candy, and drinking plenty of water may help against a dry mouth. Contact a healthcare provider if the problem persists or is severe.
- Caution should be exercised in the following:
  - Bipolar disorder or a family history of bipolar disorder
  - Diabetes
  - Heart disease
  - Liver disease
  - Electroconvulsive therapy
  - Seizures (convulsions)
  - Suicidal thoughts, plans, or attempts by patients or a family member
  - An unusual or allergic reaction to fluoxetine, other medicines, foods, dyes, or preservatives
  - Pregnancy or trying to get pregnant
  - Breastfeeding mothers who are younger than 25 years
- *Alert:* Caution should also be exercised with the following conditions: diabetes mellitus, hyponatremia, seizures, mania/hypomania, or volume depletion.

Patient and Family Education

- Store at room temperature. Take any unused medication after the expiration date to the local pharmacy on drug-giveback day. Avoid discarding the medication into the environment.

- Discuss any worsening anxiety, aggressiveness, impulsivity, or restlessness.
- Report any severe, abrupt onset or changes in symptoms to health professionals. They may be reflective of increased risk of suicidal thinking.
- There is an increased risk of suicidality in children, adolescents, and young adults with major depressive or other psychiatric disorder's especially during the first months of treatment.
- The patient must inform healthcare provider of glaucoma, hypoglycemia, or abnormal bleeding tendencies.
- Therapeutic effects may take 4 weeks to fully develop, but side effects may be noticeable.
- *Alert:* Avoid the concomitant use of NSAIDs, aspirin, warfarin, and any other drugs that alter platelets within 1 week of beginning therapy.

Special Populations

- *Older adults:* No actual contraindications exist, but due to the long half-life of the drug, it has been placed on the Beers List of Potentially Inappropriate Medications for Geriatrics.
- *Renal impairment*: No adjustment is needed for those with kidney disease.
- *Hepatic impairment*: The dose may need to be decreased in patients with liver disease.
- *Pregnancy*: category C; this is the longest-used SSRI in pregnant women. Every attempt should be made to discontinue in the third trimester secondary to development of neonatal distress on delivery.
- *Lactation*: The use of this drug is not approved for lactation and breastfeeding.
- *Children*: The drug is approved for pediatric population aged 8 years and older. Monitoring for increased suicidal ideation is critical.

FLUPHENAZINE HYDROCHLORIDE/FLUPHENAZINE DECANOATE

Classification
Antipsychotic drug, typical, first-generation, phenothiazine

Note
Previously, fluphenazine was marketed as Prolixin but is currently available only in generic form. Fluphenazine decanoate injection and fluphenazine enanthate injection are long-acting parenteral antipsychotic forms intended for use in the management of patients requiring prolonged parenteral neuroleptic therapy.

Indications
Methamphetamine-induced psychosis

Available Forms
Tablet, 1, 2.5, 5, and 10 mg; elixir, 2.5 mg/5 mL; oral concentrate, 5 mg/mL; vial, 2.5 mg/mL for injection

Dosage
- Optimal dose and frequency of administration of fluphenazine must be determined for each patient, since dosage requirements have been found to vary with clinical circumstances as well as with individual response; dosage should not exceed 100 mg; if doses >50 mg are deemed necessary, the next dose and succeeding doses should be increased cautiously in increments of 12.5 mg.
- Adult use only; not studied in pediatric patients.

Administration
- Oral solution should not be mixed with drinks containing caffeine, tannic acid (tea), or pectinates (apple juice).
- *IM decanoate*: Use dry, 21-gauge needle. May be given subcutaneously.
- Onset of action is at 24 to 72 hours after administration with significant antipsychotic actions evident within 48 to 96 hours.

Side Effects
Motor side effects from blockage of D2 in striatum; seizures, NMS, leukopenia, agranulocytosis, aplastic anemia, thrombocytopenia, elevations in prolactin from blockage of D2 in the pituitary; worsening of negative and cognitive symptoms due to blockage of D2 receptors in the mesocortical and mesolimbic dopamine pathways; sedation, blurred vision, constipation, dry mouth; weight gain; dizziness, hypotension; possible increased incidence of diabetes or dyslipidemia with conventional antipsychotics is unknown; neuroleptic-induced deficit syndrome; akathisia; EPS, parkinsonism, TD; galactorrhea, amenorrhea; sexual dysfunction; priapism; decreased sweating, depression; hypotension, tachycardia, syncope.

Drug Interactions
- It may decrease the effects of levodopa and dopamine agonists.
- It may increase effects of antihypertensive drugs except for guanethidine, whose actions may be antagonized by fluphenazine.

- Anticholinergic effects may be potentiated with concomitant atropine and fluphenazine.
- Concurrent use with CNS depressants may produce additive effects.
- Antacids may inhibit absorption. Administer the dosage at least 2 hours apart.
- Additive anticholinergic effects may occur if used with atropine or related compounds.
- Alcohol and diuretics increase the risk of hypotension.
- Some patients on neuroleptics and lithium developed an encephalopathic syndrome similar to NMS.
- Interaction with St. John's wort increases risk of photosensitivity.
- Use with epinephrine may lower BP.

Pharmacokinetics

- *Half-life:* Oral formulation, approximately 15 hours; IM formulation, approximately 6.8 to 9.6 days.
- *Peak:* PO, 30 minutes; IM decanoate, unknown; IM, 90 to 120 minutes; subcutaneous, unknown.

Precautions

- Fluphenazine differs from other phenothiazine derivatives in several respects: It is more potent on a milligram basis, it has less potentiating effect on CNS depressants and anesthetics than do some of the phenothiazines and appears to be less sedating, and it is less likely than some of the older phenothiazines to produce hypotension (nevertheless, appropriate cautions should be observed). NMS, a potentially fatal symptom complex, is associated with all antipsychotic drugs. Clinical manifestations of NMS are hyperpyrexia, muscle rigidity, altered mental status, and evidence of autonomic instability (irregular pulse or BP, tachycardia, diaphoresis, and cardiac dysrhythmias).
- Fluphenazine and epinephrine may lower BP.
- Additive anticholinergic effects may occur if used with atropine or related compounds.
- Alcohol and diuretics may increase the risk of hypotension.
- Do not use if the patient is in a comatose state.
- Do not use if there is proven allergy or sensitivity to fluphenazine.
- It may lower seizure threshold; fluphenazine has severe reactions to insulin, glaucoma, prostatic hyperplasia.

Patient and Family Education

- Inform your provider of all drug allergies.
- Take the dose exactly as prescribed by the provider. Do not take in larger or smaller amounts or for longer than recommended.
- Fluphenazine can be taken with or without food.
- Avoid becoming overheated or dehydrated during exercise and in hot weather. You may be more prone to heat stroke.
- Avoid getting up too fast from a sitting or lying position. Get up slowly and steady yourself to prevent a fall.
- Avoid drinking alcohol.
- Stop using this medication and call provider immediately if you have very stiff (rigid) muscles, high fever, sweating, confusion, fast or uneven heartbeats, tremors; feel like you might pass out; have jerky muscle movements you cannot control,

trouble swallowing, problems with speech; have blurred vision, eye pain, or see halos around lights; have increased thirst and urination, excessive hunger, fruity breath odor, weakness, nausea, and vomiting; have fever, chills, body aches, flu symptoms; or have white patches or sores inside your mouth or on your lips.
- Do not stop taking the drug suddenly without first talking to your provider, even if you feel fine. You may have serious side effects if you stop taking the drug suddenly.
- Call provider if symptoms do not improve or get worse.
- Store at room temperature away from moisture and heat.

Special Populations

- *Older adults*: Lower initial dose (1–2.5 mg/d) and slower titration in older adults. Older adults are more susceptible to adverse effects. It is not approved for treatment of older adults with dementia-related psychosis, and such patients are at increased risk of CV events and death.
- *Renal impairment*: Use with caution and with slower titration.
- *Hepatic impairment*: Use with caution and with slower titration.
- *Cardiac impairment*: CV toxicity can occur, especially orthostatic hypotension.
- *Pregnancy*: Safety during pregnancy has not been established; therefore, the possible hazards should be weighed against the potential benefits when administering this drug to pregnant patients.
- *Lactation*: Drug crosses to the infant through breast milk; dystonia, TD, and sedation have been observed in the infant. Recommend discontinuing drug or bottle-feed.
- *Children and adolescents*: Safety and efficacy of fluphenazine are not established for children and adolescents.

FLURAZEPAM (Dalmane)

Classification
Benzodiazepine (BZD)

Indications
Flurazepam is used for the treatment of insomnia.

Available Forms
Capsule, 15 and 30 mg

Dosage
Insomnia
- *Adults and children older than 15 years*: 30 mg at bedtime prn
- *Older adults*: 30 mg at bedtime prn
- *Children younger than 15 years*: not recommended

Administration
- PO with a glass of water at bedtime
- Drowsiness and/or dizziness will be exacerbated with concomitant alcohol consumption; alcohol should be avoided while taking this medication.
- Caution clients not to stop taking drug abruptly if used long term.

Side Effects
- Hallucinations; behavior changes
- Side effects that usually do not require medical attention: nausea, daytime drowsiness, headache, vomiting, dizziness, diarrhea, dry mouth, and nervousness

Drug Interactions
This medicine may interact with the following medications: antifungals; CNS depressants (including alcohol); digoxin; macrolides; phenytoin.

Pharmacokinetics
- BZD, hypnotic.
- Mechanism of action is thought to occur at the level of the GABA receptor complex.
- Highly bound to plasma proteins.
- Peak plasma levels are reached in 0.50 to 2 hours.
- The drug is metabolized by CYP450 3A4 and excreted through the urine.
- Average half-life of patent drug is 2 to 3 hours; half-life of metabolite is 40 to 114 hours.

Precautions
- See patient as often as necessary if long-term use is indicated.
- Ensure that patient is aware they are not to exceed maximum dosage.
- Instruct patient to monitor for behavior changes.
- If patient is drowsy or dizzy, patient should not drive, use machinery, or attempt to accomplish any task that requires mental alertness.
- Avoid alcohol, as concomitant use may exacerbate symptoms.

Patient and Family Education

- Store at room temperature between 20°C and 25°C (59°F and 77°F).
- Discard unused medication after the expiration date.

Special Populations

- *Older adults*: Older adults are more sensitive to hypnotics. Use lowest effective dose, maximum 15 mg. Due to sedation and increased risk of falls, all BZDs are placed on the Beers List of Potentially Inappropriate Medications for Geriatrics.
- Modify dosage accordingly in patients with hepatic function impairment, typical 15 mg maximum dose.
- *Pregnancy*: category X; absolute contraindication.
- *Lactation*: No human studies have been performed. Not recommended in breast-feeding mothers. Drug is excreted in breast milk.
- *Children*: This drug is not for use in children younger than 15 years of age.

FLUVOXAMINE (Luvox, Luvox CR)

Classification
Antidepressant, selective serotonin reuptake inhibitor (SSRI)

Indications
Fluvoxamine is used to treat OCD, social anxiety disorder, PTSD.

Available Forms
Tablet, 25, 50, and 100 mg; capsule (XR), 100 and 150 mg

Dosage
Luvox

- *Adults*: initially 50 mg at bedtime; adjust in 50-mg increments at 4- to 7-day intervals; range 100 to 300 mg/d; over 100 mg/d, divide into 2 doses giving the larger dose at bedtime.
- *Children 8 to 17 years*: initially 25 mg at bedtime; adjust in 25-mg increments over 4 to 7 days; usual range 50 to 200 mg/d; over 50 mg/d, divide into 2 doses giving the larger dose at bedtime.
- *Children younger than 8 years*: not recommended.

Luvox CR

- *Adults*: initially 100 mg once daily at bedtime; may increase by 50-mg increments at 1-week intervals; maximum 300 mg/d; swallow whole; do not crush or chew.
- *Children younger than 18 years*: not recommended.

Administration
- PO with a glass of water.
- Take the medicine with or without food. Controlled-release tablets must remain intact and not be split or crushed prior to administration.

Side Effects
- *Most common*: The most common side effects are somnolence, headache, asthenia, dizziness, sweating, dry mouth, tremor, anorexia, nervousness, anxiety, abnormal vision, change in appetite, change in sex drive or performance, diarrhea, constipation, indigestion, and nausea.
- *Less common*: The less common side effects are suicidality, worsening depression, seizures, and hyponatremia; allow 2-week washout period post-MAOI prior to initiation.
- *Tricyclic antidepressants*: Plasma levels may be increased by SSRIs, so add EPS, priapism, and acute-angle glaucoma.

Drug Interactions
Note BBWs.

Most of the interactions occur with OTC cough-and-cold preparations. This medicine may also interact with the following medications:

- Absolute contraindications include MAOIs such as phenelzine (Nardil), tranylcypromine (Parnate), isocarboxazid (Marplan), and selegiline (Eldepryl).

- Use with caution and in low doses.
- *ASA and NSAIDs:* There is an increased risk of bleeding.
- *Central nervous system depressants:* They may increase depressant effects.
- *Other selective serotonin reuptake inhibitors or serotonin antagonist and reuptake inhibitors:* They may cause serotonin syndrome in combination with other medications, such as tramadol, high-dose triptans, or the antibiotic linezolid.
- Use with caution in patients taking blood thinners (Coumadin), other antidepressants, antihistamines, lithium, TCAs, and certain antibiotics, such as erythromycin, clarithromycin, azithromycin; SNRI drugs, such as desvenlafaxine (Pristiq) and venlafaxine (Effexor); drugs with sympathomimetic properties, such as phenylpropanolamine, pseudoephedrine, St. John's wort, haloperidol; diazepam (Valium) and any other antidepressants; clopidogrel (Plavix); and lansoprazole (Prevacid); for these medications, pharmacokinetics and dynamics may change.
- Exercise caution with cold medications, NSAIDs, and drugs used for analgesia with opioid properties.
- *Alert:* This list may not describe all possible interactions. Instruct patients to provide a list of all medicines, herbs, nonprescription drugs, or dietary supplements used and state if they smoke, drink alcohol, or use illegal drugs.
- MAOIs: When this drug interacts with MAOIs, there is an extreme risk for serotonin syndrome.
- Take at regular intervals.
- Caution patients not to stop taking drug except on provider's advice.
- This drug is not prescribed for children.
- Instruct patients to take missed dose as soon as possible. If it is almost time for the next dose, advise to take only that dose.

Pharmacokinetics

- This drug is highly bound to plasma proteins and has a large volume of distribution.
- It is readily absorbed in the GI tract, metabolized in the liver, and excreted in the urine. Dosages may be decreased in patients with liver or kidney disease.
- Caution is advised for older adults.
- *Metabolism:* The liver metabolizes the drug extensively; CYP1A2, CYP2Cp, CYP3A4, CYP4501A2, 2D6 inhibitor.
- *Peak plasma levels:* Reached in 3 to 8 hours.
- *Excretion:* 85% (urine primarily); 2% unchanged.
- *Half-life:* 15.6 hours, 17.4 to 25.9 hours (older adults).

Precautions

- Adverse effects and side effects are commonly observed before therapeutic effects.
- Many side effects are dose dependent and may improve over time.
- Taper discontinuation to avoid withdrawal symptoms.
- See patients as often as necessary to ensure that the drug is working on the panic attacks, determine compliance, and review side effects.
- Make sure patients realize that they need to take prescribed doses even if they do not feel better right away. It can take several weeks before they feel the full effect of the drug.
- Instruct patients and families to watch for worsening depression or thoughts of suicide. Also watch out for sudden or severe changes in feelings, such as feeling

anxious, agitated, panicky, irritated, hostile, aggressive, impulsive, severely rest-less, overly excited, or hyperactive or not being able to sleep. If this happens, espe-cially at the beginning of antidepressant treatment or after a change in dose, patient should call the healthcare provider.

■ *Drowsiness or dizziness*: Patients should not drive or use machinery or do anything that needs mental alertness until the effects of this medicine are known.

■ Caution patients not to stand or sit up quickly, especially if older. This reduces the risk of dizziness or fainting spells. Alcohol may interfere with the effect of this medicine. Avoid alcoholic drinks.

■ Caution patients not to treat themselves for coughs, colds, or allergies without asking a healthcare professional for advice. Some ingredients can increase possible side effects.

■ *Dry mouth*: Chewing sugarless gum, sucking hard candy, and drinking plenty of water may help against a dry mouth. Contact healthcare provider if the problem persists or is severe.

■ Caution should be exercised in the following:
  ■ Bipolar disorder or a family history of bipolar disorder
  ■ Diabetes
  ■ Heart disease
  ■ Liver disease
  ■ Electroconvulsive therapy
  ■ Seizures (convulsions)
  ■ Suicidal thoughts, plans, or attempts by patients or a family member
  ■ An unusual or allergic reaction to fluvoxamine, other medicines, foods, dyes, or preservatives
  ■ Pregnancy or trying to get pregnant
  ■ Breastfeeding

Patient and Family Education

■ Antidepressant medications are used to treat a variety of conditions, including depression and other mental/mood disorders. These medications can help prevent suicidal thoughts/attempts and provide other important benefits. However, a small number of people (especially people younger than 25) who take antidepressants for any condition may experience worsening depression, other mental/mood symp-toms, or suicidal thoughts/attempts. Therefore, it is very important to talk with the clinician about the risks and benefits of antidepressant medication (especially for people younger than 25), even if treatment is not for a mental/mood condition. Tell the clinician right away if you notice worsening depression/other psychiatric con-ditions, unusual behavior changes (including possible suicidal thoughts/attempts), or other mental/mood changes (including new/worsening anxiety, panic attacks, trouble sleeping, irritability, hostile/angry feelings, impulsive actions, severe restlessness, very rapid speech). Be especially watchful for these symptoms when a new antidepressant is started or when the dose is changed.

■ The medicine should be taken about the same time every day, morning or evening, and can be taken with or without food (with food if there is any stomach upset).

■ It may start with half of lowest effective dose for 3 to 7 days and then increase to lowest effective dose to diminish side effects.

■ Administration time may be adjusted based on observed sedating or activating drug effects.

■ The drug may take up to 4 to 8 weeks to show its maximum effect at this dose, but some may see symptoms of dysthymia improving in as few as 2 weeks.

- If patient plans on becoming pregnant or is pregnant, discuss the benefits versus the risks of using this medicine while pregnant.
- As this medicine is excreted in the breast milk, nursing mothers should not breast-feed while taking this medicine without prior consultation with a psychiatric nurse practitioner or psychiatrist. Newborns may develop symptoms, including feeding or breathing difficulties, seizures, muscle stiffness, jitteriness, or constant crying.
- Do not stop taking this medication unless the healthcare provider directs. Report side effects or worsening symptoms to the healthcare provider promptly.
- The medication should be tapered gradually when changing or discontinuing therapy.
- Dosage should be adjusted to reach remission of symptoms and treatment should continue for at least 6 to 12 months following last reported dysthymic experience, duration based on number of episodes.
- Caution is advised when using this drug in older adults because they may be more sensitive to the effects of the drug. Older adults should receive a lower starting dose.
- Keep these medications out of the reach of children and pets.
- Store at room temperature. After the expiration date, take any unused medication to the local pharmacy on drug-giveback day. Avoid discarding the medication into the environment. Watch carefully for signs of suicidal ideation.

Special Populations

- *Older adults*: Older individuals tend to be more sensitive to medication side effects, such as hypotension and anticholinergic effects. They often require adjustment of medication doses for hepatic or renal dysfunction. SSRIs with shorter half-lives (e.g., paroxetine) may be more desirable for geriatric populations than SSRIs with longer half-lives (e.g., fluoxetine). SSRIs have been associated with increased risk of falls in nursing home residents and neurological effects in patients with Parkinson's disease. Older adults are more prone to SSRI-induced hyponatremia.
- *Renal and hepatic impairment*: Initial dose should be reduced in patients with severe renal and/or hepatic impairment. Titration upward should be slow and at intervals.
- *Pregnancy*: Psychotherapy is the initial choice for most pregnant patients with MDD. Most SSRIs are category C drugs, due to adverse effects; first trimester teratogenicity has been observed in animal studies. If continued during pregnancy, dosage may need to be increased to maintain euthymia due to physiological changes associated with pregnancy. Neonatal withdrawal and serotonin syndrome may occur in third trimester; persistent pulmonary HTN occurs if more than 20-week gestation.
- *Lactation*: It is generally considered safe; substantial human data show no or minimal risk to breast-milk production or to the infant.
- *Children*: Increasing doses may require more gradual increments, and discontinuation may require a more gradual taper. Monitor for suicide ideation.

GALANTAMINE HYDROBROMIDE (Razadyne, Razadyne ER)

Classification

Anti-Alzheimer; cholinesterase inhibitor

Indications

This medicine is used to treat mild-to-moderate Alzheimer's disease.

Available Forms

Tablets, 4, 8, and 12 mg; XR tablets, 8, 16, and 24 mg; oral solution, 4 mg/mL

Dosage

- Initially 4 mg BID × at least 4 weeks; usual maintenance 8 mg BID; maximum 16 mg BID

Administration

- It can be administered orally.
- Take it with food to limit drug intolerance.

Side Effects

- Nausea, vomiting, diarrhea, loss of appetite, stomach pain, heartburn, weight loss, extreme tiredness, dizziness, pale skin, headache, uncontrollable shaking of a part of body, depression, difficulty falling asleep or staying asleep, runny nose.
- *Serious side effects that require medical attention:* Difficulty urinating, blood in the urine, pain or burning while urinating, seizures.
- Bradycardia, AV block, fainting; shortness of breath; black and tarry stools; red blood in the stools; bloody vomit; vomit that looks like coffee grounds.

Drug Interactions

This medicine may interact with the following medications: cholinesterase inhibitors; conivaptan; fluoxetine; neuromuscular blockers; parasympathomimetics; paroxetine; amantadine; amiodarone; amoxapine; antiretroviral protease inhibitors; antimuscarinics; aprepitant, fosaprepitant; barbiturates; cimetidine; clarithromycin; clozapine; cyclobenzaprine; delavirdine; digoxin; disopyramide; efavirenz; erythromycin; fluconazole; fluvoxamine; general anesthetics; imatinib, STI-571; itraconazole; ketoconazole; local anesthetics; maprotiline; nefazodone; nilotinib; olanzapine; orphenadrine; phenothiazines; sedating H-1 blockers; St. John's wort; TCAs; troglitazone; troleandomycin; voriconazole; beta-blockers; bosentan; carbamazepine; phenytoin; quinidine; rifabutin; diltiazem; fosphenytoin; nevirapine; nicardipine; NSAIDs; oxcarbazepine; rifampin; rifapentine; terbinafine; verapamil; and zafirlukast.

Pharmacokinetics

- Cholinesterase inhibitor, reversible inhibitor of acetylcholinesterase.
- Peak plasma levels are reached in approximately 1 hour.
- Bioavailability is 90%.
- *Half-life:* Average 7 hours.

Precautions

- If treatment is stopped for several days with the intent to restart, then patient should be started back with the initial dose and then slowly retitrated to the highest tolerated dose.
- Use this drug with caution in patients with moderate hepatic impairment.
- Patients should be cautioned about engaging in tasks that require mental alertness, such as operating heavy machinery or driving, until reasonably certain that the drug does not affect them adversely.
- Use this drug with caution with pulmonary disease.
- Use this drug with caution in patients with cardiac disease.
- It may exacerbate symptoms of Parkinson's disease.

Patient and Family Education

Store galantamine at room temperature and away from excess heat and moisture. Throw away any medication that is outdated or no longer needed.

Special Populations

Hepatic impairment: not recommended in patients with hepatic dysfunction

Renal impairment: not recommended in patients with renal impairment

GUANFACINE HYDROCHLORIDE (Intuniv)

Classification

Antihypertensive; selective alpha-2A-adrenergic receptor agonist; centrally acting antihypertensive with alpha-2-adrenoceptor agonist properties in tablet form for oral administration

Indications

Treatment of ADHD in children and adolescents aged 6 to 17 years

Available Forms

Tablet (XR), 1, 2, and 3 mg

Dosage

- *Children 6 to 17 years:* initially 1 mg once daily; may increase by 1 mg/d at weekly intervals; usual maximum 4 mg/d
- *Children younger than 6 years:* not recommended
- *Adults:* not indicated

Administration

- Take Intuniv with water, milk, or other liquid. Do not take with a high-fat meal.
- Withdraw gradually by 1 mg every 3 to 7 days.

Side Effects

Somnolence; headache; fatigue; upper abdominal pain; nausea; irritability; dizziness; hypotension; decreased appetite; dry mouth; constipation; syncope; AV block, brady-cardia, sinus arrhythmia; dyspepsia; chest pain; asthma; emotional lability, anxiety, depression, insomnia, nightmares, and sleep changes.

Drug Interactions

- Avoid use with other CNS-depressant drugs due to increased potential for sedation.
- The administration of guanfacine concomitantly with a known microsomal enzyme inducer (phenobarbital or phenytoin) to patients with renal impairment reportedly results in significant reductions in elimination half-life and plasma concentration.
- In such cases, therefore, more frequent dosing may be required to achieve or maintain the desired hypotensive response.

Pharmacokinetics

- Guanfacine is a selective alpha-2A-adrenergic receptor agonist that has a 15- to 20-time higher affinity for this receptor subtype than for the alpha-2B or alpha-2C subtypes.
- It is a known antihypertensive agent. By stimulating alpha-2A-adrenergic receptors, guanfacine reduces sympathetic nerve impulses from the vasomotor center to the heart and blood vessels, resulting in decreased peripheral vascular resistance and a reduction in heart rate.
- Time to peak plasma concentration is 5 hours.
- *Metabolism:* liver, excreted in urine.
- *Half-life:* 18 hours.

Precautions

- Hypersensitivity to guanfacine or concomitant use with other products containing guanfacine (Tenex).
- This drug is not for use in children younger than 6 years; safety beyond 2 years of treatment has not been established.
- *Geriatric populations:* not labeled for use.
- Withdraw gradually by 1 mg every 3 to 7 days.

Patient and Family Education

- Swallow whole with water, milk, or other liquid.
- Store at room temperature.
- Do not take with a high-fat meal—plasma concentrations will increase.
- Use with caution when operating heavy equipment or machinery until response to treatment is known.
- Avoid use with alcohol.
- Avoid dehydration and becoming overheated.
- Have BP and heart rate assessed before administering drug.
- Taper dose by 1 mg/d every 3 to 7 days to discontinuing (abrupt cessation may cause increased plasma catecholamines, rebound HTN, nervousness/anxiety).

Special Populations

- *Older adults:* There is no dosing for this medication for this population.
- *Pregnancy:* category B.
- *Lactation:* safety unknown.
- *Children:* for use in ages 6 to 17 years; use with caution.

HALOPERIDOL DECANOATE, HALOPERIDOL LACTATE (Haldol, Haldol lactate)

Classification
Phenylbutylpiperadine derivative, first-generation (typical) antipsychotic

Indications
Haloperidol is used to treat psychotic disorders and control motor tics and verbal tics in adults and children who have Tourette's disorder (condition characterized by hiccups, motor or verbal tics). It is also used to treat severe behavioral problems, such as explosive, aggressive behavior, or hyperactivity, in children who cannot be treated with psychotherapy or with other medications.

Available Forms
Tablet, 0.5, 1, 2, 5, 10, and 20 mg; vial, 5 mg for IM injection, single-dose

Dosage
- *Oral*: moderate symptomology, 0.5 to 2 mg PO BID to TID; severe symptomology, 3 to 5 mg PO 2 to 3 times a day; initial doses of up to 100 mg/d have been necessary in some severely resistant cases; maintenance: After achieving a satisfactory response, the dose should be adjusted as practical to achieve optimum control.
- *Parenteral*: parenteral route of administration: prompt control of acute agitation, 2 to 5 mg IM q4h to q8h ; maintenance: Frequency of IM administration should be determined by patient response and may be given as often as every hour; maximum, 20 mg/d.

Drug Interactions
Dopamine agonists may diminish therapeutic effect. Carbamazepine increases metabolism of haloperidol. Caution must be exercised with other agents that prolong QT interval. Anticholinergics may increase glaucoma; buspirone may increase haloperidol level. Never give with lithium (acute renal insufficiency); methyldopa, may cause dementia; rifampin, decreases haloperidol level.

Administration
- Patient must stay hydrated.
- Haloperidol is frequently dosed too high. High CYP2D6 inhibitor. Doses may actually worsen negative symptoms of schizophrenia and increase EPS side effects.

Side Effects
Neuroleptic-induced deficit syndrome; akathisia; EPS, parkinsonism, TD, tardive dystonia; galactorrhea, amenorrhea; dizziness, sedation; dry mouth, constipation, urinary retention, blurred vision; decreased sweating; hypotension, tachycardia, hyperlipidemia; weight gain; rare NMS; rare seizures; rare jaundice, agranulocytosis, leukopenia; haloperidol with anticholinergics may increase intraocular pressure; reduces effects of anticoagulants; plasma levels of haloperidol lowered by rifampin; may enhance effects of antihypertensive agents; haloperidol with lithium may contribute to development of encephalopathic syndrome.

Drug Interactions

- It may decrease the effects of levodopa and dopamine agonists.
- It may increase the effects of antihypertensive drugs, except for guanethidine.
- Addictive effects with CNS depressants; dose of other should be reduced.
- It may interact with some pressor agents (epinephrine) to lower BP.

Pharmacokinetics

- *Absorption:* injection, 100%; oral, 60% to 70%
- *Onset:* IM and IV, 30 to 60 minutes
- *Duration:* 2 to 6 hours; decanoate, 2 to 4 weeks
- *Metabolism:* hepatic 50% to 60% glucuronidation
- *Half-life:* approximately 12 to 36 hours; decanoate, 3 weeks. PO, 24 hours; IM, 21 hours
- *Excretion:* urine 30%, feces 15%; PO, 3 to 6 hours; IV, unknown; IM decanoate, 3 to 9 days; IM lactate, 10 to 20 minutes

Precautions

- Keep patient recumbent for at least 30 minutes following injection to minimize hypotensive effects.
- Discontinue the use of haloperidol if patient develops symptoms of NMS.
- Use with caution in patients with respiratory depression.
- It may alter cardiac conduction and prolong QT interval.
- There is a risk of EPS and TD and hyperprolactinemia.
- Seizures.
- Excessive sedation problems.
- Avoid extreme heat exposure.
- The patient may experience rapid shift to depression if used to treat mania.
- Patients with thyrotoxicosis may experience neurotoxicity.
- Do not use this drug with Lewy body dementia or Parkinson's disease.
- Use with caution in patients with QTc prolongation, hypothyroidism, familial long-QT syndrome.
- Do not use if there is a proven allergy to haloperidol.

Patient and Family Education

- Maintain adequate hydration.
- Avoid contact (liquid) with skin; may cause contact dermatitis.
- Do not take within 2 hours of antacid.
- Take exactly as prescribed.
- Avoid getting up too fast from sitting or lying position. Get up slowly and steady yourself to prevent a fall.
- Avoid drinking alcohol.
- Stop using this medication and call provider immediately if you have very stiff (rigid) muscles, high fever, sweating, confusion, fast or uneven heartbeats, tremors; feel like you might pass out; have jerky muscle movements you cannot control, trouble swallowing, problems with speech; have blurred vision, eye pain, or seeing halos around lights; have increased thirst and urination, excessive hunger, fruity breath odor, weakness, nausea and vomiting; have fever, chills, body aches, flu symptoms, or have white patches or sores inside mouth or on lips.
- Do not stop taking drug suddenly without first talking to provider, even if you feel fine. May have serious side effects if you stop taking the drug suddenly.

- Call provider if symptoms do not improve, or get worse.
- Store at room temperature away from moisture and heat.

Special Populations

- *Older adults*: Older adults are at an increased risk for death; use with extreme caution.
- Lower doses should be used and patient monitored closely. Do not use in older adults with dementia.
- *Lactation*: Breastfeeding is not recommended.
- *Other renal impairment*: Use with caution in patients with myasthenia gravis, Parkinson's disease, and seizures.
- *Hepatic impairment*: Use with caution.
- *Cardiac impairment*: Because of risk of orthostatic HTN, use with caution.
- *Pregnancy*: category C; some animal studies show adverse effects; no controlled studies in humans. Neonates exposed during third trimester may present with EPS, withdrawal symptoms, and breathing and feeding difficulties.
- *Lactation*: category C.
- *Children and adolescents*: Safety and efficacy have not been established.

HYDROXYZINE (Atarax, Vistaril)

Classification
Anxiolytic

Indications
Hydroxyzine is used to treat anxiety.

Available Forms
Capsules, 10, 25, and 50 mg; tablets, 10, 25, and 50 mg; syrup, 10 mg/5 mL (alcohol 0.5%); oral suspension, 25 mg/mL

Dosages
- *Adults*: 50 to 100 mg PO QID; maximum 600 mg/d
- *Children older than 6 years*: 50 to 100 mg/d divided QID
- *Children younger than 6 years*: 50 mg/d divided QID

Administration
- PO: Give without regard for meals.
- Shake suspension well before giving.
- IM: Parenteral form (hydroxyzine hydrochloride) is for IM use only; use Z-track injection.
- Never give IV or subcutaneously.
- Aspirate IM injection carefully to prevent inadvertent IV injection. Inject deeply into a large muscle.

Side Effects
- *Central nervous system*: drowsiness, involuntary motor activity
- *Gastrointestinal*: dry mouth, constipation
- *Skin*: pain at IM injection site
- *Other*: hypersensitivity reactions

Drug Interactions
- *Anticholinergics*: may cause additive effects; use together cautiously.
- *Central nervous system depressants*: may increase CNS depression. Use together cautiously; may need dosage adjustments.
- *Epinephrine*: may inhibit and reverse vasopressor effect of epinephrine. Avoid using together.
- *Drug-lifestyle*: alcohol use: may increase CNS depression. Discourage use together.
- *Effects on lab test results*: may cause false increase in urinary 17-hydroxycorticosteroid level. May cause false-negative skin allergen tests by reducing or inhibiting the cutaneous response to histamine.

Pharmacokinetics
- It suppresses activity in certain essential regions of the subcortical area of the CNS. PO onset 15 to 30 minutes, peak 2 hours, duration 4 to 8 hours.
- IM onset is unknown, peak unknown, duration 4 to 6 hours. Half-life is 3 hours.

Precautions

- Contraindicated in patients hypersensitive to the drug, patients in early pregnancy, and breastfeeding women.
- Contraindicated in patients with a prolonged QT interval.
- *Overdose signs and symptoms*: hypersedation.

Patient and Family Education

- If patient is taking other CNS drugs, watch for oversedation.
- *Look alike/sound alike*: hydroxyurea, hydrogesic, or hydralazine.
- Warn patients to avoid hazardous activities that require alertness and good coordination until effects of drug are known.
- Avoid use of alcohol while taking the drug. Sugarless gum, hard candy, or ice chips may prevent dry mouth.

Special Populations

- *Pregnancy*: not recommended; warn women of childbearing age to avoid use during pregnancy and breastfeeding.
- *Pediatrics*: unknown.
- *Older adults*: Older adults may be more sensitive to adverse anticholinergic effects; monitor these patients for dizziness, excessive sedation, confusion, hypotension, and syncope.

IBUPROFEN (Motrin)

Classification
Nonsteroidal antiinflammatory drug (NSAID)

Indications
Ibuprofen is used to treat generalized pain and pain associated with opiate withdrawal.

Available Forms
Tablet, 100, 200, 400, 600, and 800 mg; chewable tablets, 50 and 100 mg; oral suspension, 100 mg/5 mL, 40 mg/5 mL

Dosage
Dose is 1,200 to 3,200 mg daily divided as follows: 300 mg QID or 400, 600, or 800 mg TID or QID; maximum, not to exceed 3,200 mg/d.

Administration
- PO with meals or milk to reduce GI upset.
- *Missed dose:* Take as soon as remembered. Skip the missed dose if it is almost time for the next scheduled dose. Do not take extra medicine.

Side Effects
The side effects of ibuprofen are heartburn, nausea, vomiting, constipation, bloating, GI ulceration, and occult blood loss.

Drug Interactions
- Heparin may prolong bleeding time.
- It may increase lithium toxicity.
- Garlic, ginger, and ginkgo may increase bleeding time.

Pharmacokinetics
- *Metabolism:* liver
- *Excretion:* eliminated in urine (50%–60%; <10% unchanged)
- *Bioavailability:* 80% to 100%
- *Onset:* 30 to 60 minutes
- *Peak:* 120 minutes (tablets); 62 minutes (chewable); 47 minutes (suspension)
- *Half-life:* 2 to 4 hours

Precautions
- Watch for toxic hepatitis, peptic ulcer disease, and anaphylaxis.

Patient and Family Education
- Notify healthcare provider immediately of passage of dark tarry stools, coffee ground emesis, or other GI distress.
- Do not take with aspirin.
- Avoid alcohol and NSAIDs.

Special Populations

- *Older adults*: There are no contraindications for the use of this drug in the older adult population.
- *Renal impairment*: Use with caution.
- *Hepatic impairment*: Use with caution; it may require smaller dosage.
- *Pregnancy*: category B.
- *Lactation*: There are no contraindications for the use of this drug in breastfeeding mothers.
- *Children and adolescents*: Whether the drug is safe to use under age 6 years has not been established.

ILOPERIDONE (Fanapt)

Classifications
Antipsychotic; dopamine and serotonin antagonist

Indication
Iloperidone is used to treat schizophrenia.

Available Forms
Tablets, 1, 2, 4, 6, 8, 10, and 12 mg

Dosage
- *Adults*: initially, 1 mg PO BID.
- Increase as needed as per dosing schedule: 2 mg PO BID on day 2; 4 mg PO BID on day 3; 6 mg PO BID on day 4; 8 mg PO BID on day 5; 10 mg PO BID on day 6; 12 mg PO BID on day 7.
- Maximum dosage is 12 mg PO BID.
- For patients taking CYP2D6 inhibitors and CYP3A4 inhibitors, reduce dosage by half.

Administration
Give drug with or without food.

Side Effects
- *Central nervous system*: somnolence, akathisia, parkinsonism, agitation, dystonia, dizziness, insomnia, anxiety, restlessness, seizures, and fatigue
- *Cardiovascular*: tachycardia
- *EENT*: blurred vision
- *Gastrointestinal*: nausea, vomiting, dyspepsia, abdominal pain, diarrhea, dysphasia, and decreased appetite
- *Metabolic*: dyslipidemia, hyperglycemia, weight gain
- *Musculoskeletal*: back pain, skin, rash, and pruritus

Drug Interactions
This medicine may interact with the following medications:
- Alpha blockers may enhance antihypertensive effects.
- Centrally acting drugs may increase CNS effects.
- Dextromethorphan may increase dextromethorphan level. Avoid use together.
- Avoid use with alcohol.
- Effects on lab test results: It may decrease hematocrit.

Pharmacokinetics
- It may antagonize dopamine type 2 and serotonin type 2.
- Onset unknown, peak 2 to 4 hours, duration unknown; half-life: 18 to 37 hours.

Precautions
- Avoid use with drugs known to prolong QT interval and in older adults with dementia-related symptoms.

- Overdose signs and symptoms are prolonged QT interval, drowsiness, sedation, tachycardia, and hypotension.
- Obtain baseline BP, monitor regularly. Life-threatening hyperglycemia may occur in patients taking atypical antipsychotics.
- Monitor CBC frequently during first few months of therapy and discontinue if WBC drops with no underlying cause.
- Monitor potassium and magnesium levels at baseline and periodically in patients at risk for electrolyte imbalance.
- Drug may lower seizure threshold in patients with history of seizures.

Patient and Family Education

- Take drug on regular basis and do not skip doses.
- Periodic blood tests will be needed to monitor tolerance to the drug.
- Monitor weight and diet.
- Tell patients to avoid alcohol, warn against driving until effects of drug are known, and immediately report sudden change in body temperature, BP, or irregular heartbeat.
- Monitor patients for TD.
- Monitor for orthostatic hypotension.
- Monitor for signs of NMS.
- Check CBC, renal function, and prolactin level periodically.
- Discontinue if severe neutropenia develops.
- Monitor for metabolic changes.
- Assess patients for risk of suicide ideation.

Special Populations

- *Older adults*: Patients with dementia-related psychosis are at increased risk for death.
- Antipsychotics are not approved for treatment of dementia-related psychosis. Use cautiously in patients with hyperlipidemia diabetes or risk for diabetes, or seizures.
- Use cautiously in patients with known CV disease and preexisting low WBC counts.
- *Pregnancy*: category C.
- *Pediatric*: Iloperidone is not indicated for use in children.

IMIPRAMINE (Tofranil, Tofranil PM, Tofranil injection)

Classification
Tricyclic antidepressant (TCA)

Indications
Imipramine is used to treat adults with depression/anxiety.

Available Forms
- *Tofranil:* Tablet, 10, 25, and 50 mg
- *Tofranil PM:* capsule, 75, 100, 125, and 150 mg; tablet, 10, 25, and 50 mg
- *Tofranil injection:* ampule, 25 mg/2 mL

Dosage
Tofranil
- *Adults and children older than 12 years*: initially 75 mg daily (maximum 200 mg); adolescents initially 30 to 40 mg daily (maximum 100 mg/d); if maintenance dose exceeds 75 mg daily, may switch to Tofranil PM for divided or bedtime dose.
- *Children younger than 12 years*: not recommended.

Tofranil PM
- *Adults and children older than 12 years*: initially 75 mg daily 1 hour before HS; maximum 200 mg.
- *Children younger than 12 years*: not recommended.

Tofranil Injection
- *Adults and children older than 12 years*: 50 mg IM; lower dose for adolescents; switch to oral form as soon as possible.
- *Children younger than 12 years*: not recommended.

Administration
- PO with a glass of water.
- Do not crush, cut, or chew XR tablets.
- Do not abruptly stop taking the medication.
- It is not prescribed for children except when used for nocturnal enuresis and depression in children as young as 6 years.
- Use lowest effective dose for shortest duration dosing.

Side Effects
The side effects of this drug are similar to those of amitriptyline.
- *More common:* Drowsiness, dizziness, constipation; nausea/vomiting, urinary retention or frequency, libido changes, weight gain, general nervousness, and galactorrhea are the most common side effects.
- *Less common:* Cardiac arrhythmias, EPS, clotting disturbances, worsening depression, suicidality, hyperthermia, and HTN are the less common side effects.
- Fatigue, sedation, and weight gain.
- Sexual dysfunction.

Drug Interactions

This medicine may interact with the following medications:

- Absolute contraindications include class 1A antiarrhythmics and MAOIs such as phenelzine (Nardil), tranylcypromine (Parnate), isocarboxazid (Marplan), and selegiline (Eldepryl).
- Avoid using with cimetidine, amiodarone, clarithromycin, haloperidol, and St. John's wort.
- *Alert:* This list may not describe all possible interactions. Instruct patients to provide a list of all medicines, herbs, nonprescription drugs, or dietary supplements used and state whether they smoke, drink alcohol, or use illegal drugs.
- MAOIs: Risk for extreme HTN.
- *CNS depressants (e.g., alcohol):* TCAs increase effects.
- *Direct-acting adrenergic agonists (e.g., epinephrine):* TCAs increase effects.
- *Anticholinergic drugs (e.g., antihistamines):* TCAs increase effects. Do not use in combination.
- *SSRIs and other medications:* serotonin syndrome.

Pharmacokinetics

- TCAs are thought to work by inhibiting reuptake of norepinephrine and serotonin in the CNS, which potentiates the neurotransmitters. They also have significant anticholinergics, antihistaminic, and alpha-adrenergic activity on the cardiac system. These classes of antidepressants also possess class 1A antiarrhythmic activity, which can lead to depression of cardiac conduction potentially resulting in heart block or ventricular arrhythmias.
- *Metabolism:* This drug is metabolized extensively by the liver to the active metabolite desipramine form by CYP450 2D6. Also metabolized by CYP450 1A2.
- *Excretion:* primarily in urine, up to <5% unchanged; also excreted in the bile/feces.
- *Peak:* 1 to 2 hours.
- *Onset:* after 2 weeks.
- *Half-life:* 6 to 18 hours.

Precautions

- See patients as often as necessary to ensure that the drug is working on the panic attacks, determine compliance, and review side effects.
- Instruct patients and families to watch for worsening depression or thoughts of suicide. Also, watch out for sudden or severe changes in feelings, such as feeling anxious, agitated, panicky, irritated, hostile, aggressive, impulsive, severely restless, overly excited, or hyperactive or not being able to sleep. If this happens, especially at the beginning of antidepressant treatment or after a change in dose, patient should call the healthcare provider.
- *Drowsiness or dizziness:* Patients should not drive or use machinery or do anything that needs mental alertness until the effects of this medicine are known. Other medications that cause drowsiness can add to the drowsiness of imipramine.
- Caution patients not to stand or sit up quickly, especially if older. This reduces the risk of dizzy or fainting spells. Alcohol may interfere with the effect of this medicine. Avoid alcoholic drinks.
- Do not abruptly withdraw this drug as it may cause headache, nausea, and malaise.
- Advise to protect skin from ultraviolet light due to increased skin sensitivity.
- Grapefruit and grapefruit juice may interact with imipramine.
- Caution should be exercised in the following:

- MDD, psychosis, or bipolar affective disorder.
- Contraindicated in patients with a recent myocardial infarction.
- Blood dyscrasias.
- Respiratory disease.
- Heart disease.
- Liver disease.
- Seizures (convulsions).
- Suicidal thoughts, plans, or attempts by patients or a family member.
- An unusual or allergic reaction to imipramine, other medicines, foods, dyes, or preservatives.
- Overdose may result in lethal cardiotoxicity or seizure.
- Use with caution in patients having a history of seizure or heart disease.
- Avoid in patients with a history of cardiac arrhythmia. Monitor with EKG.

Patient and Family Education

- Store imipramine at room temperature away from moisture and heat.
- Stopping this medication suddenly could result in unpleasant side effects.
- Take the missed dose as soon as remembered. If it is almost time for the next dose, skip the missed dose and take the medicine at the next regularly scheduled time. Do not take extra medicine to make up the missed dose.
- It should be taken about the same time every day, with or without food. It may cause prolonged sedation. Do not drive until the effect of this medication is known.
- Administration time may be adjusted based on observed sedating or activating drug effects.
- It may take up to 4 to 8 weeks to show its maximum effect, but patient may see symptoms of dysthymia improving in as few as 2 weeks.
- If patient plans on becoming pregnant, discuss the benefits versus the risks of using this medicine while pregnant.
- As this medicine is excreted in breast milk, nursing mothers should not breastfeed while taking this medicine without prior consultation with a psychiatric nurse practitioner or psychiatrist. Newborns may develop symptoms, including feeding or breathing difficulties, seizures, muscle stiffness, jitteriness, or constant crying.
- Do not stop taking this medication unless the healthcare provider directs. Report symptoms to the healthcare provider promptly.
- Drug should be tapered gradually.
- Treatment should continue for at least 6 to 12 months following last reported dysthymic experience.
- Keep these medications out of the reach of children and pets.

Special Populations

- *Older adults:* Older patients tend to be more sensitive to the medication side effects, such as hypotension and anticholinergic effects. They often require adjustment of medication doses for hepatic or renal dysfunction TCAs. Dose adjustment is necessary for geriatric patients and in patients with liver impairment
- *Pregnancy:* category D; some clinical reports of congenital malformations but no direct causal link. Not recommended in pregnancy, as there are no adequate studies showing potential for side effects during pregnancy.
- *Lactation:* This drug is excreted in human breast milk; alternative medications are recommended.
- *Children:* The drug is not recommended for children younger than 12 years old.

ISOCARBOXAZID (Marplan)

Classification
Monoamine oxidase inhibitor (MAOI)

Indications
This drug is used to treat depression and anxiety.

Available Forms
Tablet, 10 mg

Dosage
- *Adults and children older than 16 years*: initially 10 mg BID; increase by 10 mg every 2 to 4 days up to 40 mg/d; may increase by 20 mg/wk to maximum 60 mg/d divided BID to QID
- *Children younger than 16 years*: not recommended

Side Effects
- Hypertensive crisis, secondary to excessive consumption of dietary tyramine (e.g., soft cheeses, aged fish, aged meat, and avocados)
- CNS stimulation
- Orthostatic hypotension
- Sexual dysfunction

Drug Interactions
- *Selective serotonin reuptake inhibitors, serotonin-norepinephrine reuptake inhibitors, and tricyclic antidepressants*: There is a risk for extreme HTN.
- *Indirect-acting adrenergic agonists (e.g., ephedrine)*: It increases MAOI effects.
- Antihypertensive drugs may dangerously lower BP.

Pharmacokinetics
Duration of action: may last 2 to 3 weeks following discontinuation due to irreversible monoamine oxidase inhibition

Precautions
- Many drugs and foods interact with this class of drugs, so use cautiously. Should be reserved for refractory depression that has not responded to other classes of antidepressants. Concomitant use of MAOIs and SSRIs is an absolute contraindication. See manufacturer's package insert for drug and food interactions.
- Adverse effects and side effects are commonly observed before therapeutic effects.
- Dietary restrictions require substantial patient adherence.

Patient and Family Education
- This drug should be taken about the same time every day, with or without food.
- Substantial education required on dietary changes and importance of dietary adherence.
- Patient should advise all health-care providers that they are on an MAOI prior to initiating new medications.

- Administration time may be adjusted based on observed sedating or activating drug effects.
- It may take up to 4 to 8 weeks to show its maximum effect, but some may see symptoms of dysthymia depression improving in as few as 2 weeks.
- Do not take the drug in case of pregnancy or if trying to get pregnant.
- As this medicine is excreted in the breast milk, nursing mothers should not breastfeed while taking this medicine. Newborns may develop symptoms, including feeding or breathing difficulties, seizures, muscle stiffness, jitteriness, or constant crying.
- Report potential side effects to the healthcare provider promptly.
- Keep these medications out of the reach of children and pets.

Special Populations

- *Older adults*: There is a requirement for lower drug doses in adult patients over 65 years. Due to common need for polypharmacy, drug is not recommended.
- *Pregnancy*: Psychotherapy is the initial choice for most pregnant patients with MDD. This drug is generally not recommended during pregnancy.
- *Children*: It is not recommended for children younger than 16 years of age.

LAMOTRIGINE (Lamictal, Lamictal CD, Lamictal ODT, Lamictal XR)

Classification
Anticonvulsant, mood-stabilizing anticonvulsant

Indications
Used only for maintenance of bipolar I disorder, not acute phase.

Available Forms
Tablet, 25, 100, 150, and 200 mg; chewable tablet, 2, 5, and 25 mg; ODT, 25, 50, 100, and 200 mg; XR tablet, 25, 50, 100, and 200 mg

Dosage
- *Adults and children older than 12 years*: not taking an enzyme-inducing antiepileptic drug (EIAED) (e.g., phenytoin, carbamazepine, phenobarbital, primidone, valproic acid): 25 mg once daily × 2 weeks; then 50 mg once daily × 2 weeks; then 100 mg once daily × 2 weeks; then target dose 200 mg once daily; Concomitant valproic acid: 25 mg every other day × 2 weeks; then 25 mg once daily × 2 weeks; then 50 mg once daily × 1 week; then target dose 100 mg once daily; Concomitant EIAED, not valproic acid: 50 mg once daily × 2 weeks; then 100 mg daily in divided doses; then increase weekly by 100 mg in divided doses to target dose 400 mg/d in divided doses daily.
- *Children younger than 12 years*: not recommended.

Administration
- Discontinue medicine at first sign of a rash.
- This medicine should be taken as directed and is well tolerated in the recommended doses.
- Individuals taking this medicine should carry an identification card to alert medical personnel who might be caring for them.
- The potential carcinogenic, mutagenic, and fertility effects are unknown.
- This is a category C drug and should be used in pregnancy only if the potential benefit outweighs the risk. It is not known whether the drug is excreted in breast milk, so caution should be exercised when it is administered to nursing women.
- Pediatric use under the age of 18 years has not been established. Individuals taking opioid-containing medicines, such as cough-and-cold preparations, antidiarrheal preparations, and opioid analgesics with lamotrigine may not benefit from these medicines.
- Concomitant use is unknown.
- This drug does not interfere with drug testing using urine samples.

Side Effects
Dizziness, headache, diplopia, ataxia, asthenia, nausea, blurred vision, somnolence, rhinitis, rash, pharyngitis, vomiting, cough, flu syndrome, dysmenorrhea, uncoordination, insomnia, diarrhea, fever, abdominal pain, depression, tremor, anxiety, vaginitis, speech disturbance, seizures, weight loss, photosensitivity, nystagmus, constipation, and dry mouth.

Drug Interactions

See manufacturer's package insert for drug interactions, interactions with contraceptives and hormone replacement therapy, and discontinuation protocol. Avoid using the following drugs with this medicine:

- Oral progesterone contraceptives (may decrease hormonal contraceptive levels).
- Etonogestrel subdermal implant (may decrease hormonal contraceptive levels).
- Ginkgo biloba, Eun-haeng, fossil tree, ginkyo, icho, ityo, Japanese silver apricot, kew tree, maidenhair tree, salisburia, silver apricot, ginkgo (may decrease anticonvulsant efficacy).
- Medroxyprogesterone acetate (may decrease hormonal contraceptive levels).
- Acetaminophen (may decrease effects of lamotrigine).
- Valproate may decrease clearance of lamotrigine (increases lamotrigine level and decreases valproate level).
- Oxcarbazepine, phenobarbital, phenytoin, and primidone (may decrease lamotrigine level).
- St. John's wort (may decrease lamotrigine levels as clearance is increased).
- Folate inhibitors (methotrexate, sulfamethoxazole, and trimethoprim) may have an additive effect.

Pharmacokinetics

The drug is metabolized by the liver (CYP450). It is excreted in the urine (94%) and feces (2%).

- *Peak plasma:* 1 to 5 hours
- *Bioavailability:* 98%
- *Half-life:* 14.5 to 70.25 hours

Precautions

- Discontinue medicine at first sign of a rash. Incidence is 0.8% in children 2 to 6 years of age and 0.3% in adults. Most life-threatening rashes occur and may occur at any time during treatment.
- Caution should be exercised when administering this medicine to patients with suicide risk, pregnancy, hepatic impairment, renal impairment, and hypersensitivity to antiepileptic drugs.
- Individuals taking opioid-containing medicines, such as cough-and-cold preparations, antidiarrheal preparations, and opioid analgesics may not benefit from these medicines.
- This drug may cause aseptic meningitis.

Patient and Family Education

- Do not stop taking this drug suddenly; it must be tapered by your healthcare provider.
- Notify your healthcare provider immediately if your depression symptoms increase.
- High risk of nonadherence due the need to take the medication BID.

Special Populations

- *Older adults:* Caution should be exercised when administering this drug to older adults.
- *Renal impairment:* For moderate to severe impairment, decrease dose by 25%. If there is severe impairment, decrease dose by 50%.

- *Pregnancy*: category C drug. Animal studies show adverse fetal effect(s) but no controlled human studies.
- *Lactation*: It is considered unsafe for breastfeeding mothers. Medication administration requires cessation of breastfeeding.
- *Children*: It is not recommended for children younger than 12 years.

LEVOMILNACIPRAN (Fetzima)

Classification
Antidepressant; serotonin-norepinephrine reuptake inhibitor (SNRI])

Indications
Levomilnacipran is for MDD.

Available Forms
Capsule (XR), 20, 40, 80, and 120 mg

Dosage
- *Adults and children older than 12 years*: Swallow whole; initially 20 mg once daily for 2 days; then increase to 40 mg once daily; may increase dose in 40-mg increments at intervals of ≥2 days; maximum 120 mg once daily; CrCl 30 to 59 mL/min: maximum 80 mg once daily; CrCl 15 to 29 mL/min: maximum 40 mg once daily.
- *Children younger than 12 years*: not recommended.

Administration
- Swallow the XR capsule in whole.
- The medication can be taken with or without food.
- Avoid abrupt withdrawal of this drug. Slowly titrate off drug.

Side Effects
- Nausea, constipation, vomiting, hyperhidrosis, increased heart rate, erectile dysfunction, tachycardia, palpitations; HTN, urinary hesitation
- Hypersensitivity
- Suicidal thoughts and behaviors in adolescents and young adults
- Serotonin syndrome
- Elevated BP
- Elevated heart rate
- Abnormal bleeding
- Narrow-angle glaucoma
- Urinary hesitation or retention
- Activation of mania/hypomania
- Seizure
- Hyponatremia

Drug Interactions
- Use levomilnacipran with caution in patients who are on MAOIs. Allow at least 14 days after MAOI discontinuation before starting levomilnacipran.
- There is an increased risk of serotonin syndrome with other serotonergic drugs or with drugs that impair serotonin metabolism.
- There is an increased risk of bleeding with concomitant NSAIDs, aspirin, and anticoagulants; there is a need to monitor the same.
- Concomitant strong CYP3A4 inhibitors adjust dose.
- Avoid alcohol.
- Use with caution with other CNS-active drugs or drugs that can increase BP or heart rate.

Pharmacokinetics

■ The exact mechanism of action of levomilnacipran is unknown.
■ It is thought to be related to the potentiation of serotonin and norepinephrine in the CNS, through inhibition of reuptake at serotonin and norepinephrine transporters.

Precautions

■ There is an increased risk of suicidal thinking and behavior in children, adolescents, and young adults.
■ Monitor for serotonin syndrome especially if patient is on other serotonergic agents; thoroughly review patient medications for other serotonergic MAOIs, TCAs, SSRIs.
■ Use caution with patients who have history of bipolar disorder, mania, hypomania, HTN, CV disease, seizures, tachyarrhythmias, obstructive urinary disorders, seizure disorder.
■ Monitor BP and heart rate; reduce dose or discontinue if elevation persists.
■ Use of this drug can increase risk of bleeding; caution with use of NSAIDs, aspirin, or anticoagulants.
■ If patients are taking diuretics, monitor the patients' volume/electrolytes. There is an increased risk of hyponatremia.

Patient and Family Education

■ Patients should be monitored closely for changes in behavior, clinical worsening, and suicidal tendencies; this should be done during the initial 1 to 2 months of therapy and dosage adjustments.
■ The patient's family should communicate any abrupt changes in behavior to the healthcare provider.
■ Be aware of all drug interactions and notify provider if medications change.
■ Make sure patient and family are aware of all side effects.
■ Monitor CrCl in patients with existing renal impairment—moderate (CrCl 30–59 mL/min): maximum 80 mg once daily; severe (CrCl 15–29 mL/min): maximum 40 mg once daily.

Special Populations

■ *Older adults*
  ■ SSRIs and SNRIs, including Fetzima, have been associated with cases of clinically significant hyponatremia in older adults, who may be at greater risk for this adverse event.
  ■ Monitor patients' renal and liver function regularly.
■ *Pregnancy*
  ■ *Category C:* There are no adequate and well-controlled studies of Fetzima in pregnant women.
  ■ Neonates exposed to dual reuptake inhibitors of serotonin and norepinephrine (such as Fetzima) or SSRIs late in the third trimester have developed complications that can arise immediately upon delivery.
■ *Children:* not recommended in children younger than 12 years. Monitor for suicide ideation.

LISDEXAMFETAMINE DIMESYLATE (Vyvanse)

Classification
Central nervous system (CNS) stimulant

Indications
Stimulant indicated for the treatment of ADHD.

Available Forms
Capsule, 20, 30, 40, 50, 60, and 70 mg

Dosage
Dosage should be individualized according to the therapeutic needs and response of the patient. All stimulant preparations should be administered at the lowest effective dosage.

- *Adults and children older than 6 years:* 30 mg PO QAM; may increase dose 10 to 20 mg/d every week; maximum, 70 mg/d; use lowest effective dose.
- *Children younger than 6 years:* not recommended.

Administration
Swallow capsules whole with water or other liquids. If patient cannot swallow the capsule, open it and mix with water; take immediately. Follow with a drink of water or other liquid. It can be taken with or without food. Avoid afternoon doses; the drug has the potential for insomnia.

Side Effects
- Decreased appetite, dizziness, dry mouth, irritability, insomnia, upper abdominal pain, nausea and/or vomiting, weight loss, headaches, and anxiety.
- *Psychiatric events*: increase in manic states for bipolar patients, aggression, tics, and tremors.
- *Long-term growth suppression*: patients should be monitored throughout treatment; if there appears to be growth suppression, the treatment should be discontinued.
- Rash, pyrexia, palpitations, tachycardia, elevated BP, sudden death, myocardial infarction, cardiomyopathy, SJS and TEN, impotence, and libido changes.

Drug Interactions
The medication may interact with urinary acidifying agents, MAOIs, adrenergic blockers, antihistamines, antihypertensives, veratrum alkaloids, ethosuximide, TCAs, meperidine, phenobarbital, phenytoin, chlorpromazine, Haldol, lithium, norepinephrine, and propoxyphene.

Pharmacokinetics
- This drug is absorbed by the GI tract.
- The mode of therapeutic action in ADHD is not known. Amphetamines are thought to block the reuptake of norepinephrine and dopamine into the presynaptic neuron and increase the release of these monoamines into the extraneural space.

- Prodrug converted to dextroamphetamine.
- *Metabolism:* liver; mainly excreted in the urine (96%).
- *Time to peak:* 1 hour.
- *Half-life:* <0.5 hours.

Precautions

- Advanced arteriosclerosis, symptomatic CV disease, and moderate to severe HTN.
- Hyperthyroidism.
- Known hypersensitivity or idiosyncratic reaction to sympathomimetic amines.
- Glaucoma.
- Agitated states.
- *Patients with a history of drug abuse:* Amphetamines have a high potential for abuse. Administration of amphetamines for an extended period of time may lead to drug dependence. Particular attention should be paid to the possibility of patients obtaining this class of medication for nontherapeutic use or distribution to others, and the drugs should be prescribed or dispensed sparingly.
- During or within 14 days following the administration of MAOIs, hypertensive crisis may result.
- Use with caution in patients with preexisting psychosis.
- *Seizure history:* Some studies have shown the potential for lowering the seizure threshold.

Patient and Family Education

- Store the drug at room temperature, protected from light.
- Keep it out of reach of children.
- Seek medical care for any signs of heart problems (chest pain, shortness of breath), fainting, psychotic symptoms, overdose, or any other concerns.
- Routinely assess weight and BP.
- Treatment should be initiated at low doses and then titrated over 2 to 4 weeks until an adequate response is achieved or unacceptable adverse effects occur.
- If one stimulant is not effective, another should be attempted before second-line medications are considered. Although some children benefit from daily stimulant therapy, weekend and summer "drug holidays" are suggested for children whose ADHD symptoms predominantly affect schoolwork or to limit adverse effects (e.g., appetite suppression, abdominal pain, headache, insomnia, irritability, tics).

Special Populations

- *Older adults:* Use caution with polypharmacy and comorbid conditions; has not been studied for use in this population.
- *Pregnancy:* category C; based on animal data, they may cause fetal harm.
- *Lactation:* Possibly unsafe.
- *Children:* not recommended in children younger than 6 years.

LITHIUM CARBONATE (Lithobid)

Classification
First-line non-anticonvulsant mood stabilizer

Indications
This drug is used to treat mania in bipolar disorder. Initially, lithium is often used in conjunction with antipsychotic drugs as it can take up to a month for it to have an effect. Lithium is also used as prophylaxis for depression and mania in bipolar disorder. It is sometimes used for other psychiatric disorders, such as cycloid psychosis, BPD, and MDD.

Available Forms
Tablet (slow-release), 300 mg

Dosage
- *Adults and children older than 12 years:* swallow whole; usual maintenance: 900 to 1,200 mg/d in 2 to 3 divided doses
- *Children younger than 12 years:* not recommended

Administration
- Swallow whole.
- Give the drug after meals with plenty of water to minimize GI upset.
- Do not crush controlled-release tablets.

Side Effects
- Signs and symptoms of lithium toxicity include blurred vision, tinnitus, weakness, dizziness, nausea, abdominal pains, vomiting, diarrhea to (severe) hand tremors, ataxia, muscle twitches, nystagmus, seizures, slurred speech, decreased level of consciousness, coma, death.
- *CNS:* fatigue, lethargy, coma, epileptiform seizures, tremors, drowsiness, headache, confusion, restlessness, dizziness, psychomotor retardation, blackouts, electroencephalogram changes, impaired worsened mental syndrome, impaired speech, ataxia, and incoordination.
- *CV:* arrhythmias, bradycardia, reversible EKG changes, and hypotension.
- *EENT:* tinnitus and blurred vision.
- *GI:* vomiting, anorexia, diarrhea, thirst, nausea, metallic taste, dry mouth, abdominal pain, flatulence, and indigestion.
- *Genitourinary:* polyuria, renal toxicity with long-term use, glycosuria, decreased CrCl, and albuminuria.
- *Hematological:* leukocytosis with leukocyte count of 14,000 to 18,000/mm.
- *Metabolic:* transient hyperglycemia, goiter, hypothyroidism, and hyponatremia.
- *Musculoskeletal:* muscle weakness.
- *Skin:* pruritus, rash, diminished or absent sensation, drying and thinning of hair, psoriasis, acne, and alopecia.
- *Other:* ankle and wrist edema.

Drug Interactions

- Angiotensin-converting enzyme inhibitors, aminophylline, sodium bicarbonate, urine alkalizers, calcium channel blockers (verapamil), carbamazepine, fluoxetine, methyldopa, NSAIDs, probenecid, neuromuscular blockers, thiazide diuretics, and diuretics.
- Diuretics, especially loop diuretics, may inhibit lithium elimination and increase lithium toxicity.
- Caffeine may decrease lithium levels and drug effects. Advise patients who ingest large amounts of caffeine.

Pharmacokinetics

- Probably alters chemical transmitters in the CNS, possibly by interfering with ionic pump mechanisms in brain cells and may compete with or replace sodium ions. The peak action is between 30 minutes and 1 hour; XR, 4 to 12 hours.
- *Bioavailability*: 95% to 100% (immediate release/syrup); 60% to 905% (XR).
- *Excretion*: urine (95%–99%).
- *Half-life:* 18 hours (adolescents); 36 hours (older adults).

Precautions

- Signs and symptoms of lithium toxicity include blurred vision, tinnitus, weakness, dizziness, nausea, abdominal pains, vomiting, diarrhea to (severe) hand tremors, ataxia, muscle twitches, nystagmus, seizures, slurred speech, decreased level of consciousness, coma, death.
- Lithium may increase glucose and creatinine levels.
- It may decrease sodium, T3, T4, and protein-bound iodine levels.
- It may increase WBC and neutrophil counts.
- It is contraindicated if therapy cannot be closely monitored.
- Avoid using the drug in pregnant patients unless benefits outweigh risks.
- Use with caution in patients receiving neuromuscular blockers and diuretics; in older or debilitated patients; and in patients with thyroid disease, seizure disorder, infection, renal or CV disease, severe debilitation or dehydration, or sodium depletion.
- *Alert:* Drug has a narrow therapeutic margin of safety. Determining drug level is crucial to the safe use of the drug. Do not use the drug in patients who cannot have regular tests done. Monitor levels 8 to 12 hours after the first dose, the morning before the second dose is given, two or three times weekly for the first month, and then weekly to monthly during maintenance therapy.
- When the drug level is <1.5 mEq/L, adverse reactions are usually mild.
- Monitor baseline EKG, thyroid studies, renal studies, and electrolyte levels.
- Check fluid intake and output, especially when surgery is scheduled.
- Weigh patient daily; check for edema or sudden weight gain.
- Adjust fluid and salt ingestion to compensate if excessive loss occurs from protracted diaphoresis or diarrhea. Under normal conditions, patient's fluid intake should be 2.5 to 3 L daily; patient should follow a balanced diet with adequate salt intake.
- Check urine-specific gravity and report levels below 1.005, which may indicate diabetes insipidus.
- Drug alters glucose tolerance in diabetics. Monitor glucose level closely.
- Perform outpatient follow-up of thyroid and renal functions every 6 to 12 months. Palpate thyroid to check for enlargement.

Patient and Family Education

- Tell the patient to take the drug with plenty of water and after meals to minimize GI upset.
- Explain the importance of having regular blood tests to determine drug levels; even slightly high values can be dangerous.
- Warn patients and caregivers to expect transient nausea, large amounts of urine, thirst, and discomfort during the first few days of therapy and to watch for evidence of toxicity (diarrhea, vomiting, tremor, drowsiness, muscle weakness, incoordination).
- Instruct patients to withhold one dose and call the prescriber if signs and symptoms of toxicity appear, but do not stop drug abruptly.
- Warn patients to avoid hazardous activities that require alertness and good psychomotor coordination until the CNS effects of drug are known.
- Tell patients not to switch brands or take other prescription or OTC drugs without the prescriber's guidance.
- Tell patients to wear or carry medical identification at all times.

Special Populations

- *Older adults*: initial dose reduction and possibly lower maintenance doses due to age-related changes and sensitivity to side effects.
- *Pregnancy*: category D; positive evidence of fetal harm has been demonstrated.
- *Children*: It is not approved in children younger than 12 years of age; use with caution and monitor closely for side effects and suicidality. Children may experience more frequent and severe side effects.

LOPERAMIDE (Imodium, Imodium A–D)

Classification
Antidiarrheal drug

Indications
Loperamide treats diarrhea associated with opiate withdrawal.

Available Forms
Capsule, 2 mg; caplet, 2 mg; liquid, 1 mg/5 mL (alcohol 0.5%)

Dosage
Imodium
- *Adults and children older than 5 years*: 4 mg initially, then 2 mg after each loose stool; maximum 16 mg/d × 2 days
- *Children younger than 5 years*: not recommended

Imodium A–D
- *Adults*: 4 mg initially, then 2 mg after each loose stool; maximum 8 mg/d × 2 days
- *Children 9 to 11 years (60–95 lbs)*: 2 mg initially, then 1 mg after each loose stool; maximum 6 mg/d × 2 days
- *Children 6 to 8 years (48–59 lbs)*: 2 mg initially, then 1 mg after each loose stool; maximum 4 mg/d × 2 days
- *Children 2 to 5 years (24–47 lbs)*: 1 mg up to TID × 2 days
- *Children younger than 2*: not recommended

Administration
- PO with a full glass of water.
- The drug may be taken with or without food.
- *Missed dose:* Take as soon as remembered. Skip the missed dose if it is almost time for the next scheduled dose. Do not take extra medicine.

Side Effects
Anaphylactic reactions (rare); stomach pain/bloating; diarrhea that is bloody, watery, or worsening; flu-like symptoms with skin reaction/rash; dizziness; fatigue; constipation; mild stomach pain; mild skin pruritus and rash.

Drug Interactions
When given concurrently with saquinavir, the therapeutic efficacy of saquinavir should be closely monitored.

Pharmacokinetics
- *Bioavailability:* 0.3%
- *Onset:* 1 to 3 hours
- *Half-life:* 11 hours
- *Excretion:* feces (30%–40%); urine (1%)

Precautions

■ Discontinue the use of this drug if the patient has constipation, abdominal distention, or ileus develop.

Patient and Family Education

■ Do not take if stools are bloody, black, or tarry.
■ Do not use this medication to treat diarrhea caused by antibiotic use.
■ Drink extra water to prevent dehydration.
■ It may take up to 48 hours for symptoms to improve.
■ Call healthcare provider if symptoms do not improve after treatment for 10 days.
■ Exercise caution when driving or operating machinery.

Special Populations

■ *Older adults:* No dose adjustments required.
■ *Renal impairment:* No dose adjustments required.
■ *Hepatic impairment:* Use with caution; monitor for signs of CNS toxicity.
■ *Pregnancy:* category C.
■ *Lactation:* contraindicated.
■ *Children and adolescents*: Use with caution; monitor fluid and electrolyte balance. Not recommended in children younger than 2 years.

LORAZEPAM (Ativan)/LORAZEPAM INTENSOL

Classification
Benzodiazepine (BZD)

Indications
Lorazepam is used for anxiety and sedation during hypnosis.

Available Forms
Tablet, 0.5, 1, or 2 mg; oral concentrate, 2 mg/mL

Dosage
- *Adults and children older than 12 years*: 1 to 10 mg/d in 2 to 3 divided doses
- The largest dose should be taken at bedtime.
- For anxiety, most patients require an initial dose of 2 to 3 mg/d given BID or TID.
- For insomnia due to anxiety or transient situational stress, a single daily dose of 2 to 4 mg may be given, usually at bedtime.
- For older or debilitated patients, an initial dosage of 1 to 2 mg/d in divided doses is recommended, to be adjusted as needed and tolerated.
- The dosage of Ativan (lorazepam) should be increased gradually when needed to help avoid adverse effects. When higher dosage is indicated, the evening dose should be increased before the daytime doses.

Administration
- Lorazepam can be given PO, IM, or IV. Missed doses need to be given as soon as possible; however, if it is time for the next dose, do not administer a double dose.
- If a dose is missed, it should be taken as soon as possible. If it is time for the next dose, skip the missed dose and resume usual dosing schedule.

Side Effects
Dizziness, weakness, and unsteadiness; a few other side effects include nausea, constipation, fatigue, and sedation.

Drug Interactions
- Increased CNS-depressant effects when administered with other CNS depressants, such as alcohol, barbiturates, antipsychotics, sedative/hypnotics, anxiolytics, antidepressants, narcotic analgesics, sedative antihistamines, anticonvulsants, and anesthetics.
- Use caution when combining clozapine and lorazepam for they may produce marked sedation, excessive salivation, hypotension, ataxia, delirium, and respiratory arrest.
- Administration of lorazepam with valproate results in increased plasma concentrations and reduced clearance of lorazepam.
- Administration of lorazepam with probenecid may result in a more rapid onset or prolonged effect of lorazepam due to increased half-life and decreased total clearance.
- Administration of theophylline or aminophylline may reduce the sedative effects of BZDs, including lorazepam.

Pharmacokinetics

- The drug enhances GABA.
- The drug is metabolized by the liver and enhances GABA effects, which inhibits the transmission of nerve signals and thus reduces nervous excitation.
- *Bioavailability:* 90%.
- *Peak plasma:* 2 hours.
- *Half-life:* 14 hours.

Contraindications

The drug is contraindicated in patients with

- hypersensitivity to BZDs or to any components of the formulation,
- acute narrow-angle glaucoma.

Precautions

Avoid abrupt withdrawal for long-term use, use of alcohol in depressed patients, intra-arterial administration, and use in drug-abuse patients.

Patient and Family Education

- Notify healthcare provider if there are problems with the liver or kidneys, alcohol or drug consumption, glaucoma, lung problems, or if treated for psychiatric disorders.
- Herbs with sedative effects should be avoided.
- Alcoholic beverages should be avoided. Lithium with lorazepam can cause children's body temperature to drop.
- Use of CNS depressants can cause respiratory depression.
- Lorazepam should never be shared with another person, especially someone who has a history of drug abuse or addiction. Keep the medication in a secure place where others cannot get to it.
- It is dangerous to try to purchase lorazepam on the internet or from vendors outside of the United States.
- Medications distributed from internet sales may contain dangerous ingredients or may not be distributed by a licensed pharmacy.
- Samples of lorazepam purchased on the internet have been found to contain haloperidol (Haldol), a potent antipsychotic drug with dangerous side effects.
- For more information, contact the U.S. Food and Drug Administration or visit www.fda.gov/buyonlineguide.
- Store in a tightly closed container and keep at room temperature away from excess heat and moisture.

Special Populations

- *Older adults:* Caution is advised. Due to its sedative property effect and increased risk of falls, all BZDs are included on the Beers List of Potentially Inappropriate Medications for Geriatrics.
- *Renal impairment:* No adjustment is needed if using the oral form; however, dose may need to be adjusted if using the IV form.
- *Hepatic impairment:* may require decreasing the dose, and if patient has hepatic failure or impaired liver function, use should be avoided.
- *Pregnancy:* category D. This drug should not be used in women who are pregnant. Lorazepam is associated with an increased risk for birth defects.
- *Lactation:* should not be used in women who are breastfeeding.
- *Children:* Safety has not been established in children under 12 years and long-term effects are unknown; not recommended in children younger than 12 years.

LURASIDONE HYDROCHLORIDE (Latuda)

Classification
Antipsychotic; dopamine and serotonin receptor antagonist

Indications
Lurasidone hydrochloride is used to treat schizophrenia.

Available Forms
Tablet, 20, 40, 60, 80, and 120 mg

Dosage
- *Adults*: initially 40 mg once daily; usual range 40 to maximum 160 mg/d; take with food; CrCl < 50 mL/min, moderate hepatic impairment (Child-Pugh, 7–9): maximum 80 mg/d; Child-Pugh, 10–15): maximum 40 mg/d
- *Children 13 to 17 years*: initially 40 mg once daily; may titrate up to maximum 80 mg/d
- *Children younger than 13 years*: not established

Administration
This drug should be administered with food (at least 350 calories).

Pharmacokinetics
- Efficacy mediated through antagonism at the dopamine type 2 and serotonin type 2 receptors.
- Onset unknown, peaks in 1 to 3 hours, duration unknown.
- *Half-life:* 18 hours.
- *Effects on lab test results*: It may increase prolactin, total cholesterol, triglyceride, glucose, serum creatinine, AST, ALT, and creatine kinase levels. It may decrease WBC, neutrophil, and granulocyte counts.

Side Effects
- *Central nervous system*: somnolence, akathisia, parkinsonism, agitation, dystonia, dizziness, insomnia, anxiety, restlessness, seizures, and fatigue
- *Cardiovascular*: tachycardia
- *EENT*: blurred vision
- *Gastrointestinal*: nausea, vomiting, dyspepsia, abdominal pain, diarrhea, dysphasia, and decreased appetite
- *Metabolic*: dyslipidemia, hyperglycemia, and weight gain
- *Musculoskeletal*: back pain, rash, and pruritus

Drug Interactions
- Antihypertensives may increase risk of hypotension; centrally acting drugs may increase risk of adverse effects.
- Contraindicated with concomitant strong CYP3A4 inhibitors (e.g., ketoconazole, voriconazole, clarithromycin, ritonavir) and inducers (e.g., phenytoin, carbamazepine, rifampin, St. John's wort); see manufacturer's package insert if patient is taking moderate CYP3A4 inhibitors (e.g., diltiazem, atazanavir, erythromycin, fluconazole, verapamil).
- *Drug/lifestyle*: Alcohol use may increase risk of adverse effects (cognitive impairment).

Patient and Family Education

- Take drug on regular basis and do not skip doses.
- Periodic blood tests will be needed to monitor tolerance to the drug.
- Monitor weight and diet.
- Tell patient to avoid alcohol, warn against driving until effects of drug are known, and immediately report sudden change in body temperature, BP, or irregular heartbeat.
- Monitor patients for TD.
- Monitor for orthostatic hypotension.
- Monitor for signs of NMS.
- Check CBC, renal function, and prolactin level periodically.
- Discontinue if severe neutropenia develops.
- Monitor for metabolic changes.
- Assess patients for risk of suicide ideation.

Special Populations

- *Pregnancy:* category B; use cautiously in pregnant or breastfeeding women.
- *Older adults*
    - Patients with dementia-related psychosis are at increased risk for death.
    - Antipsychotics are not approved for treatment of dementia-related psychosis. Use the drug cautiously in patients with hyperlipidemia, diabetes, or risk for diabetes or seizures.
    - Use cautiously in patients with known CV disease and preexisting low WBC counts.
- *Children:* Latuda is not established for use in children younger than 13 years.

MEMANTINE HYDROCHLORIDE (Namenda, Namenda oral solution, Namenda titratio pak, Namenda XR)

Classification
N-methyl-D-aspartate (NMDA) receptor antagonist

Indications
This drug is used to treat moderate to severe Alzheimer's disease; it does not halt disease progression.

Available Forms
Tablet, 5 and 10 mg; oral solution, 2 mg/mL (sugar/alcohol free); capsule (XR), 7, 14, 21, and 28 mg; capsule, 7 × 7 mg, 7 × 14 mg, 7 × 21 mg, 7 × 28 mg/pck

Dosage
Namenda
- Initially 5 mg once daily; titrate weekly in 5-mg/d increments; week 2: 5 mg BID; week 3: 5 mg AM and 10 mg PM; week 4: 10 mg BID; CrCl 5 to 29 mL/min: maximum 5 mg BID

Namenda Oral Solution
- Initially 5 mg once daily; titrate weekly in 5-mg increments administered BID

Namenda XR
- Initially 7 mg once daily; titrate in 7-mg increments weekly; maximum 28 mg once daily; do not divide doses.

Administration
- Take the drug with or without food.
- Do not cut/divide/chew.
- The contents of the XR capsules can be sprinkled on applesauce.

Side Effects
Extreme tiredness, dizziness, confusion, headache, sleepiness, constipation, vomiting, pain anywhere in the body, especially the back, and coughing. *Serious side effects that may require medical attention:* Shortness of breath, hallucination, SJS, seizures, cataracts, conjunctivitis, cerebrovascular accident (CVA), heart failure, and suicidal ideation.

Drug Interactions
This medication may interact with dofetilide, procainamide, quinidine, acetazolamide, adefovir, alkalinizing agents, amantadine, antimuscarinics, bromocriptine, cimetidine, dextromethorphan, digoxin, entecavir, ketamine, lamivudine, levodopa, metformin, methazolamide, midodrine, morphine, pergolide, pramipexole, quinine, ropinirole, trimethoprim, trospium, vancomycin, amiloride, hydrochlorothiazide, nicotine, ranitidine, and triamterene.

Pharmacokinetics
- *Peak concentration:* immediate-release—3 to 7 hours; XR—9 to 12 hours.

■ *Bioavailability:* 100%.
■ It can be detected in the cerebrospinal fluid 30 minutes after IV infusion.
■ *Half-life:* average 60 to 80 hours.
■ *Excretion:* urine (74%).

Precautions

■ This drug should be used with caution in patients with severe hepatic disease and renal failure.
■ Memantine has not been evaluated in patients with known seizure disorders. Patients who are taking memantine and have seizures or a history of seizure disorder should be monitored closely.

Patient and Family Education

■ Do not divide, cut, or chew the capsules.
■ Contents of the capsule may be sprinkled on applesauce.
■ Store memantine at room temperature and away from excess heat and moisture.
■ Throw away any medication that is outdated or no longer needed.
■ Take the missed dose as soon as remembered. However, if it is almost time for the next dose, skip the missed dose and continue regular dosing schedule. Do not take a double dose to make up for a missed one.

Special Populations

■ *Hepatic impairment:* In patients with mild to moderate hepatic impairment, no dose adjustments are needed; however, caution is advised when using this drug in patients with severe hepatic dysfunction.
■ *Renal impairment:* In patients with CrCl 30 mL/min or greater, no adjustment is needed; if CrCl is 5 to 29 mL/min based on Cockcroft-Gault equation, a target dose of 5 mg PO BID of immediate release is recommended or a target dose of 14 mg/d of the XR capsule is recommended. Not recommended for patients with CrCl <5 mL/min.

METHADONE HCI (Dolophine, Methadose)

Classification
Partial opioid agonist

Indications
Detoxification treatment of opioid and maintenance treatment for opiate dependence

Note
Methadone administration is allowed only by approved providers with strict state and federal regulations (as stipulated in 42 CFR 8.12). BBW: Dolophine exposes users to risks of addiction, abuse, and misuse, which can lead to overdose and death. Assess each patient's risk and monitor regularly for development of these behaviors and conditions. Serious, life-threatening, or fatal respiratory depression may occur. The peak respiratory depressant effect of methadone occurs later and persists longer than the peak analgesic effect. Accidental ingestion, especially by children, can result in fatal overdose. QT interval prolongation and serious arrhythmia (torsades de pointes) have occurred during treatment with methadone. Closely monitor patients with risk factors for development of prolonged QT interval, with a history of cardiac conduction abnormalities, and taking medications affecting cardiac conduction. Neonatal opioid withdrawal syndrome (NOWS) is an expected and treatable outcome of use of methadone use during pregnancy. NOWS may be life threatening if not recognized and treated in the neonate. The balance between the risks of NOWS and the benefits of maternal methadone use should be considered and the patient advised of the risk of NOWS so that appropriate planning for management of the neonate can occur. Methadone has been detected in human milk. Concomitant use with CYP3A4, 2B6, 2C19, 2C9, or 2D6 inhibitors or discontinuation of concomitantly used CYP3A4 2B6, 2C19, or 2C9 inducers can result in a fatal overdose of methadone. Concomitant use of opioids with BZDs or other CNS depressants, including alcohol, may result in profound sedation, respiratory depression, coma, and death.

Available Forms
Tablet, 5 and 10 mg; dispersible tab, 40 mg (dissolve in 120-mL orange juice or other citrus drinks); oral solution, 5 and 10 mg/mL; oral concentrate, 10 mg/mL; syrup, 10 mg/30 mL; vial, 10 mg/mL (200 mg/20 mL multi-dose) for injection

Dosage
- *Adults and children older than 12 years*: A single dose of 20 to 30 mg may be sufficient to suppress withdrawal syndrome; narcotic detoxification: 15 to 40 mg daily in decreasing doses not to exceed 21 days; narcotic maintenance: >21 days; see manufacturer's package insert; clinical stability is most commonly achieved at doses between 80 to 120 mg/d; monitor patients with periodic EKGs (e.g., risk of lethal QT interval prolongation, torsades de pointes).
- *Children younger than 12 years:* not recommended.

Administration
- PO with a full glass of water.
- Dissolvable tablet must be dissolved in liquid prior to consumption.

- May be taken with or without food.
- *Missed dose*: Take as soon as remembered. Skip the missed dose if it is almost time for the next scheduled dose. Do not take extra medicine.

Side Effects

Dizziness, sedation; nausea, vomiting, sweating; bradycardia, palpitations; dysphoria, euphoria; respiratory depression, and pulmonary edema

Drug Interactions

Avoid CNS depressants, other agents that can cause constipation, and medications that can confound the QTc risk.

- May experience withdrawal symptoms when given opioid antagonists, mixed agonist/antagonists, and partial agonists.
- Antiretroviral agents result in increased clearance and decreased plasma levels.
- Rifampin may cause decrease in serum levels and possible withdrawal symptoms.
- Phenytoin may cause up to a 50% decrease in serum levels, leading to withdrawal symptoms.
- St. John's wort, phenobarbital, and carbamazepine may result in withdrawal symptoms.

Pharmacokinetics

- *Half-life*: 8 to 59 hours

Precautions

- Death has been reported when methadone is abused in conjunction with BZDs.
- Caution should be used when giving drugs capable of inducing electrolyte disturbance that may prolong the QT interval.
- Should not be abruptly discontinued.
- Use with caution in hypothyroidism, Addison's disease, prostatic hypertrophy, and respiratory insufficiency.
- May result in hypotension in patients who have inability to maintain stable BP.
- Use with extreme caution with head injuries.

Patient and Family Education

- Take exactly as prescribed. Do not take in larger or smaller amounts or for longer than recommended.
- Can be taken with or without food.
- Exercise caution when driving or operating machinery due to sedative effects of medication.
- Do not drink alcohol while taking methadone.
- Do not stop taking the drug abruptly.

Special Populations

- *Older adults*: Use with caution due to sedative effects.
- *Renal impairment*: Use with caution.
- *Hepatic impairment*: Use with caution.
- *Pregnancy*: category C. There are no controlled studies of methadone use in pregnant women that can be used to establish safety. NOWS is an expected and treatable outcome of methadone use during pregnancy. NOWS may be life

threatening if not recognized and treated in the neonate. The balance between the risks of NOWS and the benefits of maternal methadone use should be considered and the patient advised of the risk of NOWS so that appropriate planning for management of the neonate can occur.

- *Lactation:* Some drug is found in mother's breast milk; discontinue drug or bottle feed.
- *Children and adolescents*: not recommended in children younger than 12 years.

METHOCARBAMOL (Robaxin, Robaxin 750, Robaxin injection)

Classification
Central nervous system (CNS) depressant with sedative and musculoskeletal relaxant properties

Indications
- This drug is used to treat muscle spasms/pain.
- It is used along with rest, physical therapy, and other treatment.

Available Forms
Tablet, 500 and 750 mg; vial, 100 mg/mL (10 mL)

Dosage
Oral

- *Adults and children older than 16 years*: initially 1.5 gm QID × 2 to 3 days; maintenance, 750 mg q4h or 1.5 gm daily; maximum 8 gm/d
- *Children younger than 16 years*: not recommended

Injection

- *Adults and children older than 16 years*: 10 mL IM or IV; maximum 30 mL/d; maximum 3 days; maximum 5 mL/gluteal injection q8h; maximum IV rate 3 mL/min
- *Children younger than 16 years*: not recommended

Administration
Oral

- Dosage can usually be reduced to approximately 4 gm/d.

IM/IV

- The injectable form is hypertonic; watch to prevent vascular extravasation.
- If blood is aspirated into the syringe discard it, for it does not mix with the hypertonic solution.
- The total dosage should not exceed 30 mL (three vials) a day for more than 3 consecutive days except in the treatment of tetanus.
- Use caution in patients with seizure disorders.

Side Effects
- Anaphylactic reaction, angioneurotic edema, fever, and headache
- Bradycardia, flushing, hypotension, syncope, and thrombophlebitis
- Dyspepsia, jaundice (including cholestatic jaundice), nausea, and vomiting
- Leukopenia
- Hypersensitivity reactions
- Amnesia, confusion, diplopia, dizziness or light-headedness, drowsiness, insomnia, mild muscular incoordination, nystagmus, sedation, seizures (including grand mal), and vertigo
- Blurred vision, conjunctivitis, nasal congestion, metallic taste, pruritus, rash, and urticaria

Serious Side Effects

These side effects need to be reported immediately:

- Fever, chills, flu symptoms
- Slow heart rate
- Feeling like you might pass out
- Seizure (convulsions)
- Jaundice (yellowing of your skin or eyes)

Less Serious Side Effects

- Dizziness, spinning sensation, drowsiness
- Headache, confusion, memory problems, loss of balance, or coordination
- Nausea, vomiting, upset stomach
- Flushing (warmth, redness, or tingly feeling)
- Blurred vision, double vision, eye redness
- Sleep problems (insomnia)
- Stuffy nose
- Mild itching or rash

Drug Interactions

- Use this drug with caution in patients with myasthenia gravis receiving anticholinesterase agents.
- Using methocarbamol together with ethanol can increase nervous system side effects, such as dizziness, drowsiness, and difficulty concentrating.

Pharmacokinetics

- The plasma clearance of methocarbamol ranges between 0.20 and 0.80 L/hr/kg; the mean plasma elimination half-life ranges between 1 and 2 hours, and the plasma protein binding ranges between 46% and 50%.
- Methocarbamol is metabolized via dealkylation and hydroxylation.
- Conjugation of methocarbamol also is likely.
- Essentially all methocarbamol metabolites are eliminated in the urine.
- Small amounts of unchanged methocarbamol also are excreted in the urine.

Precautions

- Long-term studies to evaluate the carcinogenic potential of methocarbamol have not been performed.
- No studies have been conducted to assess the effect of methocarbamol on mutagenesis or its potential to impair fertility.

Patient and Family Education

- Some people may also experience impairment in thinking and judgment.
- Avoid or limit the use of alcohol while on methocarbamol.
- Avoid activities requiring mental alertness, such as driving or operating hazardous machinery, until you know how the medication affects you.
- Inform provider about all other medications, including vitamins and herbs.
- Patient needs to be reminded not to stop using this medication without first talking to provider.

Special Populations

- *Older adults*
  - Elimination half-life of methocarbamol is prolonged.
  - Fraction of bound methocarbamol is decreased in the older adults.
  - Renal clearance of methocarbamol is reduced in those with impaired renal function.
- *Pregnancy: category C*
  - It is also not known whether the drug can cause fetal harm when administered to a pregnant woman or affect reproduction capacity.
- *Nursing mothers:* It is not known whether the drug is excreted in human milk, and hence it should be used with caution.
- *Pediatric use:* not recommended for children younger than 16 years.

METHYLPHENIDATE—LONG ACTING (Concerta, Cotempla XR-ODT, Metadate CD, Metadate ER, Quillichew ER, Quillivant XR, Ritalin LA, Ritalin SR)

Classification

Methylphenidate (amphetamine derivative)

Indications

This drug is used primarily to treat narcolepsy and ADHD.

Available Forms

Capsule (XR), 10, 20, 30, and 40 mg; tablet (XR), 10 and 20 mg; SR tablet, 18, 27, 36, and 54 mg; tablet (ODT/XR), 8.6, 17.3, 25.9; chew tablets (XR), 20, 30, and 40 mg; bottle, 5 mg/mL, 25 mg/5 mL powder for reconstitution, 300 mg (60 mL), 600 mg (120 mL), 750 mg (150 mL), and 900 mg (180 mL).

Dosage

Concerta
- *Adults*: initially 18 mg QAM; may increase in 18-mg increments as needed; maximum 54 mg/d; do not crush or chew.
- *Children 13 to 17 years*: initially 18 mg daily; maximum 72 mg/d or 2 mg/kg, whichever is less.
- *Children 6 to 12 years*: initially 18 mg daily; maximum 54 mg/d.
- *Children younger than 6 years*: not recommended.

Cotempla XR-ODT
- *Adults and children older than 6 years*: initially 8.6 mg; may increase as needed and tolerated by 8.6 mg/d; daily dosage >51.8 mg is not recommended. Take consistently with or without food in the morning.
- *Children younger than 6 years*: not recommended.

Metadate CD or ER
- *Adults*: 1 capsule daily in the AM; may sprinkle on food; do not crush or chew.
- *Children older than 6 years*: initially 20 mg daily; may gradually increase by 20 mg/d at weekly intervals as needed; maximum 60 mg/d; may sprinkle on food; do not crush or chew.
- *Children younger than 6 years*: not recommended.

QuilliChew ER
- *Adults*: initially 1 × 10-mg chew tablets once daily in the AM.
- *Children older than 6 years*: initially 10 mg daily; may gradually increase by 20 mg/d at weekly intervals as needed; maximum 60 mg/d.
- *Children younger than 6 years*: not recommended.

Quillivant XR
- *Adults and children older than 6 years*: initially 20 mg once daily in the AM, with or without food; may be titrated in increments of 10 to 20 mg/d at weekly intervals; daily doses above 60 mg have not been studied and are not recommended; shake the bottle vigorously for at least 10 seconds to ensure that the correct dose is administered.
- *Children younger than 6 years*: not recommended.

Ritalin LA or SR

- *Adults*: 1 capsule daily in the AM.
- *Children older than 6 years*: Use in place of regular-acting methylphenidate when the 8-hour dose of Ritalin LA corresponds to the titrated 8-hour dose of regular-acting methylphenidate; maximum 60 mg/d.
- *Children younger than 6 years*: not recommended.

Side Effects

- Decreased appetite, dizziness.
- Palpitations, stroke, myocardial infarction, sudden death in patients with structural cardiac defects, HTN, arrhythmia, overstimulation, restlessness, seizures, infection, abnormal thinking, weight loss, somnolence, changes in libido, urticaria, dry mouth, irritability, insomnia, upper abdominal pain, nausea and/or vomiting, headaches, and anxiety.
- *Psychiatric events*: increase in manic states for bipolar patients, aggression, tics, tremors
- *Long-term growth suppression*: Patients should be monitored throughout treatment; if there appears to be growth suppression, the treatment should be discontinued.
- Rash, pyrexia, palpitations, tachycardia, elevated BP, sudden death, myocardial infarction, cardiomyopathy.
- SJS, TEN, impotence, and libido changes.
- Thrombocytopenia, purpura, and leucopenia.
- *Side effects that usually do not require medical attention*: anxiety, insomnia, diarrhea, constipation, dizziness, nausea, nervousness, rhinitis, and dry mouth.

Contraindications

Advanced arteriosclerosis, symptomatic CV disease, moderate to severe HTN, hyperthyroidism, glaucoma, history of drug abuse, agitated states, or within 14 days of MAOIs.

Drug Interactions

This drug may interact with urinary acidifying agents; the following medications are to be noted: CNS depressants (including alcohol); MAOIs; SSRIs; adrenergic blockers; antihistamines; antihypertensives; CNS stimulants; veratrum alkaloids; ethosuximide; TCAs; meperidine; phenobarbital; phenytoin; warfarin chlorpromazine; Haldol; lithium; norepinephrine; propoxyphene, caffeine.

Pharmacokinetics

- Stimulant; blocks reuptake of NE and dopamine; stimulates CNS similar to amphetamines.
- The drug is absorbed by the GI tract.
- The mode of therapeutic action in ADHD is not known. Amphetamines are thought to block the reuptake of norepinephrine and dopamine into the presynaptic neuron and increase the release of these monoamines into the extraneuronal space.
- Food prolongs time to maximum concentration by 2.5 hours.
- Peak plasma levels are reached in 6 to 8 hours.
- *Half-life*: average is 12 hours (mean half-life average shortened by 1 to 2 hours in children).
- *Metabolism*: liver, mainly excreted in the urine.
- *Half-life*: 3 to 4 hours.

Precautions

- See client as often as necessary to ensure drug is promoting positive cognitive and behavioral results.
- Advise the patient to report any new rashes immediately.

- Discontinue the drug immediately if any rash is reported.
- Advise patient of risk for transient psychotic-like symptoms (ideas of reference, paranoid delusions, and auditory hallucinations) and aggressive behaviors.
- Client may develop drug tolerance or dependence. Drug has high street value.
- Advanced arteriosclerosis, symptomatic CV disease, moderate to severe HTN.
- Hyperthyroidism.
- Known hypersensitivity or idiosyncratic reaction to sympathomimetic amines.
- Glaucoma.
- Agitated states.
- *Patients with a history of drug abuse*: Amphetamines have a high potential for abuse.
- Patients may experience transient palpitations and EKG changes.
- Avoid using in clients with left ventricular hypertrophy or mitral valve prolapse.
- During or within 14 days following the administration of MAOIs, hypertensive crisis may result.
- Use with caution in patients with preexisting psychosis.
- *Seizure history*: Some studies have shown the potential for lowering the seizure threshold.
- There is potential for growth inhibition in pediatric clients.
- Advise patient not to suddenly discontinue medication; taper off.

Patient and Family Education

- Quillivant XR must be reconstituted by a pharmacist, not by the patient or caregiver.
- Do not operate heavy machinery or equipment until reasonably certain that drug will not affect ability to engage in such activities.
- Discontinue medication immediately if rash is noted and follow up with provider.
- Store the drug at room temperature between 15°C and 30°C (59°F and 86°F). Throw away any unused medication after the expiration date.
- The patient may experience palpitations.
- Have patient monitor BP at home and notify provider of persistent BP elevations.
- Discontinue or hold medication in presence of chest pain and do not restart until reassessed by provider.
- The patient may experience transient blurred vision.
- Keep it out of reach of children.
- Seek medical care for any signs of heart problems (chest pain, shortness of breath), fainting, psychotic symptoms, overdose, or any other concerns.
- Routinely assess weight and BP.
- Treatment should be initiated at low doses and then titrated over 2 to 4 weeks until an adequate response is achieved or unacceptable adverse effects occur.
- If one stimulant is not effective, another should be attempted before second-line medications are considered. Although some children benefit from daily stimulant therapy, weekend and summer "drug holidays" are suggested for children whose ADHD symptoms predominantly affect schoolwork or to limit adverse effects (e.g., appetite suppression, abdominal pain, headache, insomnia, irritability, tics).

Special Populations

- *Older adults*: Older adults more sensitive to stimulants. Use lowest effective dose. Caution with polypharmacy and comorbid conditions.
- *Hepatic impairment*: Modify dose by one half accordingly.
- *Pregnancy*: category C; based on animal data, they may cause fetal harm.
- *Lactation*: excreted in breast milk; no human studies have been performed. It is not recommended in breastfeeding mothers (possibly unsafe).
- *Children*: For use in children 6 years of age or older.

METHYLPHENIDATE—REGULAR ACTING (Methylin, Ritalin)

Classification
Methylphenidate (amphetamine derivative)

Indications
This drug is used primarily to treat narcolepsy and ADHD.

Available Forms
Tablets, 5, 10, and 20 mg; chew tablets, 2.5, 5, and 10 mg; oral solution, 5 mg/5 mL, 10 mg/10 mL

Dosage
Methylin
- *Adults*: usual dose 20 to 30 mg/d in 2 to 3 divided doses 30 to 45 minutes before a meal; maximum 60 mg/d
- *Children older than 6 years*: initially 5 mg BID ac (breakfast and lunch); may increase 5 to 10 mg/d at weekly intervals; maximum 60 mg/d
- *Children younger than 6 years*: not recommended

Methylin
- *Adults*: 10 to 60 mg/d in 2 to 3 divided doses 30 to 45 minutes ac; maximum 60 mg/d
- *Children older than 6 years*: initially 5 mg BID ac (breakfast and lunch); may increase by 5 to 10 mg at weekly intervals as needed; maximum 60 mg/d
- *Children younger than 6 years*: not recommended

Administration
- Give drug *after* meals to reduce appetite-suppressant effects. Give last dose at least 6 hours before bedtime.

Side Effects
- Decreased appetite, dizziness.
- Palpitations, stroke, myocardial infarction, sudden death in patients with structural cardiac defects, HTN, arrhythmia, overstimulation, restlessness, seizures, infection, abnormal thinking, weight loss, somnolence, changes in libido, urticaria, dry mouth, irritability, insomnia, upper abdominal pain, nausea and/or vomiting, headaches, and anxiety.
- *Psychiatric events*: increase in manic states for bipolar patients, aggression, tics, tremors.
- *Long-term growth suppression*: Patients should be monitored throughout treatment; if there appears to be growth suppression, the treatment should be discontinued.
- Rash, pyrexia, palpitations, tachycardia, elevated BP, sudden death, myocardial infarction, cardiomyopathy.
- SJS, TEN, impotence, and libido changes.
- Thrombocytopenia, purpura, and leucopenia.
- *Side effects that usually do not require medical attention*: anxiety, insomnia, diarrhea, constipation, dizziness, nausea, nervousness, rhinitis, and dry mouth.

Contraindications

Advanced arteriosclerosis, symptomatic CV disease, moderate to severe HTN, hyperthyroidism, glaucoma, history of drug abuse, agitated states, or within 14 days of MAOIs

Drug Interactions

This drug may interact with urinary acidifying agents; the following medications are to be noted: CNS depressants (including alcohol); MAOIs; SSRIs; adrenergic blockers; antihistamines; antihypertensives; CNS stimulants; veratrum alkaloids; ethosuximide; TCAs; meperidine; phenobarbital; phenytoin; warfarin chlorpromazine; Haldol; lithium; norepinephrine; propoxyphene, caffeine.

Pharmacokinetics

- Stimulant; blocks reuptake of norepinephrine (NE) and dopamine; stimulates CNS similar to amphetamines.
- The drug is absorbed by the GI tract.
- The mode of therapeutic action in ADHD is not known. Amphetamines are thought to block the reuptake of norepinephrine and dopamine into the presynaptic neuron and increase the release of these monoamines into the extraneuronal space.
- Food prolongs time to maximum concentration by 2.5 hours.
- Peak plasma levels are reached in 6 to 8 hours.
- *Half-life:* average is 12 hours (mean half-life average shortened by 1 to 2 hours in children).
- *Metabolism:* liver, mainly excreted in the urine.
- *Half-life:* 3 to 4 hours.

Precautions

- See client as often as necessary to ensure drug is promoting positive cognitive and behavioral results.
- Advise the patient to report any new rashes immediately.
- Discontinue the drug immediately if any rash is reported.
- Advise patient of risk for transient psychotic-like symptoms (ideas of reference, paranoid delusions, and auditory hallucinations) and aggressive behaviors.
- Client may develop drug tolerance or dependence. Drug has high street value.
- Advanced arteriosclerosis, symptomatic CV disease, moderate to severe HTN.
- Hyperthyroidism.
- Known hypersensitivity or idiosyncratic reaction to sympathomimetic amines.
- Glaucoma.
- Agitated states.
- Patients with a history of drug abuse; amphetamines have a high potential for abuse.
- Patients may experience transient palpitations and EKG changes.
- Avoid using in clients with left ventricular hypertrophy or mitral valve prolapse.
- During or within 14 days following the administration of MAOIs, hypertensive crisis may result.
- Use with caution in patients with preexisting psychosis.
- *Seizure history:* Some studies have shown the potential for lowering the seizure threshold.
- There is potential for growth inhibition in pediatric clients.
- Advise patient not to suddenly discontinue medication; taper off.

Patient and Family Education

- Do not operate heavy machinery or equipment until reasonably certain that drug will not affect ability to engage in such activities.
- Discontinue medication immediately if rash is noted and follow up with provider.
- Store the drug at room temperature between 15°C and 30°C (59°F and 86°F). Throw away any unused medication after the expiration date.
- The patient may experience palpitations.
- Have patient monitor BP at home and notify provider of persistent BP elevations.
- Discontinue or hold medication in presence of chest pain and do not restart until reassessed by provider.
- The patient may experience transient blurred vision.
- Keep it out of reach of children.
- Seek medical care for any signs of heart problems (chest pain, shortness of breath), fainting, psychotic symptoms, overdose, or any other concerns.
- Routinely assess weight and BP.
- Treatment should be initiated at low doses and then titrated over 2 to 4 weeks until an adequate response is achieved or unacceptable adverse effects occur.
- If one stimulant is not effective, another should be attempted before second-line medications are considered. Although some children benefit from daily stimulant therapy, weekend and summer "drug holidays" are suggested for children whose ADHD symptoms predominantly affect schoolwork or to limit adverse effects (e.g., appetite suppression, abdominal pain, headache, insomnia, irritability, tics).

Special Populations

- *Older adults*: Older adults more sensitive to stimulants. Use lowest effective dose. Caution with polypharmacy and comorbid conditions.
- *Hepatic impairment*: Modify dose by one half accordingly.
- *Pregnancy*: category C; based on animal data, they may cause fetal harm.
- *Lactation*: excreted in breast milk; no human studies have been performed. It is not recommended in breastfeeding mothers (possibly unsafe).
- *Children*: for use in children 6 years of age or older.

METHYLPHENIDATE TRANSDERMAL (Daytrana patch)

Classification
Methylphenidate (amphetamine derivative), Central nervous system (CNS) stimulant, piperidine derivative

Indications
The drug is indicated for the treatment of ADHD in children and adults.

Available Forms
Transdermal patch, 10, 15, 20, and 30 mg

Dosage
- *Adults*: not applicable
- *Children 6 to 17 years*: initially 10-mg patch applied to hip 2 hours before desired effect daily in the AM; may increase by 5 to 10 mg at weekly intervals; maximum 60 mg/d
- *Children younger than 6 years*: not recommended

Administration
Apply same titration when converting from oral; apply to hip 2 hours before desired effect; drug effects may persist 5 hours after patch removal; rotate sites; do not alter/cut patch. Hold patch in place for 30 seconds using palm of hand, after which area is waterproof. If patch comes off, another one may be applied but not to exceed total time of 9 hr/d.

Side Effects
- Decreased appetite, dizziness, dry mouth, irritability, insomnia, upper abdominal pain, nausea and/or vomiting, weight loss, headaches, and anxiety.
- *Psychiatric events*: increase in manic states for bipolar patients, aggression, tics, and tremors.
- *Long-term growth suppression*: Patients should be monitored throughout treatment; if there appears to be growth suppression, the treatment should be discontinued.
- Rash and pyrexia.
- Palpitations, tachycardia, elevated BP, sudden death, myocardial infarction, and cardiomyopathy.
- SJS and TEN, impotence, libido changes, and skin irritation.

Drug Interactions
The drug may interact with urinary acidifying agents, MAOIs, adrenergic blockers, antihistamines, antihypertensives, veratrum alkaloids, ethosuximide, TCAs, meperidine, phenobarbital, phenytoin, chlorpromazine, Haldol, lithium, norepinephrine, and caffeine propoxyphene.

Pharmacokinetics
- The drug is absorbed by the GI tract.
- Non-catecholamine sympathomimetic amines with CNS-stimulant activity.

- The mode of therapeutic action in ADHD is not known. It is thought to block the reuptake of norepinephrine and dopamine into the presynaptic neuron and increase the release of these monoamines into the extraneural space.
- *Metabolism:* liver, mainly excreted in the urine.
- *Peak plasma:* 7.5 to 10.5 hours.
- *Onset:* 2 hours.
- *Half-life:* 3.5 hours.

Precautions

- Advanced arteriosclerosis, symptomatic CV disease, moderate to severe HTN, arrhythmias, thrombocytopenia, leukopenia, respiratory cough.
- Hyperthyroidism.
- Known hypersensitivity or idiosyncratic reaction to sympathomimetic amines.
- Glaucoma.
- Agitated states.
- Patients with a history of drug abuse have a high potential for abuse with this drug. Particular attention should be paid to the possibility of patients obtaining this class of medication for nontherapeutic use or distribution to others, and the drugs should be prescribed or dispensed sparingly.
- During or within 14 days following the administration of MAOIs, hypertensive crisis may result.
- Use with caution in patients with preexisting psychosis.
- *Seizure history:* Some studies have shown the potential for lowering the seizure threshold.

Patient and Family Education

- Store the drug at room temperature, protected from light.
- Keep it out of reach of children.
- Seek medical care for any signs of heart problems (chest pain, shortness of breath), fainting, psychotic symptoms, overdose, or any other concerns.
- Routinely assess weight and BP.
- Treatment should be initiated at low doses and then titrated over 2 to 4 weeks until an adequate response is achieved or unacceptable adverse effects occur.
- Dispose of properly, away from children or animals (remnant medication may persist on patch).
- If one stimulant is not effective, another stimulant should be attempted before second-line medications are considered. Although some children benefit from daily stimulant therapy, weekend and summer "drug holidays" are suggested for children whose ADHD symptoms predominantly affect schoolwork or to limit adverse effects (e.g., appetite suppression, abdominal pain, headache, insomnia, irritability, tics).

Special Populations

- *Adult and older adults:* not applicable.
- *Pregnancy:* category C; based on animal data, they may cause fetal harm.
- *Lactation:* possibly unsafe.
- *Children:* not recommended in children younger than 6 years.

MIDAZOLAM HYDROCHLORIDE (Versed)

Classification
Benzodiazepine (BZD), anxiolytic

Indications
This drug is used for relaxation during hypnotic sessions and preoperative procedures, to reduce anxiety and induce amnesia and somnolence.

Available Forms
Syrup (liquid), 2 mg/mL; injectable form, 1 and 5 mg/mL; preservative-free solution

Dosage
IM, IV, PO; schedule IV drug; requires a prescription with a maximum of five refills/6 months.

Procedural IV Dosing
- *Adults under 60 years:* 1 mg IV every 2 to 3 minutes with a maximum of 2.5 mg/dose; cumulative doses over 5 mg are rarely needed.
- *Over 60 years:* Maximum dose is 1.5 mg total. Cumulative doses over 3.5 mg are rarely needed.
- *Children 6 months to 5 years:* 0.05 to 0.1 mg/kg × 1; repeat every 2 to 3 minutes as needed. Maximum 0.6 mg/kg total. Cumulative dose rarely over 6 mg.
- *Children 6 to 12 years:* 0.025 to 0.05 mg/kg × 1; repeat every 2 to 3 minutes before procedure; maximum dose 0.4 mg; cumulative dose rarely above 10 mg.
- *Children over 12 years:* 0.5 to 2 mg IV × 1; repeat every 2 to 3 minutes when needed. Cumulative dose above 10 mg is rarely needed. May be mixed in same syringe with morphine sulfate, meperidine, atropine, or scopolamine. When mixing infusion, use 5-mg/mL vial and dilute to 0.5 mg/mL with D5W or normal saline.

Oral
- *Children above 6 years:* 0.25 to 0.5 mg/kg PO × 1 with a maximum of 20 mg. Give 20 to 30 minutes before procedure. Children below 6 years may need up to 1 mg/kg/dose.

IM
Note: deep IM into large muscle

- *Children above 6 years:* 0.1 to 0.15 mg/kg IM × 1 with maximum of 0.5 mg/kg total; cumulative dosing over 10 mg is rarely needed. Give 15 to 30 minutes before procedure.
- Given by slow IV administration (more than 2 minutes) with careful attention to proper venous placement to avoid extravasation.

Side Effects
Nausea, vomiting, reduced heart rate, cough, and pain at injection site. Serious side effects include difficulty breathing, irregular heart rate, allergic reactions, respiratory depression and/or cardiac arrest, airway obstruction, oxygen desaturation, apnea, and sometimes death.

Drug Interactions

- Substrate of CYP3A4 (major). Avoid concomitant use with efavirenz, protease inhibitors, fluconazole, INH, macrolide antibiotics, propofol, and certain statins. Avoid grapefruit juice with oral syrup.
- The sedative effect of IV midazolam is accentuated by any other drugs that may depress the CNS, particularly narcotics such as morphine.
- Caution is also advised when midazolam is administered concomitantly with drugs that are known to inhibit the P450 34A enzyme system, such as cimetidine (Tagamet), erythromycin, diltiazem (Cardizem), verapamil (Calan/Isoptin/Verelan), ketoconazole, and itraconazole (Sporanox).
- Both cimetidine and ranitidine increased the mean steady-state concentration of blood level for midazolam.
- Erythromycin doubled the half-life of midazolam.
- No significant adverse interactions have been noted with commonly used premedications or drugs used during anesthesia, including atropine, scopolamine, diazepam, hydroxyzine, succinylcholine, or topical local anesthetics. Grapefruit juice may increase bioavailability of oral drug; St. John's wort may decrease drug level.

Pharmacokinetics

- *Absorption:* Oral—rapid
- *Peak:* PO—45 to 60 minutes; IM—15 to 60 minutes; IV—rapid
- *Onset:* IM—15 minutes; IV—1 to 5 minutes; PO—30 to 60 minutes
- *Duration:* mean—2 hours; up to 6 hours
- *Metabolism:* hepatic via CYP3A4; 95% protein binding
- Metabolized by the liver (CYP450: 3A4 substrate) and excreted in the urine (90%) and feces (2%)
- Drug binds to BZD receptors and enhances GABA effects
- *Half-life:* 2 to 6 hours; prolonged in cirrhosis, congestive heart failure, obesity, elderly.

Precautions

- There is a possibility for loss of consciousness.
- It may cause severe respiratory depression or apnea; appropriate resuscitative equipment must be available.
- Titrate dose cautiously.
- Decrease dose by 30% if narcotics or other CNS depressants are given. Caution must be exercised in patients with compromised respiratory function or renal or hepatic impairment.
- Use the drug only in hospital/ambulatory care settings with continuous respiratory and cardiac monitoring, appropriate ventilation/intubation equipment, and personnel trained/skilled in airway management.
- One dedicated person other than practitioner performing the procedure should continuously monitor deeply sedated pediatric patients.
- Reactions such as agitation, involuntary movements, hyperactivity, and combativeness have been reported in adult and pediatric patients.
- Should such reactions occur, caution should be exercised before continuing administration.

Patient and Family Education

- Avoid use of alcohol or prescription or OTC sedatives, driving, or tasks that require alertness for a minimum of 24 hours after administration.

- There may be some loss of memory following administration.
- Tell practitioner if the patient is pregnant or a nursing mother.
- Midazolam is associated with a high incidence of partial or complete impairment of recall for the next several hours.
- Do not mix alcohol or any other depressant drug and midazolam without the healthcare provider's knowledge.
- Do not operate hazardous machinery or a motor vehicle until the effects of the drug have subsided or until 1 full day after anesthesia.

Special Populations

- *Older adults*: Glaucoma, angle closure, chronic obstructive pulmonary disease, and congestive heart failure are contraindications to the decreased sedative effects for older or debilitated patients. Due to its sedative property and increased risk of falls, all BZDs are included on the Beers List of Potentially Inappropriate Medications for Geriatrics.
- *Pregnancy:* pregnancy category D; has shown positive evidence of human fetal risk.
- *Lactation:* no breastfeeding for 24 hours after administration. Safety unknown as there is inadequate literature to assess risk.
- *Renal impairment:* The drug should be used with caution and renal function should be checked prior to beginning treatment with dose adjustment as necessary.
- *Hepatic impairment:* The drug should be used with caution and liver function should be checked prior to beginning treatment with dose adjustment as necessary.
- *Children:* Use caution in neonates, as rapid IV injection can cause severe hypotension and seizures.

MIRTAZAPINE (Remeron, Remeron SolTab)

Classification
Noradrenergic and specific serotonergic antidepressant (NaSSA), antidepressant, tetra-cyclic antidepressant

Indications
Mirtazapine is used to treat depression.

Available Forms
Tablet, 15, 30, and 45 mg; ODT, 15, 30, and 45 mg

Dosage
- *Adults and children older than 12 years:* initially 15 mg qhs; increase at intervals of 1 to 2 weeks; usual range 15 to 45 mg/d; maximum 45 mg/d
- *Children younger than 12 years:* not recommended

Administration
PO, with or without food, at bedtime

Side Effects
- *Serious:* agranulocytosis
- Anticholinergic effects; blood dyscrasias: neutropenia and agranulocytosis; ortho-static hypotension or HTN; somnolence and sedation, dizziness, tremor, confusion; increased risk for hyperlipidemia; dry mouth; significant appetite increase and weight gain (>7% body mass); asthenia; decreased appetite, hypercholesteremia, constipation, hyperglyceridemia; influenza-like symptoms; abnormal dreams, abnormal thinking; tremor; confusion; peripheral edema; myalgia; back pain; and urinary frequency.

Drug Interactions
- Serotonin agents (i.e., Linezolid)
- *Sedatives:* Effects may be exacerbated by use of other sedatives. Diazepam: Avoid use altogether.
- *Monoamine oxidase inhibitors:* risk for drug toxicity.
- Central nervous system stimulants (e.g., amphetamines)
- Given PO; regular tablet is given with water.
- To take the disintegrating tablets (RemeronolTab), keep the tablet in its blister pack until ready to use. Open the package and peel the foil from the tablet blister. Do not push a tablet through the foil or it may break the tablet. Using dry hands, remove the tablet, place in mouth, and let it dissolve. Do not swallow the tablet whole. Do not chew it. Swallow several times and flush it away with water.

Pharmacokinetics
- The drug is metabolized extensively in the liver (CYP450 1A2, 2C9, 2D6, and 3A4) and excreted in the urine (85%) and feces (15%). Prolonged half-life is 20 to 40 hours, which is increased further in patients with hepatic or renal impairment.
- *Peak plasma:* 2 hours.
- *Bioavailability:* 50%.

Precautions

- Caution should be exercised if the patient has the following conditions: bipolar disorder, hypotension, cerebrovascular diagnosis, hypovolemia, seizure threshold disorder, dehydration.
- *Anticholinergic drugs* (e.g., antihistamines): Increase effects.
- Use with caution in patients with hepatic impairment or renal impairment.
- *Patients at risk for seizure disorders:* This drug may lower seizure threshold.
- Monitor with CBC and history for signs of agranulocytosis or severe neutropenia.
- Low incidence of sexual dysfunction.
- Usually dosed at bedtime due to associated drowsiness (may be helpful in patients with insomnia or anxiety).
- It may alter liver function.
- Adverse effects and side effects are commonly observed before therapeutic effects.

Patient and Family Education

- Antidepressant medications are used to treat a variety of conditions, including depression and other mental/mood disorders. These medications can help prevent suicidal thoughts/attempts and provide other important benefits. However, a small number of people (especially people younger than 25) who take antidepressants for any condition may experience worsening depression, other mental/mood symptoms, or suicidal thoughts/attempts. Therefore, it is very important to talk with the clinician about the risks and benefits of antidepressant medication (especially for people younger than 25), even if treatment is not for a mental/mood condition. Tell the clinician right away if you notice worsening depression/other psychiatric conditions, unusual behavior changes (including possible suicidal thoughts/attempts), or other mental/mood changes (including new/worsening anxiety, panic attacks, trouble sleeping, irritability, hostile/angry feelings, impulsive actions, severe restlessness, very rapid speech). Be especially watchful for these symptoms when a new antidepressant is started or when the dose is changed.
- Take 60 to 90 minutes prior to bedtime, due to associated drowsiness. Do not drive until the effect of this medication is known.
- It may cause stomach upset or BP changes (particularly with getting up suddenly).
- This medication may increase appetite or craving for carbohydrates. Monitoring diet and exercise is important.
- It may take up to 4 to 8 weeks to show its maximum effect at this dose, but some may see symptoms of depression improving in as few as 2 weeks.
- If the patient is planning on becoming pregnant or is pregnant, discuss the benefits versus the risks of using this medicine while pregnant.
- As this medicine is excreted in the breast milk, nursing mothers should not breastfeed while taking this medicine without prior consultation with a psychiatric nurse practitioner or psychiatrist. Newborns may develop symptoms, including feeding or breathing difficulties, seizures, muscle stiffness, jitteriness, or constant crying.
- Do not stop taking this medication unless the healthcare provider directs. Report side effects or worsening symptoms to the healthcare provider promptly.
- Dosage should be adjusted to reach remission of symptoms and treatment should continue for at least 4 to 9 months following remission of symptoms.
- Avoid discontinuing the drug without tapering the dosage.
- Talk to the healthcare provider about any other medications in use. Mirtazapine is not Food and Drug Administration approved for use in the elderly because they

may be more sensitive to the effects of the drug. Older adults should receive a lower starting dose.

- Keep these medications out of the reach of children and pets.

Special Populations

- *Older adults*: Older individuals tend to be more sensitive to medication side effects, such as hypotension and anticholinergic effects. They often require adjustment of medication doses for hepatic or renal dysfunction. Recommended to begin at lower dosage.
- *Pregnancy*: contraindicated in pregnancy.
- *Children:* not recommended in children under 12 years of age. Monitor for suicide ideation.
- There is an increased risk of suicidality in children, adolescents, and young adults, especially during the first months of treatment. Mirtazapine is not approved by the FDA for use in children. Use only after consultation with psychiatric specialist.
- *Renal impairment:* Dosage has not been defined.
- *Hepatic impairment:* Dosage has not been defined.

MODAFINIL (Provigil)

Classification
Stimulant, nonamphetamine

Indications
Used primarily to treat sleep disorders that result in excessive sleepiness such as narcolepsy, obstructive sleep apnea despite use of continuous positive airway pressure (CPAP), hypopnea syndrome, and shift work sleep disorder.

Available Forms
Tablet, 100 and 200 mg

Dosage
- *Adults and children older than 16 years*: 100 to 200 mg QAM; maximum 400 mg/d
- *Children younger than 16 years*: not recommended

Administration
- PO with a glass of water.
- Take with or without food in the morning.

Side Effects
- HTN; arrhythmia; cataplexy; dysmenorrhea; dyspnea; infection; abnormal thinking; weight loss
- *Important*: Watch for SJS rash—not approved for pediatrics for any reason because of this. Discontinue at first sign of rash.
- *Side effects that usually do not require medical attention*: anxiety; back pain; diarrhea; dizziness; dyspepsia; headache; insomnia; nausea; nervousness; or rhinitis.

Drug Interactions
Modafinil may interact with the following medications: CNS depressants (including alcohol); MAOIs; macrolides; phenytoin; estrogen; antifungals that use cytochrome P450 3A4 (CYP 3A4). Modafinil is an inducer of 3A4 itself, so interactions are harder to predict.

Pharmacokinetics
- Stimulant; exact mechanism of action unknown. Believed to have similar wake-promoting actions as sympathomimetic agents.
- Rapid absorption in absence of food.
- Peak plasma levels are reached in 2 to 4 hours.
- Steady state is reached within 2 to 4 days of dosing.
- *Half-life*: Average is 15 hours once steady state is reached.

Precautions
- See client as often as necessary to ensure drug is promoting wakefulness, determine compliance, and review side effects.
- Advise patient to report any new rashes immediately.
- Discontinue drug immediately if any rash is reported.

- Advise patient of risk for transient psychosis-like symptoms (ideas of reference, paranoid delusions, and auditory hallucinations).
- May experience transient palpitations and EKG changes.
- Avoid using in clients with left ventricular hypertrophy or mitral valve prolapse.

Patient and Family Education

- Avoid alcohol.
- Do not operate heavy machinery or equipment until reasonably certain that drug will not affect ability to engage in such activities.
- Discontinue medication immediately if rash is noted and follow up with provider.
- May experience palpitations.
- Have patient monitor BP at home and notify provider of persistent BP elevations.
- Store at room temperature between 20°C and 25°C (68°F and 77°F).

Special Populations

- *Older adults*: more sensitive to stimulants. Use lowest effective dose.
- *Hepatic impairment*: Modify dose by one-half accordingly.
- *Pregnancy*: Category C.
- *Lactation*: No human studies have been performed. Not recommended in breast-feeding mothers.
- *Children*: not recommended for children younger than 16 years.

NALOXONE HYDROCHLORIDE (Evzio, Narcan, Narcan nasal spray)

Classification
Opioid antagonist and antidote

Indications
Naloxone hydrochloride is used to counter the effects of opiate overdose, for example, heroin or morphine overdose. Naloxone is specifically used to counteract life-threatening depression of the CNS and respiratory system.

Available Forms
Injection, 0.4 mg/0.4 mL, 2 mg/mL (IM/SC only); nasal spray, 4 mg/0.1 mL, single-dose (2 blister packs, each with a single nasal spray/carton); prefilled syringe, 0.4 mg/mL (1 mL), 1 mg/mL (2 mL) (IV, IM, or SC); vial/Amp, 0.4 mg/mL and 1 mg/mL

Dosage
- *Adults*: 0.4 to 2 mg; repeat in 2 to 3 minutes if no response
- *Children*: 0.01 mg/kg initially; repeat in 2 to 3 minutes at 0.1 mg/kg if response inadequate
- *Evzio*: Evzio 2 mg/0.4 mL comes with 2 autoinjectors and one trainer. This strength is indicated for the emergency treatment of known or suspected opioid overdose manifested by CNS depression. If the electronic voice instruction system does not operate properly, Evzio will still deliver the intended dose of naloxone when used according to the printed instructions on the flat surface of the autoinjector label. Evzio cannot be administered IV. Due to the short duration of action of naloxone, as compared to opioids that are longer acting, monitoring of the patient is critical as the opioid reversal effects of naloxone may wear off before the effects of the opioid.

Administration
- *Narcan nasal spray:* position supine with head tilted back; 1 spray in one nostril; if an additional dose is needed, spray into the opposite nostril.

Side Effects
Common reactions include tachycardia, HTN, hypotension, nausea, vomiting, tremor, withdrawal symptoms, diaphoresis, pulmonary edema, and irritability. Common side effects in children are seizures, ventricular fibrillation, ventricular tachycardia, and pulmonary edema (pediatric).

Drug Interactions
This medicine may also interact with the following:
- Topiramate (may increase risk of CNS depression and psychomotor impairment).
- Tramadol and tramadol/acetaminophen (may not reverse all symptoms of overdose, increase risk of seizures).
- This drug blocks effects of all opioids, including opioid-containing cough suppressants and opioid analgesics.

Pharmacokinetics

- The drug is metabolized in the liver and is excreted in the urine.
- The drug antagonizes the various opioid receptors.
- *Half-life:* 64 minutes (adults), 3 hours (neonates).
- *Peak:* parenteral—5 to 15 minutes.

Precautions

Caution is advised in patients with CV disease, opioid addiction, hepatic impairment, or renal impairment and in patients on cardiotoxic drugs.

Patient and Family Education

Stop using naloxone and call the doctor if chest pain, light-headedness, seizure, or difficulty in breathing develops.

Special Populations

- *Renal impairment:* No adjustment is needed.
- *Hepatic impairment:* Caution is advised in children with hepatic impairment; dosing not defined.
- *Pregnancy:* category B drug.
- *Lactation:* Safety in lactation is unknown. Caution is advised.
- *Children:* Dose adjustment may be required in children with renal impairment. Caution is advised in children with hepatic impairment.

NALTREXONE (ReVia, Vivitrol)

Classification
Opioid antagonist, opioid-cessation agent

Indications
Naltrexone is used primarily in the management of narcotic drug and alcohol dependence and opioid addictions.

Available Forms
Tablet, 50 mg; vial, 380 mg

Dosage
- *Adults and children older than 12 years*
  - ReVia: 50 mg daily
  - Vivitrol: 380 mg IM once monthly; alternate buttocks
- *Children younger than 12 years:* not recommended

Administration
- Take with a full glass of water.
- This drug may be taken with or without food unless stomach upset occurs.
- Do not stop taking drug without provider's advice.
- Do not take opioids while on this medicine.
- *Missed dose:* Take the medication as soon as remembered. If it is almost time for the next dose, skip the missed dose and wait until next regularly scheduled dose. Do not take extra medicine to make up the missed dose.

Side Effects
Depression, nervousness, irritability, sedation/somnolence, suicidal attempt/ideation, skin rash, pharyngitis, hepatocellular injury, aches, pains, change in sex drive or performance, feeling anxious, dizzy, restlessness, fearful, headache, loss of appetite, nausea, runny nose, sinus problems, sneezing, stomach cramps, and trouble sleeping.

Drug Interactions
This medicine may also interact with the following medications:
- CNS depressants.
- Tramadol (Rybix/Ryzolt/Ultram) and tramadol/acetaminophen may not reverse all symptoms of overdose, increase risk of seizures, or block effects of all opioids, including opioid-containing cough suppressants.
- Carry an identity card or medical identity bracelet stating that you are taking medication.
- Thioridazine may cause lethargy and somnolence with concurrent use.
- Patients may not experience significant benefit from concurrent use of opioid-containing medicines, such as cold-and-cough preparations, antidiarrheal preparations, and opioid analgesics.

Pharmacokinetics
- Opioid antagonists, such as naltrexone, are metabolized in the liver.

- They are completely absorbed from the GI tract.
- Elimination is primarily by glomerular filtration.
- Naltrexone and its metabolites may undergo enterohepatic recirculation.
- Elimination from the system takes 5 to 10 days. Initial peak is within 2 hours, followed by a second peak 2 to 3 days later.
- Measurable levels can occur for more than 1 month after initial dosing.
- Exposure is three- to fourfold higher with IM administration compared to oral administration.
- Pure opioid receptor antagonist.
- Subject to significant first-pass metabolism.
- *Half-life:* 4 hours; IM: 2 to 3 days.

Precautions

- Do not drive, operate machinery, or do anything that requires mental alertness until it is known how this drug exerts its effects.
- Caution individuals not to stand or sit up quickly, as dizziness is a side effect of this medicine.
- Check liver enzyme levels.
- Do not initiate treatment until confirmed abstinence from opioids for 7 to 10 days.
- Urine drug screen is often not sufficient proof that patient is opioid free; therefore, healthcare provider may choose to give naloxone challenge before beginning treatment and periodically thereafter.
- Tell individual not to take any medicine that contains opioids during treatment, as this could cause serious injury, coma, or death.
- Avoid pregnancy and nursing while taking this medicine.
- Attempts by patient to overcome blocking effects by using large amounts of opiates may result in life-endangering opioid intoxication.

Patient and Family Education

- *Missed dose:* Take the medication as soon as remembered. If it is almost time for the next dose, skip the missed dose and wait until next regularly scheduled dose. Do not take extra medicine to make up the missed dose.
- Use caution when driving or operating machinery.
- If stomach upset occurs, take with food.
- Wear medical identification indicating naltrexone use.
- This drug may increase sensitivity to lower doses of opioids; large doses of heroin or any other opiate may cause coma and death.
- Do not take this medicine within 7 to 10 days of taking an opioid drug.
- Exercise caution when driving or performing other tasks requiring mental alertness and coordination.
- Stop taking the medicine if any of the following develops: allergic reaction, stomach pain lasting more than a few days, white bowel movements, dark urine, or yellowing of eyes.
- Combine with psychotherapy or other counseling methods for full treatment effect.
- Notify healthcare provider if there is shortness of breath, coughing, or wheezing, as naltrexone (Vivitrol) injections may cause allergic pneumonia.
- Nausea may result after a naltrexone (Vivitrol) injection.

Special Populations

- *Older adults:* Trials of subjects over 65 years of age did not include sufficient numbers to determine the safety and efficacy in the geriatric population.

- *Hepatic impairment*: Use the drug with caution due to hepatotoxic effects. Caution is advised in children with hepatic impairment. It is contraindicated in acute hepatitis and hepatic failure.
- *Renal impairment*: Caution is advised.
- *Pregnancy*: category C; the safety and efficacy of this medicine has not been established.
- *Lactation*: Nursing mothers should not take this medicine, as it has a potential for serious adverse effects in infants. The safety and efficacy of this medicine has not been established.
- *Children*: not recommended for children younger than 12 years.

NICOTINE—TRANSDERMAL PATCH (Habitrol, Nicoderm CQ, Nicotrol step-down patch, Nicotrol transdermal, ProStep)

NICOTINE—GUM (Nicorette)

NICOTINE—LOZENGE (COMMIT, Nicorette Mini Lozenge)

NICOTINE—INHALATION PRODUCTS (Nicotrol Inhaler, Nicotrol NS)

Classification

Nicotinic receptor agonist

Indications

Used to treat tobacco nicotine dependence.

Available Forms

■ *Transdermal patch:* 7, 10, 14, and 21 mg/24 hr; 5, 10, and 15 mg/16 hr (7/pck); 11 and 22 mg/24 hr (7/pck)
■ Gum, 2 and 4 mg; lozenges, 2 and 4 mg; spray, 0.5 mg; inhaler, 4 mg; transdermal patch, 7, 14, and 21 mg/d; 5, 10, and 15 mg/d; and 11 and 22 mg/d.
■ *Gum:* 2, 4 mg (108-piece starter kit and 48-piece refill)
■ *Lozenge:* 2, 4 mg (72/pck)
■ *Inhalation products:* inhaler, 10 mg/cartridge, 4 mg delivered (42 cartridge/pck); nasal spray: 0.5 mg/spray; 10 mg/mL (10 mL, 200 doses)

Dosage

Transdermal Patch

■ *Habitrol:* adults and children older than 12 years—initially one 21 mg/24 hr patch/d × 4 to 6 weeks; then one 14 mg/24 hr patch/d × 2 to 4 weeks; then one 7 mg/24 hr patch/d × 2 to 4 weeks; then discontinue. Not recommended for children younger than 12 years.
■ *Nicoderm CQ:* adults and children older than 12 years—initially one 21 mg/24 hr patch/d × 6 weeks, then one 14 mg/24 hr patch/d × 2 weeks; then one 7 mg/24 hr patch/d × 2 weeks. Not recommended for children younger than 12 years.
■ *Nicotrol step-down patch:* adults and children older than 12 years—1 patch/d × 6 weeks. Not recommended in children younger than 12 years.
■ *Nicotrol transdermal:* adults and children older than 12 years—1 patch/d × 6 weeks. Not recommended in children younger than 12 years.
■ *ProStep:* adults and children older than 12 years—initially one 22 mg/24 hr patch/d × 4 to 8 weeks; then discontinue or one 11 mg/24 hr patch/d × 2 to 4 additional weeks. Not recommended for children younger than 12 years.

Gum

■ *Nicorette:* adults and children older than 12 years—chew one piece of gum slowly and intermittently over 30 minutes q1h to q2h × 6 weeks; then q2h to q4h × 3 weeks; then q4h to q8h × 3 weeks; maximum 24 pieces/d; 2 mg if smoked <25 cigarettes/d; 4 mg if smoked >24 cigarettes/d. Not recommended for children younger than 12 years.

Lozenge

■ *Commit Lozenge* and *Nicorette Mini Lozenge:* adults—dissolve over 20 to 30 minutes; minimize swallowing; do not eat or drink for 15 minutes before and during use;

use 2-mg lozenge if first cigarette smoked >30 minutes after waking; use 4-mg lozenge if first cigarette smoked within 30 minutes of waking; 1 lozenge q1h to q2h (at least 9/d) × 6 weeks; then q2h to q4h × 3 weeks; then q4h to q8h × 3 weeks; then stop; maximum 5 lozenges/6 hr and 20 lozenges/d. Not recommended for children younger than 18 years.

Inhalation Products

- *Nicotrol NS:* adults and children older than 12 years—0.5-mg aqueous nasal spray; 1 to 2 doses/hr nasally; maximum 5 doses/hr or 40 doses/d; usual maximum 3 months. Not recommended for children younger than 12 years.
- *Nicotrol Inhaler:* adults and children older than 12 years—10-mg inhalation system; individualize therapy; at least 6 cartridges/d × 3 to 6 weeks; maximum 16 cartridges/d × first 12 weeks; then reduce gradually over 12 more weeks. Not recommended for children younger than 12 years. Note: This system delivers nicotine but no tars or carcinogens. Each cartridge lasts about 20 minutes with frequent continuous puffing and provides nicotine equivalent to 2 cigarettes.

Administration

- Remove old patch before applying new one.
- Apply patch to non-hairy skin surface.
- Patches are heat sensitive; store at or below 30°C (86° F).

Side Effects

Headaches, dizziness, light-headedness; insomnia, irritability; tachycardia, palpitations; sore mouth, throat irritation, nausea, tingling of tongue; skin rash, pruritus; runny nose, nasal irritation, and watery eyes.

Drug Interactions

Nicotine can cause increased serum concentrations of caffeine, clozapine, olanzapine, theophylline, insulin, propranolol, and acetaminophen. Coffee and cola may decrease absorption of gum.

Pharmacokinetics

- *Half-life:* 30 to 120 minutes (3 to 4 hours for transdermal)
- *Peak plasma:* spray—4 to 15 minutes, gum—25 to 30 minutes, patch—2 to 10 hours
- *Excretion:* urine (30%)

Precautions

Contraindicated immediately postmyocardial infarction, severe angina pectoris, or in case of life-threatening arrhythmias.

Patient and Family Education

- Nicotrol Inhaler is a smoking replacement; to be used with decreasing frequency. Smoking should be discontinued before starting therapy.
- Discontinue use of patch if local skin reaction occurs.
- Smoking while using the patch increases adverse reactions.

Special Populations

- *Older adults:* Use with caution; can cause unsavory reactions.

- *Renal impairment:* No contraindications.
- *Hepatic impairment:* No contraindications known.
- *Pregnancy:* category D (nasal spray, transdermal patch); category C (gum).
- *Lactation:* Use only if benefits outweigh the risk associated.
- *Children and adolescents:* Safety and efficacy are not established; long-term effects in children/adolescents are unknown.

NORTRIPTYLINE HYDROCHLORIDE (Pamelor)

Classification
Tricyclic antidepressant (TCA)

Indications
The drug is used to treat adults with depression/anxiety and postherpetic neuralgia.

Available Forms
Capsule, 10, 25, 50, and 75 mg; oral solution, 10 mg/5 mL

Dosage
- *Adults and children older than 12 years:* -initially 25 mg TID to QID; maximum 150 mg/d.
- *Older adults:* Dose is 10 to 25 mg PO nightly and increase by 10 to 25 mg/d every 2 to 3 days; maximum, 150 mg/d. Once tolerated, may be given once per day in divided doses at bedtime. Must taper the dose gradually to discontinue.
- *Children younger than 12 years:* not recommended; BBW for use under age 16 years.

Administration
- PO with a glass of water.
- Do not abruptly stop taking the medication.
- Approved in children with enuresis and depression as young as 6 years.
- Use lowest effective dose for shortest duration.

Side Effects
- Similar to amitriptyline; cardiac arrhythmias, fatigue, sedation, and weight gain; sexual dysfunction.
- *More common:* drowsiness, dizziness, constipation; nausea/vomiting, urinary retention or frequency, libido changes, weight gain, general nervousness, galactorrhea, gynecomastia, rash, seizures, and urticaria.
- *Less common:* cardiac arrhythmias, CVA, heart block, myocardial infarction, agranulocytosis, thrombocytopenia, and hypoglycemia.
- EPS, clotting disturbances, worsening depression, suicidality, hyperthermia, and HTN.

Drug Interactions
This medicine may interact with the following:
- *Monoamine oxidase inhibitors:* risk for extreme HTN.
- *Selective serotonin reuptake inhibitor:* risk with use of clonidine.
- *Central nervous system depressants* (e.g., alcohol): TCAs increase effects.
- *Direct-acting adrenergic agonists* (e.g., epinephrine): TCAs increase effects.
- *Anticholinergic drugs* (e.g., antihistamines): TCAs increase effects with this medication.
- Absolute contraindications include class IA antiarrhythmics and MAOIs, such as phenelzine (Nardil), tranylcypromine (Parnate), isocarboxazid (Marplan), and selegiline (Eldepryl).
- Avoid using with cimetidine, amiodarone, clarithromycin, erythromycin, haloperidol, St. John's wort, evening primrose oil, and S-adenosyl-L-methionine (SAM-e).

■ *Alert:* This list may not describe all possible interactions. Instruct patients to provide a list of all medicines, herbs, nonprescription drugs, or dietary supplements used and state whether they smoke, drink alcohol, or use illegal drugs.

Pharmacokinetics

■ *Metabolism:* The drug is metabolized to an inactive form by CYP450; TCAs are thought to work by inhibiting reuptake of norepinephrine and serotonin in the CNS, which potentiates the neurotransmitters. They also have significant anticholinergic, antihistaminic, and alpha-adrenergic activity on the cardiac system. These classes of antidepressants also possess class 1A antiarrhythmic activity, which can lead to depression of cardiac conduction, potentially resulting in heart block or ventricular arrhythmias. Extensively metabolized by liver CYP 2D6 substrate.

■ *Excretion:* urine primarily, feces
■ *Peak plasma:* 7 to 8 hours
■ *Half-life:* approximately 18 to 24 hours

Precautions

■ See patients as often as necessary to ensure that the drug is working on the panic attacks, determine compliance, and review side effects, which are commonly observed before therapeutic effects.
■ Many side effects are dose dependent and may improve over time.
■ Overdose may result in lethal cardiotoxicity.
■ Monitor with routine EKG.
■ Instruct patients and families to watch for worsening depression or thoughts of suicide. Also watch out for sudden or severe changes in feelings, such as feeling anxious, agitated, panicky, irritated, hostile, aggressive, impulsive, severely restless, overly excited, or hyperactive or not being able to sleep. If this happens, especially at the beginning of antidepressant treatment or after a change in dose, patient should call the healthcare provider.
■ *Drowsiness or dizziness:* Patients should not drive or use machinery or do anything that needs mental alertness until the effects of this medicine are known.
■ Caution patients not to stand or sit up quickly, especially if older. This reduces the risk of dizziness or fainting spells. Alcohol may interfere with the effect of this medicine. Avoid alcoholic drinks.
■ Do not abruptly withdraw this drug as it may cause headache, nausea, and malaise.
■ Advise to protect skin from ultraviolet light due to increased skin sensitivity. Caution should be exercised in the following:
■ MDD, psychosis, or bipolar affective disorder
■ Contraindicated in patients with a recent myocardial infarction
■ Blood dyscrasias
■ Respiratory disease
■ Heart disease
■ Liver disease
■ Seizures (convulsions)
■ Suicidal thoughts, plans, or attempts by patients or a family member
■ An unusual or allergic reaction to imipramine, other medicines, foods, dyes, or preservatives

Patient and Family Education

■ Should be taken about the same time every day, with or without food. It may cause prolonged sedation. Do not drive until the effect of this medication is known.

- Administration time may be adjusted based on observed sedating or activating drug effects.
- It may take up to 4 to 8 weeks to show its effects, but patient may see symptoms of depression improving in as few as 2 weeks.
- If patient plans on becoming pregnant, discuss the benefits versus the risks of using this medicine while pregnant.
- As this medicine is excreted in the breast milk, nursing mothers should not breast-feed while taking this medicine without prior consultation with a psychiatric nurse practitioner or psychiatrist. Newborns may develop symptoms, including feeding or breathing difficulties, seizures, muscle stiffness, jitteriness, or constant crying.
- Do not stop taking this medication unless the healthcare provider directs. Report symptoms to the healthcare provider promptly.
- Drug should be tapered gradually when discontinued.
- Dosage should be adjusted to reach remission of symptoms and treatment should continue for at least 4 to 9 months following remission of symptoms.
- Keep these medications out of the reach of children and pets.
- Store nortriptyline at room temperature away from moisture and heat.
- Stopping this medication suddenly could result in unpleasant side effects.
- Take the missed dose as soon as remembered. If it is almost time for the next dose, skip the missed dose and take the medicine at the next regularly scheduled time. *Do not* take extra medicine to make up the missed dose.

Special Populations

- *Older adults:* Older individuals may be more sensitive to medication side effects, such as hypotension and anticholinergic effects and often require adjustment of medication doses for hepatic or renal dysfunction. The smallest effective dose is necessary for patients with melancholia, liver impairment, and unipolar depression. However, cardiac side effects and fall risk are of great concern in this population. Side effects may be more pronounced and require decreased dosage.
- *Pregnancy:* category D; not recommended in pregnancy. Some clinical reports exist of congenital malformations but no direct causal link. Alternative medications are recommended.
- *Lactation:* excreted in human breast milk; bottle-feed if possible or use with caution.
- *Children:* not recommended in children younger than 12 years.

OLANZAPINE (Zyprexa, Zyprexa Zydis)/OLANZAPINE–FLUOXETINE COMBINATION (Symbyax)

Classification
Second-generation (atypical) antipsychotic; dibenzazepine derivative

Indications
Olanzapine is used to treat schizophrenia, monotherapy, or combination therapy for acute mixed or manic episodes associated with bipolar I disorder, maintenance mono-therapy of bipolar I disorder, and agitation associated with schizophrenia or bipolar I disorder.

Available Forms
Tablet, 2.5, 5, 7.5, and 10 mg; ODT, 5, 10, 15, and 20 mg. Symbyax (olanzapine–fluox-etine combination): capsule, 3 mg/25 mg, 6 mg/25 mg, 6 mg/50 mg, 12 mg/25 mg, and 12 mg/50 mg.

Dosage
Olanzapine
- Initially 2.5 to 10 mg daily; increase to 10 mg/d within a few days; then by 5 mg/d at weekly intervals; maximum 20 mg/d

Olanzapine–fluoxetine combination
- *Adults*: initially 1 × 6/25 cap once daily in the PM; titrate; maximum 1 × 12/50 cap once daily in the PM
- *Children 10 to 17 years*: initially 1 × 3/25 cap once daily in the PM; maximum 1 × 12/50 cap once daily in the PM
- *Children younger than 10 years*: not recommended

Administration
- Tablets and combination capsules may be given with or without food.
- Advise patient to take the missed dose as soon as they remember. Skip the missed dose if it is almost time for the next scheduled dose. Do not take extra medicine to make up the missed dose.
- Store at room temperature away from moisture, heat, and light.

Side Effects
The drug can increase risk for diabetes and dyslipidemia; dizziness, sedation; weight gain; dry mouth, constipation, dyspepsia; suicide attempt, leucopenia peripheral edema; joint pain, back pain, metabolic syndrome, chest pain, extremity pain, abnor-mal gait, ecchymosis; tachycardia; orthostatic hypotension (usually during initial dose titration); hyperglycemia; increased risk of death and cerebrovascular events in elderly with dementia-related psychosis; TD (rare); rash on exposure to sunlight; NMS (rare); seizures.

Drug Interactions
- It may increase effects of antihypertensive medications and drugs that affect the QTc.

- It may antagonize levodopa and dopamine agonists.
- Antihypertensives, carbamazepine, ciprofloxacin, diazepam, and fluoxetine (even though combination formula Symbyax).
- Metoclopramide.
- There may need to be a reduced dose if given with CYP450 1A2 inhibitors (e.g., fluvoxamine).
- There may also be need to increase dose if given with CYP450 1A2 inducers (e.g., cigarette smoke, carbamazepine).
- *Alert:* This list may not describe all possible interactions. Instruct clients to provide a list of all the medicines, herbs, nonprescription drugs, or dietary supplements they use.

Pharmacokinetics

- *Metabolism:* Metabolites are inactive; through direct glycoxidation and CYP450 oxidation.
- *Peak:* 6 hours (PO), 15 to 45 minutes (IM).
- *Excretion:* urine (57%), feces (30%).
- *Half-life:* 21 to 54 hours; 30 days for XR injection.

Precautions

- Use with caution in patients with conditions that predispose to hypotension (dehydration, overheating).
- Use with caution in patients with prostatic hypertrophy, narrow angle-closure glaucoma, and paralytic ileus.
- Use with caution in patients who are at risk for aspiration pneumonia.
- Ativan often administered concomitantly in acute psychotic episodes in crisis ERs or psychiatric hospitalization.
- *Do not use if there is a proven allergy.*

Patient and Family Education

- Take exactly as prescribed by the provider. Do not take in larger or smaller amounts or for longer than recommended.
- It can be taken with or without food.
- For olanzapine ODTs, keep the tablet in its blister pack until patient is ready to take it. Open the package and peel back the foil from the tablet blister. Do not push a tablet through the foil. Using dry hands, remove the tablet and place directly on the tongue; it will begin to dissolve right away. Do not swallow the tablet whole. Allow it to dissolve in the mouth without chewing. If desired, drink liquid to help swallow the dissolved tablet.
- *If you have diabetes:* Check blood sugar levels on a regular basis while taking olanzapine.
- You can gain weight or have high cholesterol and triglycerides while taking this drug, especially if a teenager. Your blood will need to be tested often.
- Do not stop taking the drug suddenly without first talking to provider, even if you feel fine. You may have serious side effects if you stop taking the drug suddenly.
- Call provider if symptoms do not improve or get worse.
- Store at room temperature away from moisture, heat, and light.

Special Populations

- *Older adults:* BBW—in older adults, risk of CV or infection-related death. Not indicated for dementia-related psychosis.

- Older adults may tolerate lower doses better. Older adults with dementia-related psychosis treated with atypical antipsychotics are at higher risk of death and cerebrovascular events. It can increase incidence of stroke.
- *Renal impairment:* No dose adjustment is required for oral formulation. Consider lower starting dose (5 mg) for IM formulation. It is not removed by hemodialysis.
- *Hepatic impairment:* Starting oral dose is 5 mg for patients with moderate to severe hepatic function impairment; increase dose with caution. Consider lower starting dose (5 mg) for IM formulation. Check patient liver function tests a few times a year.
- *Cardiac impairment:* Use with caution because of risk for orthostatic hypotension.
- *Pregnancy:* category C; some animal studies show adverse effects. There are no controlled studies in humans. It should be used only when the potential benefits outweigh potential risks to the fetus. Olanzapine may be preferable to anticonvulsant mood stabilizers if treatment is required during pregnancy. Neonates exposed in third trimester at risk for EPS and withdrawal and severe feeding and breathing difficulty. Use only if benefits outweigh the risks.
- *Lactation:* It is not known if olanzapine is secreted in human breast milk. It is recommended to either discontinue drug or bottle-feed.
- *Children and adolescents*
    - Probably safe and effective for behavioral disturbances in this population
    - Higher risk of suicide in young adults aged 18 to 24 during first 2 months of treatment
    - Not for use under age 10 years
    - Should be monitored more frequently than adults

OXAZEPAM (Serax)

Classification
Benzodiazepine (BZD)

Indications
Oxazepam is used for the treatment of alcohol withdrawal, for sedation during hypnosis, and to treat anxiety.

Available Forms
Capsule, 10, 15, and 30 mg

Dosage
- *Adults:* anxiety: 10 to 15 mg TID to QID × 24 to 72 hours; decrease dose and/or frequency q24h to q72h; total length of therapy 5 to 14 days; maximum 120 mg/d
- *Children younger than 18 years:* not recommended
- *Older adults:* 10 to 15 mg PO TID or QID

Administration
- PO with a full glass of water.
- Oxazepam may be taken with or without food.
- Write prescription for the shortest duration possible in order to prevent potential dependence.
- *Missed dose:* Take as soon as remembered. Skip the missed dose if it is almost time for the next scheduled dose. Do not take extra medicine.
- If discontinuing the drug, healthcare provider will gradually taper.
- Dose may need to be gradually decreased to avoid side effects such as seizures.
- When used for an extended period, this medication may not work as well and may require different dosing.
- Stop smoking while taking this drug as it may decrease the effectiveness of oxazepam.

Side Effects
The side effects are clumsiness or unsteadiness, confusion, unusual risk behaviors; hyperactivity; hallucinations; jaundice; light-headedness, dizziness, drowsiness, and slurred speech; weakness; confusion; nervousness, hyperexcitability; hypersalivation, dry mouth; and hallucinations (rare).

Drug Interactions
- Increased CNS-depressive effects when taken with other CNS depressants.
- *Precautions:* BBW—not used much due to high risk of hepatic failure.
- Use with caution in patients with pulmonary impairment/disease.
- History of substance abuse increases risk of dependency; use with caution in patients with history of substance abuse.
- Some patients present with disinhibiting behaviors after administration.
- Do not use with patients with narrow-angle glaucoma.
- Some depressed patients may experience worsening of suicidal thoughts.
- Oxazepam should not be used with sodium oxybate as it may increase the risk of CNS and respiratory depression.

■ Probenecid may be used with great caution; it may increase the risk of CNS depression (aripiprazole, dexmedetomidine, and propofol). It may increase oxazepam levels and risk of toxicity. The healthcare provider needs to be notified prior to taking drugs that cause drowsiness, such as antihistamines (diphenhydramine), antiseizure drugs (carbamazepine), medicine for sleep (sedatives), muscle relaxants, narcotic pain relievers (codeine), psychiatric medicines (phenothiazines such as chlorpromazine, or tricyclics such as amitriptyline), and/or tranquilizers.

Pharmacokinetics

■ The drug is metabolized in the liver (CYP450). Enhances the GABA effects.
■ *Half-life:* 2.8 to 5.7 hours.
■ *Excretion:* urine.
■ *Peak plasma:* 3 hours.
■ *Precautions:* Monitor CBC and liver profiles. Serious reactions include leukopenia, hepatic impairment, and abuse.

Patient and Family Education

■ Take exactly as prescribed.
■ Tell the provider if treated for another psychiatric illness, such as depression.
■ Refrain from driving or operating dangerous machinery until the effect of this drug is known (sedative effects).
■ The drug can be taken with or without food.
■ Do not drink alcohol for it can cause serious problems.
■ There is a potential for dependence on the drug, so extra care is given if increasing the dose or abruptly discontinuing it.
■ If patient is pregnant during therapy or intends to become pregnant, this information should be communicated to the healthcare provider.
■ Avoid alcohol.
■ Do not abruptly stop taking this medication.

Special Populations

■ *Older adults:* Caution should be exercised and the initial dose should be the lowest possible due to the drowsiness effect. Initial dose of 30 mg in 3 divided doses: It can increase up to 60 mg/d in 3 to 4 doses if needed. Because of its sedative property and increased risk for falls, all BZDs are included on the Beers List of Potentially Inappropriate Medications for Geriatrics.
■ *Renal impairment:* Use with caution. May increase drug levels.
■ *Hepatic impairment:* Use with caution. Due to its short half-life, it is a preferred BZD for those with liver disease.
■ *Pregnancy:* category D; do not use unless benefits outweigh risks.
■ *Lactation:* Some caution is advised with breastfeeding.
■ *Children:* Drug is found in mother's breast milk; discontinue drug or bottle-feed.
■ *Children and adolescents:* not recommended for children younger than 18 years.

PAROXETINE MALEATE (Paxil, Paxil CR, Paxil suspension)

Classification
Antidepressant; selective serotonin reuptake inhibitor (SSRI)

Indications
Used primarily to treat depression but may also be used for OCD, posttrauma stress, PMDD, and social anxiety and panic disorder.

Available Forms
Tablet, 10, 20, 30, and 40 mg; table (controlled-release), 12.5, 25, and 37.5 mg; oral suspension, 10 mg/5 mL

Dosage
Paxil and Paxil Suspension
- *Adults and children older than 12 years*: initially 20 mg daily in AM; may increase by 10 mg/d at weekly intervals as needed; maximum 60 mg/d
- *Children younger than 12 years*: not recommended

Paxil CR
- *Adults and children older than 12 years*: initially 25 mg daily in AM; may increase by 12.5 mg at weekly intervals as needed; maximum 62.5 mg/d
- *Children younger than 12 years*: not recommended

Administration
- PO with a glass of water.
- Take the drug with or without food.
- Take it at regular intervals.
- It may be prescribed for children as young as 6 years of age for selected conditions (25 mg/d); *precautions do apply.*
- Instruct patients to take missed dose as soon as possible. If it is almost time for the next dose, advise to take only that dose.

Side Effects
- The drug displays some inhibition of dopamine reuptake, which may be beneficial to some patients (e.g., those experiencing hypersomnia, low energy, or mood reactivity) but problematic to others (e.g., causing overactivation in patients with panic disorder). Sertraline hydrochloride may cause more GI side effects than other drugs in its class.
- Nervousness, headache, and nausea, insomnia; serotonin syndrome; dry mouth, easy bruising, or excess perspiration; diarrhea.
- *Withdrawal syndrome (including neonatal withdrawal syndrome)*: Symptoms may include dizziness, muscle aches, headache, nausea, vomiting, gait instability, agitation, and/or "electric shock" sensations, and suicidal behavior.
  - Sexual dysfunction (more than 50% of men and women).
  - Hyponatremia (e.g., in geriatric patients taking diuretics).
  - Side effects are most common during the first or second week of therapy. Starting with a lower dosage and gradually increasing it and taking the medication with food will limit some of these side effects.

- *Most common*: dizziness, headache, insomnia, somnolence, and change in sex drive or performance.
- *Less common*: allergic reactions (skin rash, itching, or hives); swelling of the face, lips, or tongue; feeling faint or light-headed; falls; hallucination; loss of contact with reality; seizures; suicidal thoughts or other mood changes; unusual bleeding or bruising; unusually weak or tired; vomiting; change in appetite; diarrhea; increased sweating; indigestion; nausea; myalgia, and tremors.

Drug Interactions

- *Monoamine oxidase inhibitors*: extreme risk for serotonin syndrome. Allow 2-week washout period post-MAOI prior to initiation.
- *Tricyclic antidepressants:* Plasma levels may be increased by SSRIs, so add with caution in low doses.
- *Aspirin and nonsteroidal antiinflammatory drug*: increased risk of bleeding.
- *Central nervous system depressants*: It may increase depressant effects.
- *Selective serotonin reuptake inhibitors or serotonin antagonist and reuptake inhibitors*: It may cause serotonin syndrome in combination with the following medications: tramadol, high-dose triptans, or the antibiotic linezolid. Cimetidine may decrease clearance of sertraline.
- Use with caution in patients taking blood thinners (Coumadin); other antidepressants; antihistamines; ; and certain antibiotics, such as erythromycin, clarithromycin, or azithromycin.
- Absolute contraindications include MAOIs, such as phenelzine (Nardil), tranylcypromine (Parnate), isocarboxazid (Marplan), and selegiline (Eldepryl).
- Avoid using with SNRI agents, triptans, and other SSRI agents.
- Caution with aspirin, NSAIDs (e.g., ibuprofen or naproxen), COX inhibitors, other antiinflammatory drugs.
- *Alert*: This list may not describe all possible interactions. Instruct patients to provide a list of all medicines, herbs, nonprescription drugs, or dietary supplements used and state if they smoke, drink alcohol, or use illegal drugs.

Pharmacokinetics

- This drug is highly bound to plasma proteins and has a large volume of distribution.
- It is readily absorbed in the GI tract; SSRIs are metabolized in the liver and excreted in the urine. Dosages may be decreased in patients with liver or kidney disease.
- Caution advised in elderly clients.
- *Metabolism*: It is metabolized in the liver by cytochrome P450 microsomal enzymes.
- *Peak plasma levels*: 2 to 10 hours.
- *Half-life*: variable but most SSRIs have half-lives of 20 to 26 hours. They are highly bound to plasma proteins and have a large volume of distribution.
- Addition of serotonergic medications to a patient's regimen must not occur until 2 to 3 weeks after discontinuation of an SSRI (some recommend a 5-week "washout" period for fluoxetine prior to initiation of an MAOI).
- *Metabolism*: liver: CYP2D6.
- *Excretion*: urine 64% (none unchanged); feces 36% (<1% unchanged).

Precautions

- This drug may cause sedation and mental clouding.

- Use this drug with caution in patients with liver, kidney, or CV disease.
- Adverse effects and side effects are commonly observed before therapeutic effects.
- Many side effects are dose dependent and may improve over time.
- Taper discontinuation to avoid withdrawal symptoms.
- *Older adults*: Older adults may require decreased dosage.
- See patients as often as necessary to ensure that the drug is working on the panic attacks, determine compliance, and review side effects.
- Make sure patients realize that they need to take prescribed doses even if they do not feel better right away. It can take several weeks before they feel the full effect of the drug.
- Instruct patients and families to watch for worsening depression or thoughts of suicide. Also, watch out for sudden or severe changes in feelings, such as feeling anxious, agitated, panicky, irritated, hostile, aggressive, impulsive, severely restless, overly excited, or hyperactive or not being able to sleep. If this happens, especially at the beginning of antidepressant treatment or after a change in dose, patient should call the healthcare provider.
- *Drowsiness or dizziness*: Patients should not drive or use machinery or do anything that needs mental alertness until the effects of this medicine are known.
- Caution patients not to stand or sit up quickly, especially if older. This reduces the risk of dizziness or fainting spells. Alcohol may interfere with the effect of this medicine. Avoid alcoholic drinks.
- Caution patients not to treat themselves for coughs, colds, or allergies without asking a healthcare professional for advice. Some ingredients can increase possible side effects.
- For dry mouth, chewing sugarless gum or sucking hard candy and drinking plenty of water may help. Contact your healthcare provider if the problem persists or is severe.
- Caution should be exercised in the following:
  - Bipolar disorder or a family history of bipolar disorder
  - Diabetes
  - Heart disease
  - Liver disease
  - Electroconvulsive therapy
  - Seizures (convulsions)
  - Suicidal thoughts, plans, or attempts by patients or a family member
  - An unusual or allergic reaction to sertraline, other medicines, foods, dyes, or preservatives
  - Pregnancy or trying to get pregnant
  - Breastfeeding

Patient and Family Education

- Antidepressant medications are used to treat a variety of conditions, including depression and other mental/mood disorders. These medications can help prevent suicidal thoughts/attempts and provide other important benefits. However, a small number of people (especially people younger than 25) who take antidepressants for any condition may experience worsening depression, other mental/mood symptoms, or suicidal thoughts/attempts. Therefore, it is very important to talk with the clinician about the risks and benefits of antidepressant medication (especially for people younger than 25), even if treatment is not for a mental/mood condition. Tell the clinician right away if you notice worsening depression/other psychiatric conditions, unusual behavior changes (including possible suicidal thoughts/attempts), or other mental/mood changes (including new/worsening anxiety, panic attacks, trouble sleeping, irritability, hostile/angry feelings, impulsive actions, severe restlessness, very rapid speech). Be especially watchful for these symptoms when a new antidepressant is started or when the dose is changed.

- It should be taken about the same time every day, morning or evening, and can be taken with or without food (with food if there is any stomach upset).
- It may start with half of lowest effective dose for 3 to 7 days and then increase to lowest effective dose to diminish side effects.
- Administration time may be adjusted based on observed sedating or activating drug effects.
- It may take up to 4 to 8 weeks to show its maximum effect at this dose, but some may see symptoms of dysthymia improving in as few as 2 weeks.
- If patient plans on becoming pregnant or is pregnant, discuss the benefits versus the risks of using this medicine while pregnant.
- As this medicine is excreted in the breast milk, nursing mothers should not breast-feed while taking this medicine without prior consultation with a psychiatric nurse practitioner or psychiatrist. Newborns may develop symptoms, including feeding or breathing difficulties, seizures, muscle stiffness, jitteriness, or constant crying.
- Do not stop taking this medication unless the healthcare provider directs. Report side effects or worsening symptoms to the healthcare provider promptly.
- The medication should be tapered gradually when changing or discontinuing therapy.
- Dosage should be adjusted to reach remission of symptoms and treatment should continue for at least 6 to 12 months following last reported dysthymic experience.
- Caution is advised when using this drug in older adults because they may be more sensitive to the effects of the drug. Older adults should receive a lower starting dose.
- Keep these medications out of the reach of children and pets.
- Store the drug at room temperature. Take any unused medication after the expiration date to the local pharmacy on drug-giveback day. Avoid throwing the medication into the environment.
- Discuss any worsening anxiety, aggressiveness, impulsivity, or restlessness.
- Patients or families should report any severe, abrupt onset or changes in symptoms to health professionals. This may be reflective of increased risk of suicidal thinking.
- Caution for the concomitant use of NSAIDs, aspirin, and any other drugs that alter platelets.

Special Populations

- *Older adults:* Older individuals tend to be more sensitive to medication side effects, such as hypotension and anticholinergic effects. They often require adjustment of medication doses for hepatic or renal dysfunction. SSRIs with shorter half-lives or less P-450 inhibition may be more desirable (e.g., citalopram) for geriatric populations than SSRIs with longer half-lives (e.g., fluoxetine). SSRIs have been associated with increased risk for falls in nursing home residents and neurological effects in patients with Parkinson's disease. Older adults are more prone to SSRI-induced hyponatremia.
- *Hepatic impairment*: Dose adjustment is necessary.
- *Pregnancy*: Psychotherapy is the initial choice for most pregnant patients with MDD. Most SSRIs are category C drugs, due to adverse effects; risks are observed

in animal studies. Sertraline has been found to have lower cord blood levels than other SSRIs, although the clinical significance is unknown. Thus, an individual risk–benefit analysis must be done to determine appropriate treatment in pregnant women with DD. If continued during pregnancy, SSRI dosage may need to be increased to maintain euthymia due to physiological changes associated with pregnancy.

- *Lactation*: Adverse reactions have not been reported; however, long-term effects have not been studied, and the manufacturer recommends caution.
- *Children*: not recommended for children younger than 12 years. Monitoring for increased suicidal ideation using SSRI therapy in children is critical.

PERPHENAZINE (Trilafon)

Classification
Antipsychotic, phenothiazine class

Indications
Perphenazine is used to treat schizophrenia.

Available Forms
Tablets, 2, 4, 8, and 16 mg; oral concentration, 16 mg/5 mL; ampule, 5 mg/mL

Dosage
- *Adults and children older than 12 years:* 5 mg IM (may repeat in 6 hours) or 8 to 16 mg/d PO in divided doses; maximum 15 mg/d IM; maximum 24 mg/d PO
- *Children younger than 12 years:* not recommended

Administration
- Store tablets in tight, light-resistant container.
- Obtain baseline BPs before starting therapy and monitor regularly. Watch for orthostatic hypotension.

Side Effects
- *Central nervous system:* seizures, NMS, EPS, TD, sedation, drowsiness
- *Cardiovascular:* orthostatic hypotension, tachycardia, EKG changes
- *EENT:* blurred vision, ocular changes, nasal congestion
- *Gastrointestinal:* dry mouth, constipation, nausea, vomiting, diarrhea
- *Genitourinary:* urinary retention, dark-colored urine, menstrual irregularities, inhibited ejaculation; hematological: leukopenia, agranulocytosis, thrombocytopenia
- *Hepatic:* cholestatic jaundice
- *Metabolic:* weight gain
- *Skin:* mild photosensitivity reactions
- *Other:* gynecomastia

Drug Interactions
- Antacids may inhibit absorption or oral phenothiazines.
- Separate doses by at least 2 hours.
- *Atropine, phosphorus insecticides:* It may increase anticholinergic effects.
- *Barbiturates:* It may decrease phenothiazine effect.
- CNS depressants may increase CNS depression.
- Fluoxetine, paroxetine, sertraline, and TCAs may increase phenothiazine level.
- *Lithium:* This drug may increase neurological adverse effects.
- *Drug–herb:* St. John's wort: The drug my cause photosensitivity reactions. Drug–lifestyle: Alcohol use may increase CNS depression. Sun exposure may increase risk of photosensitivity reactions.

Pharmacokinetics
- Perphenazine may exert antipsychotic effects by blocking postsynaptic dopamine receptors in the brain.
- Onset, peak, and duration unknown

Precautions

- The drug is contraindicated in those with CNS depression, blood dyscrasia, bone marrow depression, and liver damage.
- Use the drug cautiously in patients with alcohol withdrawal, psychotic depression, suicidal ideation, severe adverse reactions to other phenothiazines, renal impairment, CV disease, and respiratory disorders.
- Neonates exposed to antipsychotics in the third semester of pregnancy are at risk for developing EPS and withdrawal signs and symptoms following delivery. Use the drug during pregnancy only if the benefit to the mother justifies the risk to the fetus.
- *Overdose signs and symptoms*: The signs and symptoms of perphenazine overdose are stupor, coma seizures in children, tachycardia, prolonged QRS or QT interval, AV block, torsades de pointes, ventricular arrhythmia, hypotension, and cardiac arrest.

Patient and Family Education

- Warn patients about activities that require alertness or coordination until effect of drug is known.
- Advise patients to avoid alcohol while taking this medication.
- Have patients report signs of urinary retention or constipation.
- Tell patients to wear sun block and stay hydrated if exposed to sunlight.
- Patients can relieve dry mouth with sugarless gum or hard candy. They should carry bottled water with them at all times and drink when thirsty.

Special Populations

- *Older adults*: Older adults with dementia-related psychosis treated with conventional or atypical antipsychotics are at increased risk for death. Antipsychotics are not approved for treatment of dementia-related psychosis.
- *Pregnancy*: category C.
- *Pediatric*: not for use in children under age 12 years.

QUETIAPINE FUMARATE (Seroquel, Seroquel XR)

Classification
Atypical antipsychotic (second generation); dibenzothiazepine

Indications
Quetiapine fumarate is used to treat schizophrenia, depressive episodes associated with bipolar disorder, monotherapy or combination therapy for acute manic episodes associated with bipolar I disorder, MDD, adjunctive therapy, OCD, and acute and maintenance treatment of schizophrenia.

Available Forms
Tablet, 25, 50, 100, 200, 300, and 400 mg; tablet (XR), 50, 150, 200, 300, and 400 mg

Dosage
SeroQUEL
- *Adults*: initially 25 mg BID, titrate every 2nd or 3rd day in increments of 25 to 50 mg BID to TID; usual maintenance 400 to 600 mg/d in 2 to 3 divided doses
- *Children 10 to 17 years*: initially 25 mg BID, titrate every 2nd or 3rd day in increments of 25 to 50 mg BID to TID; maximum 600 mg/d in 2 to 3 divided doses
- *Children younger than 10 years*: not recommended

SeroQUEL
- *Adults*: swallow whole; administer once daily in the PM; day 1: 50 mg; day 2: 100 mg; day 3: 200 mg; day 4: 300 mg; usual range 400 to 600 mg/d
- *Children younger than 18 years*: not recommended

Administration
- Tablets may be given with or without food.
- Advise patient to take this medicine with a full glass of water.
- Advise patient not to crush, chew, or break an XR tablet. Swallow the pill whole. Breaking the pill may cause too much of the drug to be released at one time.
- Advise patient to take the missed dose as soon as remembered. Skip the missed dose if it is almost time for the next scheduled dose. Do not take extra medicine to make up the missed dose.

Side Effects
The drug can increase risk for diabetes and dyslipidemia; dizziness, sedation, palpitations; blurred vision; dry mouth, constipation, dyspepsia, abdominal pain, weight gain; tachycardia; hyperglycemia; increased risk of death and cerebrovascular events in older adults with dementia-related psychosis; palpitations; fatigue; asthenia; somnolence; dizziness; cough; orthostatic hypotension (usually during initial dose titration); NMS (rare); and seizures (rare leukopenia).

Drug Interactions
This medicine may interact with the following:
- Alcohol and other CNS depressants may increase CNS depression.
- It my increase hypotensive effects of antihypertensives.

- The drug may increase the clearance of hepatic enzyme inducers, such as phenytoin.
- It may also decrease total free thyroxine (T4); serum levels of quetiapine may be increased.
- However, no dose adjustment is required.
- *Alert:* This list may not describe all possible interactions. Instruct clients to provide a list of all the medicines, herbs, nonprescription drugs, or dietary supplements they use.
- It may increase serum cholesterol, triglycerides, AST, alanine transaminase, WBC count, and GGT levels.
- It may produce false-positive results.

Pharmacokinetics

- *Metabolism:* Metabolites are inactive. Blocks dopamine and serotonin 5-HT2 receptors.
- *Onset:* Unknown.
- *Peak:* 1.5 hour; PO—1.5 hours, XR—6 hours.
- *Bioavailability:* 100%.
- *Metabolism:* The drug is metabolized by the liver into the metabolite N-desalkyl quetiapine. The CYP enzymes responsible for the metabolism of quetiapine are CYP2D6 and CYP3A4.
- *Excretion:* It is primarily excreted in the urine (73%) and the remaining amount of the drug is excreted in the feces (27%).
- *Half-life:* 6 to 7 hours; 6 hours for PO, 7 to 12 hours for XR.

Precautions

- Use the drug with caution in patients who are at risk for aspiration pneumonia.
- It is not approved for children under age 10 years.
- It may increase suicidal ideation in children through those aged 24 years.
- The manufacturer recommends examining for cataracts before and every 6 months after starting quetiapine.
- Use the drug with caution in patients with Alzheimer's dementia, history of breast cancer, CV disease, cerebrovascular disease, dehydration, hepatic impairment, seizures, and hypothyroidism.
- *Do not use the drug if there is a proven allergy.*
- *Contraindications:* none known.

Patient and Family Education

- Take as much drug exactly as prescribed by the provider. Do not take it in larger or smaller amounts or for longer than recommended.
- It can be taken with or without food.
- Quetiapine can cause side effects that may impair thinking or reactions. Be careful if you drive or do anything that requires you to be awake and alert.
- Quetiapine may cause high blood sugar (hyperglycemia). Talk to provider if any signs noted of hyperglycemia, such as increased thirst or urination, excessive hunger, or weakness. If diabetic, check blood sugar levels on a regular basis.
- Drink fluids often, especially during physical activity.
- Avoid becoming overheated or dehydrated during exercise and in hot weather. You may be more prone to heat stroke.
- Avoid getting up too fast from a sitting or lying position. Get up slowly and steady yourself to prevent a fall.

- *Avoid alcohol intake.*
- *Stop using this medication and call provider immediately* if you have very stiff (rigid) muscles, high fever, sweating, confusion, fast or uneven heartbeats, tremors; feel like you might pass out; have jerky muscle movements you cannot control, trouble swallowing, problems with speech; have blurred vision, eye pain, or see halos around lights; have increased thirst and urination, excessive hunger, fruity breath odor, weakness, nausea and vomiting; have fever, chills, body aches, flu symptoms; or have white patches or sores inside your mouth or on your lips.
- Do as ordered; do not stop taking the drug suddenly without first talking to the healthcare provider, even if you feel fine. You may have serious side effects if you stop taking the drug suddenly.
- Call provider if symptoms do not improve or get worse.
- Store at room temperature away from moisture and heat.
- Avoid tasks that require alertness and motor skills until response to drug is established.

Special Populations

BBW for older adults with dementia due to increased risk of death.

- *Older adults*: Generally lower dose is used (e.g., 25–100 mg BID) in older adults. Higher dose can be used if it can be tolerated. Older adults with dementia-related psychosis treated with atypical antipsychotics are at higher risk of death and cerebrovascular events.
- *Renal impairment*: No dose adjustment is required.
- *Hepatic impairment*: Dose may need to be reduced.
- *Cardiac impairment*: Use with caution because of risk of orthostatic hypotension.
- *Pregnancy*: category C; some animal studies show adverse effects. There are no controlled studies in humans. It should be used only when the potential benefits outweigh potential risks to the fetus. Quetiapine may be preferable to anticonvulsant mood stabilizers if treatment is required during pregnancy.
- *Lactation: not recommended.* It is not unknown whether the drug is secreted in human breast milk. It is recommended to either discontinue drug or bottle-feed. Infants of women who choose to breastfeed while on this drug should be monitored for possible adverse effects.
- *Children and adolescents:* SeroQUEL is not for use in children younger than 10 years; SeroQUEL XR is not for use in children. Should be monitored more frequently than adults. May tolerate lower doses better. Watch for activation of suicidal ideation. Inform parents or guardian of this risk so they can help monitor the risk. There is an increased risk of suicidal thinking and behavior in children and adolescents with MDD and other psychiatric disorders.

RISPERIDONE (Risperdal, Risperdal Consta, Risperdal M-Tab)

Classification
Atypical antipsychotic (second generation); benzisoxazole derivative

Indications
This drug is used for the treatment of schizophrenia, monotherapy, or combination therapy for acute, mixed, or manic episodes associated with bipolar I disorder, Tourette syndrome, and OCD and treatment of irritability associated with autistic disorder in children and adolescents.

Available Forms
Tablet, 0.25, 0.5, 1, 2, 3, and 4 mg; ODT, 0.25, 0.5, 1, 2, 3, and 4 mg; oral solution, 1 mg/mL (30-mL bottle); vial, 12.5-, 25-, 37.5-, and 50-mg powder for long-acting IM injection after reconstitution, single-use, with diluent and supplies.

Dosage
Risperdal
- *Adults and children older than 10 years:* tablet: initially 2 to 3 mg once daily; may adjust at 24-hour intervals by 1 mg/d; usual range 1 to 6 mg/d; maximum 6 mg/d; oral solution: do not take with cola or tea; M-tab: dissolve on tongue with or without fluid; consta: administer deep IM in the deltoid or gluteal; give with oral risperidone or other antipsychotic × 3 weeks; then stop oral form; 25 mg IM every 2 weeks; maximum 50 mg every 2 weeks.
- *Children 5 to 10 years:* initially 0.5 mg once daily at the same time each day; adjust at 24-hour intervals by 0.5 to 1 mg to target dose 1 to 2.5 mg/d; usual range 1 to 6 mg/d; maximum 6 mg/d.
- *Children younger than 5 years:* not established.

Risperdal Consta
- *Adults:* Tab: initially 2 to 3 mg once daily; may adjust at 24 hour intervals by 1 mg/d; usual range 1 to 6 mg/d; max 6 mg/d; Oral solution: do not take with cola or tea; M-tab: dissolve on tongue with or without fluid; Consta: administer deep IM in the deltoid or gluteal; give with oral risperidone or other antipsychotic × 3 weeks; then stop oral form; 25 mg IM every 2 weeks; max 50 mg every 2 weeks.
- *Children younger than 18 years:* not established

Risperdal M-Tab
- *Adults and children older than 10 years:* tablet: initially 2 to 3 mg once daily; may adjust at 24-hour intervals by 1 mg/d; usual range 1 to 6 mg/d; maximum 6 mg/d; oral solution: do not take with cola or tea; M-tab: dissolve on tongue with or without fluid; consta: administer deep IM in the deltoid or gluteal; give with oral risperidone or other antipsychotic × 3 weeks; then stop oral form; 25 mg IM every 2 weeks; maximum 50 mg every 2 weeks.
- *Children younger than 10 years:* not established.

Administration
- Give drug PO with food. Place M-Tab directly on tongue.

- Advise patient to take the missed dose as soon as remembered. Skip the missed dose if almost time for the next scheduled dose.
- Open package by peeling off foil backing with dry hands.
- Measure the liquid form of risperidone with a special dose-measuring spoon or cup, not a regular tablespoon.
- Do not mix the liquid form with cola or tea.
- Phenylalanine contents of ODTs are as follows: 0.5-mg tablet contains 0.14 mg phenylalanine; 1-mg tablet contains 0.28 mg phenylalanine; 2-mg tablet contains 0.56 mg phenylalanine; 3-mg tablet contains 0.63 mg phenylalanine; 4-mg tablet contains 0.84 mg phenylalanine.

Intramuscular

- Continue oral therapy for the first 3 weeks of IM injection therapy until injections take effect; then stop oral therapy.
- To reconstitute IM injection, inject premeasured diluent into vial and shake vigorously for at least 10 seconds. Suspension appears uniform, thick, and milky; particles are visible, but no dry particles remain. Use drug immediately or refrigerate for up to 6 hours after reconstitution. If more than 2 minutes pass before injection, shake vigorously again. See manufacturer's package insert for more detailed instructions.
- Refrigerate IM injection kit and protect it from light. Drug can be stored at temperature <77°F (25°C) for no more than 7 days before administration.

Side Effects

This drug can increase risk for diabetes and dyslipidemia, EPS (dose dependent), hyperprolactinemia (dose dependent), and dizziness. These side effects can occur at low doses with pseudolactation occurring.

- Akathisia, somnolence, dystonia, insomnia, headache, agitation, anxiety; nausea, sedation, weight gain, constipation, abdominal pain; tachycardia; sedation; sexual, parkinsonism dysfunction; hyperglycemia; increased risk of death and cerebrovascular events in older adults with dementia-related psychosis; TD; suicide attempt, dizziness, fever, hallucination, mania, impaired concentration, abnormal thinking and dreaming, tremor, hypoesthesia, fatigue, depression, nervousness, and NMS.
- Tachycardia, chest pain, orthostatic hypotension (rare, usually during initial dose, titration); NMS seizures (rare); peripheral edema, syncope, and HTN.
- Rhinitis, sinusitis, pharyngitis, and ear disorder.
- Constipation, nausea, vomiting, dyspepsia, abdominal pain, anorexia, dry mouth, increased saliva, and diarrhea.
- Urinary incontinence, increased urination, abnormal orgasm, vaginal dryness, weight gain, hyperglycemia, and weight loss.
- Arthralgia, back pain, leg pain, and myalgia.
- Coughing, dyspnea, and upper respiratory infection.
- Rash, dry skin, photosensitivity reactions, acne, and injection site pain.
- Injury and decreased libido.

Drug Interactions

- It may increase effects of antihypertensive medications.
- It may antagonize levodopa and dopamine agonists.
- Plasma levels of risperidone may be reduced if given in conjunction with antihypertensives and carbamazepine.

- Plasma levels of risperidone may be increased if given in conjunction with CNS depressants, dopamine agonists, levodopa, fluoxetine, or paroxetine.
- Plasma levels of risperidone may be increased if given in conjunction with clozapine, but no dose adjustment is required. Avoid using together as it may increase toxicity of these drugs.
- *Methadone*: This drug may decrease methadone levels.
- *Theophylline*: This drug may decrease theophylline levels.
- *Trazodone*: This drug may increase trazodone level.
- Rifampin and rifapentine may decrease ritonavir levels.
- St. John's wort may substantially reduce drug levels. Using the two together is contraindicated.
- *Oral contraceptives*: It may reduce effectiveness of contraceptive.
- *Alert:* This list may not describe all possible interactions. Instruct clients to provide a list of all the medicines, herbs, nonprescription drugs, or dietary supplements they use.

Pharmacokinetics

- *Elimination:* 7 to 8 weeks after last injection (long-acting formulation)
- *Metabolism:* Metabolites are active; the drug is metabolized by CYP450 2D6. Blocks dopamine and 5-HT two receptors in the brain
- *Half-life:* 3 to 24 hours (oral formulation); 3 to 6 days (long-acting formulation)
- *Peak action:* 2 hours
- *Excretion:* urine (70%), feces (14%)
- *Duration of effect:* Unknown

Precautions

- Use with caution in patients with conditions that predispose to hypotension (dehydration, overheating).
- It may increase prolactin level.
- It may decrease hemoglobin level and hematocrit.
- Sun exposure may increase risk of photosensitivity reactions.
- It is contraindicated in patients hypersensitive to drug and in breastfeeding women.
- Use cautiously in patients with prolonged QT interval, cerebrovascular disease, dehydration, hypovolemia, history of seizures, or conditions that could affect metabolism or hemodynamic responses.
- Use cautiously in patients exposed to extreme heat.
- Use cautiously in patients at risk for aspiration pneumonia.
- Priapism has been reported.
- *Do not use if there is a proven allergy.*
- Use IM injection cautiously in those with hepatic or renal impairment.
- *Alert:* Obtain baseline BP measurements before starting therapy and monitor pressure regularly. Watch for orthostatic hypotension, especially during first-dose adjustment.
- *Alert:* Fatal cerebrovascular adverse events (stroke, TIA) may occur in older adults with dementia. Drug is not safe or effective in these patients.
- Monitor patient for TD, which may occur after prolonged use. It may not appear until months or years later and may disappear spontaneously or persist for life, despite stopping drug.
- Life-threatening hyperglycemia may occur in patients taking atypical antipsychotics. Monitor patients with diabetes regularly.

- Monitor patient for weight gain.
- Periodically reevaluate drug's risks and benefits, especially during prolonged use.
- *Alert:* Watch for evidence of NMS (extrapyramidal effects, hyperthermia, autonomic disturbance), which is rare but can be fatal.
- *Alert:* Monitor patient for symptoms of metabolic syndrome (significant weight gain and increased body mass index, HTN, hyperglycemia, hypercholesterolemia, and hypertriglyceridemia).

Patient and Family Education

- Take exactly as prescribed by the provider. Do not take in larger or smaller amounts or for longer than recommended.
- It can be taken with food.
- You may be more sensitive to temperature extremes (very hot or cold conditions) when taking this medication. Avoid getting too cold or becoming overheated or dehydrated.
- Drink plenty of fluids, especially in hot weather and during exercise.
- Risperidone can cause side effects that may impair thinking or reactions. Be careful if you drive or do anything that requires you to be awake and alert.
- Risperidone may cause high blood sugar (hyperglycemia). Talk to your provider if any signs of hyperglycemia, such as increased thirst or urination, excessive hunger, or weakness, occur. If diabetic, check blood sugar levels on a regular basis.
- The risperidone ODT may contain phenylalanine. Talk to your provider before using this form of risperidone if you have PKU.
- *Avoid drinking alcohol.* It can increase some of the side effects.
- Do *not* mix the liquid form with cola or tea.
- *Stop using this medication and call provider immediately* if you have fever, stiff muscles, confusion, sweating, fast or uneven heartbeats, restless muscle movements in face or neck, tremor (uncontrolled shaking), trouble swallowing, light-headedness, or fainting.
- Do not stop taking the drug suddenly without first talking to provider, even if you feel fine. You may have serious side effects if you stop taking the drug suddenly.
- Call provider if symptoms do not improve or get worse.
- Store the drug at room temperature away from moisture, light, and heat. Do not freeze the liquid form of risperidone.
- Warn patient to avoid activities that require alertness until effects of drug are known.
- Warn patient to rise slowly, avoid hot showers, and use other precautions to avoid fainting when starting therapy.
- Advise patient to use caution in hot weather to prevent heatstroke.
- Tell patient to take drug with food.
- Instruct patient to keep the ODT in the blister pack until just before taking it. Use dry hands to peel a part of the foil to expose the tablet; do not attempt to push it through the foil. After opening the pack, dissolve the tablet on tongue without cutting or chewing.

Special Populations

- *Older adults:*
  - Initially, 0.5 mg PO once a day; then increase to 0.5 mg BID. Titrate once a week for doses above 1.5 mg BID.
  - *Long-acting risperidone:* 25 mg every 2 weeks. Oral administration should be continued for 3 weeks after the first injection.

- Older adults with dementia-related psychosis treated with atypical antipsychotics are at higher risk for death and cerebrovascular events. BBW for older adults with dementia.
- *Renal impairment:*
  - Initially, 0.5 mg PO BID for the first week. Increase to 1 mg BID during the second week.
  - Long-acting risperidone should not be given to patients with renal function impairment unless they can tolerate at least 2 mg/d PO.
  - Long-acting risperidone should be given 25 mg every 2 weeks. Oral administration should be continued for 3 weeks after the first injection.
- *Hepatic impairment:*
  - Initially, 0.5 mg PO BID for the first week. Increase to 1 mg BID during the second week.
  - Long-acting risperidone should not be given to patients with hepatic function impairment unless they can tolerate at least 2 mg/d PO.
  - Long-acting risperidone should be given 25 mg every 2 weeks. Oral administration should be continued for 3 weeks after the first injection.
- *Cardiac impairment:* Use with caution because of risk for orthostatic hypotension. There is a greater risk of stroke if given to older adults with atrial fibrillation.
- *Pregnancy:* category C; some animal studies show adverse effects. There are no controlled studies in humans. It should be used only when the potential benefits outweigh potential risks to the fetus. Risperidone may be preferable to anticonvulsant mood stabilizers if treatment is required during pregnancy. Effects of hyperprolactinemia on the fetus are unknown.
- *Lactation:* Drug is secreted in human breast milk. It is recommended to either discontinue the drug or bottle-feed.
- *Children and adolescents:* This drug is not for use in children under age 5.

RIVASTIGMINE TARTRATE (Exelon, Exelon oral solution, Exelon patch)

Classification
Cholinesterase inhibitor; anti-Alzheimer's

Indications
The drug is used for treatment of the following:
- Mild to moderate dementia of the Alzheimer's type
- Mild to moderate dementia associated with Parkinson's disease

Available Forms
Capsule, 1.5, 3, 4.5, and 6 mg; oral solution, 2 mg/mL; patch, 4.6, 9.5, and 13.3 mg/24 hr

Dosage
Capsule: initially 1.5 mg BID, increase every 2 weeks as needed; maximum 12 mg/d; take with food.

Oral solution: initially 1.5 mg BID; may increase by 1.5 mg BID at intervals of at least 2 weeks; usual range 6 to 12 mg/d; maximum 12 mg/d; if stopped, restart at lowest dose and retitrate; may take directly from syringe or mix with water, fruit juice, or cola.

Transdermal: Initially apply 4.6-mg/24-hr patch; if tolerated, may increase to 9.5-mg/24-hr patch after 4 weeks; maximum 13.3 mg/24 hr; change patch daily; apply to clean, dry, hairless, intact skin; rotate application site; allow 14 days before applying new patch to same site.

Administration
- *Oral:* This drug should be taken with meals in divided doses in the morning and evening. It may be swallowed directly from the syringe provided or may be mixed with a small amount of water, cold fruit juice, or soda. Oral solution and capsules may be interchanged at equal doses.
- *Patch:* Remove previous transdermal patch before placing a new one.

Side Effects
- Nausea, vomiting, loss of appetite, heartburn or indigestion, stomach pain, weight loss, diarrhea, constipation, gas, weakness, dizziness, headache, extreme tiredness, lack of energy, tremor or worsening of tremor, increased sweating, difficulty falling asleep or staying asleep, bradycardia, and confusion.
- *Serious side effects that may require medical attention:* fainting, black and tarry stools, red blood in stools, bloody vomit, vomit that looks like coffee grounds, difficult or painful urination, seizures, depression, anxiety, aggressive behavior, hearing voices or seeing things that do not exist, uncontrollable movements and muscle contractions, and SJS.

Drug Interactions
This medicine may interact with the following medications: amantadine, other cholinesterase inhibitors, neuromuscular blockers, orphenadrine, cyclobenzaprine, parasympathomimetics, disopyramide, sedating H-1 blockers, amoxapine, antimuscarinics, clozapine, digoxin, general anesthetics, local anesthetics, maprotiline, nicotine, NSAIDs, olanzapine, phenothiazines, nicotine(smoking)-may increase drug clearance, and TCAs.

Pharmacokinetics

Selective inhibitor of brain acetylcholinesterase and butylcholinesterase

Oral

- Peak plasma concentrations reached in approximately 1 hour.
- Bioavailability after a 3-mg dose is 36%, indicating a significant first pass effect.
- It should be taken with food to enhance bioavailability.
- *Half-life*: 1.5 hours.
- *Duration*: 10 hours.

Topical

- Peak plasma concentrations are typically reached in 8 hours (range 8–16 hours).
- Steady state of medication is affected by body weight.
- Approximately 50% of the drug load is released from the transdermal system over 24 hours.
- *Half-life*: 3 hours.
- *Duration*: 24 hours.
- *Excretion*: urine (97%).

Precautions

Patients with a carbamate hypersensitivity should be cautious; rivastigmine is a carbamate derivative.

Patient and Family Education

Oral

- Store at 25°C (77°F); excursions permitted to 15°C to 30°C (59°F–86°F).
- Store the drug in a tight container. Store the solution in an upright position.
- Do not place rivastigmine solution in the freezer or allow to freeze.
- When oral solution is combined with cold fruit juice or soda, the mixture is stable at room temperature for up to 4 hours.
- Throw away any medication that is outdated or no longer needed.

Patches

- Apply once daily to clean, dry, hairless, intact skin.
- It may applied to the back, chest, or upper arm.
- Rotate application sites daily. Do not apply to the same site more than once every 14 days.
- Apply patch at approximately the same time every day. Remove the old patch before replacing with a new one.
- Patch may be worn while swimming, bathing, or showering or in hot weather.
- Avoid excessive sunlight or saunas.

Special Populations

- *Older adults*: Use with caution; check liver and kidney functions.
- *Hepatic impairment*: Use with caution.
- *Cardiac impairment*: Use with caution.
- *Pregnancy*: category C; some effects on the fetus are unknown.
- *Lactation*: unknown effects.
- *Children and adolescents*: This drug is not for use in children.

SERTRALINE HYDROCHLORIDE (Zoloft)

Classification
Antidepressant; selective serotonin reuptake inhibitor (SSRI)

Indications
Sertraline is used primarily to treat depression but may also be used for OCD, personality disorders, posttrauma stress, PMDD, or social anxiety and panic disorder.

Available Forms
Tablet, 25, 50, and 100 mg; oral concentrate, 20 mg/mL (60 mL; alcohol 12%)

Dosage
- *Adults*: initially 50 mg daily; increase at 1-week intervals if needed; maximum 200 mg daily; dilute oral concentrate immediately prior to administration in 4 oz water, ginger ale, lemon-lime soda, lemonade, or orange juice.
- *Children 13 to 17 years*: initially 50 mg daily; maximum 200 mg/d
- *Children 6 to 12 years*: initially 25 mg daily
- *Children younger than 6 years*: not recommended

Administration
- PO with a glass of water.
- Take the drug with or without food.
- Take it at regular intervals.
- It may be prescribed for children as young as 6 years of age for selected conditions (25 mg/d); *precautions do apply*.
- Instruct patients to take missed dose as soon as possible. If it is almost time for the next dose, advise to take only that dose.

Side Effects
Displays some inhibition of dopamine reuptake, which may be beneficial to some patients (e.g., those experiencing hypersomnia, low energy, or mood reactivity) but problematic to others (e.g., causing overactivation in patients with panic disorder). Sertraline hydrochloride may cause more GI side effects than other drugs in its class.

- Nervousness, headache, nausea, insomnia; serotonin syndrome; dry mouth, easy bruising, or excess perspiration; diarrhea.
- *Withdrawal syndrome (including neonatal withdrawal syndrome)*: Symptoms may include dizziness, muscle aches, headache, nausea, vomiting, gait instability, agitation, and/or "electric shock" sensations, and suicidal behavior.
  - Sexual dysfunction (more than 50% of men and women).
  - Hyponatremia (e.g., in geriatric patients taking diuretics).
  - Side effects are most common during the 1st or 2nd week of therapy. Starting with a lower dosage and gradually increasing it and taking the medication with food will limit some of these side effects.
  - *Most common*: dizziness, headache, insomnia, somnolence, and change in sex drive or performance.
  - *Less common*: allergic reactions (skin rash, itching, or hives); swelling of the face, lips, or tongue; feeling faint or light-headed; falls; hallucination; loss of contact with reality; seizures; suicidal thoughts or other mood changes; unusual bleeding

or bruising; unusually weak or tired; vomiting; change in appetite; diarrhea; increased sweating; indigestion; nausea; myalgia, and tremors.

Drug Interactions

- *Monoamine oxidase inhibitors*: extreme risk for serotonin syndrome. Allow 2-week washout period post-MAOI prior to initiation.
- *Tricyclic antidepressants*: Plasma levels may be increased by SSRIs, so add with caution in low doses.
- *Aspirin and nonsteroidal antiinflammatory drug*: increased risk of bleeding.
- *Central nervous system depressants*: It may increase depressant effects.
- *Selective serotonin reuptake inhibitors or serotonin antagonist and reuptake inhibitors*: It may cause serotonin syndrome in combination with the following medications: tramadol, high-dose triptans, or the antibiotic linezolid. Cimetidine may decrease clearance of sertraline.
- Use with caution in patients taking blood thinners (Coumadin); other antidepressants; antihistamines; lithium TCAs; and certain antibiotics, such as erythromycin, clarithromycin, or azithromycin.
- Absolute contraindications include MAOIs, such as phenelzine (Nardil), tranylcypromine (Parnate), isocarboxazid (Marplan), and selegiline (Eldepryl).
- Avoid using with SNRI agents, triptans, and other SSRI agents.
- Caution with aspirin, NSAIDs (e.g., ibuprofen or naproxen), COX inhibitors, other antiinflammatory drugs.
- *Alert*: This list may not describe all possible interactions. Instruct patients to provide a list of all medicines, herbs, nonprescription drugs, or dietary supplements used and state if they smoke, drink alcohol, or use illegal drugs.

Pharmacokinetics

- This drug is highly bound to plasma proteins and has a large volume of distribution.
- It is readily absorbed in the GI tract; SSRIs are metabolized in the liver and excreted in the urine. Dosages may be decreased in patients with liver or kidney disease.
- Caution advised in older adults.
- *Metabolism*: It is metabolized in the liver by cytochrome P450 microsomal enzymes.
- *Peak plasma levels*: 2 to 10 hours.
- *Half-life*: Variable, but most SSRIs have half-lives of 20 to 26 hours. They are highly bound to plasma proteins and have a large volume of distribution.
- Addition of serotonergic medications to a patient's regimen must not occur until 2 to 3 weeks after discontinuation of an SSRI (some recommend a 5-week "washout" period for fluoxetine prior to initiation of an MAOI).
- *Metabolism*: liver: CYP 2C19, 2D6, 3A4 substrate; 2D6 (weak), 3A4 (weak) inhibitor.
- *Excretion*: urine 40% to 45% (none unchanged); feces 40% to 45% (12%–14% unchanged).

Precautions

- This drug may cause sedation and mental clouding.
- Use this drug with caution in patients with liver, kidney, or CV disease.
- Adverse effects and side effects are commonly observed before therapeutic effects.
- Many side effects are dose dependent and may improve over time.
- Taper discontinuation to avoid withdrawal symptoms.
- *Older adults*: Older adults may require decreased dosage.

- See patients as often as necessary to ensure that the drug is working on the panic attacks, determine compliance, and review side effects.
- Make sure patients realize that they need to take prescribed doses even if they do not feel better right away. It can take several weeks before they feel the full effect of the drug.
- Instruct patients and families to watch for worsening depression or thoughts of suicide. Also, watch out for sudden or severe changes in feelings, such as feeling anxious, agitated, panicky, irritated, hostile, aggressive, impulsive, severely restless, overly excited, or hyperactive or not being able to sleep. If this happens, especially at the beginning of antidepressant treatment or after a change in dose, patient should call the healthcare provider.
- *Drowsiness or dizziness*: Patients should not drive or use machinery or do anything that needs mental alertness until the effects of this medicine are known.
- Caution patients not to stand or sit up quickly, especially if older. This reduces the risk of dizziness or fainting spells. Alcohol may interfere with the effect of this medicine. Avoid alcoholic drinks.
- Caution patients not to treat themselves for coughs, colds, or allergies without asking a healthcare professional for advice. Some ingredients can increase possible side effects.
- For dry mouth, chewing sugarless gum or sucking hard candy and drinking plenty of water may help. Contact your healthcare provider if the problem persists or is severe.
- Caution should be exercised in the following:
  - Bipolar disorder or a family history of bipolar disorder
  - Diabetes
  - Heart disease
  - Liver disease
  - Electroconvulsive therapy
  - Seizures (convulsions)
  - Suicidal thoughts, plans, or attempts by patients or a family member
  - An unusual or allergic reaction to sertraline, other medicines, foods, dyes, or preservatives
  - Pregnancy or trying to get pregnant
  - Breastfeeding

Patient and Family Education

- Antidepressant medications are used to treat a variety of conditions, including depression and other mental/mood disorders. These medications can help prevent suicidal thoughts/attempts and provide other important benefits. However, a small number of people (especially people younger than 25) who take antidepressants for any condition may experience worsening depression, other mental/mood symptoms, or suicidal thoughts/attempts. Therefore, it is very important to talk with the clinician about the risks and benefits of antidepressant medication (especially for people younger than 25), even if treatment is not for a mental/mood condition. Tell the clinician right away if you notice worsening depression/other psychiatric conditions, unusual behavior changes (including possible suicidal thoughts/attempts), or other mental/mood changes (including new/worsening anxiety, panic attacks, trouble sleeping, irritability, hostile/angry feelings, impulsive actions, severe restlessness, very rapid speech). Be especially watchful for these symptoms when a new antidepressant is started or when the dose is changed.

- It should be taken about the same time every day, morning or evening, and can be taken with or without food (with food if there is any stomach upset).
- It may start with half of lowest effective dose for 3 to 7 days and then increase to lowest effective dose to diminish side effects.
- Administration time may be adjusted based on observed sedating or activating drug effects.
- It may take up to 4 to 8 weeks to show its maximum effect at this dose, but some may see symptoms of dysthymia improving in as few as 2 weeks.
- If patient plans on becoming pregnant or is pregnant, discuss the benefits versus the risks of using this medicine while pregnant.
- As this medicine is excreted in the breast milk, nursing mothers should not breast-feed while taking this medicine without prior consultation with a psychiatric nurse practitioner or psychiatrist. Newborns may develop symptoms, including feeding or breathing difficulties, seizures, muscle stiffness, jitteriness, or constant crying.
- Do not stop taking this medication unless the healthcare provider directs. Report side effects or worsening symptoms to the healthcare provider promptly.
- The medication should be tapered gradually when changing or discontinuing therapy.
- Dosage should be adjusted to reach remission of symptoms and treatment should continue for at least 6 to 12 months following last reported dysthymic experience.
- Caution is advised when using this drug in older adults because they may be more sensitive to the effects of the drug. Older adults should receive a lower starting dose.
- Keep these medications out of the reach of children and pets.
- Store the drug at room temperature. Take any unused medication after the expiration date to the local pharmacy on drug-giveback day. Avoid throwing the medication into the environment.
- Discuss any worsening anxiety, aggressiveness, impulsivity, or restlessness.
- Patients or families should report any severe, abrupt onset or changes in symptoms to health professionals. This may be reflective of increased risk of suicidal thinking.
- Caution for the concomitant use of NSAIDs, aspirin, and any other drugs that alter platelets.

Special Populations

- *Older adults:* Older individuals tend to be more sensitive to medication side effects, such as hypotension and anticholinergic effects. They often require adjustment of medication doses for hepatic or renal dysfunction. SSRIs with shorter half-lives or less P-450 inhibition may be more desirable (e.g., citalopram) for geriatric populations than SSRIs with longer half-lives (e.g., fluoxetine). SSRIs have been associated with increased risk of falls in nursing home residents and neurological effects in patients with Parkinson's disease. Older adults are more prone to SSRI-induced hyponatremia.
- *Hepatic impairment*: Dose adjustment is necessary.
- *Pregnancy*: Psychotherapy is the initial choice for most pregnant patients with MDD. Most SSRIs are category C drugs, due to adverse effects; risks are observed in animal studies. Sertraline has been found to have lower cord blood levels than other SSRIs, although the clinical significance is unknown. Thus, an individual risk–benefit analysis must be done to determine appropriate treatment in pregnant women with DD. If continued during pregnancy, SSRI dosage may need to be increased to maintain euthymia due to physiological changes associated with pregnancy.

- *Lactation*: Adverse reactions have not been reported; however, long-term effects have not been studied, and the manufacturer recommends caution.
- *Children*: not recommended for children younger than 6 years. Monitoring for increased suicidal ideation using SSRI therapy in children is critical. BBW: Only for use in children 6 years or older for OCD.

SILDENAFIL CITRATE (Viagra)

Classification

Phosphodiesterase type 5 (PDE5) Inhibitor, CGMP-Specific

Indications

Used to treat erectile dysfunction

Available Forms

Tablet, 50, 100, and 200 mg

Dosage

- One dose about 1 hour (range 30 minutes to 4 hours) before sexual activity; usual initial dose 50 mg; may decrease to 25 mg or increase to maximum 100 mg/dose based on response; maximum one administration/day

Administration

- Take with or without food.
- Do not take this medicine more than once a day. Allow 24 hours to pass between doses.
- Store at room temperature away from moisture, heat, and light.

Side Effects

- Side effects include headache, flushing, nasal congestion, rhinitis, dyspepsia, and diarrhea.
- *Serious*: heart attack symptoms—chest pain or pressure, pain spreading to jaw or shoulder, nausea, sweating, vision changes or sudden vision loss; ringing in ears or sudden hearing loss; pain, swelling, warmth, or redness in one or both legs; shortness of breath; swelling in hands or feet; light-headed feeling; erection that is painful or lasts 4 hours or longer.

Drug Interactions

- Concomitant use of nitrates in any form is contraindicated.
- Contraindicated in patients with a known hypersensitivity to sildenafil or any component of the tablet.
- Contraindicated in patients who are using a GC stimulator, such as riociguat. PDE5 inhibitors may potentiate the hypotensive effects of GC stimulators.
- If drug is coadministered with an alpha-blocker, patients should be stable on alpha-blocker therapy prior to initiating treatment; initiative at a 25-mg dose.
- The recommended dose for ritonavir-treated patients is 25 mg prior to sexual activity and the recommended maximum dose is 25 mg within a 48-hour period because concomitant administration increased the blood levels of sildenafil 11-fold.
- Consider a starting dose of 25 mg in patients treated with strong CYP3A4 inhibitors (e.g., ketoconazole, itraconazole, or saquinavir) or erythromycin. Clinical data have shown that coadministration with saquinavir or erythromycin increased plasma levels of sildenafil by about 3-fold.

Pharmacokinetics

- Metabolism: liver: CYP3A4 (major route), CYP2C9 (minor route)

- *Half-life*: 3 to 4 hours
- Feces (~80%), urine (~13%)

Precautions

- There is a potential for cardiac risk during sexual activity in patients with preexisting CV disease. Contraindicated in patients for whom sexual activity is inadvisable because of their underlying CV status. Due to system vasodilatory properties, it is not recommended for patients who have suffered a myocardial infarction, stroke, or life-threatening arrhythmia within the last 6 months; patients with resting hypotension or HTN; and patients with cardiac failure or coronary artery disease causing unstable angina.
- Use with caution in patients with anatomical deformation of the penis (such as angulation, cavernosal fibrosis, or Peyronie's disease) or in patients who have conditions that may predispose them to priapism (such as sickle cell anemia, multiple myeloma, or leukemia).
- Clinicians should advise patients to stop use of all PDE5 inhibitors and seek medical attention in the event of a sudden loss of vision in one or both eyes. Such an event may be a sign of non-arteritic anterior ischemic optic neuropathy (NAION), a rare condition and a cause of decreased vision including permanent loss of vision.

Patient and Family Education

- Advise patients to seek emergency medical help if they have signs allergic reaction—hives; difficulty breathing; swelling of face, lips, tongue, or throat—or have sudden vision loss.
- Advise patients to seek emergency medical help if they have become dizzy or nauseated or have pain, numbness, or tingling in chest, arms, neck, or jaw during sexual activity.
- Remind patients that it should be taken only when needed, about 15 to 30 minutes before sexual activity.
- Remind patients that sexual response is needed for a response to treatment. An erection will not occur just by taking a pill.
- Advise patients that drinking alcohol can increase certain side effects. Avoid drinking more than three alcoholic beverages while taking medication.
- Advise patients to avoid the use of grapefruit products.

Special Populations

- *Pregnancy*: Not indicated for use in females.
- *Older adults*: A starting dose of 25 mg should be considered in older subjects due to higher systemic exposure.
- *Hepatic and renal impairment*: A starting dose of 25 mg should be considered in any patients with hepatic or renal impairment.

TACRINE HYDROCHLORIDE (Cognex)

Classification
Cholinesterase inhibitor

Indications
For the treatment of mild to moderate dementia of the Alzheimer type

Available Forms
Capsule, 10, 20, 30, and 40 mg

Dosage
- Initially 10 mg QID, increase 40 mg/d q4w as needed; maximum 160 mg/d

Administration
Oral capsules; store at room temperature. Take prescribed doses at regular intervals between meals but take with food if GI disturbance occurs. Consistency in administration times is necessary to avoid decrease in effectiveness and increase in side effects.

Side Effects
- *Central nervous system*: dizziness and headache
- *Cardiovascular*: hypo- or HTN
- *Dermatologic*: rash
- *EENT*: rhinitis
- *Gastrointestinal*: nausea/vomiting, diarrhea, dyspepsia, and anorexia
- *Genitourinary*: urinary incontinence or frequency
- *Metabolic*: weight decrease
- *Musculoskeletal*: myalgia
- *Respiratory*: coughing

Drug Interactions
This drug may interact with cimetidine, fluvoxamine, levodopa, and theophylline.

Pharmacokinetics
- Inhibits reversible cholinesterase in CNS, leading to increased concentrations of acetylcholine.
- Absorbed after oral administration. Food decreases bioavailability by about 30% to 40%.
- The drug is metabolized by cytochrome P450 system. Elimination time is 2 to 4 hours.
- Hepatic impairment may reduce effectiveness.
- Plasma concentrations are about 50% higher in women than in men.
- Smokers get one third less effectiveness of the drug; contraindications: jaundice, rash, fever.

Precautions
Precaution must be undertaken for the following scenarios:
- Patients with history of abnormal liver function.
- Patient may be carcinogenic.

- Overdosage: cholinergic crisis.
- Transaminase levels should be checked every 3 months while taking Cognex.

Patient Education

- Effectiveness may lessen over time.
- Medication needs to be taken as directed.
- Advise patient of the usual side effects.

Special Populations

- *Pregnancy*: category C
- *Older adults*: For use older adults with mild to moderate dementia of the Alzheimer's type
- *Children*: safety and efficacy not established in any dementing illness

TADALAFIL (Cialis)

Classification
Phosphodiesterase type 5 (PDE5) Inhibitor, CGMP specific

Indications
Used to treat erectile dysfunction

Available Forms
Tablet, 2.5, 5, 10, and 20 mg

Dosage
- Initially 10 mg prior to sexual activity up to once daily; may decrease to 5 mg or increase to 20 mg based on response; maximum one administration/day; effect may last 36 hours.

Administration
- Take with or without food.
- Do not break or split a tablet. Swallow it whole.
- Store at room temperature away from moisture, heat, and light.
- Do not take this medicine more than once a day. Allow 24 hours to pass between doses.

Side Effects
- Side effects include headache, flushing, nasal congestion, rhinitis, dyspepsia, and diarrhea.
- *Serious*: heart attack symptoms—chest pain or pressure; pain spreading to jaw or shoulder, nausea, sweating; vision changes or sudden vision loss; ringing in ears or sudden hearing loss; pain, swelling, warmth, or redness in one or both legs; shortness of breath; swelling in hands or feet; light-headed feeling; erection that is painful or lasts 4 hours or longer.

Drug Interactions
- Concomitant use of nitrates in any form is contraindicated.
- Contraindicated in patients with a known hypersensitivity to tadalafil or any component of the tablet.
- Contraindicated in patients who are using a GC stimulator, such as riociguat. PDE5 inhibitors may potentiate the hypotensive effects of GC stimulators.
- Caution is advised when PDE5 inhibitors are coadministered with alpha-blockers. PDE5 inhibitors and alpha-adrenergic blocking agents are both vasodilators with BP-lowering effects. When vasodilators are used in combination, an additive effect on BP may be anticipated. In some patients, concomitant use of these two drug classes can lower BP significantly
- Not recommended in patients with CrCl < 30 mL/min.
- In patients with mild or moderate hepatic impairment, dose should not exceed 10 mg; not recommended in patients with several hepatic impairment.
- Consumption of alcohol (e.g., 5 units or greater) can increase the potential for orthostatic signs and symptoms, including increase in heart rate, decrease in standing BP, dizziness, and headache.

- Limit dose to 10 mg no more than once every 72 hours in patients taking potent inhibitors of CYP3A4 such as ritonavir, ketoconazole, and itraconazole. In patients taking potent inhibitors of CYP3A4 and tadalafil for once daily use, the maximum recommended dose is 2.5 mg.

Pharmacokinetics

- Metabolism: liver: CYP3A4 (predominantly)
- *Half-life*: 17.5 hours
- Feces (~61%), urine (~36%)

Precautions

- There is a potential for cardiac risk during sexual activity in patients with preexisting CV disease. Contraindicated in patients for whom sexual activity is inadvisable because of their underlying CV status. Due to system vasodilatory properties, it is not recommended for patients who have suffered a myocardial infarction, stroke, life-threatening arrhythmia within the last 6 months; patients with resting hypotension or HTN; or patients with cardiac failure or coronary artery disease causing unstable angina.
- Use with caution in patients with anatomical deformation of the penis (such as angulation, cavernosal fibrosis, or Peyronie's disease) or in patients who have conditions that may predispose them to priapism (such as sickle cell anemia, multiple myeloma, or leukemia).
- Clinicians should advise patients to stop use of all PDE5 inhibitors and seek medical attention in the event of a sudden loss of vision in one or both eyes. Such an event may be a sign of NAION, a rare condition and a cause of decreased vision including permanent loss of vision.

Patient and Family Education

- Advise patients to seek emergency medical help if they have signs allergic reaction—hives; difficulty breathing; swelling of face, lips, tongue, or throat—have sudden vision loss.
- Advise patients to seek emergency medical help if they have become dizzy or nauseated or have pain, numbness, or tingling in chest, arms, neck, or jaw during sexual activity.
- Remind patients that it should be taken only when needed, about 15 to 30 minutes before sexual activity.
- Remind patients that sexual response is needed for a response to treatment. An erection will not occur just by taking a pill.
- Advise patients that drinking alcohol can increase certain side effects. Avoid drinking more than three alcoholic beverages while taking medication.
- Advise patients to avoid the use of grapefruit products.

Special Populations

- *Pregnancy*: not indicated for use in females.
- *Older adults*: The greater sensitivity to medications in some older individuals should be considered.
- *Hepatic and renal impairment*: Lower doses should be used in any patients with hepatic or renal impairment.

TEMAZEPAM (Restoril)

Classification
Benzodiazepine (BZD) hypnotic

Indications
Temazepam is used for the treatment of insomnia, especially short term (7 to 10 days).

Available Forms
Capsule, 7.5, 15, 22.5, and 30 mg

Dosage
- *Adults:* 7.5 to 30 mg qhs prn; short term, 7 to 10 days; maximum 30 mg; maximum 1 month
- *Children under 18 years:* not recommended

Administration
- PO with a glass of water; take 15 to 20 minutes before bedtime.
- Drowsiness and/or dizziness will be exacerbated with concomitant alcohol consumption; alcohol should be avoided while taking this medication.
- Caution clients not to stop taking drug abruptly if used long term.

Side Effects
- Hallucinations, behavior changes
- *Side effects that usually do not require medical attention:* nausea, daytime drowsiness, headache, vomiting, dizziness, diarrhea, dry mouth, nervousness, confusion, euphoria, hangover, vertigo, anaphylaxis, angioedema, and drug dependence

Drug Interactions
This medicine may interact with the following medications:
- Antacids may decrease sedative effects.
- *Digoxin:* This drug may increase digoxin level.
- *Diphenhydramine:* It may increase effects of both drugs.
- *Probenecid:* Probenecid causes rapid or prolonged temazepam effects.
- *Theophylline:* decreases sedative effects, antifungals, CNS depressants (including alcohol).
- *Herbs:* Calendula, kava, lemon balm, and valerian may enhance sedative effect.

Pharmacokinetics
- BZD, hypnotic.
- Mechanism of action is thought to occur at the level of the GABA receptor complex; acts on limbic system, thalamus and hypothalamus.
- Highly bound to plasma proteins.
- Peak plasma levels are reached in 1.2 to 1.6 hours.
- *Half-life:* Average is 8 to 12 hours.
- *Excretion:* Urine.

Precautions
- See patient as often as necessary if long-term use is indicated.

- Ensure that the patient is aware of the fact that they are not to exceed maximum dosage.
- Instruct patient to monitor for behavior changes.
- If patient is drowsy or dizzy, patient should not drive, use machinery, or attempt to accomplish any task that requires mental alertness.
- Avoid alcohol, as concomitant use may intensify side effects of CNS depression.

Patient and Family Education

- Store the drug at room temperature between 20°C and 25°C (59°F and 77°F).
- Discard unused medication after the expiration date.

Special Populations

- *Older adults*: Older adults are more sensitive to hypnotics. Use lowest effective dose, recommended 7.5 mg/d. Due to sedation and increased risk of falls, all BZDs are placed on the Beers List of Potentially Inappropriate Medications for Geriatrics.
- *Hepatic impairment*: Modify dosage accordingly.
- *Pregnancy*: category X.
- *Lactation*: No human studies have been performed. It is not recommended in breast-feeding mothers. Drug is excreted in breast milk.
- *Children*: It is not for use in children <18 years of age.

THIOTHIXENE (Navane)

Classification
Antipsychotic, thioxanthene

Available Forms
Capsule, 1, 2, 5, and 10 mg

Indications
Thiothixene is used to treat mild to moderate to severe psychosis.

Dosages
- Mild to moderate psychosis: adults and children age 12 and older: initially 2 mg PO TID.
- Increase gradually to 15 mg daily as needed.
- Severe psychosis: adults and children age 12 and older: initially, 5 mg PO BID.
- Increase gradually to 20 to 30 mg daily as needed. Maximum dose is 60 mg daily.

Administration
- Give drug without regard to food as per dosing schedule.
- Monitor for TD, which may occur at any time but especially after prolonged use. It may persist even though the drug was stopped.
- Watch for evidence of NMS.
- Watch for orthostatic hypotension.
- Withhold dose and notify prescriber if jaundice, blood dyscrasia, or persistent EPS develops, especially in pregnant women.

Pharmacokinetics
Unknown. Probably blocks dopamine receptors in brain. Onset, peak, and duration: unknown.

Side Effects
- *Central nervous system:* NMS, seizures, extrapyramidal reactions, sedation, TD, pseudoparkinsonism, dizziness, and drowsiness
- *Cardiovascular:* orthostatic hypotension, tachycardia, dystonia, and EKG changes
- *EENT:* blurred vision, nasal congestion, and ocular changes
- *Gastrointestinal:* dry mouth and constipation
- *Genitourinary:* urine retention, menstrual irregularities, breast enlargement, and inhibited ejaculation
- *Hematological:* agranulocytosis, transient leukopenia, and leukocytosis
- *Hepatic:* jaundice
- *Metabolic:* weight gain and hyperprolactinemia
- *Skin:* mild photosensitivity reactions, allergic reactions, and exfoliative dermatitis
- *Other:* gynecomastia

Drug Interactions
- *Central nervous system depressants*: It may increase CNS depression. Use together cautiously.

■ Alcohol use may increase CNS depression.
■ The drug may increase liver enzyme levels.
■ It may increase or decrease WBC counts.
■ It may decrease granulocyte counts.
■ The drug may cause false-positive results for urinary porphyria, urobilinogen, amylase, and 5-hydroxyindoleacetic acid tests that use human chorionic gonadotropin (HCG).

Precautions

■ Contraindicated in patients hypersensitive to drug and in those with CNS depression, circulatory collapse, coma, or blood dyscrasias.
■ Use with caution in patients with history of seizure disorder and in those undergoing alcohol withdrawal.
■ Use cautiously in older or debilitated patients and in those with CV disease (may cause sudden drop in BP), hepatic disease, heat exposure, glaucoma, or prostatic hyperplasia.
■ Neonates exposed in third trimester are at risk for developing EPS and withdrawal symptoms following delivery.
■ Use in pregnancy only if potential benefit to mother justifies risk to the fetus.

Patient Education

■ Discourage use of alcohol.
■ Warn patients to avoid activities that require alertness or good coordination until effects of drug are known.
■ Drowsiness and dizziness usually subside after the first few weeks.
■ Have patient report signs of urinary retention or constipation.
■ Sun exposure may increase photosensitivity reactions.
■ Relieve dry mouth with sugarless gum or hard candy.

Special Populations

■ *Pregnancy*: category C.
■ *Older adults*: BBW: not approved for use in older adults with dementia-related psychosis.
■ *Pediatric*: not recommended for use in children below age 12 years.

TRAZODONE HCL (Oleptro)

Classification

Serotonin-2 antagonist/reuptake inhibitor; antidepressant, triazolopyridine derivative

Indications

Trazodone is used to treat MDD, depression, insomnia, and to prevent migraine.

Available Forms

Tablet, 50, 100, 150, 200, 250, and 300 mg

Dosage

- *Adults*: Initially 150 mg/d in divided doses with food; increase by 50 mg/d q3d to q4d; maximum 400 mg/d in divided doses (outpatient) and 600 mg/d (inpatient)
- *Children younger than 18 years*: not recommended

Administration

Orally, taking with food decreases some side effects and increases absorption. Scored extended-relief tablets may be broken in half but should not be crushed or chewed.

Side Effects

The side effects are sedation, hypotension, nausea; may aid patients experiencing SSRI/SNRI-induced insomnia. Rare occurrences of priapism have been reported. This should be discussed with male clients. The most common reactions to this drug include somnolence, xerostomia, headache, sedation, dizziness, nausea/vomiting, blurred vision, fatigue, diarrhea, constipation, edema, abdominal discomfort, myalgia/arthralgia, nasal congestion, weight changes, confusion, ataxia, sexual dysfunction, syncope, tremor, ocular irritation, malaise, and HTN.

Drug Interactions

SSRIs may increase plasma concentrations. It may intensify the hypotensive effects of antihypertensive agents—"decreased dosage of HTN agent may be required." Patients taking MAOIs should not take this drug.

Pharmacokinetics

The drug is metabolized by CYP450 3A4 to an active metabolite in the liver and 75% is excreted in the urine (<1% unchanged) and 20% in the feces. It inhibits CNS uptake of serotonin; not a tricyclic derivative.

- *Peak:* 1 hour (without food); 2.5 hours (with food).
- *Onset:* 6 weeks (for antidepression); 1 to 3 hours (for sleep aid).
- *Half-life:* parent drug, 7 to 8 hours; active metabolite.

Precautions

- Do not use with MAOIs.
- Use with caution in patients with history of seizures.
- Use with caution in patients at risk for undiagnosed hyponatremia, bipolar disorder, priapism bleeding risk, volume depletion, alcohol use, cardiac disease, and QT prolongation.

Patient and Family Education

Notify the healthcare provider if the patient feels more depressed after initiation of therapy. Do not use alcohol while taking this drug. Do not stop taking this drug without talking to the healthcare provider.

Special Populations

- *Older adults:* Older individuals tend to be more sensitive to medication side effects, such as hypotension and anticholinergic effects. They often require adjustment of medication doses for hepatic or renal dysfunction. Older adults may be more sensitive to side effects and require a lower dosing regimen. Use the drug with caution due to sedative effects.
- *Pregnancy:* Psychotherapy is the initial choice for most pregnant patients with mild to moderate MDD. Category C; not advised during pregnancy as there are no adequate studies (similar to nefazodone). Animal studies show adverse fetal effect(s), but no controlled human studies have been conducted.
- *Lactation:* There is limited information in animals and/or humans that demonstrates no risk/minimal risk of adverse effects to infant/breast milk production.
- *Children:* not indicated for children.
- *Renal impairment:* Renal dosing is not defined.
- *Hepatic impairment:* Caution is advised in hepatic impairment.

TRIAZOLAM (Halcion)

Note: Rarely prescribed due to high risk of abuse. Not in most formularies.

Classification
Benzodiazepine (BZD) hypnotic

Indications
Triazolam is used for the treatment of insomnia.

Available Forms
Tablet, 0.125 and 0.25 mg

Dosage
- *Adults*: 0.125 to 0.25 mg qhs prn; short term, 7 to 10 days; maximum 0.5 mg; maximum 1 month
- *Children younger than 18 years*: not recommended

Administration
- PO with a glass of water.
- Drowsiness and/or dizziness will be exacerbated with concomitant alcohol consumption; alcohol should be avoided while taking this medication.
- Caution clients not to stop taking drug abruptly if used long term.

Side Effects
- Hallucinations, behavior changes.
- *Side effects that usually do not require medical attention*: nausea, daytime drowsiness, headache, vomiting, dizziness, diarrhea, dry mouth, nervousness, light-headedness, and ataxia.

Drug Interactions
This medicine may interact with the following medications: antifungals; CNS depressants (including alcohol), digoxin, macrolides, and phenytoin.

Pharmacokinetics
- BZD, hypnotic
- Mechanism of action is thought to occur at the level of the GABA receptor complex
- Highly bound to plasma proteins
- Peak plasma levels are reached in 1 to 2 hours
- Metabolized by CYP450 3A4, glucuronic acid conjugation
- Onset: 15 to 30 minutes
- Duration: 6 to 7 hours
- Excretion: urine
- *Half-life:* Average is 1.5 to 5.5 hours

Precautions
- See patient as often as necessary if long-term use is indicated.
- Ensure that patient is aware that they are not to exceed maximum dosage.
- Instruct patient to monitor for behavior changes.

- If patient is drowsy or dizzy, patient should not drive, use machinery, or attempt to accomplish any task that requires mental alertness.
- Avoid alcohol, as concomitant use may exacerbate symptoms.

Patient and Family Education

- Store at room temperature between 20°C and 25°C (59°F and 77°F).
- Throw away any unused medication after the expiration date.

Special Populations

- *Older adults*: Older adults are more sensitive to hypnotics. Use lowest effective dose, typically 0.125 mg. Due to sedation and increased risk of falls, all BZDs are placed on the Beers List of Potentially Inappropriate Medications for Geriatrics.
- *Hepatic impairment*: Modify dosage accordingly.
- *Pregnancy*: category X; absolute contraindication.
- *Lactation*: No human studies have been performed. Not recommended in breast-feeding mothers. Drug is excreted in breast milk.
- *Children*: not for use in children younger than 18 years of age.

ZALEPLON (Sonata)

Classification
Non-benzodiazepine gamma-aminobutyric acid (GABA) receptor agonist

Indications
Zaleplon is indicated for the treatment of insomnia when a middle-of-the-night awakening is followed by difficulty returning to sleep.

Available Forms
Capsule, 5 and 10 mg

Dosage
- *Adults and children older than 12 years*: 5 to 10 mg at HS or after going to bed if unable to sleep; do not take if unable to sleep for at least 4 hours before requiring to be active again; maximum 20 mg/d × 1 month; delayed effect if taken with a meal
- *Children younger than 12 years*: not recommended

Administration
- PO with a glass of water.
- Avoid taking the drug within 2 hours of a fatty meal.
- Drowsiness and/or dizziness will be exacerbated with concomitant alcohol consumption; alcohol should be avoided while taking this medication.

Side Effects
Complex Sleep Behavior
- Hallucinations; behavior changes; SSRIs-treated patients taking zaleplon may experience impaired concentration, aggravated depression, and manic reaction; may cause amnesia. In most cases, memory problems can be avoided if zaleplon is taken only when the patient is able to get more than 4 hours of sleep before being active.
- *Side effects that usually do not require medical attention*: nausea, daytime drowsiness, headache, vomiting, dizziness, and diarrhea.

Drug Interactions
This medicine may interact with the following medications: antifungals, chlorpromazine, flumazenil, clarithromycin, rifamycin, ritonavir, SSRIs, CNS depressants (including alcohol), amiodarone, and verapamil.

Pharmacokinetics
Non-BZDs are hypnotics of the pyrazolopyrimidines class. Mechanism of action is thought to occur at the level of the GABA-BZ receptor complex.
- Peak plasma levels are reached in 1 hour.
- Bioavailability is 30%.
- *Peak*: 1 hour.
- *Duration*: shorter than zolpidem.
- *Excretion*: urine (70%), feces (17%).
- *Half-life*: Average is 1 hour.

Precautions

- Ensure that patient is aware that they are not to exceed maximum dosage.
- Patient should not take this medication unless prepared to sleep for at least 4 hours.
- Instruct patient to monitor for behavior changes.
- If patient is drowsy or dizzy, patient should not drive, use machinery, or attempt to accomplish any task that requires mental alertness.
- Avoid alcohol, as concomitant use may exacerbate symptoms.

Patient and Family Education

Store the drug at room temperature. Throw away any unused medication after the expiration date. An FDA-approved patient medication guide, which is available with the product information, must be dispensed with this medication.

Special Populations

- *Older adults*: Older adults are more sensitive to hypnotics. Use no more than 5 mg.
- *Hepatic impairment*: Modify dosage accordingly in patients with hepatic function impairment.
- *Pregnancy*: category C.
- *Lactation*: No human studies have been performed. It is not recommended in breast-feeding mothers.
- *Children*: not recommended in children younger than 12 years.

ZIPRASIDONE (Geodon)

Classification
Second-generation (atypical) antipsychotic

Indications
This drug is used for acute and maintenance treatment of mixed episodes in bipolar I disorder, as monotherapy, or as adjunct to lithium or valproic acid.

Available Forms
Capsule, 20, 40, 60, and 80 mg

Dosage
- *Adults and children older than 12 years*: Take with food; initially 40 mg BID; on day 2, may increase to 60 to 80 mg BID
- *Older adults*: Lower initial dose and titrate slowly
- *Children younger than 12 years*: not recommended

Administration
- Take this medication with a meal.
- Dosing at 20 to 40 mg BID is too low and activating, perhaps due to potent 5HT2C antagonist properties. Reduce activation by increasing the dose to 60 to 80 mg BID.
- Best efficacy in schizophrenia and bipolar disorder is at doses >120 mg/d.
- Measure body mass index monthly for 3 months, and then quarterly.
- Monitor fasting triglycerides monthly for several months in patients at high risk for metabolic complications.
- BP, fasting plasma glucose, fasting lipids within 3 months and then annually, but earlier and more frequently for patients with diabetes or who have gained more than 5% of initial weight.

Side Effects
- Nausea, constipation, dyspepsia, cough, anorexia, myalgia
- Dizziness, sedation, and hypotension, especially at high doses
- Motor side effects (rare)
- Possible increased incidence of diabetes or dyslipidemia is unknown

Drug Interactions
- It may enhance the effects of antihypertensive drugs.
- It may antagonize levodopa with dronedarone, artemether, lumefantrine, metoclopramide, nilotinib, pimozide, quinine, thioridazine, tetrabenazine, and dopamine agonists.
- It may also enhance QTc prolongation of other drugs capable of prolonging QTc interval agents.

Pharmacokinetics
- *Protein binding*: >99%.
- *Metabolism*: The drug is metabolized by CYP450 3A4. Hepatic via aldehyde oxidase; less than one third is via cytochrome P450 system.

- *Absorption*: must be given PO with food to obtain 60% bioavailability; 100% (IM).
- *Onset*: PO, 6 to 8 hours; 30 minutes to 2 hours.
- *Duration:* 2 hours.
  - Peak: 6 to 8 hours (PO), <60 minutes (IM).
  - Excretion: urine (20%), feces (66%).
- *Half-life:* 6.6 hours.

Precautions

- The drug prolongs QTc interval more than some other antipsychotics.
- Use with caution in patients with conditions that predispose them to hypotension (dehydration, overheating).
- Priapism has been reported.
- Dysphagia has been associated with antipsychotic use and should be used cautiously in patients at risk for aspiration pneumonia.
- Do not use the drug if patient is taking agents capable of prolonging QTc interval (pimozide, thioridazine, selected antiarrhythmics, moxifloxacin, sparfloxacin).
- Do not use it if there is a history of QTc prolongation, cardiac arrhythmia, recent acute myocardial infarction, or prolonged QT congenital.
- Long QT syndrome, recent myocardial infarction, uncompensated heart failure, or other QTc-prolonging arrhythmias.
- Do not use it if there is a proven allergy to ziprasidone.
- EPS, NMS, temperature regulation, dementia, and electrolyte imbalance.
- Use IM formulation with caution in patients with renal impairment due to accumulation of cyclodextrin.
- Seizures, excessive sedation.

Patient and Family Education

- Take oral formulation with a meal of a few hundred calories (e.g., turkey sandwich and a piece of fruit) to enhance the absorption.
- *Avoid becoming overheated or dehydrated during exercise and in hot weather.* You may be more prone to heat stroke.
- *Avoid getting up too fast from a sitting or lying position.* Get up slowly and steady yourself to prevent a fall.
- *Avoid drinking alcohol.*
- *Stop using this medication and call provider immediately* if you have very stiff (rigid) muscles, high fever, sweating, confusion, fast or uneven heartbeats, tremors; feel like you might pass out; have jerky muscle movements you cannot control, trouble swallowing, problems with speech; have blurred vision, have eye pain, or see halos around lights; have increased thirst and urination, excessive hunger, fruity breath odor, weakness, nausea and vomiting; have fever, chills, body aches, flu symptoms; or have white patches or sores inside your mouth or on your lips.
- *Do not stop taking* the drug suddenly without first talking to provider, even if you feel fine. You may have serious side effects if you stop taking the drug suddenly.
- Call provider if symptoms do not improve or get worse.
- Store the drug at room temperature away from moisture and heat.

Special Populations

- *Renal impairment*: No dose adjustment is necessary.
- *Hepatic impairment*: No dose adjustment is necessary.

- *Cardiac impairment*: Contraindicated in patients with a known history of QTc prolongation, recent AMI, and uncompensated heart failure.
- *Pregnancy:* category C; some animal studies show adverse effects. There are no controlled studies in humans.
- *Lactation:* It is not known whether it is secreted in breast milk. Either discontinue the use of the drug or bottle-feed.
- *Children and adolescents*: not recommended for children younger than 12 years.

ZOLPIDEM (Ambien, Ambien CR, Edluar, Intermezzo, Zolpimist)

Classification
Non-benzodiazepine gamma-aminobutyric acid (GABA) receptor agonist

Indications
This drug is used for the treatment of insomnia.

Available Forms
Tablet, 5 and 10 mg; tablet (XR), 6.25 and 12.5 mg; tablet (sublingual), 1.75, 3.5, 5, and 10 mg; oral solution spray, 5 mg/actuation (60 m actuations)

Dosage
Tablet
- *Adults*: 5 to 10 mg or 6.25 to 12.5 XR qhs prn; maximum 12.5 mg/d × 1 month; do not take if unable to sleep for at least 8 hours before requiring to be active again; delayed effect if taken with a meal
- *Children younger than 18 years*: not recommended

Sublingual Tablet
- *Adults*: Dissolve 1 tablet under the tongue; allow to disintegrate completely before swallowing; take only once per night and only if at least 4 hours of bedtime remain before planned time for awakening
- *Children younger than 18 years*: not recommended

Oral Solution Spray
- *Adults*: 2 actuations (10 mg) immediately before bedtime; older adults, debilitated, or with hepatic impairment: 2 actuations (5 mg); maximum 2 actuations (10 mg)
- *Children younger than 18 years*: not recommended

Administration
- PO with a glass of water.
- Take at least 2 hours after a meal.
- Drowsiness and/or dizziness will be exacerbated with concomitant alcohol consumption; alcohol should be avoided while taking this medication.
- Caution clients not to stop taking drug abruptly if used long term.

Side Effects
- Hallucinations, sedation; behavior changes; SSRI-treated patients taking zolpidem may experience impaired concentration, aggravated depression, and manic reaction.
- *Side effects that usually do not require medical attention*: nausea, daytime drowsiness, headache, vomiting, dizziness, and diarrhea.

Drug Interactions
This medicine may interact with the following medications: antifungals, chlorpromazine, flumazenil, imipramine, rifamycin, ritonavir, SSRIs, and CNS depressants (including alcohol).

Pharmacokinetics

- Non-BZDs hypnotic of the imidazopyridine class. Mechanism of action is thought to occur at the level of the GABA receptor complex.
- Highly bound to plasma proteins.
- Peak plasma levels are reached in 1.6 hours.
- *Half-life*: Average is 2.6 hours (PO).
- *Excretion*: urine (48%–67%), feces (29%–42%).

Precautions

- See patient as often as necessary if long-term use is indicated.
- Ensure that patient is aware that they are not to exceed maximum dosage.
- Instruct patient to monitor for behavior changes.
- If patient is drowsy or dizzy, patient should not drive, use machinery, or attempt to accomplish any task that requires mental alertness.
- Avoid alcohol, as concomitant use may exacerbate symptoms.

Patient and Family Education

- Store at room temperature between 20°C and 25°C (59°Fand 77°F).
- Discard unused medication after the expiration date.
- An FDA-approved patient medication guide, which is available with the product information, must be dispensed with this medication.

Special Populations

- *Older adults*: Older adults are more sensitive to hypnotics. Use no more than 5 mg.
- *Hepatic impairment:* Modify dosage accordingly.
- *Pregnancy*: category C.
- *Lactation*: No human studies have been performed. Not recommended in breast-feeding mothers.
- *Children*: not recommend for children younger than 18 years.

Note: For some drugs, off-label use is reported. It is the responsibility of the practitioner to evaluate the efficacy of such use.

Index

Aberrant Behavior Checklist, 335
Abilify, 370–372
Abilify Discmelt, 370–372
Abilify Maintena, 370–372
Abnormal Involuntary Movement Scale
    (AIMS), 121
absorption, 53–55
acamprosate, 359–361
acetylcholine (ACh), 40–41, 44
action potential, 39
active transport, 55
acupuncture, 191
acute hypomanic episode, 147, 159
acute mania, 65
acute manic episode, 147
acute MDE, 147
acute psychotic symptoms, 124
acute stress disorder, 9
Adderall, 290, 432–434
Adderall XR, 432–434
ADHD. *See* attention deficit hyperactivity
    disorder
adipose tissue, 56
adjustment disorders, 9
  with anxiety, 9
  with depressed mood, 9
  with disturbance of conduct, 9
  with mixed anxiety and depressed mood, 9
  with mixed disturbance of emotions and
      conduct, 9
  unspecified, 9
Adler, Alfred, 33–34
adrenergic-mediated responses, 45

advanced sleep phase type, 285
affect, 7
aggression
  behavior, 65
  CD, 328
  cyclothymic disorder, 159
  handling, 147
agitation and aggression, 65–66
agoraphobia, 9
  definition of disorder, 185–186
  demographics, 186
  diagnosis, 186–187
  etiology, 186
  medical/legal pitfalls, 187
  patient education, 187
  psychopharmacology, 187
  risk factors, 186
  treatment, 187
agranulocytosis, 120
albumin, 55, 264
alcohol
  abuse, 328
  antagonists, 87
  pharmacological treatment, 86
  withdrawal symptoms, 86
Alcoholics Anonymous (AA), 86
alcohol use disorder (AUD)
  definition of disorder, 88
  diagnosis, 88–89
  treatment, 89–90
alogia, 116
alpha-agonists, 87
alprazolam, 280, 362–364

alprostadil, 245, 365–366
alternatives investigation, 8
Ambien, 588–589
Ambien CR, 588–589
amino acids, 44
Aminoketones, 317
amitriptyline, 265, 280, 367–369
amphetamines, 65, 123, 215, 290, 317, 323, 432–434
Amrix, 421–422
AN. *See* anorexia nervosa
Anafranil, 265, 280, 408–410
analgesia, 59
Analgesic + first-generation antihistamine combination, 287
androgen and gender dysphoria, 247
animal therapy, 323
anorexia nervosa (AN), 9
  associated features, 257–258
  complications, 259
  definition of disorder and diagnostic criteria, 257
  demographics, 259
  diagnosis, 260–263
  medical/legal pitfalls, 266–267
  patient education, 266
  prevalence and etiology, 258–259
  risk factors, 260
  treatment, 263–266
Antabuse, 88, 439–441
antacids, 55
antagonists, 59
anticholinergic drugs, 87
anticholinergics, 11
antidepressants, 11, 59, 88, 106, 111, 123, 147, 149, 243, 252, 267, 273
antidiarrheal drugs, 87
antihistamines, 191, 233
anti-narcoleptic agents, 285
antinuclear antibody (ANA), 141
antipsychotic agents, 111, 120
antipsychotic medications, 101, 121
antipsychotics, 67, 147, 243, 252, 266
antisocial behaviors, 305
antisocial personality disorder (ASPD), 10
  definition of disorder, 301
  demographics, 301
  diagnosis, 302–303
  etiology, 301
  medical/legal pitfalls, 304–305

  patient education, 304
  risk factors, 302
  treatment, 303–304
anxiety disorders, 34, 80, 139–140, 191
  agoraphobia, 185–187
  anxiety disorder due to another medical condition, 193–194
  due to another medical condition, 193–194
  generalized anxiety disorder (GAD), 188–191
  panic disorder, 183–185
  phobias and social anxiety, 176–181
  selective mutism, 174–176
  separation anxiety disorder, 171–174
  social anxiety disorder, 181–183
  specific phobia, 181
  substance-/medication-induced anxiety disorder, 192–193
  unspecified anxiety disorder, 194
anxiety-related disorders, 139
anxiolytics, 11, 191, 233
Aplenzin, 395–397
Apo-Alpraz, 362–364
Apo-Alpraz Ts, 362–364
appearance, mental status examination, 6
applied behavioral analysis (ABA), 322
arbitrary inference, 25
archetypes concept, 32
Aricept, 78, 447–448
Aricept ODT, 447–448
aripiprazole, 111, 118, 124, 370–372
armodafinil, 285, 293, 373–374
aromatherapy, 191
arousal difficulties, 246
Art therapy, 323
asenapine, 111, 118, 375–377
ASPD. *See* antisocial personality disorder
Asperger's syndrome, 319
assigned sex at birth (ASAB), 248
Atarax, 480–481
Ativan, 102, 503–504
atomoxetine, 318
atomoxetine hydrochloride, 378–379
attention deficit hyperactivity disorder (ADHD), 154
  definition of disorder, 313
  demographics, 313
  diagnosis, 314–316
  etiology, 313
  hyperactivity-impulsivity symptoms, 316
  medical/legal pitfalls, 318–319

patient education, 318
risk factors, 314
treatment, 316–318
attitude/rapport, 6
atypical antipsychotics, 67, 149, 161
delusional disorder, 106
drugs, 101
atypical anxiolytics, 81
atypical (second generation) antipsychotic
drugs, schizophrenia, 117
atypical second-generation antipsychotics, 226
AUD. *See* alcohol use disorder
Autism Behavior Checklist, 321
Autism diagnostic interview, 321
Autism Screening Questionnaire, 321
autism spectrum disorder
definition of disorder, 319
demographics, 320
diagnosis, 320–322
etiology, 319
medical/legal pitfalls, 324–325
patient education, 324
risk factors, 320
treatment, 322–324
autistic disorders, 116, 319
automatic thoughts, 24
autonomic dysfunction, 68
autonomic nervous system (ANS), 43, 242
avanafil, 380–381
axonal conduction, 46

baby talk, 338
barbiturates, 123
basal ganglia, 46
B complex, 382–383
Beck Depression Inventory, 12, 132
BED. *See* binge-eating disorder
behavioral therapy, 23–24, 135
behavior therapy and cognitive therapy, 11
Benadryl, 443–444
Bentyl, 437–438
benzodiazepines (BZDs), 66–69, 87, 89–90, 97,
101, 123, 149, 173, 179, 185, 187, 191,
226, 233, 274, 280, 287, 351
benztropine, 119
betablockers, 179, 226
binge-eating disorder (BED)
definition of disorder, 275
demographics, 276
diagnosis, 277–278

etiology, 275–276
family history, 276–277
medical/legal pitfalls, 280–281
patient education, 280
pharmacotherapy, 279–280
risk factors, 276
treatment, 278–279
binge-eating/purging type of AN, 258, 275
bioequivalence, 53
biotransformation, 57
bipolar disorder, 9
Bipolar I, 146
Bipolar II, 146
definition of disorder, 137
demographics, 138
diagnosis, 141–145
etiology, 137–138
hypomanic episode, 146
major depressive episode, 145–146
manic episode, 145
medical/legal pitfalls, 151
patient education, 150–151
psychopharmacology, 149–150
rapid cycling, 146
risk factors, 138–140
treatment, 146–149
Bipolar I or II disorder, 146, 150, 154
Bipolar Spectrum Diagnostic Scale (BSDS), 142
bipolar spectrum disorders
risk factors for harm to others in, 155
risk factors for suicidal behavior in, 154
bismuth subsalicylate, 384–385
Black box warning, 318
blood-brain barrier, 44, 56
BN. *See* bulimia nervosa
body dysmorphic disorder, 10
definition of disorder, 204
demographics, 204
diagnosis, 205–206
environment, 204
etiology, 204
genetics and physiology, 204
medical/legal pitfalls, 207
patient education, 207
psychopharmacology, 206
treatment, 206
Body Dysmorphic Disorder Questionnaire, 205
Body Dysmorphic Disorder-Yale Brown
Obsessive Compulsive Scale (BDD-
YBOCS), 205

body-focused repetitive behavior disorder, 218
body mass index (BMI), 120
bone mineral density, 261
borderline personality disorder (BPD), 10
   definition of disorder, 305
   demographics, 305
   diagnosis, 306–307
   etiology, 305
   medical/legal pitfalls, 308–309
   patient education, 308
   risk factors, 306
   treatment, 307–308
brain and spinal cord, 44
breakfast, feeding and eating disorders, 263
Brexpiprazole, 111, 118
brief psychotic disorders, 10
   definition of disorder, 99
   demographics, 99
   diagnosis, 99–101
   etiology, 99
   medical/legal pitfalls, 103
   patient education, 102
   risk factors, 99–100
   treatment, 101–102
bromocriptine, 387
bromocriptine mesylate, 386–388
bulimia nervosa (BN), 9, 260
   definition of disorder, 267
   demographics, 268–269
   diagnosis, 269–271
   etiology, 268
   family history, 269
   medical/legal pitfalls, 274–275
   patient education, 274
   pharmacotherapy, 273–274
   risk factors, 269
   treatment, 271–273
buprenex, 389–391
buprenorphine, 389–394
buprenorphine HCL, 389–391
bupropion, 134, 318, 395–397
bupropion hydrobromide, 395–397
bupropion hydrochloride, 395–397
buspirone, 190
butrans, 389–391
BZD. *See* benzodiazepines

CAGE (cut down, annoyed, guilty, and eye
   opener) screening questionnaire, 85, 110
Calcium channel moderator, 190, 233

California Verbal Learning Test (CVLT), 353
Campral, 359–361
cannabis, 39, 91, 123
   definition of disorder, 91
   diagnosis, 91–92
   treatment, 92
carbamazepine, 226, 280, 398–402
Carbatrol, 398–402
cardiac arrhythmias, 264
cardiovascular/medical issues, 242
cardiovascular mortality, 148, 153
Cariprazine, 111, 118
castration complex, 29
cataplexy, 292–293
Catapres, 318, 413–414
Catapres-TTS, 413–414
catastrophizing, 25
Caverject, 365–366
Caverject Impulse, 365–366
Celexa, 405–407
cell membrane-embedded enzymes and
   transporters, 59
central nervous system (CNS), 43–45
chief complaint (CC), 6
Childhood Autism Rating Scale, 321
childhood disintegrative disorder, 319
childhood-onset fluency disorder, 325–328
   definition of disorder, 325
   demographics, 325
   diagnosis, 325–327
   etiology, 325
   medical/legal pitfalls, 328
   patient education, 327–328
   risk factors, 325
   treatment, 327
childhood sexual abuse (CSA), 305
children, gender dysphoria in, 246
Children's version of Y-BOCS (CY-BOCS),
   201
chlordiazepoxide hydrochloride, 403–404
chlorpromazine, 101
cholinergic-mediated responses, 45
cholinesterase inhibitors, 78
chronic hyperprolactinemia, 242
chronic pain, 130
chronic prostatitis/chronic pelvic pain
   syndrome (CP/CPPS), 253
chronic renal failure, 243
Cialis, 573–574
cimetidin, 74

circadian rhythm disorder (CRSD)
  definition of disorder, 283
  diagnosis, 284
  epidemiology, 283–284
  patient education, 285
  treatment, 284–285
circumstantiality, 7
cisapride, 265
citalopram, 184
citalopram hydrochloride, 405–407
CIWA-Ar Scale (Clinical Institute
    Withdrawal Assessment for Alcohol
    scale), 85, 89
classic neurotransmission, 39
client-centered therapy, 33
clinical decision making, 8
clinical neuroanatomy, 43
clinical neuropharmacology, 43
Clinical Opioid Withdrawal scale (COW),
    94–95
clinical psychopharmacology
  nervous system, 43–47
  neuropharmacology, 48–51
  neurotransmitters, 47–49
clinical reasoning and decision making, 8
Clinical Worsening and Suicide Risk label,
    267
clock-drawing test, 12, 77
clomipramine, 203, 265, 280, 408–410
clonazepam, 280, 411–412
clonidine, 226, 318
clonidine hydrochloride, 413–414
clorazepate, 415–416
clozapine, 111, 118, 120, 417–420
Clozapine, 118
Clozaril, 417–420
Clutter Image Rating (CIR), 208
cocaine, 65, 123, 130, 215
  and other stimulant use disorder
    definition of disorder, 92
    diagnosis, 93–94
    treatment, 94
  pharmacological treatment, 86
Cocaine Anonymous (CA), 86
codeine, 123
Cognex, 571–572
cognitive and personality factors, 129–130
cognitive behavioral therapy (CBT), 23, 106,
    178, 209, 264, 303
  cognitive distortions, 25

dialectical behavioral therapy (DBT), 27
  evidence-based applications, 26–27
  fundamental features, 24–25
  interactive techniques, 25–26
  psychoeducation, 25
  therapist qualities, 26
cognitive conceptualization, 25
cognitive disconnection, 228
cognitive distortions, 25
cognitive therapeutic approaches, delusional
    disorders, 108
cognitive therapy, 23, 226, 229
competitive antagonists, 60
complementary and alternative medicine
    (CAM), 191
complete blood count (CBC), 132
complete metabolic panel, 132
Composite International Diagnostic Interview
    (CIDI), 5
Comprehensive metabolic panel (CMP), 244
compulsions, 202
Concerta, 518–520
concurrent pharmacotherapy, 53
conduct disorder
  definition of disorder, 328
  demographics, 328
  diagnosis, 329–330
  etiology, 328
  medical/legal pitfalls, 331
  risk factors, 328
  treatment, 330–331
connection, clinical decision making, 8
Connor's Parent and Teacher Rating Scale,
    315
consensus guidelines, 67–68
controlled release (CR) formulations, 54
conventional (typical) antipsychotic
    medications, 101
conversion disorder, 10
corticotropin-releasing hormone (CRH), 129
cortisol hypersecretion, 153
Cotempla XR-ODT, 518–520
cotinine, 123
countertransference, 32
couple's problem, 254
CRH. *See* corticotropin-releasing hormone
CRSD. *See* circadian rhythm disorder
cyclobenzaprine, 421–422
Cycloset, 386–388
cyclothymia, 151

cyclothymic disorder, 9, 152
  cyclothymic disorder, 158
  definition of disorder, 151–152
  demographics, 153
  diagnosis, 155–157
  dysthymia, 157–158
  etiology, 152–153
  hypomanic, 158–159
  hypomanic episode, 157
  medical/legal pitfalls, 163
  patient education, 162–163
  risk factors, 153–155
  treatment, 159–162
Cymbalta, 191, 451–453
cyproheptadine, 69, 265, 423–424
cytochrome P450 (CYP), 57

Dalmane, 471–472
DAN (Defeat Autism Now!) protocol, 321
DBT. *See* dialectical behavioral therapy
decision-making process, 8
defense mechanisms, 30–31
degrees of dysfluency, 326
dehydration, 264
delayed sleep phase type, 285
delirium, 65, 68
  clinical presentation, 73
  definition of disorder, 71
  demographic, 72
  diagnostic workup, 73
  differential diagnosis, 72
  DSM-5 diagnostic guidelines, 73
  etiology, 71–72
  ICD-10 codes, 72–73
  initial assessment, 73
  medical/legal pitfalls, 74–75
  patient education, 74
  risk factors, 72
  treatment, 74
delusional disorder, 7, 65, 99, 116
  definition of disorder, 103
  demographics, 103
  diagnosis, 104–105
  etiology, 103
  medical/legal pitfalls, 108
  patient education, 108
  psychopharmacology, 106–108
  risk factors, 104
  treatment, 105–106
dementia, 20, 65
Depacon, 444–446

Depakene, 444–446
Depakote, 444–446
Depakote ER, 444–446
Depakote Sprinkle, 444–446
dependent personality disorder, 10
depersonalization-derealization syndrome, 9
  definition of disorder, 227
  demographics, 227
  diagnosis, 228–229
  etiology, 227
  medical/legal pitfalls, 230
  risk factors, 228
  treatment, 229–230
depressants, 83
depression, 20–21, 137, 267, 360
  and anxiety, 242
  symptoms in AN, 258
depression disorder (DD), 397
desensitization, 60
desensitizing agents, 254
desipramine, 425–426
desvenlafaxine, 427–429
development history, 6
Dexedrine, 290, 432–434
Dexedrine Spansule, 432–434
dexmethylphenidate, 430–431
dextroamphetamine, 290, 432–434
DextroStat, 432–434
diagnosis-specific questions, 5, 12
diagnostic encounter, phases
  body of interview, 6
  closing phase, 6
  opening phase, 5–6
diagnostic formulation, 8
dialectical behavioral therapy (DBT), 27, 118
Diastat, 435–436
Diastat acudial, 435–436
diazepam, 102, 149, 435–436
dichotomous thinking, 25
dicyclomine, 437–438
diencephalon, 44
dieting, 260
dietitian, 279. *See also* binge-eating disorder
diphenhydramine, 119
diphenhydramine hydrochloride, 443–444
disorganized speech, 99
dissociative amnesia, 9
  definition of disorder, 230
  demographics, 231
  diagnosis, 231–232
  medical/legal pitfalls, 233–234

patient education, 233
risk factors, 231
treatment, 232–233
dissociative disorders, 9
depersonalization/derealization disorder, 227–230
dissociative amnesia, 230–234
dissociative identity disorder, 223–227
specified, 234
unspecified, 234
Dissociative Experiences Scale (DES), 225
dissociative fugue, 9
dissociative identity (multiple personality) disorder, 9
definition of disorder, 223
demographics, 224
diagnosis, 224–225
etiology, 224
medical/legal pitfalls, 27
risk factors, 224
treatment, 225–227
distribution, 55–56
distrust, 4
disulfiram, 88, 439–441
divalproex sodium, 444–446
doctor shopping, 88
Dolophine, 509–511
donepezil hydrochloride, 447–448
dopamine, 40–41
antagonist, 327
receptor agonists, 298
dopaminergic neurons, 38
Down syndrome, 335
doxepin, 449–450
dream material, 31
dronabinol, 265
drug action mechanisms, 59
Drug Addiction Treatment Act (DATA) of 2000, 390
drug dissolution, 54
drug-drug interactions, 55, 60
drug-induced erectile dysfunction, 239
drug-receptor interactions, 50, 59–60
drug side effects, 59
drug-specific variables, 53
drug therapy for agitation in psychiatric emergencies, 66
DSM-5 disorders and ICD-10 Codes, 8–10
adjustment disorders, 9
dissociative disorders, 9
eating disorders, 9

impulse control disorders, 9
mood disorders, 9
personality disorders, 10
psychotic disorders, 10
sexual disorders, 9
sexual dysfunctions, 10
sleep disorders, 9–10
somatoform disorders, 10
substance disorders, 10
dual-energy X-ray absorptiometry (DXA), 261
duloxetine, 191, 451–453
dysesthetic sensations, 297
dyslexia
definition of disorder, 331
demographics, 331
diagnosis, 332–333
etiology, 331
medical/legal pitfalls, 333
patient education, 333
risk factors, 331
treatment, 333
dyspareunia, 10
dysthymic disorder, 9, 131, 157–158. *See also* persistent depressive disorder

eating disorders, 9
ECT. *See* electroconvulsive therapy
ECT, bipolar disorder, 148
EDEX, 365–366
Edluar, 588–589
efficacy, 60
ejaculation. *See* premature ejaculation
Elavil, 265, 280
electrical impulses, 39
electroconvulsive therapy (ECT), 11, 112, 135, 229
electrolyte imbalance, 264
E-medicine, 251
emotional distress, 23
emotional expressions, 4
emotional reasoning, 25
employment programs, 121
endocrine dysfunction, 242
endocrinopathies, 65
endogenous neurotransmitters, 42
enteric coating, 54
enterohepatic recirculation, 54
enzyme-linked immunosorbent assay (ELISA), 142
Epworth Sleepiness Scale, 289
Equetro, 398–402

erectile disorder
  atherosclerosis, 238
  definition of disorder, 237
  demographics, 238
  diagnosis, 238–240
  etiology, 237–238
  medical/legal pitfalls, 241
  patient education, 241
  risk factors, 238
  treatment, 240–241
  vascular disease, 238
erectile dysfunction, 239
Erectile Dysfunction Inventory of Treatment
    Satisfaction (EDITS), 239
Erikson, Erik, 33
Eros, 245
erythrocyte sedimentation rate, 261
escitalopram, 184, 454–457
Estradiol, 261
estrogen therapy, 251
eszopiclone, 458–459
euthymic, 110
evidence-based clinical decision making, 8
Evzio, 531–532
excitation-secretion coupling, 39
excoriation disorder
  definition of disorder, 212
  demographics, 213
  diagnosis, 213–214
  etiology, 212
  genetics and physiology, 213
  medical/legal pitfalls, 214
  patient education, 214
  psychopharmacology, 214
  treatment, 214
excretion, 58
Exelon, 78, 562–563
  oral solution, 562–563
  patch, 562–563
exercise therapy, 279
exhibitionism, 9
exposure and response prevention (ERP), 203
expressive therapy, 226, 229
extrapyramidal symptoms (EPS), 119
Eye Movement Desensitization and
    Reprocessing (EMDR), 226

family history (FH), 6
family-oriented therapies, 121
family therapy, 11, 124, 226, 229, 265

Fanapt, 484–485
fasting blood glucose, 120
fat-free foods, 264
faulty thinking, 23
Fazaclo, 417–420
fear and anorexia nervosa (AN), 257
Federal Drug Administration black box
    warning, 167
feeding and eating disorders
  anorexia nervosa (AN), 257–267
  binge-eating disorder (BED), 275–281
  bulimia nervosa, 267–275
female androgen insufficiency, 243
female orgasmic disorder, 10
female sexual interest/arousal disorder,
    10, 242
  definition of disorder, 241–242
  demographics, 243
  diagnosis, 243–245
  etiology, 242
  medical/legal pitfalls, 246
  patient education, 246
  risk factors, 243
  treatment, 245
Fetishism, 9
Fetzima, 494–495
Fexmid, 421–422
FH. See family history
first-degree biological relatives, cyclothymic
    disorder, 152
first-generation antipsychotics (FGAs), 60,
    111, 118
first-line therapy, 67
first-pass effect, 54
Flexeril, 421–422
flexible batteries, 15
flibanserin, 245
flight of ideas, 7
fluoxetine, 175, 184, 187, 203, 254
fluoxetine hydrochloride, 460–463
fluphenazine decanoate, 468–470
fluphenazine hydrochloride, 468–470
flurazepam, 471–472
fluvoxamine, 184, 203, 464–467
Focalin, 427–431
Focalin ER, 427–431
Focalin XR, 427–431
focused attentiveness, 26
Follicle Stimulating Hormone (FSH), 261
food-drug interactions, 55

forbidden foods, 258
forebrain, 44
forensic psychiatrists, 304
formal interview, 4
Freud, Anna, 33
Freud's Personality Theory, 27–29
    The Structural Model (ca. 1920), 28–29
    The Topographic Model (1900), 27–28
frontostriatal and temporoparietaloccipital
        circuits, 204
frotteurism, 9
functional impairment level, 143

GABAergic neurons, 38
GAD. *See* generalized anxiety disorder
galantamine hydrobromide, 473–474
gamma-aminobutyric acid (GABA), 40–42,
        48–49, 287, 298
gastric motility, 265
gastric motor activity, 274
gastroesophageal reflux disease (GERD), 321
gender dysphoria, 246–251
    in adults and adolescents, 246–247
    associated with disorder of sex
        development, 247
    in children, 246
    definition of disorder, 246
    demographics, 248
    diagnosis, 249
    etiology, 247–248
    medical/legal pitfalls, 251
    patient education, 251
    risk factors, 248
    specified gender dysphoria, 247
    treatment, 249–251
    unspecified, 247
gender identity disorder, 10
    of childhood, 249
gender reassignment surgery, 250
gene expression, 40
generalized anxiety disorder (GAD), 9
    definition of disorder, 188
    demographics, 188
    diagnosis, 188–189
    in elderly, 80–81
    etiology, 188
    family history, 188
    medical/legal pitfalls, 191
    mental health disorder, 188
    patient education, 191

stressful events in susceptible people, 188
    treatment, 190–191
genital or nongenital sensations, 242
genitourinary examination, 7
Geodon, 585–587
Gl-Lytely, 265
glucocorticoid receptor, 59
glutamate, 40, 42
glutamatergic neurons, 38
Glycolax, 265
G protein-coupled receptors (GPCRs), 59
graduate education, 26
Grandiose thinking, 146
grossly disorganized or catatonic behavior, 99
group psychotherapy, 11, 250
group therapy, 124, 167, 226, 229, 265
guanfacine, 318
guanfacine hydrochloride, 475–476
guanosine triphosphate (GTP)-binding
        protein, 59
Guided discovery, 26

Habitrol, 536–538
Halcion, 581–582
Haldol, 101, 477–479
Haldol lactate, 477–479
half-life, 58
hallucinations, 7, 99, 116
hallucinogenic use disorder, 91
hallucinogens, 83, 130, 228
haloperidol, 101, 106, 111, 118
    intramuscular (IM), 117
haloperidol decanoate, 477–479
haloperidol lactate, 477–479
Hamilton Depression Scale, 12, 110
harm to others in bipolar spectrum
        disorders, 140
heart failure, 264
heroin, 123
high lipid solubility, 55
high-potency drugs, 60
hindbrain, 45
hippocampus, 46
histamine, 44
history of present illness (HPI), 6
histrionic personality disorder, 10
HIV testing, 142
hoarding disorder
    definition of disorder, 207
    demographics, 207

hoarding disorder (*contd.*)
  diagnosis, 208–209
  environment, 207
  etiology, 207
  genetics and physiology, 207
  medical/legal pitfalls, 209–210
  patient education, 209
  psychopharmacology, 209
  temperament, 207
  treatment, 209
Hoarding Rating Scale (HRS), 208
homicidal ideation, 7
hopelessness, 64
hormone replacement therapy, 76, 240
hormone therapy, 250
Horney, Karen, 34
HPI. *See* history of present illness
Human Chorionic Gonadotrospin (HCG), 261
human leukocyte antigen (HLA)
    haplotypes, 291
Hurlbert Index of Sexual Desire, 244
hydroxyzine, 480–481
hyperprolactinemia, 243
hypersomnolence disorder
  definition of disorder, 288
  demographics, 288
  diagnosis, 289–290
  etiology, 288
  patient education, 290–291
  risk factors, 288
  treatment, 290
hyperthyroidism, 76, 149
hypnotherapy, 226, 229
hypoactive sexual desire disorder, 10
hypoalbuminemia, 56
hypochondriasis disorder, 10
hypocretin deficiency, 292
hypokalemia, 264
hypomanic episodes, 143–144, 146, 149,
    154, 157
hypophosphatemia, 264
hypothalamus, 46
hypothyroidism, 76, 138, 149, 153

ibuprofen, 482–483
illusions, 7
iloperidone, 484–485
Iloperidone, 111, 118
imipramine, 59, 486–488
Imodium, 501–502

Imodium A-D, 501–502
impulse control disorders, 9
impulsivity, 7, 64
inappropriate or overreactive affect, 116
in-depth mental status examination, 101
individualized education program (IEP), 325
Individuals with Disabilities Education Act
    (IDEA), 325
infections and violent behavior, 65
informed consent, 66
inhalant and other psychoactive substance
    (OPS) use disorders
  definition of disorder, 95–96
  diagnosis, 96
  treatment, 96–97
inpatient hospitalization, 101
insight, 7
insight-oriented therapy, 107
insomnia disorder
  definition of disorder, 285
  diagnosis, 286–287
  epidemiology, 285
  patient education, 288
  pharmacotherapy, 287
  risk factors, 285–286
  treatment, 287
insulin-dependent diabetes mellitus (DM), 258
intellectual disability
  definition of disorder, 333
  demographics, 333
  diagnosis, 334–335
  etiology, 333
  medical/legal pitfalls, 335
  patient education, 335–336
  risk factors, 334
  treatment, 335
intensive care delirium screening checklist
    (ICDSC), 73
intensive psychoanalytic psychotherapy, 311
Intermezzo, 588–589
intermittent explosive disorder, 9
International Index of Erectile Function
    (IIEF), 239
interpatient variability, 60–61
interpersonal psychotherapy, 178
interpersonal therapy, 148
intoxication, 96
intracavernosal injection of vasodilators, 240
intracellular enzymes and signaling
    proteins, 59

intramuscular (IM) administration, 54. *See also* absorption
intraurethral prostaglandin E1 pellets, 240
intravenous (IV) injection, 54–55
introversion and self-absorption, cyclothymic disorder, 158
intuitive reasoning and experiences, 8
Intuniv, 475–476
ion
    channels, 39
    trapping, 55
irregular sleep/wake patterns, 152
isocarboxazid, 184, 489–490

judgment, 7
Jung, Carl, 32

Kapvay, 413–414
ketamine, 228
kindling theory, 137, 152
kleptomania, 9
Klonopin, 280, 411–412

lactation, sexual dysfunction, 243
Lamictal, 491–493
Lamictal CD, 491–493
Lamictal ODT, 491–493
Lamictal XR, 491–493
lamotrigine, 491–493
Latuda, 505–506
lead poisoning, 322
lethargy alternates, cyclothymic disorder, 158
levomilnacipran, 494–495
Lexapro, 454–457
Librium, 403–404
life chart, 151
ligand, 59
ligand-gated ion channels, 59
limbic system, 45
lipid profiles, 120
lipid-soluble substances, 44
lisdexamfetamine dimesylate, 496–497
Lithium, 111
lithium carbonate, 498–500
Lithobid, 498–500
logical, normal thought process, 7
long-acting risperidone, 118
loose associations, 7
loperamide, 501–502
lorazepam, 102, 117, 149, 503–504

lorazepam intensol, 503–504
Lunesta, 458–459
Lurasidone, 111, 118
lurasidone hydrochloride, 505–506
Luteinizing Hormone (LH), 261
Luvox, 464–467
Luvox CR, 464–467
Lyrica, 190
lysergic acid diethylamide (LSD), 123

major depressive disorder (MDD), 9
    definition of disorder, 129
    demographics, 130
    diagnosis, 131–133
    in the elderly, 79–80
    episode, 145
    etiology, 129–130
    medical/legal pitfalls, 136–137
    patient education, 136
    psychopharmacology, 80
    risk factors, 130–131
    SSRIs as first line of drug therapy, 135–136
    treatment, 79–80, 134–135
major emergencies, 63
maladaptive, 23
maladaptive patterns of thinking, 23
male erectile dysfunction, 10, 239
male orgasmic disorder, 10
manic episode, 143, 145
MAOIs. *See* monoamine oxidase inhibitors
marijuana, 39
Marinol, 265
marked impairment in communication, 319
marked personality disorder symptoms, 154
Marplan, 489–490
Massachusetts General Hospital Hairpulling Scale (MGH-HPS), 210
MDD. *See* major depressive disorder
MDE, 144
MDQ. *See* Mood Disorder Questionnaire
mean initial sleep latency, 289
medical emergencies, 63
    delirium, 68–69
    neuroleptic malignant syndrome (NMS), 68–69
    in psychiatry, 68–69
    serotonin syndrome, 69
Medication Assisted Treatment (MAT), 95
medication noncompliance, 148, 159
melatonin receptors, hypersensitivity, 138

memantine hydrochloride, 507–508
menses resumption, 265
mental confusion alternates, cyclothymic
    disorder, 158
mental health disorder, cyclothymic
    disorder, 154
mental illness, 32, 63. *See also* psychiatric
    emergencies
mental status examination, 6–7, 101, 105, 110
mental status exam (MSE), 12
Merck Manual of Diagnosis and Therapy, 251
metabolic disorders, 65
metabolism, 56–58
metabolite, 57
Metadate CD, 518–520
Metadate ER, 518–520
methadone, 123
methadone HCL, 509–511
Methadose, 509–511
methamphetamines, 123
methocarbamol, 512–514
3,4-methylenedioxymethamphetamine
    (MDMA), 228
Methylin, 515–517
methylphenidate, 521–522
methylphenidate-long-acting, 518–520
methylphenidate-regular-acting, 515–517
methylphenidates, 290, 317, 324
metoclopramide, 265, 387
midazolam hydrochloride, 523–525
midbrain, 44
mild depressive episodes, 149
mindfulness and radical acceptance, 27
mindful strategies and meditation, 27
Mini-Cog, 12
MINI-International Neuropsychiatric
    Interview (MINI[-Plus]), 5
Mini-Mental State Examination, 12
minimization and magnification, 25
minor emergencies, 63
mirtazapine, 134, 526–528
misconceptions, 24
mixed-language disorders, 337
mixed receptive-expressive language disorder
    definition of disorder, 336
    diagnosis, 337–339
    etiology, 336–337
    patient education, 340
    treatment, 339–340
The MMPI-2, 14

modafinil, 285, 290, 529–530
Modern Western culture cultivates and
    reinforces, 259
Modified Checklist for Autism in Toddlers, 321
Modified Neurotic Excoriation Yale-Brown
    Obsessive-Compulsive scale (NE-Y-
    BOCS), 213
monoamine oxidase, 59
monoamine oxidase inhibitors (MAOIs),
    135–136, 168, 184
monoamines, 44, 178
mood, 7
Mood Disorder Questionnaire (MDQ), 142
mood disorders, 9, 123, 280
    bipolar disorder, 137–151
    cyclothymic disorder, 151–163
    major depressive disorder (MDD), 129–137
    persistent depressive disorder, 163–168
mood stabilizers, 11, 149
mood-stabilizing anticonvulsants, 149, 151,
    160, 274, 280
mood symptoms, 141
morphine, 74, 123
motivational interviewing, 209
Motrin, 482–483
multiple sclerosis (MS), 130
multiple sleep latency test (MSLT), 289
multivitamin with thiamine, 264
muscarinic activation, 45
muscarinic cholinergic neurons, 38
muscle dysmorphia, 204
music therapy, 323
myocardial contractility, 264
myocardial infarction, 130

naloxone, 392–394
naloxone HCL dihydrate, 389–391
naloxone hydrochloride, 531–532
naltrexone, 226, 533–535
Namenda, 507–508
Namenda oral solution, 507–508
Namenda titratio pak, 507–508
Namenda XR, 507–508
Narcan, 531–532
Narcan nasal spray, 531–532
narcissistic personality disorder (NPD), 10,
    309–311
    definition, 309–310
    demographics, 309
    diagnosis, 310–311

etiology, 309
 medical/legal pitfalls, 311
 patient education, 311
 risk factors, 310
 treatment, 311
narcolepsy, 9
 definition of disorder, 291
 demographics, 291
 diagnosis, 291–293
 etiology, 291
 patient education, 294
 risk factors, 291
 treatment, 293–294
narcotics, 83
Narcotics Anonymous (NA), 86
nasogastric feeding, 264
National Clearing House, 267
National Institute of Mental Health, 148
natural herbs, 266
Navane, 577–578
neoanalytical thinking, 309
neologism, 7
nervous system
 brain, 44–45
 central nervous system, 43–44
 peripheral nervous system, 43, 45
 somatic nervous system, 45–47
neurocognitive disorder (NCD), 75
 clinical presentation, 77
 definition of disorder, 75
 demographic, 75
 diagnostic workup, 76–77
 differential diagnosis, 76
 DSM-5 diagnostic guidelines, 77–78
 etiology, 75
 ICD-10 codes, 76
 initial assessment, 77
 major and mild, 75–78
 medical/legal pitfalls, 79
 patient education, 78
 relationship to other diseases, 76
 risk factors, 75–76
 treatment, 78
neurodevelopmental disorders
 attention deficit hyperactivity disorder
  (ADHD), 313–319
 autism spectrum disorder, 319–325
 childhood-onset fluency disorder, 325–328
 conduct disorder, 328–331
 dyslexia, 331–333

 intellectual disability, 333–336
 mixed receptive-expressive language
  disorder, 336–340
 oppositional defiant disorder, 340–343
 reactive attachment disorder (RAD), 343–346
 selective mutism, 347–348
 separation anxiety disorder, 349–351
 specific learning disorder, 351–354
neuroleptic malignant syndrome (NMS),
 68–69, 120
neuroleptics, 11
neurological illnesses, 65
neuromuscular junction, 46
neuropharmacology, 48–51
neuropsychological/psychological testing, 205
neuropsychological test batteries, 15
neurotransmitters, 39, 47–49, 259
 anterograde, 38–39
 in central nervous system, 38
 chemical, 38–39
 clinical psychopharmacology, 47–48
 intracellular signaling, 37
 nonsynaptic, 39
 for psychotropic drugs, 38
 receptors, 39–40
 retrograde, 39
Nexiclon XR, 413–414
Nicoderm CQ, 536–538
nicotine
 definition of disorder, 90
 diagnosis, 90
 patient education, 91
 pharmacological treatment, 86
 receptor agonists, 87–88
 replacement therapy, 87
 treatment, 91
nicotine-transdermal patch, 536–538
Nicotinic$_M$, 45
Nicotinic$_N$, 45
Nicotrol step-down patch, 536–538
Nicotrol transdermal, 536–538
nightmare disorder, 9
 definition of disorder, 294
 diagnosis, 294–295
 etiology, 294
 patient education, 296
 risk factors, 294
 treatment, 295–296
NIMH Trichotillomania Impairment Scale
 (NIMH-TIS), 210

NIMH Trichotillomania Severity Scale
(NIMH-TSS), 210
nitric oxide, 39, 245
N-methyl-d-aspartate (NMDA) receptor
antagonist, 78
NMS. *See* neuroleptic malignant syndrome
nonamphetamine, 290
nonanticonvulsant mood stabilizer, 149, 160
Non-benzodiazepine GABA receptor
agonists, 287
non-BZD anxiolytic agent, 190
noncompetitive antagonists, 60
noncompliance, 114
non-24-hour sleep-wake type, 285
non-opioids, 95
nonsteroidal anti-inflammatory drugs
(NSAIDs), 76
nonverbal communication, 4
noradrenergic and specific serotonergic
antidepressants (NaSSAs), 136, 167
noradrenergic neurons, 38
norepinephrine, 39, 41, 129
norepinephrine/dopamine reuptake
inhibitors (NDRIs), 87, 136, 167
Norpramin, 425–426
nortriptyline hydrochloride, 539–541
Novo-Alprazol, 362–364
NPD. *See* narcissistic personality disorder
NSAIDs, 87
Nu-Alpraz, 362–364
nuclear transcription factors, 59
nutritional compromise in AN, 258
Nuvigil, 285, 293, 373–374

obsessive-compulsive and related disorders
body dysmorphic disorder, 204–207
disorder due to another medical condition,
216–218
excoriation disorder, 212–214
hoarding disorder, 207–210
obsessive-compulsive disorder (OCD),
199–204
specified and Unspecified OCD and related
disorder applies, 218–219
substance/medication-induced OCD and
related disorder, 214–216
trichotillomania, 201–212
obsessive-compulsive disorder (OCD), 9
definition of disorder, 199
demographics, 200

diagnosis, 201–202
environment, 200
etiology, 199–200
genetics and physiology, 200
and related disorder symptoms, 216–218
specified and unspecified, 218–219
temperament, 200
treatment, 202–203
obsessive-compulsive tendencies, AN, 258
occupational therapy, 226, 229, 335
OCD. *See* obsessive-compulsive disorder
olanzapine, 111–112, 118, 542–544
olanzapine-fluoxetine combination,
542–544
Oleptro, 579–580
olfactory reference syndrome, 104, 218
open-ended questions, 4–5
opioids, 94–95
antagonists, 87
pharmacological treatment, 86–87
opioid use disorder
definition of disorder, 94
diagnosis, 94–95
treatment, 95
oppositional defiant disorder
definition of disorder, 340
demographics, 341
diagnosis, 341–342
etiology, 340–341
medical/legal pitfalls, 343
pharmacotherapy, 343
risk factors, 341
treatment, 342–343
oral administration, 54
oral contraceptives, 242
ovarian malignant, 251
overconfidence, 158
oxazepam, 545–546

pain disorder, 10
paliperidone, 111, 118
Pamelor, 539–541
Pandua Inventory-Washington State
University Revision (PI-WSUR), 201
panic disorder
background information, 183–184
diagnosis, 184
medical/legal pitfalls, 185
patient education, 185
psychopharmacology, 184–185

panic disorder-with agoraphobia or without Agoraphobia, 9
paranoid personality disorder, 10
paranoid stalkers, 305
parenteral nutrition, 264
Parlodel, 386–388
paroxetine, 178, 184, 203, 281
paroxetine maleate, 547–551
partial opioid agonists, 87
passive diffusion, 55
past medical history (PMH), 6
past psychiatric history, 6
pathological gambling, 9
patient-clinician relationship, 3
The Patient Health Questionnaire, 132
patient-provider relationship, 3–4
patient's body language, 4
Paxil, 267, 281, 547–551
Paxil CR, 281, 547–551
Paxil suspension, 547–551
Peabody Individual Achievement Test-Revised (PIAT-R), 353
Pediatric Autoimmune Neuropsychiatric Disorders Associated with Streptococcal Infections (PANDAS), 201
pediatric psychopharmacology, 203
pedophilia, 9
penile erections. *See* erectile disorder
peptides, 44
Pepto-bismol, 384–385
perceptions, cyclothymic disorder, 158
periactin, 69, 265, 423–424
peripheral nervous system (PNS), 43, 45
perphenazine, 552–553
persistent depressive disorder, 163–168
  definition of disorder, 163
  demographics, 164
  diagnosis, 165–166
  etiology, 164
  medical/legal pitfalls, 168
  patient education, 168
  risk factors, 164–165
  treatment, 166–168
personality disorder, 280
personality disorders, 10, 19–20, 140, 154
  antisocial personality disorder, 301–305
  borderline personality disorder (BPD), 305–309
  narcissistic personality disorder (NPD), 309–311

personalization, 25
personal therapy, 120
pervasive development disorder (PDD), 319
Pervasive Development Disorders Screening Test, 321
P-glycoprotein, 44
pharmacodynamic principles
  drug action mechanisms, 59
  drug-drug interactions and side effects, 60
  drug-receptor interactions, 59–60
pharmacogenetics, 60
pharmacokinetic principles
  absorption, 53–55
  distribution, 55–56
  excretion, 58
  metabolism, 56–58
pharmacotherapy, 50, 134, 226, 230, 266
phencyclidine (PCP), 65, 123
phenelzine, 178, 184
phenobarbital, 123
phobias and social anxiety
  definition of disorder, 176
  demographics, 177
  diagnosis, 180–181
  etiology, 176–177
  medical/legal pitfalls, 179
  patient education, 179
  risk factors, 177–178
  treatment, 178–179
phosphodiesterase-5 (PDE5) inhibitors, 240–241, 245
physical examination, 7
physical restraints, 114
pica, 322
pimozide, 106
plasma protein binding, 55–56
plateau, 58
pleasure center, 45
PMH. *See* past medical history
poisoning, 65
polymorphisms, 60
polypharmacy, 106
polysomnography, 289
Positive and Negative Symptoms Scale (PANSS), 110
postsynaptic neurons, 39
posttraumatic stress disorder (PTSD), 9, 139
Prazosin, 226
pregabalin, 190
pregnancy, sexual dysfunction, 243

pregnant mothers with MDD, 130
premature ejaculation, 10
    definition of disorder, 251–252
    demographics, 252
    diagnosis, 253–254
    etiology, 252
    medical/legal pitfalls, 254
    patient education, 254
    risk factors, 252
    severity, 251–252
    treatment, 254
presynaptic neuron, 39
prilocaine/lidocaine cream, 254
primary hypersomnia, 9
primary insomnia, 9
problematic behaviors, 23
progressive muscle relaxation training, 23
prolactin, 253, 261
Propulsid, 265
prostaglandin E1, 241
ProStep, 536–538
Provigil, 285, 290, 529–530
Prozac, 187, 460–463
Prozac weekly/Sarafem, 460–463
pseudoephedrine, 74
pseudoparkinsonism reaction, 119
psychiatric assessment, 142
psychiatric consultation, 397
psychiatric emergencies
    agitation and aggression, 65–66
    consensus guidelines, 67–68
    definition, 63
    diagnostic workup, 66
    drug selection for, 67
    drug therapy for agitation in, 66
    etiology, 63
    incidence, 64
    medical/legal pitfalls, 66–67
    suicidal state, 64–65
    violent behavior, 65
psychiatric history, 6, 84, 100, 105
psychiatric impairments and active
        observation, 4
psychiatric interview
    clinical decision making, 8
    diagnostic encounter, phases of, 5–6
    diagnostic evaluation, 12
    diagnostic formulation, 8
    DSM-5 disorders and ICD-10 Codes, 9–10
    investigations, 7–8
    mental status examination, 6–7
    nonverbal communication, 4
    patient-provider relationship, 3–4
    physical examination, 7
    psychiatric history, 6
    psychological testing, 13–15
    structured interviews, 5
    treatment modes, 11
    treatment planning, 10–11
    verbal communication, 4–5
psychoanalysis
    Freud, Sigmund, 27
    The Freudians, 32–34
    Freud's Personality Theory, 27–29
    Psychosexual Stages of Development,
        29–32
    unconscious role, 32
psychoanalytic psychotherapy, 225–226, 309
psychodynamic psychotherapy, 249
psychodynamic therapy, 167, 178
psychoeducation, 25, 149
Psychological and Interpersonal Relationship
        Scales (PAIRS), 239
psychological testing, 13–15
    issues in, 14
    measures, 15
    The MMPI-2, 14
    neuropsychological test batteries, 15
    patients types, 13–14
    referral sources, 15
    The Rorschach, 15
    self-report instruments, 15
    time to complete, 14
    types, 13
    The WAIS-IV, 14
psychologic therapy, 240, 254
psychomotor agitation or retardation, 110
psychopathy, 301
psychosexual energy, 29
psychosexual forces, 33
psychosexual stages of human development,
        29
psychosis, 102
psychotherapeutic management
    disorders, 19–21
    initial interview, 18
    philosophy of, 17
    record and standard of care, 19
    standards of care in, 17–18
psychotherapeutic treatment modalities, 124

psychotherapy techniques, 106, 124, 225–226, 229–230, 264, 340
psychotic disorders, 10, 21, 101, 112
psychotropic medication, 134
purines, 44

quetiapine, 111, 118
quetiapine fumarate, 118, 554–556
Quillichew ER, 518–520

RAD. *See* reactive attachment disorder
random plasma glucose (RPG), 142
Rank, Otto, 33
rapid calming, 66
rapid cycling, 146
rapid eye movement (REM)
    period latency, 152
    sleep, 289
rational emotive therapy, 24
Razadyne, 473–474
Razadyne ER, 473–474
reactive attachment disorder (RAD)
    definition of disorder, 343
    demographics, 344
    diagnosis, 344–346
    etiology, 344
    medical/legal pitfalls, 346
    patient education, 346
    risk factors, 344
    treatment, 346
receptive-expressive language disorder, 336–337
receptors, 59
    binding, 47
    specific to psychopharmacology, 39–40
reduced skin conductance, 153
Reglan, 265
Reiss Scales, 335
reliability, 7
Remeron, 526–528
Remeron SolTab, 526–528
Reminyl, 78
repressed conflicts, 32
reserve IM injections, 68
respiratory sedation, 59
restless leg syndrome
    definition of disorder, 296
    diagnosis, 297–298
    epidemiology, 296
    patient education, 298

pharmacotherapy, 298
    risk factors, 296–297
    treatment, 298
Restoril, 575–576
retrograde neurotransmitters, 39
Revia, 533–535
review of systems (ROS), 6
reward-based measures, 24
Risperdal, 335, 557–561
Risperdal Consta, 557–561
Risperdal M-Tab, 557–561
risperidone, 111–112, 118, 123, 335, 557–561
Ritalin, 290, 515–517
Ritalin LA, 518–520
Ritalin SR, 518–520
rivastigmine tartrate, 562–563
Robaxin, 512–514
Robaxin 750, 512–514
Robaxin injection, 512–514
The Rorschach, 15
ROS. *See* review of systems

salvia and tetrahydrocannabinol, 228
Saphris, 375–377
SARIs. *See* selective alpha-2a-adrenergic receptor agonist
Saving Inventory-Revised (SIR), 208
Schedules for Clinical Assessment in Neuropsychiatry (SCAN), 5
schizoaffective disorder, 10, 111
    definition of disorder, 108
    demographics, 109
    diagnosis, 109–111
    etiology, 108–109
    family history, 109
    medical/legal pitfalls, 114
    patient education, 113
    psychopharmacology, 111–113
    risk factors, 109
    treatments, 111
schizophrenia, 10, 65
    definition of disorder, 114
    demographics, 114–115
    diagnosis, 115–117
    etiology, 114
    medical/legal pitfalls, 121
    patient education, 121
    psychopharmacology, 118–121
    risk factors, 115
    treatment, 117–118

schizophreniform disorder, 10
  definition of disorder, 122
  demographics, 122
  diagnosis, 122–123
  etiology, 122
  family history, 122
  medical/legal pitfalls, 125
  patient education, 124–125
  risk factors, 122
  treatment, 123–124
SCOFF questionnaire, 279
seasonal affective disorder (SAD), 395
second-generation (atypical) APS, 111
second-line treatment, schizoaffective
    disorder, 111
second messengers, 42
sedative hypnotics, 11
seizure disorders, 110
selective alpha-2a-adrenergic receptor agonist
    (SARIs), 317, 324
selective mutism, 347–348
  definition of disorder, 174
  demographics, 174
  etiology, 174
  medical/legal pitfalls, 176
  patient education, 176
  psychopharmacology, 175
  risk factors, 174–175
  treatment, 175
selective norepinephrine reuptake inhibitors
    (SNRIs), 317, 324
selective-serotonin reuptake inhibitors
    (SSRIs), 69, 79–80, 134–135, 167, 173,
    179, 185, 190, 203, 209, 214, 233, 254,
    265–266, 274, 280, 351
self-actualization, 34
self-confidence, 158
self-defeating, 23
self-destructiveness, 23, 32
self esteem, 280, 309
Self-Esteem and Relationship (SEAR)
    questionnaire, 239
Self-help groups, 229
self-reported excessive daytime sleepiness,
    288
self-report instruments, 15
sensory integration, 322
separation anxiety disorder, 171–172
  definition of disorder, 171, 349
  demographics, 172, 349
  diagnosis, 172–173, 349–350

  etiology, 171–172, 349
  medical/legal pitfalls, 174, 351
  patient education, 174, 351
  psychopharmacology, 173
  treatment, 173, 350–351
Serax, 545–546
Seroquel, 554–556
Seroquel XR, 554–556
serotonergic neurons, 38
serotonin, 39–40, 129, 265
  1A agonist, 185
  5-HT transporter, 61, 259
  syndrome, 60, 69
serotonin-2 antagonist/reuptake inhibitors
    (SARIs), 136, 167
serotonin-norepinephrine reuptake inhibitors
    (SNRIs), 79–80, 136, 167, 179, 185, 190,
    209, 233
sertraline, 173, 178, 184, 187, 203, 254
sertraline hydrochloride, 564–568
sex hormone therapy, 251
sex therapy, 254
sexual arousal, 241
sexual aversion disorder, 10
sexual desire, 241–242
Sexual Desire Inventory Questionnaire, 244
sexual disorders, 9
sexual dysfunctions, 10
  erectile disorder, 237–241
  female sexual interest/arousal disorder,
    241–246
  gender dysphoria, 246–251
  premature ejaculation, 251–254
Sexual Encounter Profile (SEP), 239
Sexual Interest and Desire Inventory-Female,
    244
sexually transmitted diseases (STDs), 248
sexual masochism, 9
sexual response, 242
sexual sadism, 9
SH. *See* social history
shared decision making, 8
shared psychotic disorder, 10
shift work type, CRSD, 285
short-acting benzodiazepine, 117–118
short allele polymorphism, 61
short-term assessment of risk and treatability
    (START), 142
Shubo-kyofu (excessive fear of having a
    bodily deformity), 218
shyness, 174

signal transduction, 40
  endogenous neurotransmitters, 42
  gene expression, 40
  second messengers, 42
  synaptogenesis, 40
sildenafil, 245
sildenafil citrate, 569–570
Sinequan, 449–450
Skin Picking Scale, 213
sleep deprivation, 138
sleep disorders, 9–10, 133
  circadian rhythm disorder (CRSD),
    283–285
  hypersomnolence disorder, 288–291
  insomnia disorder, 285–288
  narcolepsy, 291–294
  nightmare disorder, 294–296
  restless leg syndrome, 296–298
sleep terror disorder, 9
sleepwalking disorder, 10
SLP. See speech/language pathologist
SMAST (Short Michigan Alcoholism
    Screening Test) screening tool, 85
SN-Ran, 191
SNRIs. See selective norepinephrine reuptake
    inhibitors; serotonin-norepinephrine
    reuptake inhibitors
social anxiety disorder, 176
  diagnostic criteria, 181–182
  differential diagnosis, 182–183
  psychopharmacology, 183
  subtype, 181
social history (SH), 6
social phobia, 9
social rhythm therapy
  bipolar disorder, 148
  cyclothymic disorder, 161
social skills training, 23, 120
Society for Adolescent Medicine, 266
sociopathy, 301
Socratic method, CBT, 26
sodium oxybate, 293
soft bipolar spectrum disorder., 151
somatic delusions, 106
somatic nervous system, 43
  axonal conduction, 46
  basal ganglia, 46
  hippocampus, 46
  hypothalamus, 46
  receptor binding, 47
  synaptic transmission, 47

termination of transmission, 47
transmitter release, 47
transmitter storage, 47
transmitter synthesis, 47
somatization disorder, 10, 133
somatoform disorders, 10
Sonata, 583–584
SPARI, 191
specific learning disorder
  definition of disorder, 351–352
  diagnosis, 352–353
  etiology, 352
  medical/legal issues, 354
  patient education, 354
  treatment, 353–354
specific phobia, 176, 181
specified dissociative disorders, 234
specified gender dysphoria, 247
speech, 7
speech/language pathologist (SLP), 327
SSRIs. See selective-serotonin reuptake
    inhibitors; selective serotonin reuptake
    inhibitors
state-mandated criteria, 8
Stendra, 380–381
stereotyped patterns of behavior, 319
stimulants, 83, 130, 290, 293
stop-start or squeeze-pause technique, 254
Strattera, 318, 378–379
Strengths and Weaknesses of ADHD
    Symptoms and Normal Behavior
    (SWAN) Rating Scale, 315
stress management and lifestyle changes,
    135, 167
The Structural Model (ca. 1920), 28–29
Structured Clinical Interview for DSM-5
    disorders (SCID), 5
Structured Clinical Interview for DSM-5
    Dissociative Disorders (SCID-D),
    225
structured interviews, 5
subcutaneous (SC) administration, 54. See also
    absorption
Suboxone, 389–394
substance abuse, 10, 20, 87–88, 121, 130
substance dependence, 10
substance disorders, 10
substance-induced persisting dementia, 115
substance-induced psychotic disorder, 115
substance-/medication-induced anxiety
    disorder, 192–193

substance/medication-induced OCD and
    related disorder
  definition of disorder, 214–215
  demographics, 215
  diagnosis, 215–216
  etiology, 215
  medical/legal pitfalls, 216
  patient education, 216
  treatment, 216
substance use disorders (SUD), 140
  classes, 83
  clinical presentation, 85
  cyclothymic disorder, 154
  definition of disorder, 83
  demographics, 83–84
  diagnosis, 84
  diagnostic workup, 84
  DSM-5 diagnostic guidelines, 85
  etiology and risk factors, 83
  ICD-10 codes, 84
  initial assessment, 84–85
  medical/legal pitfalls, 88
  patient education, 88
  treatment, 86–88
Subutex, 389–391
SUD. See substance use disorders
sudden refeeding syndrome, 264
suicidal behavior in bipolar spectrum
    disorders, 140
suicidal ideation, 7
  cyclothymic disorder, 159
  depressed patients with, 134
  handling, 147
  homicidal, 110
suicide, 109, 130, 274
  bipolar disorder, 148
  mental health disorder, 266–267
  risk, 102
  schizophrenia attempt and, 115
  state, 64–65
superego, 28–29
Swedish Council on Technology Assessment
    in Health Care, 78
Symbyax, 542–544
synapse, 38
synaptic transmission, 47
synaptogenesis, 40

tacrine hydrochloride, 571–572
tactile hallucinations, 104
tadalafil, 573–574

tangentiality, 7
tardive dyskinesia (TD), 118
Tegretol, 280, 398–402
Tegretol XR, 398–402
telencephalon, 44
temazepam, 575–576
temperature disturbances, 65
termination of transmission, 47
testosterone, 253, 261
therapeutic alliance, 4
therapeutic drug monitoring, 57
therapeutic effects, 59
thiamine hydrochloride, 382–383
thioridazine, 118
thiothixene, 577–578
Thorazine, 101
thoughts, 158
  blocking, 7
  process, 7
thyroid function studies, 132
thyroid hormone receptor, 59
Thyroid Stimulating Hormone (TSH), 261
tobacco use disorder. See nicotine
Tofranil, 486–488
Tofranil injection, 486–488
Tofranil PM, 486–488
token economies, 24
Topamax, 280
topiramate, 280
The Topographic Model (1900), 27–28
tranquilization, 65–66
transdermal administration, 54. See also
    absorption
transferrin and iron, 277
transferritin and iron, 261
transmitter. See also neurotransmitters
  release, 47
  storage, 47
  synthesis, 47
transsexualism, 247, 249
transvestic fetishism, 9
Tranxene, 415–416
tranylcypromine, 184
trazodone HCL, 579–580
treatment and education of autistic and
    related communication-handicapped
    children (TEACCH), 322
triazolam, 581–582
trichotillomania
  definition of disorder, 210
  demographics, 210

diagnosis, 210–211
etiology, 210
genetics and physiology, 210
medical/legal pitfalls, 212
patient education, 212
psychopharmacology, 212
treatment, 211
tricyclic antidepressants (TCAs), 135–136,
168, 179, 184–185, 190, 203, 209, 212,
233, 265–266, 274, 280, 351
trifluoperazine, 118
trihexyphenidyl, 119
Trilafon, 552–553
25-hydroxyvitamin D (25[OH]D), 261

unconscious, 28, 32
unexplained tearfulness alternates,
cyclothymic disorder, 158
unspecified dissociative disorders, 234
unspecified gender dysphoria, 247
utero drug distribution, 56

vaginal lubrication, 242
vaginismus, 10
Valium, 102, 435–436
Valium injectable, 435–436
Valium intensol oral solution, 435–436
Valium oral solution, 435–436
valproate, 111–112
Vancouver Obsessional Compulsive
Inventory, 201
vascular endothelial growth factor (VEGF),
240
venlafaxine, 134
venlafaxine XR, 184
verbal communication, 4–5
Viagra, 569–570
Violence Screening Checklist (VSC), 142
violent behavior, 65
Vistaril, 480–481
vital exhaustion, 153
Vitamin B1, 382–383
vitamins, 65, 87–88
Vivitrol, 533–535

voltage-sensitive potassium channels, 39
voltage-sensitive sodium channels, 39
voyeurism, 9
Vyvanse, 496–497

WAIS-IV, 14
Wechsler Intelligence Scale for Children
(WISC-III), 353
weight-oriented sports or occupations, 260
Wellbutrin, 318, 395–397
Wellbutrin SR, 395–397
Wellbutrin XL, 395–397
Western Blot test, 142
white matter hyperintensities, 138
Woodcock-Johnson Psychoeducational
Battery, 353

Xanax, 280
Xanax/Xanax Xr/Niravam, 362–364
Xyrem, 293

Yale-Brown Obsessive-Compulsive Scale-
Trichotillomania (Y-BOCS-TM), 210
Yale-Brown Obsessive-Compulsive Scale
(Y-BOCS-II), 201
Young Mania Scale, 110
yo-yo dieting, 259

zaleplon, 583–584
Zestra, 245
zinc supplementation, 265
ziprasidone, 111, 118, 124, 585–587
Ziprasidone (Geodon) IM, 117
Zohar-Fineburg Obsessive-Compulsive
Screen, 201
Zoloft, 187, 564–568
zolpidem, 588–589
Zolpimist, 588–589
Zonegran, 280
zonisamide, 280
Zung Self-Rating Scale, 132
Zyban, 395–397
Zyprexa, 542–544
Zyprexa Zydis, 542–544

Printed in the United States
by Baker & Taylor Publisher Services